Women's Health in Africa

This edited book includes new policy-relevant research on women's health issues in Africa. Scholars explore critical topics from different disciplinary traditions using a variety of research methodologies and data sources. The contributors include African scholars with in-depth knowledge of their home contexts, who can furnish nuanced interpretations of local health issues and trends; international researchers who bring vigorous comparative viewpoints; emerging scholars adding to scientific knowledge; and more established researchers with a deep global knowledge of women's health issues.

The range of women's health issues is vast, including the HIV epidemic and its impacts; domestic violence; the persistence of homebirths; and abortion. In addition, the book investigates emerging health concerns such as CVDs and cancers. Readers will learn that, while old health issues have persisted and assumed new dimensions, newer concerns have materialized and are now gaining momentum. The inability of health systems to tackle these issues complicates matters in Africa, creating a sense of desperation that can only be successfully confronted through strong political will and strategic planning, grounded in further research.

The chapters in this book were originally published in the journal *Health Care for Women International*.

Chimaraoke O. Izugbara is Director of the Research Capacity Strengthening Division and Head of Population Dynamics and Reproductive Health at the African Population and Health Research Centre, Nairobi, Kenya.

Eleanor Krassen Covan is Professor Emerita in the School of Health and Applied Human Sciences at the University of North Carolina, Wilmington, USA. She is the Editor-in-Chief of *Health Care for Women International*.

Elizabeth Fugate-Whitlock is Interim Coordinator of the Gerontology Program at the University of North Carolina, Wilmington, USA. She is the Managing Editor of *Health Care for Women International*.

Women's Health in Africa

Issues, challenges and opportunities

Edited by
Chimaraoke O. Izugbara,
Eleanor Krassen Covan and
Elizabeth Fugate-Whitlock

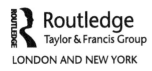

Routledge
Taylor & Francis Group

LONDON AND NEW YORK

First published 2015
by Routledge

2 Park Square, Milton Park, Abingdon, Oxon OX14 4RN
711 Third Avenue, New York, NY 10017, USA

Routledge is an imprint of the Taylor & Francis Group, an informa business

First issued in paperback 2017

British Library Cataloguing in Publication Data
A catalogue record for this book is available from the British Library

ISBN 13: 978-1-138-85498-7 (hbk)
ISBN 13: 978-1-138-08279-3 (pbk)

Typeset in ITC Garamond
by RefineCatch Limited, Bungay, Suffolk

Publisher's Note
The publisher accepts responsibility for any inconsistencies that may have arisen during the conversion of this book from journal articles to book chapters, namely the possible inclusion of journal terminology.

Disclaimer
Every effort has been made to contact copyright holders for their permission to reprint material in this book. The publishers would be grateful to hear from any copyright holder who is not here acknowledged and will undertake to rectify any errors or omissions in future editions of this book.

Contents

CONTENTS

Part VIII: Aging Issues

Citation Information

The following chapters were originally published in the journal *Health Care for Women International*. When citing this material, please use the original volume and issue information and page numbering for each article, as follows:

Chapter 1
Editorial: Research on Women's Health in Africa: Issues, Challenges, and Opportunities
Chimaraoke O. Izugbara and Eleanor Krassen Covan
Health Care for Women International, volume 35, issues 7–9 (2014)
pp. 697–702

Chapter 2
The Whales Beneath the Surface: The Muddled Story of Doing Research with Poor Mothers in a Developing Country
Lou-Marie Kruger
Health Care for Women International, volume 35, issues 7–9 (2014)
pp. 1010–1021

Chapter 3
Gender Differences in the Experiences of HIV/AIDS-Related Stigma: A Qualitative Study in Ghana
Gladys B. Asiedu and Karen S. Myers-Bowman
Health Care for Women International, volume 35, issues 7–9 (2014)
pp. 703–727

Chapter 7
Experiences of Emotional Abuse Among Women Living With HIV and AIDS in Malawi
Winnie Chilemba, Neltjie van Wyk and Ronell Leech
Health Care for Women International, volume 35, issues 7–9 (2014)
pp. 743–757

* * * *

All other chapters had, at the time of publishing this book, only been published online. When citing these eight chapters, please do be sure to cite the original source journal, *Health Care for Women International*, along with the article's DOI, as follows:

Chapter 4

Management of Conflicts Arising From Disclosure of HIV Status Among Married Women in Southwest Nigeria
Oladapo T. Okareh, Onoja M. Akpa, John O. Okunlola and Titilayo A. Okoror
DOI: 10.1080/07399332.2013.794461

Chapter 5

Universal Access to HIV Treatment in the Context of Vulnerability: Female Farm Workers in Zimbabwe
Sandra Bhatasara and Manase Kudzai Chiweshe
DOI: 10.1080/07399332.2013.810220

Chapter 6

Stories of African HIV+ Women Living in Poverty
Samaya VanTyler and Laurene Sheilds
DOI: 10.1080/07399332.2013.862797

Chapter 8

Association Between Domestic Violence and HIV Serostatus Among Married and Formerly Married Women in Kenya
Elijah O. Onsomu, Benta A. Abuya, Irene N. Okech, David L. Rosen, Vanessa Duren-Winfield and Amber C. Simmons
DOI: 10.1080/07399332.2014.943840

Chapter 14

What Are the Factors That Interplay From Normal Pregnancy to Near Miss Maternal Morbidity in a Nigerian Tertiary Healthcare Facility?
Ikeola A. Adeoye, Omotade O. Ijarotimi and Adesegun O. Fatusi
DOI: 10.1080/07399332.2014.943839

Chapter 18

Modernization and Development: Impact on Health Care Decision-Making in Uganda
Debra Anne Kaur Singh, Jaya Earnest and May Lample
DOI: 10.1080/07399332.2013.798326

Chapter 20

Gender Equality as a Means to Improve Maternal and Child Health in Africa
Kavita Singh, Shelah Bloom and Paul Brodish
DOI: 10.1080/07399332.2013.824971

Chapter 27

South African Mothers' Coping With an Unplanned Caesarean Section
Samantha van Reenen and Esmé van Rensburg
DOI: 10.1080/07399332.2013.863893

Please direct any queries you may have about the citations to
clsuk.permissions@cengage.com

Introduction

Research on Women's Health in Africa: Issues, Challenges, and Opportunities

CHIMARAOKE O. IZUGBARA

African Population and Health Research Center, Nairobi, Kenya; Department of Social Work, University of Gothenburg, Gothenburg, Sweden; School of Public Health, University of Witwatersrand, Johannesburg, South Africa; and Department of Sociology & Anthropology, University of Uyo, Uyo, Nigeria

ELEANOR KRASSEN COVAN

School of Health and Applied Human Sciences, University of North Carolina, Wilmington, North Carolina, USA

As we approach 2015—the target year for achieving the Millennium Development Goals (MDGs)—several facets of women's health remain insufficiently tackled. Urgent and concerted attention to these facets is crucial for several reasons. Advances in the health care of women and girls are powerfully central to the overall wellbeing of households, communities, and societies. Women's health status is a foremost barometer of development levels in a society (World Health Organization, 2012). Transformations in the health status of women often mirror deeper systematic impacts of development processes in the everyday lives of people and communities. Poor health among women has the potential to upset societal progress and eclipse development and wellbeing. Investing intentionally and purposefully in protecting and safeguarding women's health will secure current levels of progress and guarantee future potentials for societal growth and advancement.

In more recent decades, women's health has become a global priority, enjoying both worldwide attention and massive political support (Institute for Women's Health, 2013). While the international prioritization of women's health has delivered far-reaching benefits for women, and indeed society at large, significant gaps remain in our knowledge of the drivers and dynamics of several of the health issues that face women; the interventions for addressing these issues; pathways for consolidating the gains of existing health actions; and strategies for forestalling the emergence of new diseases and the resurgence of old ones. In many instances, these gaps continue to trigger massive reversals in gains made in women's health in several parts of the world, extending health inequalities in and among societies and impeding health development (Chen et al., 2004).

In Africa, women's health indicators are vastly deplorable. Progress towards the attainment of the MDGs that directly concern women's health and wellbeing has been slowest in Africa. The region hosts only 12% of the world's population but currently contributes 50% of all global maternal deaths (Africa Progress Panel, 2010). It is also in Africa that the modest gains realized in women's health in recent decades are witnessing the briskest reversals. Health services that are basic and essential for women in other parts of the world remain unavailable to millions of women in Africa. Globally, Africa governments continue to rank among the sloppiest in the formulation and execution of policies and programs to deliver quality health services to women. It is clearly against this backdrop that Africa has also become the world's current largest laboratory for trying out policies and interventions to advance women's health. Curiously, while only a small minority of these interventions is driven by rigorous scientific evidence, they continue to attract massive funding support from several donors. The scope and focus of these interventions are also particularly interesting; they range from small-scale programs that "bribe" in-school young girls to postpone their sexual debuts; national programs that teach women to use female condoms and challenge community norms that affect their health and welfare; interventions that use religious leaders and ministers to promote women's use of family planning services; and schemes that teach older women to fight off rapists—to projects seeking to boost female sex workers' capacity to navigate client violence and hostile prostitution laws.

Critical social, cultural, political, economic and environmental issues drive Africa's tragic women's health profile (Izugbara & Afangideh, 2005). The bulk of people who live below the poverty line in Africa are women. Most of these women lack access to basic health essentials and services, which exposes them to poor sexual and reproductive health outcomes including unsafe abortion and maternal morbidity and mortality (African Population and Health Research Center, Ministry of Health [Kenya], Ipas, & Guttmacher Institute, 2013). Worsening livelihoods have increased women's susceptibility to violence (Izugbara & Ngilangwa, 2010). There is also rising evidence that African men who are unable to attain popular manhood markers due to growing marginalization are increasingly resorting to heightened sexism, sadism, and sexual aggression towards women to assert themselves (Izugbara, 2011; Izugbara, Tikkanen, & Barron, 2014; Silberschmidt, 1999, 2001). Pervasive poverty and feelings of alienation and exclusion have also cultivated religious and other forms of fundamentalism hinged on practices that degrade women's health. Historic power imbalances between Africa and high-income countries continue to promote local policies that have little bearing on domestic realities, expand the imperial interests of developed countries, advance women's oppression, and weaken health systems.

Intractable wars, terrorism, and political instability continue to devastate the health and safety of women and girls in Africa, as most recently demonstrated by the abduction of school girls in Northern Nigeria by the extremist group, Boko Haram. Corruption and weak local and global accountability arrangements are responsible for much of the inefficiency that diverts scarce resources meant to improve public health in Africa. The unceasing incapacity of most African political leaders to realistically contradistinguish between their personal, political goals and the everyday realities of citizens' lives has frustrated actions targeting crucial areas of women's health. For instance, despite the rising incidence of cancer among women in Africa, specialized oncology care has yet to be prioritized by many African governments. Most women cancer patients in Africa are thus currently diagnosed very late, resulting in acute sufferings and mortalities (Pezzatini, Marino, Conte, & Catracchia, 2007).

Climate change and environmental depletion have increased poverty, food shortages, and livelihood insecurity for women. Famines, conflicts over land, crop failures, and droughts have forced young vulnerable African women to migrate into cities where they are exposed to poor health (Izugbara, 2012). Given the deplorable economic fortunes of and poor governance arrangements in these cities, the bulk of these migrant women end in congested informal urban settlements, commonly called slums (Izugbara, Kabiru, & Zulu, 2009; Kimani-Murage & Ngindu, 2007; Parks, 2014). For instance, in Nairobi, Kenya, about 60% of the residents (mainly women and girls) live in slums characterized by substandard social services, insecurity, unhealthy environments, and poor housing as well as deplorable social and other outcomes. These conditions fuel infections and diseases among women, aggravate national indicators and delay progress towards the Millennium Development Goals (Izugbara, Ezeh, & Fotso, 2009). Widespread illiteracy, high dependence on men, limited access to education and poor employment and economic opportunities among women in Africa are key drivers of large family sizes, poor reproductive health, and unsafe abortion in Africa (Izugbara & Ezeh, 2010). Currently, several women in Africa survive through livelihood activities and relationships that render them vulnerable to unwanted pregnancies, HIV and poor health outcomes (Izugbara & Egesa, 2014; Izugbara, Ochako, & Izugbara, 2011). Due to weak social protection and insurance systems, the bulk of the region's women also continue to pay out-of-pocket for essential medical services, further intensifying household poverty and straining family incomes. There is also globalization which, among other things, has unleashed far-reaching lifestyle changes that have exposed women and girls to new health issues, including cardiovascular diseases (CVDs), cancers, and early sexual activity etc.

Research can unlock the drivers of health in Africa, support the design and delivery of effective interventions to address current health issues, and lay the foundation for preventing poor health in future generations of Africans. Our aim in preparing this special issue was to assemble original research articles that offer insights on, and strengthen our understanding of the dynamics of women's health in Africa. Grounding African policy and programmatic responses to women's health issues in robust research will improve health planning and save lives and resources. Through research, we can learn from past health interventions in Africa in order to strengthen current efforts and plan future programs. Research will not only illuminate the origins and enormity of women's health challenges in Africa, it will also unveil prospects for improving wellbeing sustainably. Without prioritizing research, the roots and triggers of ill-heath among women in Africa will continue to be misinterpreted, the soundest interventions for addressing them will stay unarticulated, and the strategies for optimizing the effectiveness of health actions will remain elusive.

In this special issue of the *HCWI*, we bring together important new and policy-relevant research on a variety of women's health issues and from a number of African countries. The studies published here cover an assortment of critical topics that are explored by authors from different disciplinary traditions and who use a miscellany of research methodologies and data sources. The range of women's health issues covered in this volume is astoundingly outstanding, and includes traditional and longstanding women's health challenges such as the persistence of homebirths, policy frameworks for ensuring women's health, the HIV epidemic and its impacts, abortion, and sexual violence as well as emerging health concerns including CVDs and cancers. In reading these articles, it is obvious that while old health issues of women have persisted and assumed new dimensions, newer concerns have materialized and are gaining momentum. Weak health system capacity to tackle these myriad issues complicates matters in Africa and creates a sense of despondency and desperation that can only be successfully confronted through strong political will and strategic planning. The blend of authors in this collection is also striking: African scholars with in-depth knowledge of their home contexts and who can furnish nuanced interpretations of local health issues and trends; international investigators who bring vigorous comparative viewpoints; emerging scholars raring to add to scientific knowledge and build their profiles; and more established researchers with deep global knowledge of women's health issues.

At this decisive moment in human history, it is a pleasure to offer readers of *HCWI*, and indeed all those interested in women's health, this rich and stimulating menu of important research on women's health in Africa. It is also particularly exciting to see the work of these many African scholars on such an important issue as women's health in a truly international, widely-read and reputable scholarly health journal. Research by Africans on

Africa's development questions can support scientific and technological innovations that are sensitive to the cultures, aspirations, and levels of progress in the region (Fonn, 2006). However, weak local capacity for research has remained the bane of quality knowledge production on the continent. Unlike many other parts of the world, sub-Saharan Africa continues to experience massive deficits in highly-skilled scientists and researchers (Kabiru, Izugbara, Wairimu, Amendah, & Ezeh, 2014). In reviewing articles for this issue, we rejected several potentially important articles; some had relied on flawed methodologies, were poorly written, or did not show familiarity with the state of debate and knowledge in their research problems. Supporting health research capacity in Africa is key to filling the knowledge gaps on women's health in Africa. African and Africanist researchers as well as research and teaching institutions in the region need sustained support to deliver on their obligations to provide timely and robust evidence for policy formulation and program implementation. Policy-makers and program executors in the region also need to be appropriately armed with the tools and skills to enable them locate, understand, evaluate and deploy quality research evidence in their everyday work.

Taken together, the articles published in this collection hold forth a solid optimism for a healthier future for women and girls in Africa. Indeed, while the authors clearly recognize that Africa is disadvantaged in terms of women's health, they also unswervingly show that solutions are both possible and urgent. The ball, it appears, is now decisively in the court of all those truly committed to women's health in Africa and the expectation is that they will coordinate their efforts better and more purposefully.

REFERENCES

African Population and Health Research Center, Ministry of Health [Kenya], Ipas, & Guttmacher Institute. (2013). *Incidence and complications of unsafe abortion in Kenya: Key findings of a national study*. Nairobi, Kenya: African Population and Health Research Center.

Africa Progress Panel. (2010). *Maternal health: Investing in the lifeline of healthy societies and economies*. Geneva, Switzerland: Africa Progress Panel Secretariat. Retrieved from http://www.who.int/pmnch/topics/maternal/app_maternal_health_english.pdf

Chen, L., Evans, T., Anand, S., Boufford, J. I., Brown, H., Chowdhury, M., . . . Elzinga, G. (2004). Human resources for health: Overcoming the crisis. *The Lancet, 364*(9449), 1984–1990.

Fonn, S. (2006). African PhD research capacity in public health: Raison d'etre and how to build it. *Global Forum Update on Research for Health, 3*, 80–83.

Institute for Women's Health. (2013). *Global women's health*. Retrieved from http://www.womenshealth.vcu.edu/outreach/global/index.html

Izugbara, C. O. (2011). Poverty, masculine violence and the transformation of men: Ethnographic notes from Kenyan slums. In K. Pringle, E. Ruspini, J. Hearn &

B. Pease (Eds.), *Men and masculinities around the world: Transforming men's practices* (pp. 236–246). New York, NY: Palgrave Macmillan.

Izugbara, C. O. (2012). Client retention and health among sex workers in Nairobi, Kenya. *Archives of Sexual Behavior, 41*, 1345–1352.

Izugbara, C. O., & Afangideh, A. I. (2005). Urban women's use of rural-based health care services: The case of Igbo women in Aba city, Nigeria. *Journal of Urban Health, 82*(1), 111–121. doi: 10.1093/jurban/jti013

Izugbara, C. O., & Egesa, C. (2014). The management of unwanted pregnancy among women in Nairobi, Kenya. *International Journal of Sexual Health, 26*, 100–112.

Izugbara, C. O., Ezeh, A., & Fotso, J.-C. (2009). The persistence and challenges of homebirths: Perspectives of traditional birth attendants in urban Kenya. *Health Policy and Planning, 24*(1), 36–45.

Izugbara, C. O., & Ezeh, A. C. (2010). Women and high fertility in Islamic northern Nigeria. *Studies in Family Planning, 41*, 193–204.

Izugbara, C. O., Kabiru, C. W., & Zulu, E. M. (2009). Urban poor Kenyan women and hospital-based delivery. *Public Health Reports, 124*, 585–587.

Izugbara, C. O., & Ngilangwa, D. P. (2010). Women, poverty and adverse maternal outcomes in Nairobi, Kenya. *BMC Women's Health, 10*(1), 33.

Izugbara, C. O., Ochako, R., & Izugbara, C. (2011). Gender scripts and unwanted pregnancy among urban Kenyan women. *Culture, Health & Sexuality, 13*, 1031–1045.

Izugbara, C. O., Tikkanen, R., & Barron, K. (2014). Men, masculinity, and community development in Kenyan slums. *Community Development, 45*(1), 32–44.

Kabiru, C. W., Izugbara, C. O., Wairimu, J., Amendah, D., & Ezeh, A. C. (2014). Strengthening local health research capacity in Africa: The African Doctoral Dissertation Research Fellowship Program. *The Pan African Medical Journal, 17*(Suppl. 1), 5–7.

Kimani-Murage, E. W., & Ngindu, A. M. (2007). Quality of water the slum dwellers use: The case of a Kenyan slum. *Journal of Urban Health, 84*, 829–838.

Parks, M. J. (2014). Urban poverty traps: Neighbourhoods and violent victimisation and offending in Nairobi, Kenya. *Urban Studies, 51*, 1812–1832. doi: 10.1177/0042098013504144

Pezzatini, M., Marino, G., Conte, S., & Catracchia, V. (2007). Oncology: A forgotten territory in Africa. *Annals of Oncology, 18*, 2046–2047. doi: 10.1093/annonc/mdm523

Silberschmidt, M. (1999). *"Women forget that men are the masters": Gender antagonism and socio-economic change in Kisii District, Kenya.* Stockholm, Sweden: Nordiska Afrikairstitutet.

Silberschmidt, M. (2001). Disempowerment of men in rural and urban East Africa: Implications for male identity and sexual behavior. *World Development, 29*, 657–671.

World Health Organization. (2012). *Addressing the challenge of women's health in Africa: Report of the Commission on Women's Health in the African Region.* Brazzavile, Republic of the Congo: WHO Regional Office for Africa.

The Whales Beneath the Surface: The Muddled Story of Doing Research With Poor Mothers in a Developing Country

LOU-MARIE KRUGER

Department of Psychology, Stellenbosch University, Cape Town, South Africa

In this article I attempt to show how research ideals of social change and usefulness can lead to "research paralysis." I also argue that if there is sufficient reflexivity about the research process itself, paralysis is not inevitable, and useful knowledge can indeed be generated. I substantiate this by illustrating how the same interview data can be analyzed on multiple levels, rendering it useful in different ways in different contexts. I thus argue that reflexivity is essential in the Community Psychologist's struggle for usefulness: it is in reflecting on the complexity of the research task (the demands of different contexts and different communities) that the Community Psychologist can engage strategically and productively with the possibilities and the limits of her usefulness. The data that are the focus of this article were generated in a long-term qualitative research project focusing on low-income, Black mothers from a semirural community in South Africa.

The White Rabbit put on his spectacles. "Where shall I begin, please your Majesty?" he asked. "Begin at the beginning," the king said, very gravely, "and go on till you come to the end: then stop." —*Lewis Carroll (1865, Chapter XII)*

Such indeed, is the conditions of things ... I do know that however long I did so, I would not get anywhere near to the bottom of it. Nor have I ever gotten anywhere near the bottom of anything I have ever written about. Cultural analysis is intrinsically incomplete. And, worse than that, the more deeply it goes the less complete is. It is a strange science whose most telling assertions are its most tremulously based, in which to get somewhere with the matter at hand is to intensify the suspicion, both your own and that of others, that you are not getting it quite right. —*Clifford Geertz (1973, p. 29)*

For my part, it has struck me that I might have seemed a bit like a whale that leaps up to the surface of the water disturbing it momentarily with a tiny jet of spray and lets it be believed, or pretends to believe, or wants to believe, or himself does in fact indeed believe, that down in the depths where no one sees him any more, where he is no longer witnessed or controlled by anyone, he follows a more profound, coherent and reasoned trajectory. —*Michel Foucault (1980, p. 79)*

Although there is no single definition of Community Psychology, it can be said that Community Psychology compels the researcher to pay attention to do research that is orientated toward social change. It is thus concerned with the usefulness of the research to communities themselves (Flax, 1993). Research can be useful in direct and in indirect ways. It can be indirectly useful in that knowledge that is useful can be generated; that is, the results can be useful. It can also be indirectly useful in that the process of knowledge construction can be useful as well. If it is clear that research is conducted "to be of use," it can also be stipulated what the standard is against which to measure research: Community Psychologists work with a moral imperative and with political designs. In research where there is an emphasis on social change and usefulness, the idea that advocacy and scholarship are not compatible is of central importance. In such research, "Knowing will be judged by ethical as well as epistemological ideals. I evaluate ways of knowing and the knowledge they produce in the light of the good to which they lead and that they yield" (Ruddick, 1996, p. 267).

My research is about marginal maternities—I look at the impact of poverty and race on the emotional experience of motherhood. The data that are the focus of this article were generated in a long-term multifaceted qualitative research project conducted in one low-income semirural community in the Western Cape, South Africa. Although a clinical psychologist by training, in a research context I think of myself as a psychoethnographer. As an ethnographer I am interested in the maternal body; the practices, rituals, and myths related to pregnancy, birth, and motherhood; the experiences of women becoming mothers, in how these "seemingly natural processes of swelling, bearing and suckling, the flows of blood, semen and milk are constituted and fixed not just by the force of cultural conception but by the coagulation of power" (Jolly, 1998, p. 2). I want to understand how these rituals and practices, at once very personal, very local, and very ideological, impact on women: how do they themselves experience pregnancy, birth, and motherhood? As a clinician I am interested in how these reproductive experiences shape the nature and the articulation of psychological distress and psychological resilience, hoping to use this knowledge toward the designing of policies and planning of services that can address the distress while utilizing the resilience. I struggle with the binary oppositions of individual and society and am interested exactly in the murky place where the individual internalizes the social or where the individual constructs the social.

It is in these identifications of myself that it is already possible to discern the inevitable tension between the desire to know and the longing to help, the schism between epistemology and action/ethics/politics.

Let us consider extracts from an interview with Elize, a 33-year-old "Coloured"[1] farmworker. At the time of this interview Elize's third child, a girl, was 6 months old. The Protestant church group that she joined before the baby's birth insisted that Elize marry her long-time partner—before that they had been living together for about 13 years. The couple lives with their three children in a small house in a semirural town in the Western Cape. The total weekly household income is R340.00 (U.S. $34). The family's staple food is "*pap*" (a stiff porridge made from maize), which Elize flavors with custard powder and milk. Elize reported in every interview that her husband is a heavy drinker and a womanizer and that he beats her regularly. When she gave birth to her baby in the busy local hospital, she was by herself, with nursing staff only attending to her about 15 minutes after the baby's birth. She starts the interview with the following disclaimer:

> But I want to ask is it good, should I. ... It feels to me that I complain that I only complain to you about my problems. Can I talk about them? ... It feels to me, yes, as if it is about my problems that I come and talk about and that is not the actual thing that you really want to talk about. If maybe it is only about the baby.

The interviewer reassures her and she continues:

> Yes, there were many times that I thought, wow, with whom is there not someone to whom I can open my heart? Can take my problems to. Because you can't with everyone. ... But I mean if our welfare people and them ... he will probably ... they will probably frighten him. He will probably get a bit of head for them.

She then talks about her baby being sick and her concern for her children and the lack of support from her husband. She continues with a rather long narrative:

> He then lost it totally and while I was writing up my groceries for the Friday and Saturday I felt him hitting me on my mouth; my jaw hurt. Then I thought there is only one way, because before that I boiled water for the child's bottle, so I took the water and he realized and he followed

me and he took my chair to throw it at me, but then I took the kettle just like that with the water and I gave him a shot of the water. That water then broke him down. That was the only way in which I could defend myself. . . . But I really don't know what to do with the man.

In the next section of the interview she talks about the church and her frustration with not being able to participate fully in church activities, as her husband does not support her:

Many days I think this is probably the way it should be. They say if there is not a struggle, there is not victory.

In the rest of the interview there is much more said about her husband, his womanizing, his drinking, his spending, his sexual demands, and his violence. She also reveals that she is worried about diseases because he sleeps with women who are rumored to have diseases. When the interviewer asked her about the possibility of leaving her husband that she expressed as a fantasy in the previous interview, Elize explains why she stays:

Now the church people, the priests, they say if you are married, only death, only death can set us apart. It does not exist with them the possibility that you can get divorced; then death should separate you. Now they say if they pray, they pray the Lord should take that person away so that I can get rid of him. Look he is they say he stands in my way. I want to continue with things, the work of the Lord, but he stands in my way.

The challenge for me and my research team is then to show that the collecting of personal narratives of pregnancy, birth, and motherhood is useful, that it can serve as the basis for the construction of useful knowledge. Stories can be useful in different ways on different levels. In other words, they can be analyzed on different levels: this notion of different levels of analysis is present in most good qualitative research, be it narrative analysis or discourse analysis. My analyses of the interviews therefore constitute a constant movement between levels.

Analysis on a First Level: Narratives as Acts of Self-Presentation

On a first level people tell stories simply to recapitulate the past. On a very basic level, then, the narratives of the respondents can be understood as their stories—as acts of self-presentation. On this level of analysis, the assumption is that the text can be autonomous and that it does represent "reality." What participants say about their lives in their personal narratives would thus be believed to, in a transparent and authentic way, reflect their experiences.

If we consider Elize's narrative on this level, we have a story of a woman whose violent and disloyal husband constantly threatens her and undermines her, so that one day in self-defense she throws some boiling water at him.

She does not express guilt or regret about her action. The only emotion that is articulated is fear: she is afraid of his retaliation. For the researcher listening to Elize's story in the here and now, there might be enough evidence that what she is hearing is the truth so that she decides to actually act to at least try to ensure Elize's safety.

Analysis on a Second Level: Narratives as a Social Act

As suggested above, however, narratives "are used not only *in* talk, but *to* talk, not only to recapitulate past events but to negotiate present and future events" (Langellier, 1989, p. 261). Narratives as events are functional for the narrators in their specific contexts. Storytelling happens between social actors under particular social constraints (Langellier, 1989; Riessman, 1993). This inevitably leads to the question of *how* storytelling functions in the larger social context. In other words, "Under what conditions do particular individuals tell particular stories to particular listeners?" In such an analysis, the stories that the participants tell are analyzed not as objects, but as events that do something or accomplish something as discourse in the social world. More specifically, how are their narratives functional for themselves in the interview situation?

If we consider the interview with Elize, it is clear from her introduction that she is aware of the fact that I as the interviewer (a White clinical psychologist attached to an academic institution) have expectations, expectations that she might not be meeting. She also states, however, that she has hopes that someone can hear her story and do something. Given this preamble to the interview, one can interpret Elize's story as an attempt to show how desperate she is and how desperate the measures are that she has to take. As such, the whole story can be understood as an appeal for help or support from the researcher.

Analysis on a Third Level: Narratives as Political Acts

The next question is about how the personal narrative functions politically (Langellier, 1989; Phoenix, 2000; Riessman, 1993). Even as a social event, narrative cannot be isolated from a wider political context. This means that an analysis of stories should involve an attempt to determine which ideologies or myths are the ones that are reproduced/supported or undermined/contested. In such an analysis, it may be found, as in the current study, that there is important common ground among women in different locations (Walby, 2000). Harding (2001) warns against the danger of remaining "preoccupied with women's voices, important as these nevertheless are, and [to] fail to examine the cultural discourses through which women's experiences are framed and continuously reframed" (p. 518). Such an examination will illuminate that some narratives can be seen as supportive of the existing status quo, while others have subversive potential.[2] Individual narratives can be an arena of political struggle (Langellier, 1989).

If it is acknowledged that individual stories are socially situated and are grounded in the material conditions of existence, this implies that psychologists, when they do analyze individual narratives, have to pay attention to the material and ideological conditions that shape the lives of individual storytellers. This attunement to material and ideological conditions will enable the researcher to try to understand why a person would have a specific narrative. Stories are informed not only by personal intrapsychic factors (such as its own very infantile experiences), but they are also determined by factors such as class, race, religion, sexuality, and culture (Collins, 1994; Glenn, 1994). All experiences are overdetermined on many levels (Bassin, Honey, & Kaplan, 1994). The researcher thus does not only take into account the subjects' social environments, but focuses upon "that metaphysical place where the social gets transformed into the psychological—where individuals construct meaning of their experience in the world" (Wolf, 1987, p. 217).

In terms of politics, Elize's narrative certainly is informed by a larger gender discourse that states that women can or should not have agency. For instance, they are not able to leave their men, even if the men are very abusive. Elize expresses the belief, like many other women in other contexts, that she has very little choice with regards to how to cope with her situation. She states that she has to accept that this is the way things are and that "there will be no victory if there is no struggle." She is extremely poor and she is exhausted and sometimes depressed, but she does go to church work every evening. Interestingly, however, despite this lip service to a dominant gender ideology (actively advocated by her church), Elize does resist in very physical ways. One cannot help thinking that on an unconscious level she might think that she is doing God's work by attacking her husband. After all, her pastor is praying for him to die.

It is in this process of making sense that the importance of theory is highlighted: the researcher needs theory or to theorize in order to understand how the personal narrative is related to the material and ideological conditions within which it is constructed (Walby, 2000). The researcher also needs theory if she wants to explain how the narrative functions for this particular individual with this particular personal history. It would, for instance, be interesting to understand Elize's attachment to the church in more psychoanalytic terms: in terms of her own personal history where there have been no consistent good attachment relationships.

Analysis on a Fourth Level: Narrative and the Need for Closure

On yet another level, it is important, even while trying to hear different voices and to expose essentialist tendencies in personal narratives, to make sense of this essentialist tendency. In the final instance, it is important for feminists to study and understand the need for narrative, that is, the quest for closure and coherence. In the words of Jane Flax, "Feminist theories ... should encourage us to tolerate and interpret ambivalence, ambiguity, and multiplicity as well as to expose our needs for imposing order and structure no matter how arbitrary and oppressive these needs may be" (1990, p. 56).

If Elize's narrative was to be analyzed on this level, it would be necessary to look at how this gender discourse functions in this community. In the context of the current study, this would mean further exploring the dominant gender discourse, its current functioning, and its history. Foucault elaborates: "how these phenomena of repression and exclusion possessed their instruments and their logic, in response to a certain number of needs" (1980, pp. 100–101).[3] What is important for the purposes of this article, however, is that by asking questions on this political level new possibilities for study are opened, such as the one that I have shown. These possibilities can be exciting, but can also feel paralyzing: there are no final answers, no complete analysis—always another level to go to.[4]

CONCLUSION

Different Levels of Analysis for Different Contexts

Given that the narratives we work with can be analyzed in different ways, such as the four or more that I have highlighted above, one can ask how a researcher decides which analytic level she should be working on and how a particular analysis can become valid. This brings one back to the notion of usefulness, that is, what kind/level of analyses will be most useful in a particular context.

Another way to ask this question is to ask to whom the analysis should be useful. Here, Jane Flax's idea that "to be useful, requires communities" (1993, p. 4) is an important one. She expands: "Communities provide one with puzzles to address; theoretical frames to appropriate, purposes to evaluate, adopt, or reject" (1993, p. 5). One can then ask whether a certain analysis is useful to a specific respondent herself, to the community of which she is a member, to the academic community, to a community of health care workers or mental health care workers, to the students one is trying to make more politically and socially aware, or to policy-making bodies.

Communities[5] open up possibilities for knowledge and action, but they also provide the limits and boundaries of usefulness (Flax, 1993). They put the brakes on for scholars and academics who tend to be grandiose and overly idealistic. A research project therefore can have different uses for different communities. The researcher's challenge is to engage with the different communities that she is involved in as conversation partners. In these dialogues she can say things, write things, know things; she can take positions; she can have beliefs.

There can be a basis for action (social action, political action, even research action). Such positions constitute what Squire has called "strategic essentialism" (1998, p. 86) or Goldberger, Tarule, Clinchy, and Belenky, "commitment within relativism" (1996, p. 17). In these conversations or dialogues a certain flexibility is required, but also a commitment to assess the appropriateness and utility of a particular way of knowing given the moment, situation, cultural and political imperatives, and relational and ethical ramifications (Flax, 1993). The researcher has to evaluate the usefulness of her work within those specific frameworks, with those specific purposes in mind, with those specific puzzles to solve. She has to understand that sometimes what constitutes useful knowledge in one community may not be so useful in another community, what is a puzzle in one community may not be a puzzle in another, and what is a useful process for one community may not be useful for another. Geertz (1973) warns against cultural analysis that loses touch "with the hard surfaces of life" (p. 30) and states that the only defense against drifting hopelessly into relativism is analyses that are is context sensitive and experience near. Relativism can be avoided if analyses stay specific and contextual. There can be claims about the world (knowledge, specific and more general) or there can be critique, but for either to be valid it has to be useful.

In considering our research project, it feels clear that doing research is a complicated process of moving between communities, carefully considering what kind of knowledge or process of knowledge is useful in a particular community. This means that the feminist researcher has to be skilled at splitting up what she knows and finding the appropriate language within which to convey this knowledge. It means that sometimes she simply retells a story. At other times, she shows how the story functions for this particular respondent in this particular context. In other contexts it may be appropriate to put on the agenda the fact of the stories themselves—the fact that people on the margins of society tell stories that either entrench dominant discourses or subvert them. All of these levels of analyses may be interesting or important, but all of them will not be useful in all contexts and for all communities. Rather than becoming paralyzed by the complexity of her work, the feminist committed to knowledge and ethics should become a conscious strategist.[6]

I have attempted to show that the very ideal to do research that is useful can result in many points of paralysis for the researcher. On the one hand, she may find that the process of doing research is not directly beneficial to the respondent in the ways that she and the respondent expected it to be. This may lead to disillusionment and paralysis. On the other hand, the researcher may also find that the results of her research (i.e., the knowledge and critiques that are constructed through her research) are also not satisfying in that it is impossible to represent the lives of others in ways that are useful in all contexts, that is, useful in any universal sense of the word. To write up findings in a useful way, the researcher has to always bracket certain things that she found out, therefore having the experience of not fully or adequately representing her respondent. Given the fragmentation of modern society (academic world, political world, and professional world; academic disciplines; paradigms within one discipline, etc.) and the fact that the researcher is thereby almost forced to pluck out different aspects of her research in different contexts, she may feel fragmented, muddled, and incoherent. She might feel a yearning for a coherent story that has a beginning, a middle, and an end, a story that gets to the bottom of things (Geertz, 1973), a story that tells of a "more profound, coherent and reasoned trajectory" (Foucault, 1980, p. 79). Instead, one feels compelled to tell a more ambiguous story—a rather melancholic one.

This is why we as researchers always begin and end with reflexivity: reflecting on what we really are doing, how we are doing it, what we are finding out, and what we are doing with what we are finding. In such reflections about our research, the links between different levels of analyses are illuminated: one can begin to see that the chasms are not in the knowledge but in society, and that a notion of partially situated knowledge is not necessarily related to "retreatism" (Walby, 2001, p. 486) or "a defensive stance" (p. 485), but has to do with strategic choices of how to present your work in order for it to be useful.

It is, then, a "struggle with responsibility under conditions of disenchantment, disorder, and imperfection" (Flax, 1993, p. xiii). It is a recognition that the empiricist or modernist desire for order, certainty, and total control of both the process and results of research is impossible—it is the giving up of innocence. These seemingly endless reflexive endeavors[7] of community psychologists can highlight the melancholia, can feel the paralysis, but if the researcher persists, it can also be enabling, as in the words of Myerhoff and Ruby (1992):

> We can never return to our former easy terms with a world that carried on quite well without our administrations. We may find ourselves like Humpty-Dumpty, shattered wrecks unable to recapture a smooth, seamless innocence, or like the paralyzed centipede that never walked again once he was asked to consider the difficulty in manipulating all those legs. Once we take into account our role in our own productions, we may be led into new possibilities that compensate for this loss. We may achieve a greater originality and responsibility than before, a deeper understanding at once of ourselves and of our subjects. (p. 1)

NOTES

1. We are mindful of the fact that the use of racial categories in South African scholarship is controversial. Such categories are socially constructed, however, and carry important social meanings. As such, we believe that, following the argument presented by Jewkes and colleagues (1998), it is impossible to conduct a meaningful analysis of our findings within the context of postapartheid South Africa without

making reference to previous racial classifications, since these still inform existing power relations. In this article the category of "Coloured" will be used to refer to South Africans said to be of diverse and mixed racial origins; designated under Apartheid racial classification as "Coloured."

2. Foucault (1980) articulates something about the agency of the seemingly powerless in the midst of social constraint. He says, "Power is employed and exercised through a net-like organisation. And not only do individuals circulate between its threads; they are always in the position of simultaneously undergoing and exercising this power. They are not only its inert or consenting target; they are always the elements of its articulation. In other words, individuals are the vehicles of power, not its points of application."

3. Foucault highlights the social researcher's task to understand the need for closure as follows:

What needs to be done is something quite different. One needs to investigate historically, and beginning from the lowest level, how mechanisms of power have been able to function. In regard to the confinement of the insane, for example, or the repression and interdiction of sexuality, we need to see the manner in which, at the effective level of the family, of the immediate environment, of the cells and most basic units of society, these phenomena of repression and exclusion possessed their instruments and their logic, in response to a certain number of needs. We need to identify the agents responsible for them, their real agents. ... We need to see how these mechanisms of power, at a given moment, in a precise conjuncture and by means of a certain number of transformations, have begun to become economically advantageous and politically useful. I think that in this way one could easily manage to demonstrate that what the bourgeoisie needed, or that in which its system discovered its real interests, was not the exclusion of the mad or the surveillance and prohibition of the infantile masturbation, but rather, the techniques and procedures themselves of such an exclusion. It is the mechanisms of that exclusion that are necessary, the apparatuses of surveillance, the medicalization of sexuality, of madness, of delinquency, all the micro-mechanisms of power, that came, from a certain moment in time, to represent the interests of the bourgeoisie. (Foucault, 1980, pp. 100–101)

4. It is Geertz's well-known story that seems to best capture the incompleteness of cultural analysis: "There is an Indian story—at least I heard it as an Indian story—about an Englishman who, having been told that the world rested on a platform which rested on the back of an elephant which rested in turn on the back of a turtle, asked (perhaps he was an ethnographer; it is the way they behave), what did the turtle rest on? Another turtle. And that turtle? 'Ah, Sahib, after that it is turtles all the way down' " (1973, pp. 28–29).

5. I am well aware of the controversy around using the term "community" (Harding, 2001; Walby, 2001). The ideal of community has been very central in feminism (see, for instance, Goldberger et al., 1996). Young states: "Community is an understandable dream, expressing a desire for selves that are transparent to one another, relationships of mutual identification, social closeness and comfort" (1990, p. 300). This positive orientation toward community can be understood in the light of Tonnies' (1957) analysis of *Gemeinschaft* and *Gesellschaft*. With the advent of capitalism and industrialization, smaller and more concrete communities of face-to-face contact (corresponding with the preindustrial community or Gemeinschaft) were replaced by larger more abstract social collectives (Gesellschaft). Paradoxically, Tonnies (1957) states, the need for community is a feature of the impersonal Gesellschaft. It is exactly because the word community evokes such romantic fantasies of internal consensus, shared norms, and separateness that makes it appropriate to use in this context: the use of this word highlights the idea that knowledge is validated by groups of people with interests and agendas. Walby (2001) proposes the use of the word "network" instead. I agree with Harding (2001, p. 517) that the use of the word "network" can deemphasise the politics of knowledge.

6. In her argument about story telling, Walby (2000) states that even if story telling is good for feminist politics, it is not necessarily good for feminist theory. She says that she is reluctant to equate feminist politics with feminist theory and states that feminist theory is not advanced by story-telling (Walby, 2000). While it is very difficult to define what counts as "feminist theory," it seems that in reviewing different discussions of feminist theory, one always find some kind of analysis of power relations (domination and subordination) and some notion of liberation, emancipation, and social transformation. Feminist theories therefore always include some explicit or implicit reference to political strategy. I would go so far as to say that to engage in feminist theory is to be a political activist. In fact,

as Foucault has argued, to engage in any theory is a political act. This should not paralyze us into not using theory. It should, however, make us more self-aware.

7. When there is such an emphasis on reflexivity, an insistence on looking at the personal stories of women on so many different levels, the question of where the researcher herself stands when doing all this reflection arises. Harding (2001) says that while no one can ever get completely outside their culture's assumptions, "only a small amount of alienation or separation from some such assumptions is necessary to create the possibility of bringing it into critical focus" (p. 518).

REFERENCES

Bassin, D., Honey, M., & Kaplan, M.-M. (1994). Introduction. In D. Bassin, M. Honey, & M.-M. Kaplan (Eds.), *Representations of motherhood* (pp. 1–25). New Haven, CT: Yale University Press.

Caroll, L. (1865). *Alice's adventures in wonderland*. London, UK: Macmillian.

Collins, P. H. (1994). Shifting the center: Race, class, and feminist theorizing about motherhood. In E. N. Glenn, G. Chang, & L. R. Forcey (Eds.), *Mothering: Ideology, experience, and agency* (pp. 45–66). London, England: Routledge.

Flax, J. (1990). *Thinking fragments: Psychoanalysis, feminism and post-modernism in the contemporary West*. Berkeley, CA: University of California Press.

Flax, J. (1993). *Disputed subjects. Essays on psychoanalysis, politics and philosophy*. London, England: Routledge.

Foucault, M. (1980). *Power/knowledge. Selected interviews and other writings 1972–1977*. Sussex, England: Harvester Press.

Geertz, C. (1973). *The interpretation of cultures*. New York, NY: Basic Books.

Glenn, E. N. (1994). Social constructions of mothering: A thematic overview. In E. N. Glenn, G. Chang, & L. R. Forcey (Eds.), *Mothering: Ideology, experience, and agency* (pp. 1–32). London, England: Routledge.

Goldberger, N. R., Tarule, J. M., Clinchy, B. M., & Belenky, M. F. (1996). *Knowledge, difference, and power: Essays inspired by women's ways of knowing*. New York, NY: Basic Books.

Harding, S. (2001). Comments on Walby's "Against epistemological chasms: The science question in feminism revisited: Can democratic values and interests ever play a rationally justifiable role in the evaluation of scientific work?" *Signs: Journal for Women in Culture and Society, 26*, 511–536.

Jewkes, R., Abrahams, N., & Mvo, Z. (1998). Why do nurses abuse patients? Reflections from South African obstetric services. *Social Science & Medicine, 47*, 1781–1795.

Jolly, M. (1998). Introduction. Colonial and postcolonial plots in histories of maternities and modernities. In K. Ram & M. Jolly (Eds.), *Maternities and modernities: Colonial and postcolonial experiences in Asia and the Pacific* (pp. 1–25). Cambridge, England: Cambridge University Press.

Langellier, K. M. (1989). Personal narratives: Perspectives on theory and research. *Text and Performance Quarterly, 9*, 243–276.

Myerhoff, B., & Ruby, J. (1992). *Remembered lives: The work of ritual, storytelling and growing older*. Ann Arbor, MI: University of Michigan Press.

Phoenix, A. (2000). Response to Sylvia Walby's "Beyond the politics of location: The power of argument in a global era." *Feminist Theory, 1*, 230–235.

Riessman, C. K. (1993). *Narrative analysis*. Newbury Park, CA: Sage.

Ruddick, S. (1996). Reason's "femininity": A case for connected knowing. In N. R. Goldberger, J. M. Tarule, B. M. Clinchy, & M. F. Belenky (Eds.), *Knowledge, difference, and power: Essays inspired by women's ways of knowing* (pp. 248–270). New York, NY: Basic Books.

Squire, C. (1998). Women and men talk about aggression: An analysis of narrative genre. In K. Henwoord, C. Griffin, & A. Phoenix (Eds.), *Standpoints and differences. Essays in the frontiers of feminist psychology* (pp. 65–90). London, England: Sage.

Tonnies, F. (1957). *Community and society.* New York, NY: Harper & Row.

Walby, S. (2000). Beyond the politics of location: The power of argument in a global era. *Feminist Theory, 1,* 189–206.

Walby, S. (2001). Against epistemological chasms: The science question in feminism revisited. *Signs: Journal of Women in Culture and Society, 26,* 485–509.

Wolf, B. H. (1987). *Low-income mothers at risk: Psychological effects of poverty-related.* (Unpublished doctoral thesis.) Graduate School of Education, Harvard University, Cambridge, MA.

Young, I. M. (1990). The ideal of community and the politics of difference. In L. J. Nicholson (Ed.), *Feminism/postmodernism (thinking gender)* (pp. 300–324). London, England: Routledge.

Gender Differences in the Experiences of HIV/AIDS-Related Stigma: A Qualitative Study in Ghana

GLADYS B. ASIEDU and KAREN S. MYERS-BOWMAN

School of Family Studies and Human Services, Kansas State University, Manhattan, Kansas, USA

Globally more women have been diagnosed with HIV/AIDS and are more likely to be stigmatized than men, especially in male-dominant societies. Gender differences in the experience of HIV-related stigma, however, have not been extensively explored. Researchers investigate the gender differences in HIV/AIDS-related stigma experiences here. Interviews were conducted with eight HIV patients and their nine discordant family members in Ghana. Our findings include gender differences in disclosure and response to HIV/AIDS diagnosis. The negative impact of HIV-related stigma was found to be more extensive for women than for men. Our findings may be used to facilitate an awareness and understanding through which supportive interventions can be implemented.

In our article we address an issue of global health importance—the AIDS crisis and its resulting stigma. We focused this study specifically on the gender differences of HIV/AIDS-related stigmas in Ghana, a male-dominant society. We examined the phenomenon through the theoretical lens of symbolic interactionism (SI) and employed phenomenological qualitative research methods in interviews with individuals diagnosed as HIV positive and their family members. We believe that our study sheds new light on HIV/AIDS-related stigma and its gendered nature and that other scholars will recognize implications for societies around the globe that share this health crisis.

Gladys B. Asiedu is now affiliated with the Department of Health Sciences Research, Division of Health Care Policy & Research, Mayo Clinic.

Since the identification of the first Human Immunodeficiency Virus (HIV)/Acquired Immune Deficiency Syndrome (AIDS) case, the disease has had a gendered dimension to it. According to the Joint United Nations Programme on HIV/AIDS (UNAIDS, 2012), globally 34 million people were living with HIV/AIDS at the end of 2011, with sub-Saharan Africa being the most severely affected, accounting for 69% of the global estimate. More than half (63%) of the sub-Saharan HIV/AIDS cases are women (UNAIDS/World Health Organization [WHO]/UNICEF, 2011).

Ghana was one of the first countries to acknowledge that HIV/AIDS had been identified in certain communities in the mid-1980s. The government responded to this by establishing the Ghana AIDS Commission (GAC) and subsequently the National HIV/AIDS Policy (Agyei-Mensah, 2006) to reduce new HIV transmission and the impact of its related vulnerability, morbidity, and mortality. Since then, HIV prevention and treatment programs have been working aggressively to combat the AIDS epidemic, and the HIV prevalence rate in Ghana decreased from 3.6% in 2003 to 2.3% in 2005 (Akumatey & Darkwa, 2009). Reports from the United Nations Integrated Regional Information Networks (IRIN) on Africa, however, indicated that the Ghanaian government's HIV/AIDS program is in danger of failure due primarily to stigmatization (IRIN, 2005). In fact, the GAC estimates that about 95% of Ghanaians are aware of HIV/AIDS; however, stigmatization of persons living with HIV/AIDS (PLHAs) remains the biggest challenge to the fight against the disease (GAC, 2004). This hinders all efforts to prevent the spread of the virus and mitigate the social and economic impacts of the epidemic (GAC, 2004).

Women face more stigma than men. In Ghana, the disease was initially considered to be a women's disease, and AIDS was explained as standing for "**A**kosua **I**s **D**ying **S**lowly"[1] (Ampofo, 2003) because of the overwhelming number of women (80% of PLHA) who were diagnosed with the disease in the late 1980s. More recent data show that the uneven diagnosis rates continue. Out of the 600,000 PLHAs in Ghana, 61% are females and 39% are males (Akumatey & Darkwa, 2009).

Women with HIV/AIDS in many areas around the world (including India [Aggleton, 2000]; Vietnam [Hong, Van Anh, & Ogden, 2004]; Ethiopia, Tanzania, and Zambia [Nyblade et al., 2003]; and Latin America and the Caribbean [Anderson, Marcovici, & Taylor, 2002]) are blamed and stigmatized more than their male counterparts. Nyblade and colleagues (2003) found that the reasons given for blaming women versus men for being responsible for bringing HIV infection into a partnership, home, or community are intricately tied to socially accepted norms regarding gender-specific roles, responsibilities, and sexuality. Both men and women who transgress these norms may face blame.

---

[1] Akosua is a name among the Akan tribe in Ghana given to a female born on Sunday.

When men in male-dominated cultures are blamed (by women or by men), however, it is with an underlying assumption that the misbehavior is to be expected and tolerated, because of social perceptions of men's proclivity for multiple sexual partners. Similarly, a study in Vietnam (Hong et al., 2004) highlighted that the family is at the center of Vietnamese culture and one is meant to act in ways that support and reinforce the well-being of one's family. Those who violate this norm are often harshly criticized and are simply not tolerated. These norms do not, however, apply to men and women equally. This is reflected in many Vietnamese proverbs, such as: "No matter how wise, she is still a woman; no matter how silly, he is still a man." A female participant in the Vietnamese study expressed this cultural sentiment:

> I think it is no problem for a man to get HIV/ AIDS and he could be talked with, but people hate a woman who gets infected. I say the truth. Why is that so? Because work is available for women—they should have good employment [keep busy]. So if a woman indulges in play too much, people would hate it. For example, people do not hate a drug-addicted man nearly as much as a drug-addicted woman. To say frankly, if men are still young and they indulge in play and get [HIV] infected, that's the general story of the society. If a girl gets this disease, no one would like to get close to her, because it is a problem of her conduct and her morality. It is not tolerated in females compared to males. (Nyblade et al., 2003, p. 34)

Thus, as part of their social functions, women are expected to do all the household chores and take care of their husbands and the rest of the family. Simply put, there is no time for a woman to engage in "play" that will result in getting infected with HIV/AIDS. HIV is regarded as evidence that women have failed to fulfill this important social function.

Ignored in these arguments are the many factors that contribute to women's high levels of vulnerability to HIV/AIDS infection. The WHO (2004) indicated that biological differences make women more susceptible than men in any given heterosexual encounter. Women have a greater area of mucous membrane exposed during sex. This mucous membrane is a soft tissue in the female reproductive tract that can tear easily during intercourse. This produces an easy transmission route for HIV. Also, during sexual intercourse more fluids are transferred from men to women than from women to men. Finally, male sexual fluids have a higher viral content than vaginal fluids. Vaginal tissue absorbs fluids easily, including semen, which remains in the vagina for hours following intercourse. This combination of factors leads to the estimations that male-to-female transmission of the disease is eight times more likely than female-to-male transmission.

Also, several researchers have looked at the social factors that make women more vulnerable to HIV/AIDS than men (Dunkel et al., 2004), particularly Ghanaian women (Akumatey & Darkwa, 2009; Mill, 2003; Oppong & Agyei-Mensah, 2004). Most of these social factors result from the lower status and power of women when compared with men. They include the acceptance of violence against women, the privileging of men within families, and laws or customs in patrilineal societies that prevent females from inheriting land and property. These factors relegate women to second-class status. Furthermore, there are common practices among several tribes in Ghana that could make them susceptible to HIV/AIDS (Nukunya, 1992, cited in Perry, 1997). Polygyny, the marriage of one man to two or more women, is commonly practiced. Also extramarital affairs by husbands are common, while extramarital affairs by wives are prohibited and often prompt and justify divorce (Nukunya, 1992, as cited in Perry, 1997). These social relationship factors keep women in relationships with men who may have multiple sex partners. It also highlights the opportunity for one man to spread HIV to multiple women.

High illiteracy rates among women also have been recognized as a factor that adds to women's burden of risk for HIV/AIDS in Ghana (Seager, 2009). Girls are less likely than boys to complete secondary or higher education because of social economic factors, such as early marriage, pregnancy, and care duties at home. For example, 2006 statistics show that equal proportions of males (93%) and females (94%) enrolled in basic primary education; however, at the university level women made up only 34% of the students (Seager, 2009). On the whole, more women (about 50%) were uneducated as compared with 34% of males in Ghana in 2006 (Seager, 2009). These high levels of undereducation leave a majority of women working in farming and other low-wage activities (such as trading, vending) with few women found in higher paying administrative and managerial jobs. This creates economic dependency for women as they seek relationships with men, including sex and the risk of HIV/AIDS, for the necessary money and other resources to live. Women end up depending heavily on their male partners for their own survival and that of their children.

Although there has been an overwhelming amount of research around the world that testifies to the greater vulnerability of women than men to HIV/AIDS (Anderson et al., 2002; Brewer et al., 1998; Giffin & Lowndes, 1999; Gupta & Selvaggio, 2007; ICRW, 2006; Mane & Aggleton, 2001; UNAIDS, 2002), only a few researchers have examined the *stigma* that relates to gender explicitly (Sandeowsky, Barroso, & Voils, 2009). Considering that Ghanaian women outnumber the men in diagnoses and are at risk for contracting HIV/AIDS from their husbands (due to low social status, polygyny, and extramarital affairs), it is imperative to understand the gendered experiences of stigma. Therefore, the main research question for this study is, What are the HIV/AIDS-related stigma experiences of PLHAs in Ghana? Specifically, we examined how those experiences impact women's lives. This particular study is a component of a larger project that was designed to document the concept/definition of HIV/AIDS-related stigma, ways it is expressed, factors influencing it, and the impact is has on both those living with HIV/AIDS and their family members in Ghana.

THEORETICAL FRAMEWORK

SI provided the theoretical framework for this study. SI is a sociological perspective based on the work of George H. Mead (1934) and Charles H. Cooley (1902). According to SI, meaning is an important aspect of human behavior that cannot be ignored (Ingoldsby, Smith, & Miller, 2004). People act according to the meaning something has for them. That meaning is learned through interaction with others, and people interpret things according to what they learn through their experiences (Ingoldsby et al., 2004). The importance of meaning in SI is reflected in the saying that situations are real if their consequences are perceived as real (White & Klein, 2002).

There are several unexplored issues related to gender differences in the experience of HIV/AIDS-related stigma in Ghana that can be understood by applying this framework. These include the meaning of stigma and the interpretation associated with an HIV/AIDS diagnosis and the notion that HIV/AIDS is a woman's disease. For instance, if people see HIV/AIDS as a woman's disease that results from improper behavior, then it follows that women will be stigmatized more than men.

Goffman (1963) defined stigma as an "attribute that is deeply discrediting" and reduces the bearer "from a whole and usual person to a tainted, discounted one" (p. 3). While Goffman's definition focused on the individual aspects of stigma, Parker and Aggleton (2003) offered a framework that emphasizes stigma as a social process that produces and reproduces relations of power and control. Stigma is used by dominant groups to legitimize and perpetuate inequalities, such as those based on gender. Dominant groups effectively limit the ability of stigmatized groups and individuals to resist subordination because of their entrenched marginal status. Furthermore, stigmatized individuals and groups often accept the norms and values that label them as having negative differences (Goffman, 1963). As a result, stigmatized individuals or groups may accept that they deserve to be treated poorly and unequally, making resistance to stigma and its resulting discrimination even more difficult.

HIV/AIDS-related stigma has been defined in many ways and has been expressed as a complex social process resulting from the interactions between social and economic factors in the environment that create unfavorable attitudes, beliefs, and policies directed toward people perceived to have HIV/AIDS as well as toward their families, close associates, social groups, and communities (Brimlow, Cook, & Seaton, 2003; Ogden & Nyblade, 2005). It can result in PLHAs and those associated with them being rejected from their community, shunned, discriminated against, or even physically hurt.

In this study, SI provided a conceptual framework within which to explore the meanings of HIV/AIDS-related stigma, especially as experienced by women. It provided the lens through which we viewed the phenomenon. We focused specifically on the meaning and personal experiences of women's encounters with HIV/AIDS-related stigma as we created the research questions, conducted the analyses of the data, and interpreted the results.

METHODS

Qualitative methods were used to gain an in-depth understanding of HIV/AIDS-related stigma in Ghana. In Ghanaian culture, family members of PLHAs also experience a high level of stigmatization even if they do not have HIV/AIDS (Brimlow, Cook, & Seaton, 2003; ICRW, 2006; Nyblade et al., 2003; Ogden & Nyblade, 2005; Parker & Aggleton, 2003). Therefore, the study included those who have been diagnosed with HIV/AIDS and their family members. A context-sensitive form of interpretive inquiry, phenomenology (van Manen, 1990), was employed to explore the lived experiences of these individuals and how HIV/AIDS-related stigma impacted their lives. Phenomenologic inquiry is qualitative descriptions eliciting explorative questioning about a particular phenomenon from which underlying patterns and structures of meanings may be drawn (van Manen, 2012). This method is used to open and explore possible human experience—in this case, the stigma experiences of PLHAs and their family members. This approach led us to gather rich information from those who have experienced it directly and intensely.

Research procedures were reviewed and approved by the Internal Review Board for Research on Human Subjects (IRB) at Kansas State University and the Health Research Unit of the Ghana Health Service. Permission to conduct the study also was obtained from appropriate local authorities in Ghana, the Eastern Regional AIDS Project (RAP), and the Eastern Regional Association of PLHA (ERAP). Two representatives from RAP and ERAP (who facilitated recruitment) underwent the Kansas State University IRB training and agreed to abide by the regulations. This process ensured that the rules regarding the ethical treatment of participants in the project were followed in an appropriate manner. This was especially important because of the sensitive nature of the information we were discussing.

Data Collection

The data were gathered in 2010 in the eastern region of Ghana that has been identified as having the highest HIV prevalence in the country. We employed criterion homogeneous sampling techniques (Patton, 2002). This means that individuals were invited to participate in the study only if they met a standard set of conditions. The criteria were chosen to help recruit participants who could provide rich information about the phenomenon under investigation: the PLHA must have been diagnosed a minimum of 5 years prior, he or she must have told his or her serostatus to at least one family member, and he or she must have at least one family member participate in the study who is aware of his or her serostatus.

Recruitment was facilitated by the RAP and the ERAP. Representatives of each organization made initial contacts and presented information about the study to potential participants at their regional and district meetings with PLHAs. Individuals were asked to contact the RAP if they were interested in the study. The interviewer then followed up with participants after they had expressed an interest to participate. Twenty-four PLHAs showed interest in the study and were asked if they would be willing to include their family members. Nine of the PLHAs indicated that their family members were not aware of their diagnosis. Because they did not meet the eligibility criteria, they were not included in the study. Eight out of the remaining 15 PLHAs agreed to participate in the study together with their family members (four females and four males). Two of the female PLHAs included their mothers in the study, one her sister, and one her son. One male participated with both of his parents, one with his cousin, one with his wife, and one with his sister.

A total of 17 people participated in the study, eight PLHAs (four males and four females) and nine of their family members (three males and six females; one PLHA had both parents participate). The PLHAs ranged in age from 27 to 54, with the mean age of 41.1 years ($SD = 8.9$). Mean age at diagnosis was 33.8. One male was married, one female was separated from her husband, and one male was widowed. Four PLHAs were single (including three females). All PLHAs had at least an eighthgrade education. Five of them were self-employed, with two unemployed. Family members ranged in age from 22 to 63 with the mean age of 46.1 years ($SD = 14.7$). The PLHAs lived in several different towns in rural areas with their family members. Participants were all from discordant families: the PLHAs' family members had not tested positive for HIV. All PLHAs were receiving antiretroviral treatment (ART).

Interview Procedure

Before each interview, participants were provided with information about the nature and purpose of the study and data handling protocol. They were informed that participation was voluntary and that they could withdraw from participating at any time. Participants were assured of the confidentiality of any information they provided, and all participants were given pseudonyms to protect their identities.

Interviews were conducted at various locations, such as participants' homes, local restaurants, and workplaces. The PLHAs and their family members chose the locations based on their own preferences. The interviews were conducted in the local language of their choice (either Twi or Ga, both of which the interviewer, a native of Ghana, speaks fluently). All interviews were audio recorded. Participants were given the option to interview together as a family or individually. All of them opted to be interviewed separately.

A standardized open-ended interview guide was used to ensure that all participants had the opportunity to answer the same questions throughout the process. Probes were used when needed to elicit further details of the incidents described. Two specific interview protocols were prepared to serve as guides, one for interviewing PLHAs and another for family members with wording appropriate for each role. For example, PLHAs were asked the following: Do you feel men and women are treated differently when they have AIDS? Please explain. What are your experiences as a woman/man who has AIDS? What are your experiences as mother/wife, father/mother? How is your experience different from your husband/wife/mother/father/sister/brother/etc.? Has your role as mother/wife, father/husband changed? If yes, please explain. How do you think people see you as a woman/man or as mother/wife or as father/husband who has AIDS? What do you think are the factors that contribute to gender differences with regards to stigmatization? Family members were asked the following: Do you feel there are gender differences in the way people are stigmatized? Please explain. How do you think people see women/men who have AIDS? What do you think are the factors that contribute to gender differences with regards to stigma?

After interviewing 17 people, data saturation was achieved, so recruitment ended. Data saturation is the point in data collection when the interviewer determines that later interviews include similar information to previous interviews and are not adding new themes. After the interviews, each participant received 30 Ghanaian Cedis as compensation for his or her time.

Data Analyses

Data were transcribed and then translated from Twi or Ga into English by the interviewer. Another individual fluent in all three languages then translated the interviews back into the original language. When the back translation did not match the original words and ideas of the participants, adjustments were made to the English translation. This process insured that the English transcripts accurately represented the participants' voices.

Data analyses were conducted in an inductive fashion. New themes and categories were created as they emerged from the data, without the restraints imposed by structured methodologies (Thomas, 2006). To begin, each interview was read and reread several times in order to find answers to each of the research questions within the participants' words. Important passages were highlighted within each interview for ease in locating them again. This led to the identification of preliminary themes within individual interviews. Once this initial step was completed for all interviews, we began cross-case comparison. We looked for similarities in the themes across the participants. When we identified that several participants had provided related answers, we compiled those answers into one theme. The next step included combining themes into broader categories. These categories joined the themes that fit together in a theoretical or logical way.

Both coauthors participated in the analysis process in order to produce credible findings. This triangulation of analysis helped to assure that the data were examined from more than one perspective. We discussed the themes and categories at length in order to come to consensus on the final results. Here we provide information about ourselves to aid the readers in understanding our backgrounds and perspectives.

Gladys B. Asiedu: I was the interviewer and am a native of Ghana. This project was conducted as the dissertation for my doctoral program. Prior to the data collection I had worked with PLHA in Ghana several years before relocating to the United States. During my doctoral program I took several classes in qualitative methods and worked on qualitative research projects. Since completing my dissertation, I have been involved in several qualitative studies involving African immigrant and refugee women as well as cancer patients.

Karen S. Myers-Bowman: I am a native of the United States. I served as the major professor for Gladys Asiedu's doctoral work. I have conducted qualitative research studies for over 20 years and teach the qualitative series of courses in the Family Studies and Human Services graduate program at Kansas State University. I have never been to Ghana, but I have traveled internationally throughout my life. I have worked in the area of human sexuality since the 1980s, including providing direct educational and counseling services about HIV/AIDS.

RESULTS

This study was a phenomenological inquiry into gender differences in the experiences of HIV/AIDS-related stigma. Because we applied an SI lens, participants' perceptions and understandings of gender differences regarding HIV-related stigmas were central to this study. Three major categories were identified as differences between men and women in the experiences of

HIV-related stigma: disclosure, response to disclosure, and attributed reasons for the diagnosis related to social norms.

Disclosure

All PLHA expressed that disclosure of their serostatus was the beginning of their stigmatizing experiences. Disclosure of the serostatus of PLHA took four forms: voluntary self-disclosure, involuntary disclosure, implied or perceptible disclosure, and third-party disclosure.

Voluntary self-disclosure.   Voluntary self-disclosure took place when a PLHA chose to disclose his or her status out of her or his own free will. The decision to disclose one's status on one's own terms depended on how one perceived the reaction of the person to whom the information would be revealed and its impact. Usually it was to receive some kind of support, as a female PLHA shared:

> I went to my supervisor and informed her of the situation, so that she can help me out or tell me what to do. So, she took me to the authorities, but they refused and let me go, but at that time I didn't have much education about this disease and I didn't even know my rights. So what they gave me was 1-month salary and they released me.

Another female PLHA related her experience:

> So I was there when my sister came to me and asked what was wrong. I told her, "It's nothing," but I was still crying. So she consoled me, encouraged me, comforted me, and so I eventually told her. So I told her that "This is the problem, so right now I am dead, I am going to die," and she told me not to say that.

Involuntary disclosure.   Involuntary disclosure was forced upon the PLHA. It occurred when a PLHA was asked by health workers to share his or her status with one other relative (who served as a guarantor) as a requirement of receiving ART for HIV. Having a guarantor was mandatory in an attempt to ensure that the medications would be taken correctly, as expressed by a female PLHA:

> Part of the rules is that if a person is diagnosed with HIV/AIDS, he or she has to come with a relative or friend for support and also as a witness who will make sure that the patient adheres to his or her medications.

Sometimes, however, the family members refused to serve in that role and provide guarantees of their support. For instance, one participant discussed how her husband initially refused to serve as a guarantor and she had to plead with him:

He said this disease is a supernatural disease, so he refused for me to accept the medication from the hospital. And so that first day I had to beg him to be my witness before the medication was given to me.

Implied disclosure.   Implied or perceptible disclosure took place when the PLHA's status was inferred from his or her poor health, physical appearance, or weight loss. In this form of disclosure, the true status of the PLHA was not known for sure, and she or he sometimes chose not to affirm people's suspicions even when confronted. One male PLHA shared how his friends became suspicious of his diagnosis:

> I don't know, I have not told them, but I know they are suspicious. That is why they are not on talking terms with me. You know, I have been sick on and off, so they suspect that disease. None of them have been able to ask me anything, but they are not talking to me and don't visit as they used to do.

An interesting effect of the introduction of ART is that it has helped PLHAs gain weight and has thus confounded many people's assumptions about physical appearance as a sign of one's status. This may reduce the number of PLHAs whose status is disclosed in this way.

Third-party disclosure.   Sometimes, other persons shared the status of a PLHA with others, creating the final category of third-party disclosure. Medical workers, religious leaders, PLHAs' friends, coworkers, and family members could do this. Like perceptible or implied disclosure, however, with third-party disclosure the true status of the PLHA was not known for sure and he or she could decide to affirm it or deny it. Two PLHAs shared how disclosure of their diagnoses snowballed in their families:

> Yes, the man that I trusted, he [PLHA's brother] went to tell my father that this is what is happening. In fact, I was very sad . . . so my father also went and told the rest of the family that I have gone for the bad disease so they should come and look at me.

> So when I informed my mother, she also informed my uncle about it [HIV diagnosis]. I guess she did that for sympathy. Out of "okra mouth" my uncle also spread the "news" to everyone we knew in their community.

Another female PLHA shared how a health worker disclosed her diagnosis:

> My colleagues did not know what went on, but the nurse who was in the consulting room with the doctor was the one who spread the news that I have this disease and that is why I don't come to work.

One of the major differences between men's and women's stigma experiences was how their serostatus was disclosed. Most participants expressed that women were stigmatized more than men because women often voluntarily disclosed their status, whereas men did not. Participants expressed that most men do not voluntarily disclose their status and therefore are not stigmatized. For example, one participant, a female PLHA, shared that she would not have disclosed her status if she were a male: "But the thing is, most men don't tell. So probably I wouldn't have told anybody."

Data from this study suggest that women disclosed their status to receive support financially and emotionally, whereas men were too proud to disclose or did not see the need because they had the resources they needed, as stated by a female PLHA:

> Well, maybe they have the money to buy the medications or maybe they think it's a disgrace to let other people know of their status. And you know how men are, proud. And you know how men are able to keep secrets [better] than women.

Similarly, when asked whether there are differences between men and women regarding HIV/AIDS-related stigma, a male PLHA answered in the affirmative and gave a probable reason for that:

> Well, I think it depends on how they tell other people about their status. In our association, for instance, there was a lady who sells "koko" (cornmeal porridge). She told people about her status; so eventually she lost all her customers. You know, I believe women talk much more than men. Maybe that is why they are stigmatized more.

While women were thought to share their diagnoses easily, ironically they concealed their spouses' diagnoses. Men, on the other hand, concealed their own diagnoses, but revealed their spouses' diagnoses. A female PLHA recounted how her husband disgraced her by revealing her status:

> For me, if it hadn't been my husband who had disgraced me all over this place, I would never be ashamed if I am in public. But he has disgraced me so much that I don't visit many places.

When men disclose their spouse's status to family members in Ghana, it provides legal or social justification to dissolve the marriage or to find another woman, as one woman described:

> He even told his family members about my situation during one of our (family) meetings to dissolve the marriage. ... The problem is when women have it, they tell their husbands. Because their husbands too, for

one reason or another, will want to go in for other women, they inform their family members just so they can have their support for going in for another woman. And the family members too when they hear that, oh my goodness, they will say all sorts of nasty things about you and sometimes evict you from your marital home.

Responses to HIV/AIDS Disclosure

Once serostatus had been disclosed, PLHAs encountered the reactions of others to their diagnosis. When examining the differences between men and women's experiences, two main themes emerged: gendered marital expectations and public shaming or name-calling.

Gendered marital expectations. A major difference between women's and men's experiences concerns the reactions or responses of others to the HIV/AIDS diagnosis, either one's own diagnosis or when a spouse had been diagnosed. Our data suggest that people reacted to women's diagnoses differently than to men's. According to the participants, when men are diagnosed with HIV/AIDS, their wives are forgiving, compassionate, and supportive of them, but men, on the other hand, lack compassion and often are not supportive when their wives test positive for HIV/AIDS, as one female PLHA said:

> Well, I think that when a married woman gets this [HIV], she is neglected by her husband and most of the time the men even leave the children with the women, knowing very well that they [women] would not have money to take care of them. But when it is the man who has the disease, the woman will stay with him no matter what and take care of him.

We suggest that women in this study support their spouses when the men are diagnosed with HIV more than husbands support their wives. This was expressed by a female PLHA whose diagnosis led to her husband leaving her:

> Now I don't have a husband. But if he was the one who had the disease, I would have stayed with him ... because we women think of the children more than anything, and when you leave, that will be it. He will not take care of the children. I would have stayed. I would have stayed.

Another woman said,

> I also think when men are sick the women stay with them and take care of them. But what kind of a husband will stay with his wife and nurse her? No, they won't do that; they would rather go for another woman.

One of the female participants asserted that it is also easier for a man to find someone other than his wife to care for him than it is for a woman to find another man. This made her keep her status a secret from men:

> Because they will always get someone to care for them, their wives or mothers or sisters or some woman. Now, I think most of us are learning from them; that is why I don't want to tell any man I meet about my condition.

When a male PLHA was asked his opinion on the differences between men's and women's experiences, he also attributed it to the good character-istics of women:

> You know, naturally women have more compassion than men. Women are very sympathetic, so they tend to stay in the marriage to care for their husbands.

One male PLHA's wife asserted that her husband would have left her if she were the one who was HIV positive, as she expressed:

> Do you think if I were the one who has the disease, he would have gone through what I went through for him? No way! I believe he would have left me long ago.

When asked why, she replied:

> Because that is what men do. They are not compassionate like women. Only few women will leave their husbands, but most men will go find other women.

Public shaming/name-calling. As part of women's blame for their serostatus, they were labeled, called names, and received insults. Many Ghanaians called them "ashawo," meaning whores or prostitutes, as one female PLHA said:

> Well, in this society, hmmm you know, in my situation when I got it people started saying that I am a prostitute, I have had a bad life, that I have slept with many men. That is why I got it. But if it were a man, well, they will insult him, but it wouldn't be so much as they did to me.

For one female PLHA, people's perceptions of her were described as, "One thing—prostitute. Multiple partners, that's it and nothing will convince them that their thoughts are wrong." According to her, if men were labeled at all, they were simply called "men."

Yet others indicated that women were blamed more than men because there are more women than men who are diagnosed with HIV/AIDS. A male PLHA recounted, "But you see, in this society, if you have this disease, then it means you have had multiple partners and there are more women than men, so . . ." Thus the dominance of women in terms of the number infected made it easier for them to be blamed.

Based on our data we suggest that although men were sometimes called "womanizers," this is seldom talked about. The wife of a PLHA said, "You see, a woman cannot be a prostitute because it is not acceptable; but a man can be a womanizer because it is acceptable."

When asked what people think of men who have AIDS, a father of a male PLHA said, "People think he's also had multiple partners or he is a womanizer. But, you see, in the case of the man, people don't really talk about it." He went on to contrast the situation of men to that of women:

> *Father*: Honestly, I am a man, but I will say this, "I think there is nothing wrong with it when a man has multiple partners, but when a woman has multiple partners, hmm it's not good."

> *Interviewer*: Why is it not good, if you can have multiple partners, why can't a woman?

> *Father*: If you are a woman, you don't have to do that, otherwise you will not get a husband and people will not respect you. Even some men will take advantage of that and come and propose to you, but they won't marry you. They will want to sleep with you and leave you.

> *Interviewer*: So what is the difference between men and women?

> *Father*: I think people accept men more easily than women because, you see, it is believed that when you have this disease then you have not done something right. And when men sleep with many women, there is nothing wrong; but if it is the other way, people will never forgive you.

> *Interviewer*: So do you think it's okay?

> *Father*: No, it's not okay, but what I am saying is it's not a big deal. I can have multiple women and choose one to marry. But for a woman, if you do that you may not have a husband.

Reasons for Stigma

When asked whether there were differences in the experience of stigma between men and women, most participants initially said they did not believe there were. When they were asked to share their perceptions on stigma for the opposite gender, however, they explained that women experience stigma more than men and shared some of the reasons for the differences – acceptable sexual norms and women as caregivers.

Acceptable sexual norms. Participants expressed strong beliefs about the reasons women experience more stigma, blame, and shame than men when they have AIDS. In fact, similar to the last theme, most of the reasons participants gave for the differences are related to the gendered perceptions of moral and immoral sexual behavior. When women and men have AIDS, it was attributed to having multiple sexual partners. In Ghanaian culture, however, men are assumed to have a natural propensity to have multiple partners, while it is unacceptable for women to do so, as a participant whose sister was living with HIV/AIDS expressed:

> Oh, but madam [addressing interviewer], all men are promiscuous. How many men in this world will stick to their wives only? I believe there is no man. So, somehow we already know that all men have multiple partners. But that is what it is. There is nothing wrong with it [said sarcastically]. Why do we say that when a married woman sleeps with another man, she has committed adultery; but if a married man does it, no one thinks of it as adultery? It's the norm.

Asked whether he would have experienced the same rejection from his friends if he were a woman, a male PLHA, who said he is a virgin and does not know how he contracted HIV, replied the following:

> Oh that would have been worse, worse, worse. ... A woman? Hmm, I don't think even my parents would have believed me if I told them I were a virgin. You know, when a woman has this disease her situation is worse because people think she did more than double what the man did.

Even when men had HIV/AIDS, women were seen as the ones to blame, as a female PLHA explained:

> And, you know, I can tell you that there are many men who have this disease, but they always say it's a women's disease. ... You see, we don't see men having multiple partners as a new thing; but if it's a woman, oh God, everybody will hear it. In the same way, when a man has the disease, even though people will believe that he had had multiple partners, they don't usually refer to that fact or even say it in public. Sometimes they will even say, "It is so-and-so woman who gave it to him."

Similarly, two participants who were mothers of PLHAs affirmed that when men have AIDS, they make reference to where they contracted it (usually from a woman):

Interviewer: I see, so what do you think people think of a woman who has AIDS?

Mother 1: She has led an unacceptable life.

Interviewer: What if it's a man?

Mother 1: He got it from one of his multiple partners and, you see, naturally men always have multiple partners, but if you are a woman you cannot do that; otherwise people will not respect you.

Interviewer: So what do you think people think of women who have AIDS?

Mother 2: Maybe they had multiple partners, prostitutes.

Interviewer: What about men?

Mother 2: Maybe they got it from a prostitute or maybe they also had multiple women.

The caregiving role.   The reasons given for blaming and stigmatizing women more than men were intertwined with social roles regarding gender-specific roles and responsibilities. When a woman (depending on her age) has HIV/AIDS and is unable to perform her social role of caregiver, then it means she has violated a norm and may not be forgiven. In cases where the infected woman is married, it becomes difficult for the husband to accept his new role as a caregiver. Therefore, he may choose to neglect his wife, as described by one female PLHA:

And one thing that I also notice is that being a woman itself is a problem because women are the ones that take care of everyone. We take care of children and men. So, if a man has this disease, it is not a new thing that a woman takes care of him; but if the woman becomes sick, then who takes care of her? So I believe people ask why they should be taking care of you when according to the norm you should be taking care of them.

When a young woman is diagnosed with HIV/AIDS and is being taken care of by her parents, it is also a violation of the caregiving norm that adult children care for their aging parents. This is a significant role change that Ghanaian society frowns upon, as one female PLHA who used to support her family financially expressed:

Since I was not able to supply anymore, my family started looking down on me. My role as a daughter who cared for her parents, like everyone expects, changed. And I was no more a daughter, but a burden to my mother. For my sister, I believed she did not respect me because, maybe in her mind, she thinks I have led a bad life. That is why I have this disease.

Traditionally, in Ghana, men are the breadwinners and heads of household, and so when they are sick and are not able to provide for the family, it is a big change for the family, but their wives are expected to find other avenues or take on multiple jobs to replace their husbands' income to support the family. When a male PLHA was asked whether his role as a father has changed, he responded, "No. I don't know what will happen if my children know, but for now they don't know, so everything is normal." His wife gave a similar response:

Well, I don't think so, because my husband is still my husband and he is the same father to his kids. But, well, I think in terms of caring for the family financially, it changes because, like my husband, he was the main breadwinner, and so when he became sick, things were tough. But apart from that, I don't see any changes. No matter what, that respect is there, even if the person is sick. It doesn't make him less of a husband.

Thus, for both men and women, caregiving roles are violated, but the consequence are considered more disruptive for women than men. Also it is socially expected that a wife must stay with her ill husband and take care of him. This was expressed by one participant whose husband has HIV: "But since he is the one who has the disease, his family expects me to take care of him."

DISCUSSION

In this study we highlight some of the differences between men and women's experiences of HIV/AIDS-related stigma in Ghana. We suggest that women are more negatively affected by this stigma than men. The reasons given are related to HIV diagnosis disclosures and are also intricately tied to socially accepted norms regarding gender-specific roles, sexual behavior, and responsibilities.

SI provides a helpful theoretical lens through which to view and interpret these findings. Specifically, in the Ghanaian culture HIV/AIDS has been symbolized as a women's disease. In the context of this assumption, women are regarded as the transmitters of HIV/AIDS; hence, when they test positive for HIV/AIDS, they are blamed more than their male counterparts.

HIV/AIDS has been regarded as a symbol of moral impropriety because it is assumed that one has had multiple sexual partners (Aggleton, 2000; Belsey, 2005; Brooks, Etzel, & Hinojos, 2005; Ogden & Nyblade, 2005; Parker & Aggleton, 2003). As a result of this, PLHA are seen as personally responsible for their diagnosis. This seems to invoke anger and resentment in the person attributing responsibility, which then turns into social rejection and stigma (Breitkopf, 2004). Within the Ghanaian culture extramarital affairs by husbands are common and acceptable but are prohibited for wives and often lead to divorce (Nukunya, 1992, as cited in Perry, 1997). According to SI, because we live in a world that is socially constructed, some behaviors are rewarded and respected while others are condemned or punished (Ingoldsby et al., 2004: White & Klein, 2002). Thus, the diagnosis of HIV/AIDS renders the meaning that women, but not men, have violated a norm and should be punished.

This fundamental double standard (that is not unique to Ghana), makes men more likely be exposed to a whole host of sexually transmitted infections (STIs), including HIV. Women, on the other hand, are expected to be sexually faithful, "proper," and not engage in any "improper" behaviors. Considering that extramarital affairs are acceptable for men, it is ironic to blame women more than men when they test positive for HIV. It is very likely that, because men are the ones who have multiple partners, they are the ones who are contracting HIV outside the marital relationship and are infecting their wives (and other sexual partners).

Although most participants in the study initially said that they did not believe there were differences in the stigma experiences of men and women, when asked what the experiences would have been if they were the opposite gender, most of them expressed that stigma experiences are worse for women than men. As much as it may seem contradictory, it is probable that most participants shared the same beliefs and values of society about gender roles and responsibility, as well as the meaning of HIV/AIDS diagnosis, so that, while there are obvious differences, they seem normal to them. This finding may have implications for other male-dominant cultures that include gender inequality.

Gendered caregiving expectations explain why women experienced blame more than men in the male-dominant society of Vietnam (Hong et al., 2004). Similarly, in Ghana women are expected to be the caregivers, nurturing men, children, and the elderly. Because of the exhaustive effects of HIV/AIDS and medications, often women are unable to execute their proscribed domestic duties or participate in a normal active life, which also changes their role as care *givers* to care *receivers*. This corroborates the findings of an earlier study (Hong et al., 2004) that HIV provides evidence that women are considered to have failed society when they cannot fulfill their important social function of caregiver, when instead they themselves require care.

The men in our study with HIV/AIDS receive care and support from their wives and other family members, while HIV-positive women are ill-treated by their husbands and relatives. Regardless of HIV status, women in Ghana are considered to be of lower social status and are often marginalized relative to men in their families and communities. One female participant explained how her diagnosis resulted in a divorce. In the Ghanaian context, the stigma she experienced is multilayered because she is a woman and has HIV, which means she is considered a prostitute. She was rejected by her husband, which implies that she has failed as a "proper" woman. Being rejected by a husband is a huge problem for many Ghanaian women because most of them depend on their husbands financially (Nukunya, 1992, as cited in Perry, 1997). It also means that the children (if any) will be taken care of solely by the woman, sometimes with little or no help from the husband, which leads to negative consequences for the children.

Some of the findings about disclosure of this study are contrary to an earlier study (Ulasi et al., 2009) in which males were more likely to be in favor of disclosure of HIV-positive status than females. A significant aspect of gender-related stigma in the current study is the issue surrounding disclosure of PLHAs' serostatus. Participants expressed that women experience more stigma than men because they disclose their status more often than men. Thus, even though men may report favoring the idea of disclosing one's serostatus more than women do (Ulasi et al., 2009), women are the ones who disclose their status more often.

The major reason for voluntary self-disclosure as expressed by participants in this study is for financial support. Men often do not disclose their status because they have the economic means to afford basic necessities as well as their medications and treatment. Hence, there is an implied relationship between gender and poverty with regards to HIV/AIDS-related stigma that needs to be addressed. Similar to our findings several scholars have emphasized how poverty plays a role in driving people to disclose their status and depend on their families for sustenance (Nyblade et al., 2003; Ogden & Nyblade, 2005). Most of the members of the ERAP are women. The ERAP is a local government organization that provides education to the public about HIV/AIDS and support to PLHAs by offering them counseling and referring them to the appropriate organizations for financial support. Being diagnosed with HIV or another life-threatening disease, compounded with abandonment from their husbands, can be quite devastating; hence, the use of public or governmental assistance (which also means revealing one's status) is very common for women.

Because of the stigmatization associated with the disclosure of HIV/AIDS and the impact it has on women, many women are adopting the nondisclosure method used by their male counterparts. Women in this study indicated that other women in their support groups do not disclose their status to their husbands and, in fact, some of the participants were not prepared to share their status to their future/aspiring husbands because of the fear of partner rejection. While this mechanism may provide some kind of relief for women diagnosed with HIV/AIDS, it does not help in the prevention and the fight against HIV/AIDS. Nondisclosure often results in the spread of HIV, thus diminishing the objectives of public health. The challenge of keeping records of PLHAs also poses a challenge. Unfortunately, in Ghana there is no proper record keeping on individuals and so there is no way of tracking PLHAs who may relocate or do not disclose their serostatus. There remains so much to be done in finding a balance between disclosure and nondisclosure to minimize the experience of stigma as well encouraging people to disclose their status for public health reasons. It is not surprising that stigmatization of PLHAs still remains one of the most significant challenges in developing countries for all HIV/AIDS programs, across the continuum of prevention and care.

Implications for Research

We learned from this study that there are several challenges and questions that arise regarding gender and stigma in Ghana that need to be addressed. For example, how do we explain to the Ghanaian community that HIV/AIDS is not a women's disease? How do we make Ghanaian men feel responsible for caring for their ailing wives and children when policies that address those issues do not work? How do we encourage women to stand up for themselves in the midst of HIV/AIDS and poverty? How can we reduce the stigma attached to a positive HIV status so that individuals will share their status with sexual partners and reduce the spread of the disease?

In order to fully understand HIV and its related stigma, we must gain more knowledge about its path through society. For example, is its prevalence in Ghana related to the tendency of men to have multiple partners? To answer this question, a more complete and rigorous tracking system of HIV/AIDS would be required than is currently practiced in Ghana. This highlights one of the fundamental challenges encountered by professionals interested in reducing the spread of the disease—in order to understand HIV/AIDS-related stigma, we must comprehend how the disease is spread; however, the stigma prevents honest cooperation and disclosure, making it difficult to track the path of HIV. This conundrum must be explicitly addressed if we are to gain a full understanding of HIV/AIDS.

Future research also is necessary to explore the relationships among cultural expectations and both internalized and externalized stigma. Before we can reduce the negative effects of HIV/AIDS-related stigma, especially on women, we must explore the bidirectional connections between gendered social roles and a diagnosis of HIV.

Limitations of the Current Study

While the inclusion of family members enriched our understanding of HIV/AIDS-related stigma, undoubtedly, it limited participation in the study. There was general reluctance of PLHAs to include their family members. This may have been either because most of their family members were not aware of their status or would not approve of their status. Participants in this study were from rural settings in the Eastern Region of Ghana and were of low socioeconomic status. Therefore, findings may not reflect perspectives from other areas of the country or from diverse socioeconomic backgrounds.

CONCLUSION

The uniqueness and the major contribution of this study is its focus on the differences between women and men's experiences of HIV/AIDS-related stigma. While there are many studies on HIV, gender differences in the stigma experience and the inclusion of family members have been given little attention, which highlights the complexity of the phenomenon and emphasizes the importance of the disclosure aspect as a point of intervention for those working to reduce the spread of HIV/AIDS and its negative consequences. Finally, this study indicates that more research is essential to build an understanding of this phenomenon in different social environments and in areas around the world, especially those in which HIV/AIDS-related stigma is high.

ACKNOWLEDGMENTS

The authors are grateful to all participants in this study and to the Eastern Regional AIDS Project and the Eastern Regional Association of People Living with HIV/AIDS. Also, many thanks to Joan Jurich for her feedback and assistance with the manuscript.

FUNDING

The study was supported by a travel grant from the West Africa Research Association.

REFERENCES

Aggleton, P. (2000). *HIV and AIDS-related discrimination, stigmatization and denial*. Geneva, Switzerland: UNAIDS. Retrieved from http://data.unaids.org/Publications/IRC-pub02/JC587-India_en.pdf

Agyei-Mensah, S. (2006). Poverty and HIV prevalence in Ghana: A geographical perspective. *GeoJournal, 66*, 311–324.

Akumatey, B., & Darkwa, A. (2009). *Gender norms, domestic violence and women's vulnerability to HIV/AIDS. Report of a national study*. Ghana, Africa: Gender Studies and Human Rights Documentation Centre.

Amnesty International. (2004). *Women, HIV/AIDS and human rights*. Retrieved from http://www.amnesty.org/en/library/asset/ACT77/084/2004/en/1358d0af-d55f-11dd-bb24-1fb85fe8fa05/act770842004en.pdf

Ampofo, A. (2003). The sex trade, globalization and issues of survival in sub-Saharan Africa. *Ghana Studies, 6*, 59–90.

Anderson, H., Marcovici, K., & Taylor, K. (2002). *The UNGASS, gender and women's vulnerability to HIV/AIDS in Latin America and the Caribbean*. Washington, DC: Pan-American Health Organization.

Awusabo-Asare, K., & Marfo, C. (1997). Attitudes to and management of HIV/AIDS among health workers in Ghana: The case of the Cape Coast municipality. *Health Transition Review, 7*, 271–280.

Belsey, M. A. (2005). *AIDS and the family: Policy options for a crisis in family capital*. New York, NY: United Nations.

Breitkopf, C. R. (2004). The theoretical basis of stigma as applied to genital herpes. *Herpes, 11*, 1–7.

Brewer, T., Hasbun, J., Ryan, C. A., Hawes, S. E., Martinez, S, Sanchez, J., ... Holmes, K. K. (1998). Migration, ethnicity and environment: HIV risk factors for women on the sugar cane plantation of the Dominican Republic. *AIDS, 12*, 1879–1887.

Brimlow, D. L., Cook, J. S., & Seaton, R. (2003). *Stigma and HIV/AIDS: A review of the literature*. Rockville, MD: U.S. Department of Health and Human Services.

Brooks, R. A., Etzel, M. A., & Hinojos, E. (2005). Preventing HIV among Latino and African American gay and bisexual men in a context of HIV-related stigma, discrimination and homophobia: Perspectives of providers. *AIDS Patient Care and STDs, 19*, 737–744.

Cooley, C. H. (1902). *Human nature and the social order*. New York, NY: Scribner's.

Dunkel, K. L., Jewkes, R. K., Brown, H. C., Gray, G. E., McIntryre, J. A., & Harslow, S. D. (2004). Gender-based violence, relationship power, and risk of HIV infection in women attending antenatal clinics in South Africa. *Lancet, 363*, 1415–1421.

Ghana AIDS Commission (GAC). (2004). *HIV/AIDS in Ghana, current situation, projections, impacts and interventions* (4th ed.). Accra, Ghana: Author. Retrieved from http://www.policyproject.com/pubs/countryreports/HIVAIDS_IN_GHANA_CURRENT%20SITUATION.pdf

Giffin, K., & Lowndes, C. (1999). Gender, sexuality and the prevention of sexually transmissible diseases: A Brazilian study of clinical practice. *Social Science and Medicine, 48*, 283–292.

Goffman, E. (1963). *Stigma: Notes on the management of spoiled identity*. Englewood Cliffs, NJ: Prentice-Hall.

Gupta, G. R., & Selvaggio, K. (2007). *It can be done: Addressing gender in the AIDS epidemic through PEPFAR programs*. Washington, DC: ICRW. Retrieved from http://www.icrw.org/files/publications/It-Can-Be-Done-Addressing-Gender-in-the-AIDS-Epidemic-through-PEPFAR-Programs.pdf

Hong, K. T., Van Anh, N. T., & Ogden, J. (2004). *Because this is the disease of the century: Understanding HIV and AIDS-related stigma and discrimination in Vietnam*. Washington, DC: ICRW. Retrieved from http://www.icrw.org/docs/vietnamstigma_0204.pdf

Ingoldsby, B. B., Smith, S. R., & Miller, J. E. (2004). *Exploring family theories*. Los Angeles, CA: Roxbury.

Integrated Regional Information Networks (IRIN). (2005, August, 17th). Ghana: AIDS treatment on rise, but stigma still around. *Integrated Regional Information Networks*. Retrieved from http://www.irinnews.org/report/38899/ghana-aids-treatment-on-rise-but-stigma-still-around

International Center for Research on Women (ICRW). (2006). *HIV/AIDS stigma: Finding solutions to strengthen HIV/AIDS programs*. Washington, DC: Author. Retrieved from http://www.icrw.org/docs/2006_stigmasynthesis.pdf

Mane, P., & Aggleton, P. (2001). Gender and HIV/AIDS: What do men have to do with it? *Current Sociology, 49*, 23–37.

Mead, G. H. (1934). *Mind, self & society (Charles W. Morris)*. Chicago, IL: The University of Chicago Press.

Mill, J. E. (2003). Shrouded in secrecy: Breaking the news of HIV infection to Ghanaian women. *Journal of Transcultural Nursing, 14*, 6–16.

Nyblade, L., Pande, R., Mathur, S., MacQuarrie, K. Kidd, R., Banteyerga, H., … Bond, V. (2003). *Disentangling HIV and AIDS stigma in Ethiopia, Tanzania and Zambia*. Washington, DC: ICRW. Retrieved from http://www.icrw.org/files/publications/Disentagling-HIV-and-AIDS-Stigma-in-Ethiopia-Tanzania-and-Zambia.pdf

Ogden, J., & Nyblade, L. (2005). *Common as its core: HIV-related stigma across contexts*. Washington, DC: ICRW. Retrieved from http://www.icrw.org/files/publications/Common-at-its-Core-HIV-Related-Stigma-Across-Contexts.pdf

Oppong, J. R., & Agyei-Mensah, S. (2004). HIV/AIDS in West Africa: The case of Senegal, Ghana and Nigeria. In E. Kalipeni, S. Craddock, J. R. Oppong, & J. Ghosh (Eds.), *HIV/AIDS in Africa: Beyond epidemiology* (pp. 58–69). Malden, MA: Blackwell.

Parker, R., & Aggleton, P. (2003). HIV and AIDS related stigma and discrimination: A conceptual framework and implications for action. *Social Science & Medicine, 57*, 15–24.

Patton, M. Q. (2002). *Qualitative research and evaluation methods* (3rd ed.). Thousand Oaks, CA: Sage.

Perry, T. E. (1997). *The lived experience with Ghanaian women living with HIV/AIDS: A phenomenological study*. (Unpublished doctoral dissertation). University of Alabama, Tuscaloosa, AL.

Sandeowsky, M., Barroso, J., & Voils, C. I. (2009). Gender, race/ ethnicity, and social class in research reports on stigma in HIV-positive women. *Health Care for Women International, 30*, 273–288.

Seager, J. (2009). *The penguin atlas of women in the world* (4th ed.). New York, NY: Penguin Books.

Thomas, D. (2006). A General inductive approach for analyzing qualitative evaluation data. *American Journal of Evaluation, 27*, 237–246.

Ulasi, C. I., Preko, P. O., Baidoo, J. A., Bayard, B., Ehiri, J. E., Jolly, C. M., & Jolly, P. E. (2009). HIV/AIDS-related stigma in Kumasi, Ghana. *Health & Place, 15,* 255–262.

UNAIDS. (2002). *Report on the global HIV/AIDS epidemic.* Geneva, Switzerland: Author. Retrieved from https://www.unaids.org/en/media/unaids/contentassets/dataimport/pub/report/2002/brglobal_aids_report_en_pdf_red_en.pdf

UNAIDS. (2012). *Global report: UNAIDS report on the global AIDS epidemic.* Geneva, Switzerland: Author.

UNAIDS/World Health Organization (WHO)/UNICEF. (2011). *Global HIV/AIDS Response epidemic update and health sector progress towards universal access. I (Progress report).* Geneva, Switzerland: Author.

van Manen, M. (1990). *Researching lived experience: Human science for an action sensitive pedagogy.* London, ON, Canada: Althouse.

van Manen, M. (2012). Carrying: Parental experience of the hospital transfer of their baby. *Qualitative Health Research, 22*(2) 199–211.

White, J. M., & Klein, D. M. (2002). *Family theories* (2nd ed.). Thousand Oaks, CA: Sage.

World Health Organization (WHO). (2004). *World health report 2004: Changing history.* Retrieved from http://www.who.int/whr/2004/en/report04_en.pdf

Management of Conflicts Arising From Disclosure of HIV Status Among Married Women in Southwest Nigeria

OLADAPO T. OKAREH

*Department of Environmental Health Sciences, Faculty of Public Health,
University of Ibadan, Ibadan, Oyo State, Nigeria*

ONOJA M. AKPA

*Department of Epidemiology, Medical Statistics, and Environmental Health,
Faculty of Public Health, University of Ibadan, Ibadan, Oyo State, Nigeria*

JOHN O. OKUNLOLA

*Department of Peace and Conflict, Institute of African Studies, University of Ibadan,
Ibadan, Oyo State, Nigeria*

TITILAYO A. OKOROR

*Department of Health and Kinesiology; and African American Studies Research Center,
Purdue University, West Lafayette, Indiana, USA*

This study examined if disclosure to their spouses by married women living with HIV/AIDS resulted in conflicts. Fifty-seven women completed a questionnaire on conflict indicators. While 93% disclosed their status within 6 months of diagnosis, 12.3% did so through a third party. More than thirty-six percent (36.8%) confirmed that disclosure led to conflict. Although 19.3% had their conflicts resolved through a third party, 10% suffered separation. Marital status and fear of stigma significantly influence time to disclose ($p < .01$ and $p < .05$), while type of marriage strongly influences whether status will be disclosed ($p < .01$).

The authors are grateful to I. O. Albert, Director of the Institute for African Studies, University of Ibadan. We are also grateful to the principal investigator, APIN Plus Adeoyo Maternity Hospital, the management of the Adeoyo Maternity Hospital, all the health workers and counselors at the Grace Foundation support group, and finally, the participants in this study, for defiling the prevailing societal barriers to participating in a study of this nature.

Programs for women with HIV should consider conflicts that may arise from disclosure.

Although new cases of HIV infection in many developed countries have been very low in recent years, sub-Saharan Africa continues to bear a disproportionate share of the global HIV burden. In mid-2010, about 68% of all people living with HIV resided in sub-Saharan Africa, a region with only 12% of the global population (World Health Organization [WHO], 2011). According to recent estimates, 76% of all HIV positive women live in sub-Saharan Africa (UNAIDS, 2010). Women in sub-Saharan Africa account for over 60% of people living with HIV/AIDS in the region, and young women especially (ages 15–24) remain disproportionately affected. In fact, for every 10 men infected with HIV in sub-Saharan Africa, 13 women are infected. This highlights the need to address gender inequity and harmful gender norms as a central component of the global response to HIV (National Agency for the Control of AIDS [NACA], 2011; UNAIDS, 2010; WHO, 2011).

It has been reported that the high prevalence of HIV/AIDS in sub-Saharan Africa is largely due to some misconceptions that have made voluntary counseling and testing (VCT) as well as HIV-positive status disclosure (in many countries) much more difficult if not impossible (Akpa, Adeolu-Olaiya, Olusegun-Odebiri, & Aganaba, 2011; Bhagwanjee, Petersen, Akintola, & George, 2008). In order to reduce HIV seroprevalence, emphasis is always placed on the importance of HIV status disclosure (particularly to sexual partners) within HIV counseling and testing programes among HIV infected clients. This has made disclosure an important public health issue in that, in addition to facilitating access to treatment by people living with HIV and AIDS (PLWHA), disclosure may motivate sexual partners to seek HIV testing, change behaviors, and ultimately decrease the transmission of HIV (Galvan, Bing, & Bluthenthal, 2000; Group VH-CaTES, 2000; Vergerout, Reiser, Krchnavek, Druckenmiller, & Davis, 1998).

Despite these crucial essences of disclosure, it has been reported that infected individuals and couples in particular are usually unwilling to disclose their HIV status to friends, family members, and, most importantly, their spouses or sexual partners (Gielen, O'Campo, Faden, & Eke, 1997; Group VH-CaTES, 2000; Lester, Partridge, Chesney, & Cookee, 1995). Actually, the level of economic burden of HIV infection, mental depression arising from a family member being HIV positive, stigmatization, and so on, have made HIV/AIDS a very important societal problem in human relationships, rather than just a viral disease, particularly in Nigeria. Also, fears of rejection, abandonment, verbal abuse, physical assault, discrimination, and maltreatment have complicated the issue in some situations. In most cases, women have been reported to be the most affected with the consequences of disclosing their HIV status to their sexual partners or spouses (Gielen, McDonnell, Burke, & O'Campo, 2000; Simbayi et al., 2007).

Past studies have shown that between 25% and 66% of women living with HIV and AIDS (WLWHA) who disclosed their HIV status to their family members (or sexual partners) were violently maltreated (Gielen et al., 1997; Simbayi et al., 2007; Vlahov et al., 1998). Consequently, most WL-WHA (particularly in developing countries) would choose not to disclose their HIV status even to family members or their sexual partners due to fear of violence, abuse, and maltreatment (Crepaz et al., 2006; Medley, Garcia-Moreno, McGill, & Maman, 2004; Simbayi et al., 2007). It is worth mentioning that none of the reviewed literature (above) reported how conflicts or other unfriendly attitudes due to disclosure of HIV status were managed among couples, nor is there a published study on such a subject in Nigeria located during literature searches.

Therefore, in addition to providing tools for policymakers on issues of interventions among married women living with HIV and AIDS (MWLWHA), the present study seeks to bridge the gap in knowledge. Although largely descriptive, the present study seeks to understand if the disclosure of HIV status by MWLWHA to their spouses resulted in conflicts (or any form of unfriendly attitudes) between them and their spouses, and how such conflicts were resolved. We also explored why many women may not want to disclose their HIV status to their spouses, in addition to methods employed in disclosing their HIV status. Associations of some HIV related attitudes and indicators of conflicts following HIV status disclosure with selected sociodemographic characteristics of MWLWHA were also assessed.

METHODS

Study Design, Population, and Sampling Techniques

We carried out the study among married women attending a support group at the Adeoyo Maternity Hospital, Ibadan North Local Government (INLGA), Ibadan in Oyo State, Nigeria. The group was selected due to ongoing collaborative efforts between the hospital and the Grace Foundation, a religious-based organization that provides funding for programs geared toward PLWHA, especially women. In addition, this is the only known religious-based support group in Ibadan. The focus was to study the topic of conflict resolution following HIV disclosure among MWLWHA in the support group. Prior to data collection, we visited the group on several occasions to acquaint the members with the intention to carry out a study among them and to also provide some voluntary counseling and care services to the patients. Although obtaining the exact number of MWLWHA in Ibadan INLGA is difficult, as at the time of this study, the support group under study had 57 married women, all of whom participated in this study after giving verbal consent. Since some MWLWHA do not attend support group meetings for fear of being identified as having HIV infection and reaching them through a cross-sectional survey will be a waste of effort (particularly in the area covered by the study), every effort (ethically permissible) was made to appeal to all the women in the support group to participate in the study.

Description and Analysis of the Study Instruments

The research instrument for this study was a pretested, structured questionnaire designed (in a simple or easy-to-understand form) to elicit relevant responses from the participants. The questionnaire was divided into two sections, with section one containing questions on selected sociodemographic characteristics of the respondents ranging from age and religion to the type of employment in which they engage. The second section consisted of questions regarding HIV related attitudes and indicators of conflicts as well as its management following HIV status disclosure among couples (see Tables 1 and 2 for details). The reliability of the instrument was established through a pretest survey with a retest done 2 weeks after the initial test and the reliability coefficient was found to be 0.73. We corrected identified errors and limitations of the questionnaires before the final data collection exercise.

Data Collection and Exclusion Criteria

Prior to data collection, we explained the concept and the importance of HIV disclosure as well as the purpose of this study to the participants. We

TABLE 1 Sociodemographic Characteristics of MWLWHA

Variable	Frequency	Percentage
Age		
≤30	27	47.4
31–40	19	33.3
>40	11	19.3
Religion		
Islam	30	52.6
Christianity	27	47.4
Marital status		
Married	51	89.5
Widowed	4	7.0
Separated	2	3.5
Education		
Primary	37	64.9
Secondary	12	21.1
Tertiary	8	14.0
Type of marriage		
Monogamous	27	47.4
Polygamous	30	52.6
Employment		
Employed	24	42.1
Self-employed	33	57.9

TABLE 2 Distribution of MWLWHA According to HIV Related Attitudes and Indicators of Conflicts Following Disclosure of HIV Status

HIV related attitudes and indicators of conflicts	Frequency	Percentage
When did you know your HIV status?		
During antenatal	27	47.4
VCT	18	31.6
During illness	12	21.1
How long did it take you to disclose your current HIV status to your spouse?		
≤6 months	53	93.0
>6 months	4	7.0
How did you disclose your HIV status to your spouse (if you have)?		
Self	50	87.7
Third party	7	12.3
Has disclosing your status to others changed your relationships with them?		
Yes	49	86.0
No	8	14.0
What was your spouse's initial reaction toward your current HIV status?		
Supportive	40	70.2
Quarrelsome/abusive	17	29.8
What was your spouse's subsequent attitude toward your current HIV status?		
Supportive	44	77.2
Quarrelsome/abusive	13	22.8
Did disclosure of your current HIV status cause any conflict in your marriage?		
Yes	21	36.8
No	36	63.2
What could prevent you from disclosing your HIV status to your spouse?		
Stigma/discrimination	30	52.6
Fear of divorce	27	47.4
How did the society treat you after disclosing your current HIV status?		
With care and love	30	52.6
With rejection	27	47.4
From your experiences, should MWLWHA disclose their status to their spouses?		
Yes	48	84.2
No	9	15.8

administered the questionnaires at the monthly meeting of PLWHA at the Adeoyo Maternity Hospital, Ibadan. We administered the questionnaires on a one-on-one basis to ensure confidentiality, and we provided assistance to any participant having difficulty with the questionnaires item(s). All categories of MWLWHA as well as women who had never been married attending the support group were excluded from this study. Relatives of MWLWHA who accompanied then to the meeting and the caregivers (and other health professionals) were also excluded from the study.

Ethical Approval

Initial approval to carry out this study was sought from the directorate of the Institute of African Studies, Peace and Conflict Studies Programme, University of Ibadan. In addition to consent given by the individual participants, management of the Grace Foundation Support Group (GFSG) and the Adeoyo Maternity Hospital also gave approval that the study met their ethical conditions.

Data Management, Presentations, and Analysis

Responses of the participants were coded and input into the computer. The input data were edited for every possible errors and inconsistencies. Because we were performing a quantitative study, we employed frequency distribution tables, graphs, and percentages to provide descriptive analysis of data. The Pearson chi-square test of independence was used to assess the associations of selected HIV related attitudes and indicators of conflicts arising from HIV status disclosure with selected sociodemographic characteristics of MWLWHA. The Statistical Package for Social Sciences (SPSS), version 20, was used for the data analysis.

RESULTS

Sociodemographic Characteristics of MWLWHA

As seen in Table 1, almost half (47.4%) of the participants in this study were less than 31 years old, while 11 (19.3%) were older than 40 years. Also, the majority of the participants (30/52.6%, 51/89.5%, and 33/57.9%) were Muslim, married, and self-employed. Similarly, while more than half (37/64.9%) of the participants had completed only primary education, and only 8 (14.0%) had completed tertiary education. In addition, most of the participants (52.6%) were in a polygamous marriage (i.e., their husbands have more than one wife).

HIV Related Attitudes, Indicators of Conflicts, and Management Following HIV Status Disclosure

As shown in Table 2, out of the 57 MWLWHA who participated in this study, 27 (47.4%) learned of their current HIV status during an antenatal visit to a health center, while 18 (31.6%) discovered their current HIV status through a VCT, and 12 (21.1%) found out about their status on a visit to a hospital during an ailment. Although an overwhelming 93% of the MWLWHA reported to have disclosed their current HIV status to their spouse within 6 months of diagnosis (only 7% of them told their spouse after 6 months of

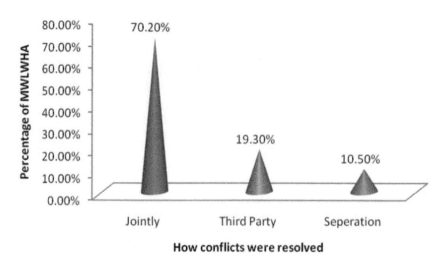

FIGURE 1 Distribution of MWLWHA according to how conflicts arising from HIV status disclosures were resolved.

diagnosis), 12.3% of the participants were only able to disclose their current HIV status to their spouses through a third party.

Similarly, while most MWLWHA reported that their spouses were supportive both at the break of the news of their current HIV status (70.2%) and thereafter (77.2%), 36.8% of the participants actually confirmed that the disclosure of their current HIV status led to conflicts between them and their spouses. As shown in Figure 1, although most of them had their conflicts resolved with their spouses without any mediator, 19.3% of the women had theirs resolved through a third party, while the marriages of more than 10% of the women suffered separation (or divorce). Furthermore, while fear of unknown phenomena, like divorce, for example, kept some (47.4%) of the WMLWHA from disclosing their HIV status to their spouses over a period of time, 52.6% of them reported that the fear of stigma and discrimination were their major hindrances. Also, 52.6% of the women reported that people around them treated them with care after disclosing their current HIV status, but 47.4% of them indicated that the community treated them with rejection, while 15.8% concluded from their own experiences that women diagnosed with HIV should not disclose their status to their spouse.

Results of Inferential Statistical Data Analysis

The results of testing the independence of selected HIV related attitudes and indicators of conflicts arising from HIV status disclosure with selected sociodemographic characteristics of MWLWHA are presented in Table 3. The results presented were only for situations where the test results yielded a significant relationship. The employment status of women was found to

TABLE 3 Factors Associated With Selected HIV Related Attitudes and Indicators of Conflict Following HIV Status Disclosure

Dependent variable	Independent variable	Chi-square test		
		df	Test value	p
How current HIV status was diagnosed	Employment status	2	6.22	.040
Time to disclosure of HIV status (in months)	Marital status	2	12.23	.002
	Hindrances to disclosing HIV status	1	4.78	.030
Spouse's initial reaction to current HIV status	Employment status	1	5.08	.020
Should HIV status be disclosed to spouse	Type of marriage	1	7.39	.007

df: degrees of freedom.

influence how their current HIV status was diagnosed ($p < .05$), while marital status and fear of stigma/discrimination were found to significantly influence time to disclosure of HIV status by the participants ($p < .01$ and $p < .05$, respectively). Furthermore, employment status was also found to influence spouses' initial reaction to HIV status of their wives ($p < .05$). Whether HIV status should be disclosed to spouses was strongly related to the type of marriage the woman was in ($p < .01$), based on the experiences of the MWLWHA.

DISCUSSION

In this article, we reported HIV related attitudes and indicators of conflicts following disclosure of HIV status among MWLWHA in Ibadan north Local Government Area (LGA), Ibadan, Nigeria. Although detailed inferential analyses were not carried out, attention was focused on MWLWHA and the possible consequences of disclosing their HIV status to their spouses. We also explored the fears and experiences of MWLWHA following the disclosure of their HIV status to their spouses as well as how these issues were managed. It was found that the majority of the participants were less than 31 years old, while less than 20% of the participants were over 40 years old. In some studies conducted among PLWHA in Nigeria and other part of the world, the majority of PLWHA were younger and in their active/productive age (Akpa et al., 2011; Gielen et al., 2000; Kalipeni, 2008; Monjok, Smesny, & Essien, 2009; Rahangdale et al., 2010; Simbayi et al., 2007). Having over 80% of the participants in their active reproductive age could have serious consequences for their spouses (if great care and counseling is not taken) and mother-to-child transmission of HIV infection in the study area; even more, the majority of them are still married to their spouses.

Also, the participants in this study largely had only a primary school education; primary school education is the minimum level of formal education obtainable in Nigeria. In a study conducted among PLWHA in Nigeria, it was found that most PLWHA coming for treatment in some states either had no formal education or only a primary school education (Akpa et al., 2011). Although the results of the above study and the present one may not be sufficient to conclude that HIV infection in Nigeria is of the less educated, there is evidence from past studies supporting a strong correlation between level of education and HIV infection (Atilola, Akpa, & Komolafe, 2010; Merrigan et al., 2011; Moses & Chama, 2009). The highly educated tend to be more aware of the infection and to adopt HIV related protective/preventive measures than the less educated. Furthermore, we observed that most MWLWHA who participated in this study were self-employed. We are not be able to say whether they lost their employment after disclosing their current HIV status, but in Nigeria there has been evidence of PLWHA losing their employments after being diagnosed with HIV infection (Akpa et al., 2011). In fact, Akpa and colleagues (2011) reported that the employment of over 20% of PLWHA was affected after being diagnosed to be HIV positive.

Voluntary counseling and testing (VCT) for HIV (though recommended by many stakeholders in HIV prevention) has not been popular in Nigeria due to the general attitude of the populace and the fear of being diagnosed to be HIV positive. Hence, most people only get tested for HIV when they are compelled to do so by their situations. Most participants in this study confirmed that they learned about their HIV status during antenatal visit to a hospital. Together, over 60% of the participants discovered their HIV status either during an antenatal visit to a hospital or during an illness. Poor attitude toward VCT is perhaps one of the most implicative potentials for the future of the HIV pandemic in any country (Galvan et al., 2000; Group VH-CaTES, 2000; Maman et al., 2002).

While most participants disclosed their status to their spouses within 6 months of diagnosis, it was found that some of them did so 6 months after they were diagnosed; and others could only disclose their HIV status to their spouses through a third party for fear of conflicts. The question that may remain unanswered is whether the spouses of these women were having sexual relations with them during this period. If they were, there was a likelihood that they did so without any form of protection, which could result in HIV infection. Actually, it is not unlikely that MWLWHA would be sexually involved with their spouses who were unaware of their HIV status. Simbayi and colleagues (2007) reported that 56% of WLWHA had sex with partners who were not aware of their HIV status.

We also found that the initial reactions and subsequent attitudes of some spouses of the MWLWHA who participated in this study were abusive. Specifically, while close to 30% of them were initially nonsupportive, close to 20% of the women continue to face quarrels and abuse in their marriages due to their current HIV status. This is consistent with the reports in past studies where women were physically, emotionally, and sexually abused because of their HIV status (Dunkle et al., 2004; Gielen et al., 2000; Holt-Lunstad, Smith, & Layton, 2010; Silverman, Decker, Kapur, Gupta, & Raj, 2007). In Nigeria, it is likely for a man to be stigmatized or rejected (in some ways) because he has a HIV positive wife. Perhaps the later behaviors of their spouses were due to the frustrations and the economic burden being incurred by the family due to caring for an HIV patient.

In addition, because all the participants faced some forms of stigmatization/discrimination, divorce, and rejection, some of them concluded that it was unwise for any married woman diagnosed with HIV to disclose their status to their spouses. Although it may sound wicked and unbelievable, past studies in South Africa have shown that not only did WLWHA refuse to disclose their HIV status to their partners, they were sexually involved with their partners without telling them their HIV status (Simbayi et al., 2007). Imagine a polygamous marriage where the husband has up to three or four wives in their active reproductive age. If a women who is HIV positive refuses to disclose her status to her husband for fear of the unknown, she becomes the reservoir for distributing the virus to other members of that union and, in some occasions, to an unborn baby through mother-to-child transmission.

Although great efforts were made to report comprehensive data in this study, it must be mentioned that the quality of results presented would have been enhanced if more MWLWHA had participated, thereby increasing the sample size. Also, although GFSG was the only comprehensive group considered in this study, a more robust finding certainly requires comparison of results between groups. In addition, there appears to be inconsistency in the number of women who suffered separation in their marriages following the disclosure of their HIV status. When asked of their marital status, barely 4% of the MWLWHA indicated that they have separated from their spouses, while over 10% claimed to have fixed their conflict by separation.

Nevertheless, this study has added another dimension to gender based research focusing on HIV/AIDS infections. Because infection with HIV continues to generate conflicts and unfriendly attitudes from spouses of PLWHA, managing such conflicts are crucial to the management and delivery of health care packages to patients, especially women. Programs geared toward assisting MWLWHA must take into account conflicts that may arise from disclosure.

REFRENCES

Akpa, O. M., Adeolu-Olaiya, V., Olusegun-Odebiri, C. A., & Aganaba, D. (2011). HIV/AIDS-related stigma and access to HIV treatments by people living with HIV/AIDS: A case study of selected states in North-West Nigeria. *HIV & AIDS Review, 10,* 19–25.

Atilola, G. O., Akpa, O. M., & Komolafe, I. O. O. (2010). HIV/AIDS and the long-distance truck drivers in south-west Nigeria: A cross-sectional survey on the knowledge, attitude, risk behaviour and beliefs of truckers. *Journal of Infection and Public Health, 3,* 166–178.

Bhagwanjee, A., Petersen, I., Akintola, O., & George, G. (2008). Bridging the gap between VCT and HIV/AIDS treatment uptake: Perspectives from a mining-sector workplace in South Africa. *African Journal of AIDS Research, 7,* 271–279.

Crepaz, N., Lyles, C. M., Wolitski, R. J., Passin, W. F., Rama, S. M., Herbst, J. H., … Stall, R. (2006). Do prevention interventions reduce HIV risk behaviors among people living with HIV? A meta-analytic review of controlled trials. *AIDS, 20,* 1430–157.

Dunkle, K. L., Jewkes, R. K., Brown, H. C., Gray, G. E., MCintyre, J. A., & Harlow, S. D. (2004). Gender based violence, relationship power, and risk of HIV infection in women attending antenatal clinics in South Africa. *The Lancet, 363*(9419), 1415–1421.

Galvan, F. H., Bing, E. G., & Bluthenthal, R. (2000). Accessing HIV testing and care. *Journal of Acquired Immune Deficiency Syndromes, 25*(Suppl. 2), S151–S156.

Gielen, A. C., McDonnell, K. A., Burke, J. G., & O'Campo, P. (2000). Women's lives after an HIV-positive diagnosis: Disclosure and violence. *Maternal and Child Health Journal, 4*(2), 111–120.

Gielen, A. C., O'Campo, P., Faden, R. R., & Eke, A. (1997). Women's disclosure of HIV status: Experiences of mistreatment and violence in an urban setting. *Women & Health, 25*(3), 19–31.

Group VH-CaTES. (2000). Efficacy of voluntary HIV-1 counselling and testing in individuals and couples in Kenya, Tanzania and Trinidad: A randomised trial. *The Lancet, 356*(9224), 103–112.

Holt-Lunstad, J., Smith, T. B., & Layton, J. B. (2010). Social relationships and mortality risk: A meta-analytic review. *PLoS Medicine, 7*(7), e1000316. doi:10.1371/journal.pmed.1000316.

Kalipeni, E. (2008). HIV/AIDS in women: Stigma and gender empowerment in Africa. *Future HIV Therapy, 2,* 147–153.

Lester, P., Partridge, J. C., Chesney, M. A., & Cookee, M. (1995). The consequences of positive prenatal HIV antibody test for women. *Journal of Acquired Immune Deficiency Syndromes, 10,* 341–349.

Maman, S., Mbwambo, J. K., Hogan, N. M., Kilonzo, G. P., Campbell, J. C., Weiss, E., & Sweat, M. D. (2002). HIV positive women report more lifetime partner violence: Findings from a voluntary counselling and testing clinic in Dar Es Salaam, Tanzania. *American Journal of Public Health, 92,* 1331–1337.

Medley, A., Garcia-Moreno, C., McGill, S., & Maman, S. (2004). Rates, barriers and outcomes of HIV sero-disclosure among women in developing countries:

Implication for prevention of mother-to-child transmission programmes. *Bulletin of the World Health Organisation, 82*, 299–307.

Merrigan, M., Azeez, A., Bamgboye, A., Chabikuli, O. N., Onyekwena, O., Eluwa, G., . . . Hamelmann, C. (2011). HIV prevalence and risk behaviours among men having sex with men in Nigeria. *Sexually Transmitted Infections, 87*, 65–70.

Monjok, E., Smesny, A., & Essien, E. J. (2009). HIV/AIDS-related stigma and discrimination in Nigeria: Review of research studies and future directions for prevention strategies. *African Journal of Reproductive Health, 13*(3), 21–35.

Moses, A. E., & Chama, C. (2009). Knowledge, attitude and practice of ante-natal attendees towards prevention of mother to child transmission (PMTCT) of HIV infection in a Tertiary Health Facility, North-East Nigeria. *The Internet Journal of Third World Medicine, 8*, 1.

National Agency for the Control of AIDS (NACA). (2011). *Factsheet 2011: Women, girls and HIV in Nigeria by the National Agency for the Control of AIDS*. Retrieved from http://naca.gov.ng/index2.php?option=com_content&do_pdf=1&id=419

Rahangdale, L., Banandur, P., Sreenivas, A., Turan, J. M., Washington, R., & Cohen, C. R. (2010). Stigma as experienced by women accessing prevention of parent-to-child transmission of HIV services in Karnataka, India. *AIDS Care, 22*, 836–842.

Silverman, J. G., Decker, M. R., Kapur, N. A, Gupta, J., & Raj, A. (2007). Violence against wives, sexual risk and sexually transmitted infection among Bangladeshi men. *Sexually Transmitted Infections, 88*, 211–215.

Simbayi, L. C., Kalichman, S. C., Strebel, A., Cloete, A., Henda, N., & Mqeketo, A. (2007). Disclosure of HIV status to sex partners and sexual risk behaviours among HIV-positive men and women, Cape Town, South Africa. *Sexually Transmitted Infections, 83*, 29–34. doi:10.1136/sti.2006.019893.

UNAIDS. (2010). *UNAIDS global report fact sheet: Sub-Saharan Africa*. Retrieved from http://www.unaids.org/en/media/unaids/contentassets/documents/factsheet/2010/20101123_FS_SSA_em_en.pdf

Vergerout, J. M., Reiser, W. J., Krchnavek, K. A., Druckenmiller, J. K., & Davis, J. (1998). Meeting the challenge of early identification of HIV infection in primary care. *Wisconsin Medical Journal, 97*, 52–61.

Vlahov, D., Wientge, D., Moore, J., Flynn, C., Shumann, P., Schoenbaum, E., & Zier Ler, S. (1998). Violence among women with or at risk for HIV infection. *AIDS Behavior, 2*, 53.

World Health Organization (WHO). (2011). *Global HIV/AIDS response epidemic update and health sector progress towards universal access: Progress report 2011*. Retrieved from http://whqlibdoc.who.int/publications/2011/9789241502986_eng.pdf

Universal Access to HIV Treatment in the Context of Vulnerability: Female Farm Workers in Zimbabwe

SANDRA BHATASARA

Sociology Department, University of Zimbabwe, Harare, Zimbabwe

MANASE KUDZAI CHIWESHE

Sociology Department, Rhodes University, Grahamstown, South Africa

In this study we extend the theoretical and empirical debate on gender justice regarding universal access to antiretroviral therapy. In many circumstances, debates about human rights and HIV/AIDS are premised on the view that universal access to primary health care improves the multiple health burdens of those infected by the epidemic. We argue that "universal access" does not always benefit those in marginalized positions in society. Female farm workers living in rural, marginalized spaces at the intersection of systems of social inequality and oppression shape the way in which they experience access to antiretroviral drugs.

Universal access to antiretroviral drugs (ARVs) has created enormous debate and controversy in developing countries (Ciccio, 2004). In this article we examine how rural women farm workers in Zimbabwe living with HIV and AIDS experience "universal access" to HIV treatment using Crenshaw's (1994) intersectionality approach. These women occupy multiple marginalized spaces emerging from and in relation to their historical context, including their health status, their rural location, their class, and their gender in Africa's most struggling postcolonial economy in the geopolitical South (Crenshaw, 1994). The authors utilize qualitative methods to highlight how the intersection of global and local factors influences access to treatment for vulnerable groups in Zimbabwe. Interviews and focus group discussions offered a nuanced understanding of women's circumstances and ensured their voices were captured. This article is important in that there is little work that shows the complex interplay of forces and localized structures in impacting the everyday experiences of people in the developing world. We avoid a reductionist view in explaining lack of universal access to HIV medication but rather offer an explanation of how intersecting and mutually reinforcing systems of inequality at international and national levels operate to deny access to certain groups.

FARM WORKERS IN ZIMBABWE

The farm worker community, in general, has remained at the margins of mainstream Zimbabwean society. Schou (2000) has described them as "quasi-citizens" and outsiders living within. The government of Zimbabwe over the years has remained suspicious of farm workers, often accusing them of being foreigners. It is their connection to White farmers as farm workers that the ruling party mistrusts, and they have faced persecution during elections since 2000. As West and Rutherford (2005, p. 399) highlight, "This construct and the perceptions embedded within it, further alienated farm workers from the inner political and social circles of the community and the state." These interactions between structural factors and farm workers' lived experiences in relation to HIV medications have been largely underexplored in policy and academic discourses. The key thrust of this article is therefore to explore the gender, location, and class of infected women in relation to structural factors that exist and inhibit accessible means of health care and affordable ARVs.

ACCESS TO HIV TREATMENT

A Worldview

Universal access is defined as treatment coverage of around 80% of the population. In the case of HIV and AIDS, universal access is often equated with access to ARVs. Access to treatment is also often defined in terms of accessibility, affordability, and availability of treatment. At the end of 2007, 3 million (31% of people in need) were receiving antiretroviral therapy (World Health Organization [WHO], 2009). Universal access itself is predicated on drug markets and market economies informed by profit motives that are known to not work for so-called developing world populations (Bond, 2006). Globally, only one-third of people who need treatment are on it. HIV testing is underutilized—most people still find out that they are HIV positive when they develop clinical symptoms of AIDS. Antiretroviral therapy is not homogeneous in cost, effectiveness, or tolerability.

In 2009, an estimated 5 million people living with HIV in low- and middle-income countries are receiving treatment, up from about 400,000 in

2003—a more than 12-fold increase in 6 years. Despite progress, the global coverage of antiretroviral therapy remains low (UNAIDS, 2009). For every two people newly on treatment, five more become newly infected. In 2008, the vast majority of adults (98%) and children (97%) surveyed in 43 high burden countries were receiving first line antiretroviral regimens. The reported proportion of adults on second line regimens remained low, amounting to no more than 2% of those on antiretroviral therapy (Renaud, Nguimfack, & Vitoria, 2007). In low- and middle-income countries the average annual cost of the mostly widely used first line drug treatments was U.S. $143 per person in 2008, a price reduction of 48% since 2004; however, second line regimens continue to be expensive (WHO, 2009).

In 2004, the Zambian government was able to dramatically reduce the monthly cost of ART from $64 to $8 per month after receiving support from the Global Fund to Fight AIDS, Tuberculosis and Malaria. Given that well over half—some reports put it as high as 70%—of the 870,000 Zambians living with HIV/AIDS are women, officials expected to see a majority of women receiving ART. Instead, men began showing up in much greater numbers. In one rural town, of the 40 people on ART, only three were women. Zambian women reported various reasons for not accessing treatment:

- *Discrimination:* Where money was limited, families often chose to pay for medication for the men in the household rather than the women;
- *Property rights:* One couple, who could only afford treatment for one of them told reporters that if the husband died, his family would inherit his land and his wife would have no way to support their children. If the wife died, he would still have the land;
- *Poverty:* More women than men lacked the money to pay for monthly medication (IRIN/PlusNews, 2004).

In July 2005, leaders of the Group of Eight (G8) countries announced their intention to work with WHO, UNAIDS and other international bodies to develop and implement a package for HIV prevention, treatment and care, with the aim of as close as possible to universal access to treatment for all those who need it by 2010. All United Nations Member States subsequently endorsed this goal at the High-Level Plenary Meeting of the 60th Session of the United Nations General Assembly in September 2005 (WHO, 2006). The major problem with all these commitments and UN documents on HIV treatment is that they are silent on the operations of multinational drug companies. They do not question the existing status quos of patents and rights. The discussions center on funding and treatment approaches whilst there is total silence on the profiteering of drug cartels.

HIV Medication and International Drug Companies

Warren (2000) notes, "AIDS policy is now a key world commodity right up there with shiploads of computers, crude oil and wheat" (para. 16). He suggests that global pharmaceutical companies place great emphasis on profits at the expense of human lives. As an example of this social pattern, on July 19, 2000, the Export-Import Bank of the United States offered $1 billion per year for 5 years in loans to Sub-Saharan Africa to finance the purchase of U.S. HIV/AIDS medications and related equipment and services from U.S. pharmaceutical firms. Three southern African countries, Namibia, South Africa, and Zimbabwe, rejected the offer, however, because the loans would further the dependency and debt of African countries, while American pharmaceutical corporations would benefit (Shah, 2009). This donation for profit pattern is not new. In 1997, 39 U.S. corporations took the South African government to court for passing a law that would allow them to make generic ARVs. The corporations dropped the case in April 2001 but at the cost of 400,000 lives that were lost during that period (Kasper, 2001). In this profit-driven HIV medication arena, treatment that has transformed HIV from a death sentence to chronic illness is becoming more out of reach for the majority of vulnerable groups, especially rural women in Africa, who remain the major victims of the pandemic.

The control of ARVs has meant that the corporations have a monopoly of the market and can thus charge exorbitant prices. Drug companies justify the need for high drug prices by arguing that the profits support further research and development. A report by the consumer health organization, Families USA, in 2000, however, refutes the pharmaceutical industry's claim that high and increasing drug prices are needed to sustain research and development. The report suggests that drug companies are spending more than twice as much on marketing, advertising, and administration than they do on research and development, and that drug company profits, which are higher than all other industries, exceed research and development expenditures. Bond (2006) notes that even in a relatively prosperous South Africa, an early death for millions was the outcome of state and employer reactions to the AIDS epidemic. With cost–benefit analyses demonstrating that keeping most of the country's five to six million HIV-positive people alive through patented medicines costs more than the people were worth.

Wagenberg (2009) notes that about one-third of the world's population (roughly two billion people) lack even the most basic access to essential medicines. Each year an estimated 25 million individuals, 10 million of them children, die of treatable and preventable diseases. A large share of those deaths could be averted by low-cost access to pharmaceuticals developed and patented by U.S. universities. University patents are found in a quarter of HIV and AIDS drugs and a fifth of high-impact drugs approved between 1988 and 2005. In 2001, a group of Yale students learned that d4T (Stavudine), an HIV antiretroviral drug patented by Yale and licensed to Bristol-Myers Squibb, was being sold at exorbitant prices overseas, preventing access for HIV patients living in South Africa and other developing countries. Troubled that Yale-developed drugs were being priced out of reach for HIV patients, the students joined in a publicity campaign that eventually pressured the university and pharmaceutical company into reducing the price of the drug and making it available for generic production in South Africa.

The cost of drugs and health care continues to be an obstacle to universal access to HIV treatment. Walker (2005) argues that in South Africa the cost of ARVs can exceed U.S. $10,000 per patient per year. This cost plays a role in the limited access HIV-infected South Africans have to the medications especially when only 19% of the people have medical insurance (Kaiser Family Foundation, 1999). The coverage of AVR treatment in Africa stood at 28% in 2005 (Walker, 2005). The numbers do not reflect the qualitative experiences of family losses such as breadwinners dying prematurely and children who are orphaned and trapped in poverty without any hope for the future.

The Antiretroviral Therapy Program in Zimbabwe

The United Nations General Assembly Special Session (UNGASS, 2010) Report on Zimbabwe noted that there was an estimated 1,187,822 adults and children who were living with HIV and AIDS in 2009 in the country. The report states that more than half were women, and 17.1% of them were pregnant. Of the total number of persons who need ARVs to fight AIDS, only 38% are receiving them. Sixty-seven percent of pregnant women receive ARVs under the government's Prevention of Mother to Child Transmission program.

The Ministry of Health and Child Welfare (MoHCW) introduced the Antiretroviral Therapy (ART) Programme in April 2004 and "Plan for the Nationwide Provision of ART" was finalized in December 2004 covering the period 2005 to 2007. As part of its strategy to scale up ART services toward universal access to HIV treatment in 2010, the MoHCW commissioned a review of the ART program. According to the Review of the National HIV and AIDS Treatment and Care Programme (ART) 2004–2007, coverage increased from about 5,000 to over 100,000 (29%) by December 2007. Findings of this review contributed tremendously to the development of the "Plan for the Nationwide Provision of Antiretroviral Therapy 2008–2012." Through this plan the United Nations Children's and Educational Fund, the U.S. government, Clinton Foundation, and the National AIDS Council procure the ARVs. Once the drugs are gathered and arrive in the country, NatPharm delegates the distribution of the drugs to the MoHCW AIDS and Tuberculosis Logistics Sub-Unit. The numbers of adults and children accessing ART were 148,144

(39.7%) in December 2008 and 215,109 (56.8%) in November 2009 (UNGASS, 2010).

Guiding the scale up of pediatric ART is the detailed plan for pediatric HIV and AIDS care that was finalized in the last quarter of 2006. The number of children accessing ART was 8,627 (24.8%) in 2007, 13,287 (38.7%) in 2008, and 20,003 (57.1%) in 2009. This trend has been attributed to the scale up and decentralization of the ART program associated with an increase in ART initiation and follow up as well as training of health care workers. The government of Zimbabwe has also made efforts to subsidize local manufacture of ARVs through provision of foreign currency for purchase of raw materials and waiver of duty on raw materials for local production of ARVs and imported ARVs in 2008. Nevertheless, by end of 2007, 17% of people living with HIV and AIDS were receiving ART (United States Agency for International Development [USAID], 2010). Using the WHO recommendations of less than 350 CD4 criteria, adult patients in need of ART increased from 317,894 to 500,857 in 2009 (UNGASS, 2010). As observed here, universal access to ARVs is still very problematic in the country.

A number of challenges have been observed such as lack of funding for the high number of people not accessing ARVs. Differentiation in terms of gendered access between men and women has also been quantitatively documented. For example, the MoHCW (2008) observed that as of March 2008, 55,737 women, 31,417 men, and 9,287 children were receiving free government ARVs. The concept of universal access has not been problematized, however, in relation to women occupying various sociospatial positions in Zimbabwe.

Conceptual Framework

Intersectionality theory provides useful insights into our understanding of the gendered dimensions of universal access to ART. Using Crenshaw's (1994) thesis of intersected oppressions, we highlight how the perception of the experience of HIV-infected women can be enhanced by understanding the differentiated nature of women across the continent. Crenshaw (1994) provides a theoretical orientation that explains the interplay of various factors in explaining an individual's position. The theoretical basis of intersectionality approach involves viewing societal knowledge as being located within an individual's specific geographic and social location. This approach also analyzes how various social and culturally constructed categories interact on multiple levels to manifest themselves as inequalities within society. Race, gender, and class mutually shape forms of oppression in society. In the case of female farmworkers in Zimbabwe, our concern was how their access to ART is mediated by an intersection of multinational drug companies' monopoly of medicines and local exclusion of female workers.

To reduce analysis of women's lives to gender alone is to strip them of racial and class historical antecedents that characterize their marginal position within most African societies. The intersectionality approach is of the view that difficulties arise due to the many complexities involved in making multidimensional conceptualizations that explain the way in which socially constructed categories of differentiation interact to create a social hierarchy. For example, intersectionality holds that knowing that a woman lives in a sexist society is insufficient information to describe her experience; instead, it is also necessary to know her race, sexual orientation, class, as well as her society's attitude toward each of these memberships. It is only through analyzing how these complex concepts intertwine and interlink that we are able to understand gendered experiences of both men and women in different contexts.

METHODOLOGY

We employed a qualitative methodology that involved in-depth interviews, focus group discussions, and key informant interviews. The study was conducted in Mazowe, a district in Mashonaland Central in Zimbabwe. The district is located in the Mashonaland Central province of Zimbabwe and 60 kilometers from the capital city, Harare. The district is divided into 32 ward, with 13 wards in Chiweshe communal areas and the rest in new resettlement areas that are formally White-owned commercial farming areas. The study concentrated on female farm workers living in the newly resettled areas. The newly resettled areas were borne out of the fast track land reform implemented in 2000 by the government of Zimbabwe. When White farmers were removed from their farms, their workers remained living in the compounds.

Access to female farm workers was negotiated through a local HIV and AIDS support group called *Tsungirirai* and through members of home-based care initiatives. Women farm workers infected and affected by HIV and AIDS were purposefully sampled, and 20 in-depth interviews were conducted on 14 farms. Four focus group discussions were conducted with 36 different women in the farm compounds. This was done to include as many women as possible in the study. The purpose of this study is not to generate findings that can be generalized over the whole farm worker community in Zimbabwe. There are varied realities facing women farmer worker populations not only in Mazowe but in the whole country. Through this study, however, a common vulnerability in failing to access treatment is highlighted. Key informant interviews were conducted with staff at a local hospital and the Ministry of Gender and with women conducting home-based care and council officials.

The interviews and group discussions were conducted in local language (Shona), tape recorded, then transcribed and translated into English. Thematic analysis was used to analyze the data. Common themes were drawn from the data and grouped together. This was done through the pairing and sieving of data, without which ideas or experiences as generated by the respondents would have been meaningless. Ethical questions were important in this study given that the participants gave access into their private lives and thoughts. No names or addresses were taken in this study and thus anonymity was maintained. The research ensured informed consent by first explaining the purpose of the research to the respondents who were given the chance to decline being interviewed. No farm names are mentioned in this article to ensure that farm workers are not victimized and that their identity is protected. No financial incentives were given to respondents in soliciting for participation in the study.

FINDINGS

Social Differentiation of Female Farm Workers in Mazowe

This section outlines the demographic characteristics of female farmworkers who participated in the study. Our sample included 56 purposively sampled women ranging from 15 to 62. The majority of the respondents were aged between 23 and 36. All the respondents were involved in sexual relations, with the majority living with a man. All the respondents had at least one child, and from the interviews it was clear that the majority have lived with more than one partner. Changing of sexual partners was highlighted as a recurrent phenomenon that complicates sexual networks. Out of the 56, participants, only 20 had Zimbabwean identity papers with the rest finding it difficult to access the papers as they were considered to be foreigners. At the time of research the workers were not attached to any farmer but offered their services on a part-time basis. None of the women had gone beyond primary school due to the poor nature of farm schooling. Their livelihood options were thus limited by their lack of education, location, citizenship, and class.

Women Farm Workers and Land Reform

Women in the former commercial farming areas in Zimbabwe face multiple challenges. The fast track land reform changed many dynamics in the livelihoods of farm workers generally. Much has been written in the literature around the negative impacts of the program on farm workers (Magaramombe, 2004; Marongwe, 2002; Masiiwa & Chigejo, 2003; Sachikonye, 2003). Marongwe (2002) highlights that land reform led to loss of jobs and income, while provision of services such as health and sanitation,

HIV counseling, and home-based care (HBC) and the construction of Blair toilets by advocacy nongovernmental organizations such as the Farm Community Trust of Zimbabwe were curtailed. The farm worker community in the region where the current research was conducted is predominantly female with over 30% being of foreign descent. These are mostly second- or third-generation immigrants whose parents or grandparents had moved to Zimbabwe (or the former Rhodesia prior to independence in 1980) as migrant laborers from Malawi, Zambia, or Mozambique.

Prior to the introduction of the Citizenship Amendment Act (2001), many of these "foreign" farm workers had been entitled to Zimbabwean nationality under the country's constitution and the Citizenship of Zimbabwe Act. Indeed, many of them had lived in Zimbabwe their entire lives and had no formal links with the countries of their ancestral origin (Ridderbos, 2009). This lack of citizenship makes it impossible for them to obtain national identity cards or birth certificates, which are required to register into treatment programs. The marginalization of these communities from HIV treatment has to be understood not only from the internal dynamics of governance but also from the international workings of the pharmaceutical companies. Female farm workers thus face vulnerability because of their gender, citizenship, and location in the third world. Such vulnerable groups are those who are worst affected by the cost of HIV treatment.

HIV and AIDS Prevalence and Health Delivery Among Female Farm Workers

HIV/AIDS remains a highly emotive and sensitive issue that raises distrust when it is discussed in rural communities. The actual prevalence rate of HIV among farm workers in this district is hard to disaggregate. Officials at an HIV/AIDS treatment program, however, highlighted that the prevalence of the whole district is estimated at 22%. It is not known how many of that percentage are female farm workers. One official at the clinic indicated that there are not many female farm and believes that most are not seeking treatment due to lack of knowledge, fear of stigma, and transportation costs. The hospital is located in the Chiweshe communal areas; thus farm workers in the newly resettled areas, have to foot transport bills to receive medication. Apart from the local hospital, the health care system in newly resettled areas is in a decrepit state. The government in Zimbabwe employed a "resettle first and services later" approach, which meant that the huge movement of people into the newly resettled areas was not met with a similar upgrading in social service infrastructure (Chiweshe, 2008). After settlement, the local District Council tried to redress the situation by opening six clinics at various farms in the district. This was done by renovating farm houses into treatment rooms and accommodation for clinic staff.

These clinics are set up at various farms and in many ways become the property of the residents since they contributed labor and money in starting the clinics. This also makes it difficult for farm workers who were not involved in fundraising to gain access to services. While they can use the clinics, they have to pay a fee that women and children often do not have. Even if they can pay, health care services are not adequate and are characterized by low bed capacity; inadequate medical equipment; absence of essential drugs; insufficient staff; with each clinic having on average one primary care nurse and nurse aides; poor pricing of health services, which does not allow for cost recovery; and poor access to water and sanitation in some clinics. The clinics lack access to critical life saving medicines and at best offer little palliative care. ARVs never reach such areas, and the majority of rural people in Zimbabwe who are infected suffer with no hope.

Experiences of Being HIV Positive Among Women Farm Workers

Experiencing HIV and AIDS is a difficult situation for any human being. The multiplicity of exertions facing women in the farm worker community makes the experience of being infected and affected by the pandemic more painful than it should be, as one woman related:

> Contracting HIV within the farm compounds is a death sentence. Prayer will not save you. You cannot do anything because you are poor. Only the rich can afford this disease because they can buy the pills [antiretroviral drugs].

This is because women lack any means or support to acquire the life-prolonging ARVs. The women have resigned to the fact that death will come, and most indicated that they do not use protection because the men do not like condoms, as one girl indicated:

> We are not afraid of AIDS because it like our daily bread. After all, we will all die. That is the reason why we do not get tested. Why bother with the testing if there is no cure and you cannot get pills? Testing is a waste of time and knowing your status will only stress you and make you die quicker. Not knowing will not kill you.

This resignation of hope is most apparent in infected women who have given up on life and any hope of getting better. Without medication and access to a good diet, HIV becomes a death sentence.

Women living with HIV live in abject conditions. The farm compounds do not offer a hygienic or clean environment for their inhabitants. Farm compound houses on most farms are in a dilapidated state, and dirt is part of everyday life for farm workers. Housing for farm workers has always been poor even before the land reform program. The housing conditions have continued to deteriorate as now the workers cannot depend on farm owners to repair or improve conditions. The living conditions impede the care for the sick and leave the infected vulnerable to death, as an interview with a woman highlighted:

> We stayed in dirty conditions and we cannot afford cleaning materials. We do not have any protective clothing to help those caring for the sick. Our houses do not have proper floors. Plus when you are sick you are unable to fetch water to clean. With the use of American dollars, we can no longer afford to buy soap. Without money, farm workers cannot improve their living conditions.

Another part of experiencing HIV on the farms is the stigma and discrimination that accompanies the condition. Stigma and discrimination in the newly resettled areas tend to follow gender and class lines. The most marginalized group in the hierarchy—female farm workers—are blamed and accused for causing and spreading the pandemic. Stigma associated with the disease tends to prevent women from getting tested because they fear gossip and discrimination. Lack of access to drugs increases stigma and makes testing irrelevant to the people. Treatment might contribute to prevention because people would be more likely to seek blood tests and lessen discrimination toward those living with the disease (AIDS Law Project, 2001). Treatment will create new opportunities for prevention because it will create a larger demand and infrastructure for HIV testing and create settings for counseling. Those who are suspected to have the disease are shunned, and in the end most are socially isolated. This leads to a loss of the only social network that farm workers have.

Within the farm worker community there are girls as young as 14 who are already mothers and wives. These young mothers and wives, because of their age, appear to be more vulnerable to HIV because they are physically and economically less powerful than all other groups. They cannot negotiate for safe sex, and their livelihoods depend on men who use this to their advantage, as one such young wife indicated:

> My husband is the one who decides when and how we have sex. I got married when I was 12, 4 years ago. I do not know the age of my husband, but I think he is 40 years old. When he wants sex there is nothing I can do even if I have heard stories of him sleeping with other women in the compound. You do as you are told.

Any discussions of condoms or safe sex among spouses are not tolerated. Older women noted that they have known young women who have been beaten up for demanding safe sex. Whilst there are a multiplicity of issues affecting vulnerability and lack of access to treatment of farm worker women, the lack of access to ART remains an important factor.

Access to HIV Treatment for Female Farm Workers

In 2003 the local hospital opened a clinic to administer tuberculosis treatment. In 2004 the clinic started to offer HIV antiretroviral treatment to a limited number of patients. In 2008, 500 out of a possible 50,000 eligible patients were receiving treatment. The criteria for accessing the program are based on the waiting list, which means that patients have to wait for someone to die to receive medication. The clinic depends on donors and well wishers, and they cannot afford the cost of treatment for all those who need it. Most female farm workers encountered in this research knew about the treatment program but did not know how to join it. They seemed to view it as something meant for others and not them. Officials at the clinic noted that very few female farm workers are on the program or visit the clinic for information. Through home-based care programs among farm workers, however, the clinic has tried to educate them about its work.

The clinic is forced to concentrate more on palliative care because it cannot afford to give treatment to all. Access to treatment is based on a waiting list of which most infected female farm workers are unable to come and register due to transport cost and some for not possessing a national identity card as they are regarded as foreigners. The burden of HIV on women is felt in multiple ways. For instance, in the home-based care program very few men are involved, which leaves women with a heavy domestic burden of caring for the sick and finding work to feed the family. The complexity of the predicament facing married women is that if the husband is infected too, they are expected to care for him. Unlike the new farmers who have relatives and kin networks in the communal and urban areas to care for them when ill, for most female farm workers such networks are nonexistent. There are thus cases of infected women who have died because of lack of care in terms of hygiene and food.

DISCUSSION

The Myth of Universal Access

Evidence from the field in this district provides a reflection of life for people living beyond the margins. After all the rhetoric of universal access to treatment, the most affected groups are still marginalized in Zimbabwe. Donors are unwilling to work in the newly resettled areas because they do not agree with the land reform program. The most vulnerable group within the newly resettled areas are farm worker women who are infected by HIV. In Asia, many HIV services for women and children living with HIV are available only in large urban centers, and women who lived in rural villages experienced significantly more discrimination than women in urban areas (Women's Working Group of the Asia Pacific Network of People Living With HIV, 2009). They occupy a marginalized space, which means that their basic human rights are not respected. Government policy over the years has tended to look at farm workers as aliens who do not deserve the same rights given to citizens. The workers are thus caught between a donor community that is anti-land reform and a government that does not fully care about their welfare.

The rhetoric of universal treatment and the numbers shown of an increase in access by the WHO around the world fails to highlight the stories of women struggling with a difficult existence in the former commercial farming areas in Zimbabwe. The root cause for the lack of drugs has always been the cost associated with acquiring them. The female workers are reluctant to get tested because, for them, it changes nothing knowing whether they are infected or not.

Under the global neoliberal system in which profits appear to be more important than human life, drug companies may decide who lives or dies; where skin color or being born on the "wrong" continent could be a death sentence (Craddock, 2000; Jones, 2004). Drugs patented by multinational pharmaceutical corporations have been shown to be far more expensive than genetically manufactured drugs (Panos, 2000). The poor cannot access these drugs because of the high prices; thus contracting HIV becomes a hopeless situation. In other contexts, studies on migrant and seasonal farm workers relating to HIV/AIDS indicate a high degree of risk and inadequate access to testing and care in the United States (Statewide AIDS Service Delivery Consortium Advisory Group, 2007).

The Zimbabwean government has tried to increase access to ARVs in national hospitals, but still female farm workers do not have access due to the competition involved in accessing these programs. They have neither the social nor economic capital to buy their way into such schemes. Human rights discourses under neoliberalism have a bias toward civil and political rights rather than social and economic rights. Jones (2004, p. 389) notes, "Human rights having been commandeered by [this] liberal project in order to lend support to free market economics and the freedom to create wealth, as embodied in the values of the World Trade Organization." Access to lifesaving medicines and care for people living with HIV and AIDS has been largely determined by race, class, gender, and geography. AIDS thus points to more fundamental global inequalities than those involving a single disease, illuminating centuries-old patterns of injustice. Indeed, today's international political economy, in which undemocratic institutions systematically generate economic inequality, should be described as "global apartheid" (Booker & Minter, 2001).

HIV and AIDS in Africa are gendered. Kofi Anan in 2002 lamented that AIDS in Africa has a woman's face. Women are affected in different ways, however, due to age, race, religion, citizenship, class, and ethnicity. Female farm workers are a particular type of women who shares the experience of having no access to land, depends on their labor, and lives under a compound system that leaves them vulnerable to sexual exploitation by men. The orphans she leaves behind have no extended family systems to depend on and the circle of abuse and poverty continues with them. In the field we came across children (as young as 12 or 13) who already have babies and are caring for families. The stories of such young mothers are rarely told. These are the women who need the treatment the most and whose rights are seldom advocated. In Kenya, Kimbwarata (2010) observed that rural women living with HIV often face oppression in their relationships with male partners and within the wider community because of their gender, HIV status, and economic (and social) marginalization. Women living with HIV in rural areas in the United States often have considerably less access to care than their counterparts in urban and suburban settings (Centre for Disease Control and Prevention, 2011).

Large pharmaceutical companies operate behind the guise of a free market that protects their monopoly of a product that could save millions of lives. Trade rules on patents negotiated under the World Trade Organization make it impossible for developing countries to make generic drugs, which leaves major pharmaceutical companies with huge market shares. They protect these market shares and profits regardless of how many lives are lost. Thomas states, "Despite the denials of pharmaceutical companies, the fact is that differential access to ARV drugs because of cost contributes to the uneven global experience of HIV/AIDS" (2002, pp. 252–253).

Jones (2004) argues that although ARVs have been shown to extend life and were considered by the WHO Action Programme as "essential" and an integral dimension of fulfilling the right to health, Western donor policy on HIV and AIDS in 2003 remained largely silent about their provision and much more preoccupied with preventative programs. The stories of hopelessness among female farm workers provide a suffering human face to this tragic quest for profits and market shares. If we hold national governments accountable for human rights abuses that cost lives, then we should also hold these companies accountable for every life lost due to a lack of treatment.

CONCLUSIONS

Women farm workers are a marginalized group in Zimbabwe who have little access to treatment, especially with regards to HIV and AIDS. It is groups living beyond the margins such as female farm workers who bear the worst brunt of AIDS. We ask why the human rights discourse has avoided questioning drug companies responsible for the expensive medication and governments that are at best uncaring and at worst blatantly discriminatory. Poor women are paying the price for expensive medication. HIV and AIDS have become death sentences, and hopelessness has gripped those without any means to get medicine.

In such a context, questions are also raised over whether a human rights framework is able to ensure universal access to treatment given that multinational companies seem to place more emphasis on profits as well. The system of inequality that exists between the geopolitical North and South is likely to adversely affect those groups living beyond the margins of society such as women farm workers in Zimbabwe. The human suffering of millions of children and women should be more important than patent rights and profit margins.

REFERENCES

AIDS Law Project. (2001). *HIV and AIDS and the law.* Witwatersrand, South Africa: Wits University.

Anan, K. (2002). *In Africa, AIDS has a woman's face.* Retrieved from http://www.un.org/News/ossg/sg/stories/sg-29dec-2002.htmn

Bond, P. (2006). *Looting Africa: The economics of exploitation.* Pietermaritzburg, South Africa: UKZN Press.

Booker, S., & Minter, W. (2001). *Global apartheid, the nation.* Retrieved from http://www.thenation.com/article/global-apartheid

Centre for Disease Control and Prevention. (2011). *Rural HIV infected women's access to medical care: Ongoing needs in California.* Atlanta, GA: Author.

Chiweshe, M. K. (2008). *Education and skills development in the newly resettled areas in Mazowe.* Report Submitted under the Ruzivo/Oxfam Land and Livelihoods Programme in Mazowe and Mangwe, Zimbabwe.

Ciccio, L. (2004). ARV treatment in poor settings: State of the art. *Health Policy and Development, 2*(1), 52–61.

Craddock, S. (2000). Disease, social identity, and risk: Rethinking the geography of AIDS. *Transactions, 25,* 153–168.

Crenshaw, K. (1994). Mapping the margins: Intersectionality, identity politics, and violence against women of color. In M. Fineman & R. Mykitiuk (Eds.), *The public nature of private violence* (pp. 93–118). New York, NY: Routledge.

Families USA. (2000). *Off the charts: Pay, profits and spending by drug companies.* Retrieved from http://www.familiesusa.org/assets/pdfs/offthecharts6475.pdf

IRIN/PlusNews. (2004). *Zambia: The ultimate sacrifice.* Retrieved from www.plusnews.org/webspecials/womensday/zam040305.asp

Jones, P. S. (2004). When "development" devastates: Donor discourses, access to HIV/AIDS treatment in Africa and rethinking the landscape of development. *Third World Quarterly, 25,* 385–404.

Kaiser Family Foundation. (1999). *The second Kaiser Family Foundation survey of health care in South Africa.* Washington, DC: Author.

Kasper, T. (2001, April 30). Developing countries must stand firm on people over patents. *South Centre Bulletin, 11*, 3–5.

Kimbwarata, J. (2010). *Kenya—Devastating impact of HIV/AIDS on rural women.* Nairobi, Kenya: Institute of Policy Analysis and Research.

Magaramombe, G. (2004). The impact of land redistribution on commercial farm workers. In M. Masiiwa (Ed.), *Post-independence land reform in Zimbabwe: Controversies and impact on the economy.* Harare, Zimbabwe: GM and S Printers.

Marongwe, N. (2002). *Conflicts over land other natural resources in Zimbabwe.* Harare, Zimbabwe: ZERO.

Masiiwa, M., & Chigejo, O. (2003). *The Agrarian reform in Zimbabwe: Sustainability and empowerment of rural community.* Harare, Zimbabwe: University of Zimbabwe Publications.

Ministry of Health and Child Welfare (MoHCW). (2008). *PMTCT Programme 2008 annual report, AIDS & TB Unit, Harare.* Harare, Zimbabwe: Author.

Mutangadura, G. (2005). Gender, HIV/AIDS and rural livelihoods in Southern Africa: Addressing the challenges. *JENda: A Journal of Culture and African Women Studies, 7*, 1–19.

Panos, A. (2000). *Beyond our means?* Retrieved from http://www.panos.org.uk/aids

Renaud, T. F., Nguimfack, B. D., & Vitoria, M. (2007). Use of antiretroviral therapy in resource limited countries in 2006: Distribution and uptake of first and second line regimens. *AIDS, 21*, S89–95.

Ridderbos, K. (2009). *Stateless former farm workers in Zimbabwe.* Retrieved from http://www.fmreview.org/

Sachikonye, L. M. (2003, April). *Land reform for poverty reduction? Social exclusion and farm workers in Zimbabwe.* Paper presented at "Staying Poor: Chronic Poverty and Development Policy" Conference, Manchester, UK.

Schou, A. (2000). The adaptation of quasi-citizens to political and social marginality: Farm workers in Zimbabwe. *Forum for Development Studies, 1-2000*, 43–63.

Shah, A. (2009, November). AIDS in Africa. *Global Issues.* Retrieved from http://www.globalissues.org/article/90/aids-in-africa

Statewide AIDS Service Delivery Consortium Advisory Group. (2007). *Migrant and seasonal farmworkers: Health care access and HIV/AIDS in this population.* New York, NY: Author. Retrieved from http://www.health.ny.gov/diseases/aids/reports/migrant_farmworkers/docs/heatlhcareaccess.pdf

Thomas, C. (2002). Trade policy and the politics of access to drugs, *Third Word Quarterly, 23*, 251–264.

UNAIDS. (2009). *Treatment 2.0.* Retrieved from http://data.unaids.org

United Nations General Assembly Special Session (UNGASS). (2010). *Zimbabwe country report on HIV and AIDS reporting period: January 2008 to December 2009.* Harare, Zimbabwe: Author.

United States Agency for International Development (USAID). (2010). *Zimbabwe health system assessment, 2010, health systems 20/20 project.* Pretoria, South Africa: Author.

Wagenberg, M. (2009, December 4). Harvard's patent policy limits access to drugs by world's poor. *Harvard Law Record.* Retrieved from http://hlrecord.org/?p=11592

Walker, M. (2005). Assessing the barriers to universal antiretroviral treatment access for HIV/AIDS in South Africa. *Duke Journal of Comparative and International Law, 15*, 193–214.

Warren, P. N. (2000, June 27). AIDS and the World Bank: Global blackmail? *A&U Magazine*. Retrieved from http://www.alternet.org/story/9360/aids_and_the_world_bank%3A_global_blackmail

West, A. R., & Rutherford, B. (2005). Zimbabwe's new clothes: Identity and power among displaced farm workers. *Sarai Reader 2005: Bare Acts*, 398–411.

Women's Working Group of the Asia Pacific Network of People Living With HIV. (2009). *A long walk: Challenges to women's access to HIV services in Asia.* Bangkok, Thailand: Author.

World Health Organization (WHO). (2006). *Progress on global access to HIV antiretroviral therapy: A report on 3 by 5 and beyond.* Geneva, Switzerland: Author.

World Health Organization (WHO). (2009). *Transaction prices for antiretroviral medicines and HIV diagnostics from 2008 to October 2009—A summary report from the global price reporting mechanism.* Geneva, Switzerland: Author.

Stories of African HIV+ Women Living in Poverty

SAMAYA VANTYLER

Department of Interdisciplinary Studies, University of Victoria, Victoria, British Columbia, Canada

LAURENE SHEILDS

School of Nursing/School of Public Health and Social Policy, Faculty of Human and Social Development, University of Victoria, Victoria, British Columbia, Canada

In this study researchers explored the daily experiences of HIV+ women living in Kibera, Kenya. Using a convergence of narrative, feminist, and indigenous approaches, we engaged in individual in-depth interviews with nine HIV+ women. Interpretive storylines include the following: Being an African woman; If I sit there, that 10 bob won't come; If I die, who will take care of my children?; I am stigma; They just come to you; Being up, feeling down, and stress-up; and Living with HIV is a challenge. We present our findings to provide evidence-based insights to better support HIV+ women living in poverty.

It was another one of those stifling hot midafternoons in the summer of 2005, and I (first author) was walking with five women on one of the earth-trodden paths in Kibera. Having read much on the Internet about this international "mega slum" and listened to my Kenyan friends speak angrily and sadly about the deplorable living conditions there, I wanted to see for myself.

As we walked I looked around, absorbing sights and smells that were strange and unusual for a privileged White woman. Live electrical wires hung loosely over and between the corrugated tin roofs of many of the wattle and mud buildings. Goats, dogs, and the occasional pig were foraging in the mounds of garbage strewn around, while children played nearby, stopping now and again to stare at me or follow, shouting out repeatedly the friendly greeting in Kiswahili, "Habari gani? Habari gani?" which means, "How are you?" in English.

I had been warned before we started to tread carefully, to watch out for black polythene bags that lay on the ground or flew through the air now and again. Because the numbers of pit latrines are not enough to meet the needs of Kibera's population, the menace of "flying toilets" continues. Those who have no money to pay to use a private latrine or who do not feel safe to venture out any distance at night to the latrines use a plastic bag to relieve themselves. Then they tie and throw them through the air or merely dump them outside their homes.

We were walking to see the view from the railway line that cuts through the middle of the settlement; the railway track runs from Mombasa to Uganda. Four of the women walked ahead of me, one stayed close by my side, pointing to holes in the ground or pieces of cement, garbage, and animal and human waste that may have caused me to stumble. They watched out for me and included me at every turn as we meandered in and out of the narrow throughways in the slum settlement. I observed silently as I listened to the sounds; I heard the heaviness of our solid tread as we moved together forward, and the vibrations began to echo in my head resonating like a steady drum beat with the rhythm of my heart. The grinding poverty so evident in the environment and the rampant spread of disease which I knew existed belied the incredible ingenuity it must take to survive day to day in such surroundings. I admire these women. I sensed an enormous capacity for survival and wanted to explore what life is like for HIV+ women who are widows, heads of households, and who live and participate in community life in Kibera, Kenya.

LITERATURE REVIEW

The HIV/AIDS phenomenon is now in its fourth decade; the rampant spread of the disease has robbed countries of resources and capacity on which both community security and development depend. Twenty-five years ago, HIV/AIDS was more generally depicted and analyzed as an infectious disease and less understood as a human rights crisis. Within the last decade, more attention has been given to the links among HIV/AIDS, human rights, and gender issues (Gruskin & Tarantola, 2000, 2001, 2005; Tallis, 2002; UNAIDS, 2004, 2010). UNAIDS (2011) reported that the viral epidemic was accompanied by a social phenomenon of comparable proportions and that fear, ignorance, and social disapproval of groups heavily affected by the virus had led to an epidemic of stigma and discrimination. While the numbers of new HIV infections have been falling since the late 1990s, and the overall growth of the global HIV/AIDS epidemic appears to have stabilized, the levels of new infections are still considered high (UNAIDS, 2010). Two-thirds of all people living with HIV are in sub-Saharan Africa, although this region contains little more than 10% of the world's population (UNAIDS, 2008). Large variations exist in the patterns of the spread of HIV in between and within African countries. In some countries HIV prevalence is still growing, as in South Africa, while in other countries such as Zimbabwe the HIV prevalence trend appears to have stabilized.

Kenya is one of the hardest-hit countries for HIV infection, and women are disproportionately impacted by economic, legal, cultural, and social disadvantages that in turn increase their vulnerability (UNAIDS, 2004). In Kenya, the HIV epidemic was not declared a national emergency until 2001, by which time 140,000 people had died (UNAIDS, 2004). By 2007 the number of AIDS related deaths in Kenya had decreased by 29%, and within the African context, Kenya was seen as making progress in the fight against the disease (UNAIDS, 2010). The impact of HIV remains significant, however, with an estimated 6.30% of Kenya's adults (aged 15–49) living with HIV/AIDS (Central Intelligence Agency, 2012). Much of the progress in the reduction of deaths is attributed to the introduction and availability of free antiretroviral drugs (ARVs) to HIV+ adults announced by President Kibaki in June 2006. This was obviously a progressive step, but cost was only one of several reasons why 60,000–200,000 eligible Kenyans were not taking ARVs (British Broadcasting Company, 2006). The high levels of poverty and frequent food shortages mean that many living as HIV+ individuals are unable to eat a healthy, balanced diet (Integrated Regional Information Networks, 2009). "Evidence shows that malnourished people are less likely to benefit from antiretroviral treatment and are at a higher risk of quicker progression to AIDS. In addition, taking treatment without food can be very painful" (UNGLASS, 2010, p. 6). Many of those infected with HIV receiving antiretroviral therapy start treatment late, which further limits the overall impact of HIV+ treatment programs (UNAIDS, 2010).

A significant reduction in mortality rates equates to an increase in the number of people living with HIV worldwide. Those who live in poverty are far more susceptible than others to secondary disease and opportunistic infections such as tuberculosis, and therefore it is not surprising that the HIV/AIDS pandemic continues to be the most serious of infectious disease challenges to public health (UNAIDS, 2010). Women and girls are disproportionately affected by the virus, and HIV/AIDS is largely a woman's burden in Kenya (Kako, Stevens, & Karani, 2011). UNGLASSS (2010) reports in 2008/2009 that women had an HIV prevalence rate of 8% compared with 4.3% for men. This disparity is even greater for young woman between the ages of 15 and 24 years who are four times more likely to become infected with HIV than men of the same age. Societal traditions that favor male dominance and long-standing patterns of sexism, racism, and other systems of oppression negatively affect the health of women (Kako et al., 2011; Sen, Ostlin, & George, 2007; Torpy, Lynn, & Glass, 2003). Women's vulnerability to HIV in sub-Saharan Africa stems from not only their likelihood of heterosexual transmission, but also from the severe social, legal, and economic disadvantages they often confront (UNAIDS, 2009). A possible contributing factor to the high incidence of HIV among women is the high rate of violent sexual contact reported by women. In 2003, a Kenyan nationwide survey showed that almost half of the women reported experiencing sexual violence and one in four women between the ages of 12 and 24 had been raped and lost their virginity by force (UNGLASS, 2008). In 2009, UNAIDS reported an estimate of 760,000 Kenyans living as HIV+ women.

The vulnerability and inequality of women worldwide has placed HIV firmly in the center of feminist debate (Edries & Trigaardt, 2004; Lather & Smithies, 1997; Lewis, 2006; UNFPA, 2006). Women, especially women in developing countries such as Kenya, bear a disproportionate burden of the world's poverty; it has been estimated that 70% of the world's poor are women (Aveggio, 2011). Within Kenya the incidence of poverty is extremely high despite the Millennium Development Goals for eradication of poverty by 2015; moreover, the geographical variation in the prevalence is considerable, with the majority of urban poor living in slum settlements such as Kibera (International Monetary Fund, 2004/2005). The impact of poverty as a determinant to health and well-being of women is immense. Poor women disproportionately suffer from hunger, disease, and environmental degradation (Chant, 2006; Chen et al., 2005; Day & Brodsky, 1998; Donner, 2002; McDonald & McIntyre, 2002; Thibo, Lavin-Loucks, & Martin, 2007; United Nations [UN], 1995a; Wilson, 1988; World Economic Forum, 2005; World Health Organization [WHO], 2008). Further compounding these issues, the HIV pandemic has resulted in a profound increase in female headed households (FHHs) as widows, grandmothers, and older sisters take on the responsibilities of caring for their own and others' children (Bongaarts, 2001; Chant, 2003; Momsen, 2002; Schatz, Madhaven, & Williams, 2011). In the late 1980s, prepandemic, it was estimated that FHHs constituted 17%–28% of the world's households with concomitant higher levels of poverty due to lack of income and resources (Horrell & Krishnan, 2007; Todaro, 1989). Although it is true that FHHs may not, by default, be impoverished, the highest absolute poverty rates are in households headed by single women (UN, 1995b). In Kenya the estimated prevalence of FHHs is 30%–40% (Moghadam, 2005; UN, 1995b). Moghadam (2005) further explicates that FHHs in urban areas were poorer than otherwise similar households. Bodewes (2005) concluded that FHH households in Kibera were as high as 70%–80%. While the population of FHHs may be diverse (elderly widows, widows with children, single women, women whose husbands are "absent"), the disproportionate number of FHHs within Kibera starkly illuminates the vulnerability to poverty (Morrison, Raju, & Sinha, 2007) as well as the potential exposure to other forms of gendered violence including harassment, intimidation, and rape (Amnesty International, 2010).

In this study, researchers explored the experienced realities of nine HIV+ women living in poverty conditions in Kibera. These women are all widows, heads of their households, and responsible for the care of 36 children.

METHODS

This is a narrative inquiry informed by feminist, indigenous, and neocolonial perspectives. Methodological convergence with a decolonizing intent was used to provide inclusive spaces for diverse perspectives when viewing and understanding the world (Loppie, 2007). This intersectionality of three methodologies enabled a blending of multiple voices of nine African women and a Western female researcher (Kincheloe, 2001). This research was conducted in Kibera, a sprawling shanty town in the east African country of Kenya with an estimated population of 800,000 people (UN Habitat, 2003). Internationally recognized as the largest slum in all of sub-Saharan Africa (Matrix, 2002), it spreads over 110 hectares of land and its density is considered to be two to three times greater than the normal measure for adequate space in refugee camps (Bodewes, 2005). Overcrowding, poor sanitation, lack of clean drinking water, and overall weak infrastructure begets malnutrition and poor health for those who live there (Bocquier et al., 2011; Davis, 2006; Kimani-Murage et al., 2011).

Over a 5-year period, I (first author) developed relationships within Kibera and in keeping with indigenous methodologies carried out this research working closely with a respected community leader (Winnie). Communication with a community contact was not only critical in the selection and recruitment of nine women, it was vitally important for every aspect of the research process in the slum settlement, guiding it in ways that were culturally sensitive, relevant, respectful, responsive, equitable, and reciprocal (Canadian Institutes of Health Research, 2007; Kovach, 2009; Smith, 1999). All aspects of this study were reviewed and approved by the University of Victoria's Human Research Ethics Board as well as under a Kenyan research permit from the Kenya National Council of Science and Technology, which is necessary for non-Kenyans.

Winnie, our community contact, identified nine potentially suitable women who met criteria for the study, and all nine were recruited successfully. Two, in-depth, semistructured conversations were the primary mode of collecting data and took place at a time that was mutually agreeable, and did not interfere with women's community activities for generating incomes. These times were usually in the early morning before the local markets were open and the sun was working its way overhead. Several women indicted that they wanted me to talk with them in their homes, yet after three home visits, Winnie became concerned for my safety. Further conversations took place in the secured compound in which Winnie had her office and working space where she taught tailoring skills to young women.

Each participant was interviewed and recruited on an individual basis. Issues of confidentiality and anonymity were explained during the initial meeting and again when asking for signatures on the "Participant Consent Form." Only two women chose pseudonyms; the other seven as well as our community contact expressed the desire to use their own names. One of the ethical considerations was that participation in the study could expose women to the risks of identification as an HIV+ woman and any potential stigma/discrimination that may ensure. In contrast, however women openly acknowledged me whenever and wherever we met in Kibera. I was invited to homes and to community functions. The narrative analysis process used in this study was informed by Riessman's (2008) dialogical/performance analysis in which the researcher becomes an active presence in the text. This acknowledges that story and story-telling are expressive, shaped by the relationship of the contextual, reciprocal interaction of teller and listener.

FINDINGS

Nine women chose to participate in the study, each a participant in a community-based nongovernment organization. The women are all adults, widows, female heads of families, and range in age from 32 years to 43 years with an average age of 37 years. They belong to five different African ethnic groupings; Nubian, Kamba, Kikuyu, Kalenji, and Balulya. Four women were born and have lived all their lives in Kibera; five were born in rural areas outside of Nairobi and still have relatives and contacts in villages away from the urban informal settlement. All women speak and understand at least three languages: their mother tongue, Kiswahili, and English, the language used for data collection. The average time length of knowing their HIV+ status was 5 years. Five women reported that their husbands died from AIDS; two reported husbands' deaths due to accidents, one husband died from tuberculosis, and another died from unknown causes. These nine women are responsible for the care of 36 children. Four each have three children and as well care for grandchildren. Two women have four children each; one woman has five children and one widow has one child. One woman has five children of her own, and cares for the four children of her dead sister and brother-in-law.

Seven storylines were identified and serve as subplots for the overall stories told by the nine women:

- Being an African woman,
- If I sit there, that 10 bob won't come,
- If I die, who will take care of my children?,

- I am stigma,
- They just come to you,
- Being up, feeling down, and stress-up, and
- Living with HIV is a challenge.

Being an African Woman

These women live alone with their children and told stories of gender inequalities that have shaped their lives and continue to shape their lives and the lives of their children. Zakia spoke of being female in Africa:

> When you are living as a woman...you have to be strong. Because in Africa, you are supposed to be strong....A woman is there to stand for everything. When you don't...give yourself courage...everything will go apart, because you are there for your children....If you don't advocate for your rights...who will advocate...for you?

Zakia remembered being physically disciplined by some men for speaking out of turn too loudly to make her needs known; "But you are not there to talk loud. If you talk loud, . . . they will even cane you."

Within this particular community in Kibera, women supported other women living with HIV. Amina A. lives with her children, mother, and sister. When she was too sick to care for her children, Amina B. called her sister who travelled to Kibera and took her back to her rural village where she stayed until strong enough to return home and resume caring for herself and her children. Zuhura's widowed mother, although poor herself, cooks a regular evening meal of ugali (maize) and sumawki (green vegetables) in her Kibera home for her daughter and grandchildren. No woman spoke of any support, financial or otherwise, received from adult men in their lives.

If I Sit There That 10 Bob Won't Come

Women were ingenious and diligent in providing for their families. Days revolve around being able to find adequate resources for their family (food, shelter), and access to school for children. Only one woman had a steady job, which was keeping house 3 days a week for another woman who lived outside Kibera. Others earn money by doing casual work such as washing, braiding hair, making and selling soap, custom crocheting, and catering at community functions when invited. Since becoming HIV+, several women stopped working at regular jobs because they no longer have the stamina or were afraid of being fired. Penninah no longer had the strength to walk to the retail market in Nairobi and return carrying large bundles of vegetables on her shoulders to sell in the local markets in Kibera. Zuhura stopped working in a well-known tourist hostel because she was afraid of being fired. It is illegal in Kenya for an employee to be fired because they are HIV+. Stories abound, however, of employers who do fire HIV+ workers. Employers know that few employees can afford court costs to challenge dismissal, as Zuhura commented:

> My life was very different because I was working. . . . You find a good job. . . . They want to take your blood and test you first so that they can pay you this good money to work there. And now you are afraid to continue the work. . . . You come back and stay in the house.

Loise spoke of walking around the villages in Kibera to sell tomatoes, onions, and recycled hard soap she makes from collecting unused soap from the industrial areas outside of Nairobi. There is no guarantee of making a sale by sitting on the roadside, as she observed:

> You can even stay there for even a day without selling. Maybe you sell what is not enough for you for the day. . . . I just go. I don't care whether—because, if I sit there, that 10 bob won't come. So I better take for you that—Yeah.

If I Die, Who Will Take Care of My Children?

Each woman is painfully aware of their sole responsibility for their children. They fear dying before children are old enough to care for themselves. This is reflected vividly in Amina B.'s remark:

> Oh, my God, if I die, who will take care of my children? Oh, my God, just give me strength to take care of my kids because there is nobody else. . . . Just give me life. . . . I'm afraid of . . . dying and leaving my children when they're still very young. I'm praying so much . . . so that I can stay until they become big and then . . . what comes after, at least they know to support themselves outside there.

Before the HIV/AIDS pandemic brought about social disruption and profound changes to the microcontexts of community and family that sustained the fabric of African life, children may have traditionally been raised within the context of a multigenerational community. These African women told stories of little or no relationships with immediate or extended family members. Lucy spoke of being shunned by her mother when she was hospitalized because of HIV+ complications; Zakia remembers her mother telling her, "You bring . . . us a lot of problems. . . . I want you to move out of my house. . . . You can go and live with other people who are HIV. I don't want to see you in my house." Loise's in-laws acted as if she was going to die when she was hospitalized for the first time before being diagnosed as HIV+. "Actually, they (in-laws) thought I was just going to die the very week. Even they had decided, taking my properties....Even the blankets, they were carrying—they saw me as I was just useless."

I Am Stigma

Women experienced stigmatization ranging from malicious gossip to actual threats. Although there is increased community-based information available regarding HIV/AIDS, there is still a great deal of ignorance surrounding the subject and a great deal of stigmatization within Kibera. Loise described well what many think when they hear that someone is HIV+ in Kibera:

> They [husband's family] knew I'm HIV. Yet, myself I had not...gone for the test. Even they had decided, they knew I was going to die....Maybe...they will keep on spreading the news, "That one got HIV, she takes big, big drugs, you know." You see, they will start talking badly....So, they think that, when you have...AIDS, you are not supposed to move near a friend or do something to somebody. You see, if I give somebody food and she or he knows that I am HIV, he thinks maybe [laughs] my disease is got...in the food which I have given him....You see, when you have rashes, people will look at you as if you are no more, yeah? So—I thinks. Make people to eliminate you.

Amina A. has been on ARVs for almost 10 years, the longest of the women in the study group, and recognizes that, if she had not been tested and had not started drug treatment, in all likelihood, she would have died. She now holds the belief that, because ARV medication is free, it is stigma that is causing the deaths of many HIV individuals and remarked, "And the thing that killing people is stigma, stigma."

They Just Come to You

Each woman is a mother; each one the female head of a household, and each have single-parent responsibilities. Zuhura commented, "And the children come to you with their problem because they don't have anybody else to tell their problem. They just come to you...me who is responsible for them."

If children are sick and cannot be left alone, mothers are unable to go into the community to work for money to buy food, water, and other necessary supplies. The days when a woman feels "down," not strong enough to leave her home, her children may be thirsty and go hungry. There are days when these women wake up feeling ill and would like to stay on their beds sleeping, resting, restoring energy, yet they get up to face the day, as Loise' described:

> Living with HIV and also just a widow...you see, whenever you feel hurt, you must wake up because you are the only person home the children are looking to. Even at times you wake up feeling very bad—a child asks you, "Mum, how are you feeling?" You just say, "I'm O.K.," because you don't want to make them worried. They know when Mum is not here, they cannot eat.

Being Up, Feeling Down, and Stress-Up

The women talked of experiences that cause them stress. They described emotional response to feelings of stress as "feeling down" or "stress-up." When they feel well, they describe themselves as "being up." Having acknowledged that ARVs are keeping her alive, Amina A. remarked:

> You have AIDS, you have nothing to eat; you have a lot of stress. You have no medication, maybe the children are there, they are waiting for you, everyone's waiting for you, plus then you—you feel, you become so down, you feel stress-up, you become sick, you have nothing to eat. That's when you can die very easily but with AIDS, you can live for some times.

Experiences of health and diagnosis of disease conceptually differ. Women associated being sick with lying on a hospital bed or being unable to work: They did not consider themselves sick merely because they were HIV+. One woman reflected, "Stress, I think stress is the biggest thing that...that make people go down." She continued:

> The medication is free. But the problem is, how will you get the food?...The biggest stress is now the food, school fees, the house, the shelter, yeah.... This is the biggest problem....About HIV, it's not the big issue for me because I have the drugs; I am taking the drugs, yeah.

Living With HIV Is a Challenge

Day-to-day life in Kibera presents many challenges; living as HIV+ women is just one. Attending support groups where the women feel safe, free from stigma and discrimination is helpful, as Penninah observed:

> My courage?—from other peoples, when we are talking, When I tell somebody I am weak in this side, she tell me, "Do this," and me, I find the way.... They (other women in the group) help me and because we

are in this support group, we are there, we are like twins, we are like friends, we are like the childrens of parents, one – one person. Because we share stories for helping. . . . I feel happy when we are together. . . . we discuss more, without mens there. . . . I have something that is hurting me, I tell them, then she tell me what I am going to do. . . . That supporting group is helping me.

The women do not have much trust in government or local nongovernment organizations who arrange for trucks to enter Kibera to distribute food supplements to HIV+ individuals. Loise drew attention to the waste of time it is to line up:

We don't [get] from the government. . . . Even if you go with the doctors' letter . . . they says, "finish," nothing is there. Actually, . . . me have never got anything from—I always say it is a waste of time, because when you go . . . are always very many, even though who are not HIV.

All the women without exception spoke of a trust and a belief in a God from whom they draw hope, comfort, and strength. As Amina A. said, "I stay in God's hands, let me pray to God. God will help me." She continued with a very realistic view of life and mortality:

Because death is there. . . . If you have HIV, if you don't have HIV, death is there. You will die, one day, one time, yeah [Laughs]. Yeah. When me is ready, when the day—ah me, I'm praying to God, I'm telling my God help me to raise my children to get good . . . education, to get to college, to get work to get their wives, to get their grandchildren. I have to succeed them, yeah, yeah.

After a full day of work, attending support groups, participating in community activities, exchanging news when talking with friends, and going for medical check-ups, these mothers generally return to their homes to have an evening meal with their children, help with homework in some households, and then to sleep. For morning comes early for these HIV+ mothers who, when feeling well, often begin their day as or before the sun rises. They rise up to face each and every day empowered by an inner strength and determined to provide for themselves and their children amidst the stark realities of poverty in the Kibera slum. Yet, their ingenuity, creativity, and courage is never enough to sustain a quality of life that so many take for granted; what they so badly lack is access to basic human resources and opportunity.

DISCUSSION

Women in this study live in a country in sub-Saharan Africa, a region of the world more heavily affected by HIV/AIDS than any other. Their daily struggle to survive is exacerbated by the abject poverty conditions in Kibera, a global mega slum, where they live and raise their children. Systemic gender inequalities, reminiscent of colonial days, continue to impact heavily on their lives and push them into the margins of society. The combined effects of stigma and discrimination, lack of access to services, plus punitive laws may have a profound influence, making the pandemic worse (UN-AIDS, 2010). Their voices have become lost in the dominant male stream of gendered privilege; human rights violations occur at an alarming rate and level, riding tandem with issues of social justice. Women in Kibera live many days in a place of despair and hunger within a world of great promise and hope. Nelson Mandela pointed out that more money is spent annually on weapons than for the support of the millions infected by HIV. "Overcoming poverty is not a gesture of charity; it is an act of justice" (Nolen, 2007, p. 353). HIV/AIDS has become a manageable disease, yet it remains difficult to overlook the magnitude and effects of poverty in Kibera when listening to voices of HIV+ women speak of their daily experiences. This study demonstrates how access to the basic prerequisites of health such as shelter, food, education, and safe environments are essential to the effective management of the HIV/AIDS pandemic. Women, particularly women who are widows, heads of households, and sole providers for their children, are and will continue to be profoundly impacted by this disease if the underlying factors of poverty and access to basic resources for human life remain unattended. The treatment of HIV must be shifted to encompass an equity lens where these broader determinants of health become integral to creating approaches that effectively mitigate these factors and treat disease.

And yet, these women must go on. In the face of disease and untenable disparities, women use their ingenuity to carve out an existence, a life, for themselves and their children. They all believe in a God and participate in at least one support group. By attending HIV+ support groups, their circle of friends has become wider. They make new friends by listening and sharing resonating stories of living positively with disease; they go to sleep after a long, full day struggling to survive and hope the next day they will feel well enough to leave their home, go into the community, and earn the money necessary to keep themselves and their children alive.

REFERENCES

Amnesty International. (2010). *Insecurity and indignity: Women's experiences in the slums of Nairobi, Kenya.* London, England: Amnesty International Publications.

Aveggio, M. T. (2011). *Reduce gender inequities: Reduce poverty.* Retrieved from http.//www.undp-povertycentre.org/pub/lPCOnePager73.pdf

Bocquier, P., Beguy, D., Zulu, E. M., Muindi, K., Konserga, A., & Yé, Y. (2011). Do migrant children face greater health hazards in slum settlements? Evidence from Nairobi, Kenya. *Journal of Urban Health, 88,* 266–281.

Bodewes, C. (2005). *Parish transformation in urban slums: Voices of Kibera, Kenya.* Nairobi, Kenya: Paulines Publications.

Bongaarts, J. (2001). Household size and composition in the developing world in the 1990s. *Population Studies: A Journal of Demography, 55,* 263–279.

British Broadcasting Corporation. (2006, June 2). Kenya to provide free AIDS drugs [Television Broadcast]. *BBC.* Retrieved from http://www.news.bbc.co.uk/2/hi/Africa/5040240

Canadian Institutes of Health Research. (2007). *CIHR guidelines for health research involving aboriginal people.* Ottawa, Ontario, Canada: Author.

Central Intelligence Agency. (2012). *The world fact book.* Retrieved from http://www.cia.gov//library/publication/the-world-factbook/rankorder//2155rank.html.

Chant, S. (2003). *Female household headship and the feminization of poverty: Facts, fiction and forward strategies.* Retrieved from http://www.eprints.lse.ac.uk/574

Chant, S. (2006). Re-thinking the feminization of poverty in relation to aggregate gender indices. *Journal of Human Development, 7,* 202–220.

Chen, M., Vanek, J., Lund, F., Heintz, J., Jhabvala, R., & Bonner, C. (2005). *Women, work and poverty.* Geneva, Switzerland: United Nations Development Fund for Women.

Davis, M. (2006). *Planet of slums.* London, England: Verso.

Day, S., & Brodsky, G. (1998). *Women and equality deficit: The impact of restructuring Canada's social programs.* Ottawa, Canada: Status of Women.

Donner, L. (2002). *Women, income and health in Manitoba: An overview and ideas for action.* Winnipeg, Canada: Women's Health Clinic.

Edries, S., & Triegaardt, M. (2004). The feminization of HIV/AIDS. *The African Renaissance, 1,* 121–124.

Gruskin, S., & Tarantola, D. (2000). Health and human rights. In R. Detels, J. McEwan, R. Beaglehole, & H. Tanaka (Eds.), *The Oxford textbook of public health* (4th ed., pp. 311–336). New York, NY: Oxford University Press.

Gruskin, S., & Tarantola, D. (2001). HIV/AIDS, health and human rights. In P. Lampley, H. Gayle, & P. Mane (Eds.), *HIV/AIDS prevention and care programs in resource–constrained settings: A handbook for the design and management of programs* (pp. 661–678). Arlington, VA: Family Health.

Gruskin, S., & Tarantola, D. (2005). Human rights and children affected with HIV/AIDS. In G. Foster, C. Levine, & S. Williamson (Eds.), *A generation at risk: The global impact of HIV/AIDS on orphans and vulnerable children* (pp. 134–156). New York, NY: Cambridge University Press.

Horrell, S., & Krishnan, P. (2007). Poverty and productivity in female-headed households in Zimbabwe. *The Journal of Development Studies, 43,* 1351–1380.

Intergrated Regional Information Networks. (2009). *Urban poverty and vulnerability in Kenya.* Retrieved from http://www.jvinnes.org/pd/Urban_Poverty_and_Vulnerability_in-Kenya

International Monetary Fund. (2004/2005). *Kenya: Poverty reduction strategy paper.* Retrieved from http://www.imf.org/external/pubs/ft/scr/2005/cr0511.pdf

Kako, P. M., Stevens, P. E., & Karani, A. K. (2011). Where will this illness take me? Reactions from HIV diagnosis from women living with HIV in Kenya. *Health Care for Women International, 32,* 278–299.

Kimani-Murage, E., Holding, P., Fotso, E., Madise, N., Kalurani, E., & Zulu, E. (2011). Food security and nutritional outcomes among urban poor orphans in Nairobi, Kenya. *Journal of Urban Health, 88*(Suppl. 2), S266–S288.

Kincheloe, J. (2001). Describing the bricolage: Conceptualizing a new rigor in qualitative research. *Qualitative Inquiry, 7,* 679–692.

Kovach, M. (2009). *Indigenous methodologies: Characteristics, conversations, and contexts.* Toronto, Canada: University of Toronto Press.

Lather, P., & Smithies, C. (1997). *Troubling the angels: Women living with AIDS.* Boulder, CO: Westview.

Lewis, S. (2006). *Stephen Lewis to continue fight against AIDS after UN envoy term ends.* Retrieved from http://www.stephenlewisfoundation.org

Loppie, C. (2007). Learning from the grandmothers: Incorporating indigenous principles into qualitative research. *Qualitative Health Research, 17,* 276–284.

Matrix Development Consultants. (2002). *An overview of informal settlements in Nairobi.* Nairobi, Kenya: Author.

McDonald, K., & McIntyre, M. (2002). Women's health, women's health care: Complicating experience, language and ideologies. *Nursing Philosophy, 3,* 260–267.

Moghadam, V. (2005). *The feminization of poverty and women's human rights.* Retrieved from http://www.unesco.org/shs/gender

Momsen, J. H. (2002). Myth or math: The waxing and waning of the female-headed household. *Progress in Development Studies, 2,* 145–151.

Morrison, A., Raju, D., & Sinha, N. (2007). *Gender equality is good for the poor.* Policy Research Working Paper 4349. Washington, DC: The World Bank.

Nolen, S. (2007). *28 Stories of AIDS in Africa.* Toronto, Canada: Knopf Canada.

Riessman, C. K. (2008). *Narrative methods for the human sciences.* London, England: Sage.

Schatz, E., Madhaven, S., & Williams, J. (2011). Female-headed households contending with AIDS-related hardship in rural South Africa. *Health Place, 17,* 598–605.

Sen, G., Ostlin, P., & George, A. (2007). *Unequal, unfair, ineffective and inefficient gender inequality in health: Why it exists and how we can change it* (Final Report to the WHO Commission on Social Determinants of Health.) Retrieved from http://www.who.int/social_determinants/.../wgekn_final_report_07.pdf

Smith, L. T. (1999). *Decolonizing methodologies: Research and indigenous peoples.* New York, NY: Palgrave.

Tallis, V. (2002). *Gender and HIV/AIDS.* Retrieved from http://www.bridge.ids.ae.uk

Thibo, M., Lavin-Loucks, D., & Martin, M. (2007). *The feminization of poverty.* Dallas, TX: The J. McDonald Williams Institute.

Todaro, M. P. (1989). *Economic development in the third world.* London, England: Longman.

Torpy, J. M., Lynn, C., & Glass, R. M. (2003). Men and women are different. *The Journal of the American Medical Association, 289,* 510.

UNAIDS. (2004). *The global coalition on women and AIDS.* Retrieved from http://www.womenandaids.unaids.org

UNAIDS. (2008). *Report on the global AIDS epidemic*. Geneva, Switzerland: Author.

UNAIDS. (2009). *Annual report*. Retrieved from http://www.unaids.org/en.../report/.../2009_report_en

UNAIDS. (2010). *Global report: UNAIDS report on the global AIDS epidemic*. Geneva, Switzerland: Author.

UNAIDS. (2011). *AIDS at 30: Nations at the crossroads*. Geneva, Switzerland: Author.

UNFPA. (2006). *Annual report*. Retrieved from http://www.unfpa.org/public/publications/pd/413

UNGLASS. (2008). *Country report—Kenya*. Nairobi, Kenya: Office of the President. Ministry of Special Programmes.

UNGLASS. (2010). *HIV and AIDS in Kenya*. Retrieved from http://www.avert.org/hiv-aids-kenya.htm

United Nations (UN). (1995a). *Report of the World Summit for Social Development*. Copenhagen, Denmark, March 6–12. (Sales No. E. 96.IV.8).

United Nations (UN). (1995b). *Second review and appraisal of the implementation of the Nairobi forward-taking strategies for the achievement of women* (Report of the Secretary General). New York, NY: Author.

United Nations (UN) Habitat. (2003). *Housing rights, land and tenure, land and housing*. Geneva, Switzerland: Author.

Wilson, J. B. (1988). Women and poverty: A democratic overview. *Women and Health*, *12*(3 & 4), 21–40.

World Economic Forum. (2005). *Women's empowerment: Measuring the global gender gap*. Geneva, Switzerland: Author. Retrieved from http://www.weform.org

World Health Organization (WHO). (2008). *Closing the gap in a generation: Health equity through action*. Geneva, Switzerland: Author.

Experiences of Emotional Abuse Among Women Living With HIV and AIDS in Malawi

WINNIE CHILEMBA, NELTJIE VAN WYK, and RONELL LEECH

Department of Nursing Science, University of Pretoria, Pretoria, South Africa

Our aim for this study was to describe emotional abuse as it is experienced by women living with HIV and AIDS in Malawi. The study was conducted in the Lilongwe district in Malawi and used a descriptive phenomenological approach. Twelve women from two public health care clinics under the Lilongwe District Health Office were interviewed. Violating experiences that scarred the personhood and inherent value of being human were found to be the essence of their emotional abuse. Their husbands, family, and community members were responsible for the humiliation, abandonment, and blaming that caused them to feel hopeless.

BACKGROUND

Globally, 33 million people were living with HIV as of 2008, of whom 30.8 million were adults and 2.2 million were children (Joint United Nations Programme on HIV/AIDS [UNAIDS], 2008). The worst-affected region was sub-Saharan Africa, with 22 million people living with HIV/AIDS. Women accounted for 50% of all adults with HIV infection worldwide, 59% of whom lived in sub-Saharan Africa (UNAIDS, 2008). In Malawi, HIV prevalence among adults aged 15–49 years was 11% in 2011 (National Statistics Office [NSO] & ICF Macro, 2011).

Being diagnosed with HIV is a traumatic event that involves emotional distress (Theuninck, Lake, & Gibson, 2010). The distress is aggravated when abuse is experienced from those whose support is required by the person who has been diagnosed. Violence and HIV infection are often linked in a complex relationship (Van Rensburg, 2007). Researchers have shown that women who are in abusive relationships are more likely to be HIV infected, while HIV infection increases the likelihood of being abused by husbands/partners (Campbell, Baty, Ghandour, Stockman, Francisco, & Wagman, 2008; Ramachandran, Yonas, Silvestre, & Burke, 2010). The disclosure of HIV/AIDS often results in emotional abuse (Medley, Kennedy, Lunyolo, & Sweat, 2009). Women are also often blamed for bringing HIV/AIDS into the family (Ndinda, Chimbwete, McGath, & Pool, 2007), particularly if they are the ones who are tested first, usually through programs for the prevention of mother-to-child transmission of HIV.

Women in Malawi bear the burden of HIV/AIDS more than their male counterparts. They have little access to formal education and income-generating opportunities, are financially dependent on their partners/husbands, and are often forced as a result of their inferior status in society into unprotected sex (Kathewera-Bandaet et al., 2005). The Malawian society to a large extent is permissive of multiple and concurrent sex partners for men and condones the exploitation of women by tolerating gender-based violence (Ministry of Women and Child Development, 2005). Low education levels for girls in Malawi lead to early marriages and multiple pregnancies, which contribute to the high fertility rate (of 5.7 children per woman) in the country (NSO & ICF Macro, 2011).

Malawi is a low-income country characterized by a heavy burden of communicable diseases and high levels of child and adult mortality, with noncommunicable diseases on the increase (Zere, Moeti, Kirigia, Mwase, & Kataika, 2007). The life expectancy is only 44 years (NSO & ICF Macro, 2011). The HIV prevalence rate for men 15 to 49 years is 8%, and the HIV prevalence rate for women 15 to 49 years is 13% (World Health Organisation [WHO], 2011). More women than men in Malawi have HIV/AIDS. Women who are dependent on their partners/husbands for financial means are powerless to reject their partner's risk behavior of having concurrent multiple sex partners (Jewkes & Morrell, 2010) and to negotiate the use of condoms (Kaufman, Shefer, Crawford, Simbayi, & Kalichman, 2008). When girls get married at very young ages, their husbands are usually many years their senior (Higgins, Hoffman, & Dworkin, 2010). The discrepancy in age increases their risk of infection, as their husbands are likely to be already infected with the virus from previous sex partners (Higgins et al., 2010).

The low societal status of women in Malawi contributes to their vulnerability to HIV/AIDS and exposure to abuse. Physical abuse leaves signs that can easily be detected by doctors and nurses, while emotional abuse leaves hidden scars. There is also very little information on how women living with HIV/AIDS experience emotional abuse from partners/husbands, family, and community members. Very little research has been done regarding women living with HIV/AIDS in Malawi. Only two recent articles could be sourced. One of the studies focused on sexual violence and women's vulnerability to

HIV infection (Kathewera-Banda et al., 2005) and the other on techniques to be used in research on women living with HIV in Malawi (Mkandawire-Valhmu & Stevens, 2010). This article contributes to the literature by exploring the experiences of Malawian women who live with HIV/AIDS and who suffer abuse. The women in this study had the opportunity to share their personal stories of painful experiences of emotional abuse.

METHODS

In this qualitative inquiry, we used a descriptive phenomenological research approach. Female patients from two clinics of the Lilongwe District Health Office in Malawi that provide primary health care to communities from both rural and urban settings were involved in the study. Due to budgetary constraints, patients had very limited access to counseling and other psychosocial support at the clinics. Care was mainly focused on the physical needs of the patients.

Female patients who used services for antiretroviral treatment at the two clinics and who had reported episodes of emotional abuse to the nurses, who were 18 years and older, who had been in a relationship, who had been known to be living with HIV/AIDS for at least 1 year, and who were willing to describe their experiences of emotional abuse were invited through the nurses at the clinics to take part in the study. Once they had agreed to participate, they were introduced to the first author who explained to them what the research was about. Informed consent to the research was obtained from each participant.

In-depth unstructured individual interviews in the local language (Chichewa) that lasted an average of 45 minutes were conducted by the first author with 12 participants in a private venue at the clinics after the women had consented to participate in the research. The participants were invited to tell the first author about the emotional abuse that they had experienced. The first author used probing questions to encourage participants to give a comprehensive description of what they were exposed to. Data were collected over a period of 1 month in 2011, and all the interviews were audiotaped with the permission of the participants. The data collection was terminated when no new information was obtained.

The recorded interviews were transcribed and translated into English. A colleague of the first author conversant in both Chichewa and English checked the translation to ensure that there was no loss of meaning in the translation.

Data analysis was guided by the processes described by Collaizi (cited in Streubert & Carpenter, 2011) and Dahlberg, Dahlberg, and Nyström (2008). The transcriptions of the interviews were analyzed to identify the essence of the experience and the associated constituents (Dahlberg et al., 2008).

Much time was spent reading and rereading the transcriptions to get a clear overall understanding of the experiences of the participants (Holloway & Wheeler, 2010), which phenomenologist researchers refer to as the "initial whole" of all the experiences of all the participants (Carlsson, Dahlberg, Lützen, & Nyström, 2004). The data were thereafter divided into meaning units, clustered together according to similar meanings and summarized in the essence that constituted the "new whole" of the experiences (Dahlberg et al., 2008).

Through eidetic reduction, the natural dimension of the experiences of the participants (the concrete way abuse happened) was replaced by the phenomenological dimension (an understanding) of the experiences (Finlay, 2002). Eidetic reduction refers to the process through which researchers look beyond what is observed to identify the meaning of what has been observed (Zahavi, 2003). The researchers remained susceptible to the reality of the experiences of the participants to get the feeling of what it would be like to go through similar experiences (Wojnar & Swanson, 2007). Through intuiting, we managed to get a sense of what it must be like to be in their position (Kumar, 2012) because intuiting urges researchers to pay attention to what is immediately given to them in the situation (Hintikka, 1995). The researchers bracketed all preunderstanding and their own perspectives about the phenomenon (Giorgi, 1997). We started with a concrete example of the phenomenon (emotional abuse of women living with HIV/AIDS) and imaginatively varied it in every possible way to identify the features that are incidental and those that are essential (Wertz, 2005) to describe the essence of the phenomenon.

Trustworthiness of the Findings

The researchers used bracketing of their preunderstanding of the emotional abuse that women living with HIV/AIDS are exposed to and ensured throughout the interviews and data analysis that the essence of the experiences of the participants was revealed as it was experienced by them (Flood, 2010). Once the essence and supporting constituents were formulated, "unbracketing" enabled the researchers to reintegrate the findings into the study context and the existing literature (Gearing, 2004). Quotations from the verbatim transcription of the interviews were used to substantiate the constituents that support the essence of the experiences.

Ethical Considerations

The Research Ethics Committee of the Faculty of Health Sciences of the University of Pretoria and the Research and Ethics Committee of the University of Malawi approved the study protocol (documents 199/2010 and

P.01/11/1028). Written permission from the responsible officer to conduct the research in clinics of the Lilongwe District Health Office was obtained and all the participants gave informed consent to take part in the research and to have the interviews audiorecorded.

RESULTS

The oldest participant was 35, and the youngest 24 years old at the time of the interviews. Eight participants had completed primary school education, and four participants had completed secondary school education. Only one participant was divorced, while the others were married but had been deserted by their husbands.

The essence of the emotional hardship of the participants is best described as "violating experiences" that originated from husbands, family, and community members. The women had to endure unacceptable treatment by their loved ones and communities. The emotional violations scarred their personhood, and they felt that they had lost the inherent value of being human. They were excluded from friendship and supporting family relations. Family and community rejection was repeatedly reinforced and gave rise to their sense of marginalization and left them vulnerable. Instead of others helping them to build a sense of self-worth, the participants experienced incidents that curtailed the same.

The majority of the violating experiences appeared in the women's close interpersonal relationships. They made them feel insecure and without any positive future expectations. The support that they required for emotional survival was withheld, and they doubted whether they would be able to cope with HIV/AIDS.

The constituents that substantiated the essence were the humiliation, abandonment, and blaming that the participants experienced and the hopelessness that they developed.

Humiliation

Family members often initiated the humiliation that the participants experienced from other people by either showing the participants' antiretroviral medication to their friends: "He takes the medicine and shows it to them" or by telling others about the participants' positive HIV status: "They started publicising to others outside our household." Irrational fears of contagion by the family members caused severe humiliation: "They say it is important not to share food with them (HIV-positive women)," while some family members wanted them to leave: "Tell her to go; we don't want her here."

The participants' husbands humiliated them by rejecting them as sex partners: "He even brings prostitutes in our house when I am there" and as carers of the family: "Every time I serve food for him he would break the plates, throwing away the food." These demeaning experiences were extended to suspicions that the participants were unfaithful to their husbands and had had sexual relationships with other men: "He was saying I am a whore and it is because of that, that I got infected."

In the community, alliances were created against the participants. Everyday activities, such as going to the communal water point, turned into difficult tasks because the community members found such activities to be an opportune time to verbally attack them: "They make comments that are hurtful." Others were warned not to interact with them: "Don't chat with so and so because she has got HIV." Visible activities that may be linked to having HIV/AIDS such as bottle-feeding of babies were often the cues that neighbors used to start rumors. When one of the participants decided not to continue breastfeeding her baby, her neighbors started gossiping about her: "The problem that I was experiencing is from the neighbours who said this one must have the virus." The humiliation that the participants experienced violated their sense of belonging to a family and community.

Abandonment

Contrary to the expectation of being supported, the participants found that their husbands attempted to distance themselves from the situation and stated that they have nothing to do with the participants who have HIV/AIDS: "That is your problem; it does not concern me." The men were not willing to be involved with the participants in any way. The participants' health status was not their problem or concern. When they became aware of the participants' HIV/AIDS status, their initial response was to leave them: "His first reaction when I told him about my (HIV) status was to end the marriage." The participants were deserted and left to fend for themselves: "The same month he left our house to marry another wife." Their former husbands did not continue to support them and their children financially and they were left without money to buy food and clothes: "When the money had run out, I started living a difficult life." Without the money that they had previously received from their husbands, they could not access food or shelter. "Living a difficult life" meant for them that they had to struggle to meet their very basic needs.

The participants could not turn to their own families, as the disclosure of their HIV/AIDS status had resulted in abandonment by their families: "At my father's village, they said that they did not want anybody with HIV. Even when I go to the village, nobody shows happiness to see me." Their families rejected them. When they required support from their families, it was not forthcoming: "Even when I was admitted at the hospital, none of my relatives came to see me."

Traditionalist African families in Malawi pay a bride price (*lobola*) to the family of the bride when the marriage is arranged, and thereafter the married woman becomes a member of her husband's family (Mwambene, 2010). In the case of one of the participants, her family used this cultural practice to abandon her. When she wanted to return to her family after her husband has chased her away, they did not welcome her return to them: "They told me that because they received *lobola*, I cannot stay." She was pushed from one place to the other: "The abuse that I am facing is of not having a place." One of the participant's major concerns was the welfare of her children when she were too sick to take care of them. Their husbands deserted them and their family members did not want to be involved: "When I was sick, there was nobody to help me with looking after the child."

The participants could also not rely on their in-laws because none of them experienced any support from their in-laws. Instead, the in-laws discriminated against them: "My in-laws discriminate against me." When they tried to show to their in-laws their need to belong to their family, they were told that they would "give them the disease (HIV/AIDS)." When the families-in-law were approached to help to solve intramarital problems, they did not respond: "I went to his aunt and told her, but she didn't do anything." Their in-laws abandoned them.

Blaming

When a person is diagnosed with HIV/AIDS, the newly diagnosed person often becomes a scapegoat. The participants were thus accused of infecting their husbands. Such allegations were made without any proof to substantiate them: "I think he blamed me for being the one who infected him with the virus." The women are blamed only because they are usually the first in the relationship to go for HIV testing. Men are reluctant to get tested even though they may be the ones engaging in risky sex behaviors: "He is always talking about me and where I got the virus from; when I tell him to go for testing, he refuses." The blame added to the emotional turmoil experienced by the participants. They had to come to terms with their husbands' accusations and they had to carry the burden of having HIV/AIDS without their support.

The participants were also forced to blame themselves for having HIV/AIDS as well as for being emotionally abused. The self-blame was a result of unfair comments that were made about them. They internalized the blame from others and started using it against themselves and held themselves responsible for other people's actions. Eventually they were not able to stand up for themselves because they felt helpless and at fault: "I might be found to be in the wrong."

Hopelessness

As a coping mechanism, the participants hoped that the end of their lives was not imminent. They had the unfortunate circumstances of dealing with people who destroyed such hopes by making statements that insinuated that the women's lives were over: "He told me since you have the disease you are already dead." Instead of adding to the voices of reason and instilling hope in the participants to live positively with HIV, they were constantly reminded of how they were dependent on medication to stay alive: "They say that we are alive because of ARVs (antiretroviral medication). We are just waiting for the day to die." Comments like these destroyed the participants' hope of having any meaningful future, where plans could be made and realized: "I can't see the future; I just live one day at a time."

The participants saw themselves as doomed to death and that there was nothing they could do about it. Feelings of hopelessness developed and made them see no future and to consider suicide as an only option: "What I want is to throw myself in the well."

The desperation of the situation and the sense of having no escape from it, compounded by the emotional abuse, prompted suicidal ideation among the participants. In these cases, suicidal ideation provided a comfort zone where the participants imagined that their suffering might be resolved. They were troubled, however, by the fact that they were contemplating suicide. Taking one's own life is considered to be evil in African culture. It went against their beliefs:

> This is very difficult and it can make me tempted (to commit suicide); maybe if they continued to abuse me I would think evil. (I would think) about taking poison. . . . Now if I don't pray for a long time, how can I defeat the devil? How can I be strong?

Seemingly, relying on prayer is thought to be important in defeating the temptation of considering suicide. In contrast, it is the lack of support and insensitivity of the people surrounding the women that drive them to consider suicide as an option for dealing with their problems.

DISCUSSION

Through humiliation, people's dignity becomes violated (Statman, 2000) and stripped away (Killmister, 2009), leaving them feeling disrespected (Malterud & Hollnagel, 2007). When the humiliation happens as a result of the betrayal of husbands, family, and community members. The detrimental impact on the self-esteem of the victims becomes worse (Parse, 2010). People's personal sense of worth is greatly shaped by what other people think of them, what they say about them, and how they treat them (Statman, 2000). When people are degraded, devalued, or are perceived to be unworthy of the love of others, they isolate themselves from others (Reyles, 2007) in order to protect themselves from further humiliation. Significant others may also abandon them through acts of rejection (Malterud & Hollnagel, 2007), which leaves the victims without support (Reyles, 2007).

Abandonment, as it has been experienced by the participants in this study, was a threat to their survival as human beings because of the importance of social ties and connectedness for psychological well-being (Eisenberger & Lieberman, 2004). Supportive relationships act as buffers to emotional hardship. The sharing of problems with significant others helps people to find solutions to problems and it lowers their anxiety levels, as they do not feel alone in the situation (Vanderhorst & McLaren, 2005). They have a support system on which to rely. When people are abandoned and ostracized, their sense of belonging is damaged by the disconnectedness with significant others (Barroso & Powell-Cope, 2000). When the soothing presence of others is lost, distress and pain are experienced (Eisenberger, Lieberman, & Kipling, 2003).

The participants were abandoned by their husbands, family, and community members to fend for themselves. For women living with HIV/AIDS, abandonment results in the loss of reliable sources of economic support and love, which is seriously needed when one is dealing with the physiological challenges associated with having HIV/AIDS (Carr & Gramling, 2004). Inadequate resources have negative repercussions. Abandoned women may not be able to meet the demands required to sustain healthy living, such as healthy nutrition, good living conditions, and adherence to treatment (Liamputtong, Haritavorn, & Kiatying-Angsulee, 2011).

Abandonment could also result in a loss of identity. The participants' identity as wives and the social status associated with being a wife could be compromised. This loss of identity and status may be severe when a woman is defined by being partnered or is dependent on her husband (De Sousa, 2010). The participants lost their status as wives in their community because their husbands had deserted them. This loss of status equates to suffering disgrace, humiliation, and shame. It becomes difficult to survive psychologically as a result of the loss of attachment that provides support (Adshead, 2010). Abandoned women therefore tend to mourn the loss of such relationships in addition to worrying about future losses that may occur in potential relationships because of having HIV/AIDS and enduring the stigma associated with it (Peterson, 2010).

Abandonment is a form of social exclusion. Persons are made to feel that they are not welcome or that they do not belong. The participants were made to believe that their families, their families-in-law, or their communities did not want to be associated with them. In this case, severe harm was sustained by their unmet needs for social connectedness (Eisenberger et al., 2003). When people become isolated from their significant others, they develop poor self-esteem and feel worthless (Klein, 1991) to the extent that they believe that they cannot control their circumstances (Teitelman, Seloilwe, & Campbell, 2009). The participants in this study were made to feel that they were not only worthless, but that they were also to be blamed for their negative interpersonal experiences.

In many contexts, having HIV/AIDS is associated with sexual promiscuity. The affected person is blamed and shamed, which implies that they are perceived to have been involved in what is considered deviant and unacceptable behavior (Nepal & Ross, 2010). The emotional abuse that the participants suffered from their family and friends might have been a part of shaming and blaming. Women who live with HIV/AIDs are often called names and are told that they are worthless (De Sousa, 2010) and blamed for becoming burdens to their families (Maman et al., 2009). The participants were blamed for having brought the virus to the family and were perceived as sources of infection for their husbands and other members of the family. The blame culture that women with HIV/AIDS experience from their husbands is often related to the broader social and cultural context of their societies (Thapar-Bjorkert & Morgan, 2010).

Blaming of other people often relates to the "othering" dynamic in cultures and societies (Petros, Airhihenbuwa, Simbayi, Ramlagan, & Brown, 2006). People assume that what happens to other groups cannot apply to them. In the context of HIV/AIDS, this "othering" could present as placing blame on certain people for being high-risk groups, for potentially being infected with HIV, and for being responsible for spreading the virus to others. Women are easily blamed and "othered" because they are the weaker sex and they are predominantly dependent on their male partners for support (Petros et al., 2006). It is also believed that the disproportional occurrence of HIV/AIDS in females compared with males (WHO, 2011) adds to the "othering," as women may be considered dirty and immoral. It is the blaming and "othering" that lead to their abuse and public shaming (Maman et al., 2009).

When people feel powerless, such as the participants of this study, they tend to develop self-blame. When the people with the power—who considered themselves to be healthy in this case and therefore even more powerful—blamed the participants, they started to believe the "powerful" people (Laverack, 2009) and started blaming themselves. They became "blameworthy" and took the responsibility of their abuse while their family, friends, and community were not held accountable for their actions.

Self-blame involves a feeling of being responsible for the negative actions of other people (Coffey, Leitenberg, Henning, Turner, & Bennet, 1996). Theories of control and counterfactual thinking can be used to explain the self-blame of the participants (Miller, Markman, & Handley, 2007). They experienced a sense of loss of control over themselves and their behavior, although the incidents of abuse by others were not in any way related to their behavior. Owing to not feeling in control, participants assumed that they could have contributed to the abuse. Their counterfactual thinking linked them to the abuse as if they had caused it. They resorted to "if only" utterances, which only perpetuated and convinced them that they were indeed to be blamed for the abuse. According to Miller and colleagues (2007), people who blame themselves are more likely to relinquish their attempts at control of their circumstances in order to guard against future negative incidents. Our participants might have lived with hope for a bright future if they had not abandoned controlling the life circumstances that developed from the HIV/AIDS diagnosis.

People with hope have a sense of meaning and purpose in life and they know that they can cope with disruptive events (Tutton, Seers, & Langstaff, 2009) and that life is worth living in the present and in the future (Kylma, Vehvilainen-Julkunen, & Lahdevirta, 2001). When people's hope is violated, they are left without the option of making their own choices (McClement & Chochinov, 2008), as they do not believe that their actions can have positive outcomes (Kneisl & Trigoboff, 2009); neither can they mobilize the energy that it takes to make decisions and to execute these decisions (Carpenito, 2000). Hopeless people have given up on life and no longer try to improve their circumstances (Kylma et al., 2001). People's hope can be violated through the harsh and uncaring treatment of others (Dunn, 2005), such as in the case of emotional abuse. The hope of survival of the participants was destroyed when their families and communities rejected them and told them that they did not have a future. Participants were made to expect negative outcomes concerning their lives through the comments of other people that their death was imminent because they had HIV/AIDS. Participants believed these pronouncements and concluded that they had no future to look forward to, as there was nothing they could do to change their situation for the better.

Suicidal ideas are nurtured when people are not supported by their significant others, when they do not foresee a future for themselves, and when they do not believe that their circumstances can change for the better (Preeau, Bouhnik, Peretti-Watel, Obadia, & Spire, 2008). The participants considered suicide because they believed that they had no solutions to their problems. Their families and communities did not support them, and they were blamed for their hardship. They also suffered severe financial problems when their families rejected them. According to Vanderhorst and McLaren (2005), women who are lonely and have financial challenges often consider suicide as a solution. The financial insecurity that the participants suffered, in addition to the ongoing abuse that they were exposed to, made them feel hopeless and want to end their misery through suicide.

CONCLUSION

In this study, women living with HIV/AIDS encountered violating emotional experiences from their husbands, families, and communities. They were exposed to humiliation, abandonment, and blaming and were made to feel hopeless to the extent that they considered suicide. Their abuse was linked to their position of being females in male-dominated societies and the ignorance of people about the spread of HIV. They were considered as different from their family members and they became the "others" who could be blamed for their own misery and for bringing "the virus" to the family.

LIMITATIONS AND STRENGTHS

The study participants were drawn from a specific area in Lilongwe district; therefore, the results may not be generalized to portray the experiences of all women living with HIV/AIDS in Malawi. The findings of this study might be useful for health care teams who render services for women living with HIV/AIDS in Africa to identify the occurrence of emotional abuse of their patients.

REFERENCES

Adshead, G. (2010). Commentary: Till we have faces on humiliation. *The American Academy of Psychiatry and Law, 38*(2), 205–208.

Barroso, J., & Powell-Cope, G. M. (2000). Meta-synthesis of qualitative research on living with HIV infection. *Qualitative Health Research, 10*(3), 340–355.

Campbell, J. C., Baty, M. L., Ghandour, R. M., Stockman, J. K., Francisco, L., & Wagman, J. (2008). The intersection of intimate partner violence against women and HIV/AIDS: A review. *International Journal of Injury Control and Safety Promotion, 15*(4), 221–231.

Carlsson, G., Dahlberg, K., Lützen, K., & Nyström, M. (2004). Violent encounters in psychiatric care: A phenomenological study of embodied caring knowledge. *Issues in Mental Health Nursing, 25,* 191–217.

Carr, R. L., & Gramling, L. F. (2004). Stigma: A health barrier for women with HIV/AIDS. *Journal of the Association of Nurses in AIDS Care, 15*(5), 30–39.

Coffey, P., Leitenberg, H., Henning, K., Turner, T., & Bennet, R. (1996). Mediators of the long term impact of child sexual abuse: Perceived stigma, betrayal, powerlessness and self blame. *Child Abuse and Neglect, 20*(5), 447–455.

Dahlberg, K., Dahlberg, H., & Nyström, M. (2008). *Reflective lifeworld research* (2nd ed.). Lund, Switzerland: Studentlitteratur.

De Sousa, R. (2010). Women living with HIV: Stories of powerlessness and agency. *Women's Studies International Forum, 33,* 244–250.

Dunn, S. L. (2005). Hopelessness as a response to physical illness. *Journal of Nursing Scholarship, 37*(2), 148–154.

Eisenberger, N., & Lieberman, D. M. (2004). Why rejection hurts: A common neural alarm system for physical and social pain. *Trends in Cognitive Sciences, 8*(7), 294–300.

Eisenberger, N., Lieberman, D. M., & Kipling, W. D. (2003). Does rejection hurt? An fMRI study of social exclusion. *Science, 302*(5643), 290–296.

Finlay, L. (2002). "Outing" the researcher: The provenance, process, and practice of reflexivity. *Qualitative Health Research, 12*, 531–544.

Flood, A. (2010). Understanding phenomenology. *Nurse Researcher, 17*(2), 7–15.

Gearing, R. E. (2004). Bracketing in research: A typology. *Qualitative Health Research, 14*, 1429–1452.

Giorgi, A. (1997). The theory, practice and evaluation of phenomenological method as a qualitative research procedure. *Journal of Phenomenological Psychology, 28*(2), 235–260.

Higgins, J. A., Hoffman, S., & Dworkin, S. L. (2010). Rethinking gender, heterosexual men and women vulnerability to HIV/AIDS. *American Journal of Public Health, 100*(3), 435–445.

Hintikka, J. (1995). The phenomenological dimension. In B Smith & D. W. Smith, *Cambridge companion to Husserl* (pp. 79–105). Cambridge, England: Cambridge University Press.

Holloway, I., & Wheeler, S. (2010). *Qualitative research in nursing and health care* (3rd ed.). Oxford, England: Wiley-Blackwell.

Jewkes, R., & Morrell, R. (2010). Gender and sexuality: Emerging perspectives from the heterosexual epidemic in South Africa and implications for HIV risk and prevention. *Journal of the International AIDS Society, 13*(6), 1–11.

Joint United Nations Programme on HIV/AIDS (UNAIDS). (2008). *Epidemiological fact sheet on HIV and AIDS. Core data on epidemiology and response.* Available from http://www.who.int /globalatlas/predefinedReports/EF 2008_MW pdf

Kathewera-Banda, M., Gomile-Chindyaonga, F., Hendricks, S., Kachika, T., Mitole, Z., & White, S. (2005). Sexual violence and women's vulnerability to HIV transmission in Malawi: A rights issue. *International Social Science Journal, 57*, 649–660.

Kaufman, M. R., Shefer, T., Crawford, M., Simbayi, L. C., & Kalichman, S. C. (2008). Gender attitudes, sexual power, HIV risk: A model for understanding HIV risk behaviour of South African men. *AIDS Care, 20*(4), 434–441.

Killmister, S. (2009). Dignity not such a useless concept. *British Medical Journal.* Retrieved from http://www.jme.bmj.com

Klein, D. C. (1991). The humiliation dynamic: An overview. *Journal of Primary Prevention, 12*(2), 93–121.

Kneisl, C. R., & Trigoboff, E. (2009). *Contemporary psychiatric-mental health nursing* (2nd ed.). London, UK: Pearson Education Inc.

Kumar, A. (2012). Using phenomenological research methods in qualitative health research. *International Journal of Human Sciences, 9*(2), 790–804.

Kylma, J., Vehvilainen-Julkunen, K., & Lahdevirta, J. (2001). Hope, despair, and hopelessness in living with HIV/AIDS: A grounded theory study. *Journal of Advanced Nursing, 33*(6), 764–775.

Laverack, G. (2009). *Public health: Power, empowerment and professional practice* (2nd ed.). New York, NY: Palgrave Macmillan.

Liamputtong, P., Haritavorn, N., & Kiatying-Angsulee, N. (2011). Living positively with HIV/AIDS in Central Thailand. *Qualitative Health Research, 22*(4), 441–451.

Malterud, K., & Hollnagel, H. (2007). Avoiding humiliations in the clinical encounter. *Scandinavian Journal of Primary Care, 25*, 69–74.

Maman, S., Abler, L., Parker, L., Lane, T., Chirowodza, A., Ntogwisaangu, J., . . . Fritz, K. (2009). A comparison of HIV stigma and discrimination in five international sites: The influence of care and treatment resources in high prevalence settings. *Social Science & Medicine, 68*, 2271–2278.

McClement, S., & Chochinov, H. M. (2008). Hope in advanced cancer patients. *European Journal of Cancer, 44*, 1169–1174.

Medley, A. M., Kennedy, C. E., Lunyolo, S., & Sweat, M. D. (2009). Disclosure outcomes, coping strategies and life changes among women living with HIV in Uganda. *Qualitative Health Research, 19*(2), 1744–1754.

Miller, A. K., Markman, K. D., & Handley, I. M. (2007). Self blame among sexual assault victims prospectively predicts re-victimization: A perceived socio-legal context model of risk. *Basic and Applied Social Psychology, 29*(2), 129–136.

Ministry of Women and Child Development. (2005). *Women, Girls and HIV/AIDS: Programme and National Plan of Action 2005–2010.* Lilongwe, Malawi: Ministry of Women and Child Development.

Mkandawire-Valhmu, L., & Stevens, P. E. (2010). The critical value of focus group discussions in research with women living with HIV in Malawi. *Qualitative Health Research, 20*(5), 684–696.

Mwambene, L. (2010). Marriage and African customary law in the face of the Bill of Rights and international human rights standards in Malawi. *African Human Rights Law Journal, 10*, 78–105.

National Statistical Office (NSO) and ICF Macro. (2011). *Malawi Demographic and Health Survey 2010.* Zomba, Malawi: Author.

Ndinda, C., Chimbwete, C., McGath, N., Pool, R. (2007). Community attitudes towards individuals living with HIV in rural Kwa-Zulu Natal, South Africa. *AIDS Care, 19*(1), 92–101.

Nepal, V. P., & Ross, M. (2010). Issues related to HIV stigma in Nepal. *International Journal of Sexual Health, 22*(1), 20–31.

Parse, R. (2010). Human dignity: A human becoming ethical phenomenon. *Nursing Science Quarterly, 23*93, 257–263.

Peterson, J. L. (2010). The challenges of seeking and receiving support for women living with HIV. *Health Communication, 25*(5), 470–479.

Petros, G., Airhihenbuwa, C. O., Simbayi, L., Ramlagan, S., & Brown, B. (2006). HIV/AIDS "othering" in South Africa: The blame goes on. *Culture, Health & Sexuality: An International Journal for Research, Intervention and Care, 8*(1), 67–77.

Preeau, M., Bouhnik, A. D., Peretti-Watel, P., Obadia, Y., & Spire, B. (2008). Suicidal attempts among people living with HIV in France. *AIDS Care, 20*(8), 917–924.

Ramachandran, S., Yonas, M. A., Silvestre, A. J., & Burke, J. (2010). Intimate partner violence among HIV positive persons in an urban clinic. *AIDS Care, 22*(12), 1536–1543.

Reyles, D. Z. (2007). The ability to go about without shame. A proposal for internationally comparable indicators of shame and humiliation. *Oxford Poverty and Human Development Initiative (OPHI) working paper no. 3.* Oxford, UK: Oxford University Press.

Statman, D. (2000). Humiliation, dignity and self-respect. *Philosophical Psychology, 13*(4), 523–540.

Streubert, H. J., & Carpenter, D. R. (2011). *Qualitative research in nursing: Advancing the human imperative* (5th ed.). Philadelphia, PA: Lippincott Williams & Wilkins.

Teitelman, A. M., Seloilwe, E. S., & Campbell, J. C. (2009). Voices from the frontlines: The epidemics of HIV/AIDS and violence among girls. *Health Care for Women International, 30*(3), 184–194.

Thapar-Bjorkert, S., & Morgan, K. J. (2010). But sometimes I think … they put themselves in the situation: Exploring blame and responsibility in interpersonal violence. *Violence Against Women, 16*(1), 32–59.

Theuninck, A., Lake, N., & Gibson, S. (2010). HIV-related posttraumatic stress disorder: Investigating the traumatic events. *AIDS Patient Care and Sexually Transmitted Diseases, 24*(8), 485–491.

Tutton, E., Seers, K., & Langstaff, K. (2009). An exploration of hope as a concept for nursing. *Journal of Orthopaedic Nursing, 13,* 119–127.

Vanderhorst, R. K., & McLaren, S. (2005). Social relationships as a predictor of depression and suicidal ideation in older adults. *Adults & Mental Health, 9*(6), 517–525.

Van Rensburg, M. S. J. (2007). A comprehensive programme addressing HIV/AIDS and gender-based violence. *Journal of the Social Aspects of HIV/AIDS, 4*(3), 695–706.

Wertz, F. J. (2005). Phenomenological research methods for counselling psychology. *Journal of Counselling Psychology, 52*(2), 167–177.

Wojnar, D. M., & Swanson, K. M. 2007. Phenomenology: An exploration. *Journal of Holistic Nursing, 25*(3), 172–180.

World Health Organization (WHO). (2011). *Cooperation strategy at a glance.* Retrieved from http://www.Measuredhs.com/pubs/pdf/PR4/PR4.pdf

Zahavi, D. (2003). *Husserl's phenomenology.* Stanford, CA: Stanford University Press.

Zere, E., Moeti, M., Kirigia, J., Mwase, T., & Kataika, E. (2007). Equity in health care in Malawi: Analysis of trends. *British Medical Council Public Health, 7,* 78. doi:10.1186/1471-2458-7-78

Association Between Domestic Violence and HIV Serostatus Among Married and Formerly Married Women in Kenya

ELIJAH O. ONSOMU

Division of Nursing, Winston-Salem State University, Winston-Salem, North Carolina, USA

BENTA A. ABUYA

Education Research Program, African Population and Health Research Center (APHRC), Nairobi, Kenya

IRENE N. OKECH

Department of Research and Policy, Imbako Public Health, Alpharetta, Georgia, USA; and Imbako Public Health, Nairobi, Kenya

DAVID L. ROSEN

Gillings School of Public Health, University of North Carolina at Chapel Hill, Chapel Hill, North Carolina, USA

VANESSA DUREN-WINFIELD

Department of Healthcare Management, Winston-Salem State University, Winston-Salem, North Carolina, USA

AMBER C. SIMMONS

Arnold School of Public Health, University of South Carolina, Columbia, South Carolina, USA

The prevalence of both domestic violence (DV) and HIV among Kenyan women is known to be high, but the relationship between them is unknown. Nationally representative cross-sectional data from married and formerly married (MFM) women responding to the Kenya Demographic and Health Survey 2008/2009 were analyzed adjusting for complex survey design. Multivariable logistic regressions were used to assess the covariate-adjusted associations between HIV serostatus and any reported DV as well as *four constituent DV measures: physical, emotional, sexual, and aggravated bodily harm, adjusting for covariates entered into each model using a forward stepwise selection process. Covariates of a priori interest included those representing marriage history, risky sexual behavior, substance use, perceived HIV risk, and sociodemographic characteristics. The prevalence of HIV among MFM women was 10.7% (any DV: 13.1%, no DV: 8.6%); overall prevalence of DV was 43.4%. Among all DV measures, only physical DV was associated with HIV (11.9%; adjusted odds ratio: 2.01, p < .05). Efforts by the government and women's groups to monitor and improve policies to reduce DV, such as the Sexual Offences Act of 2006, are urgently needed to curb HIV, as are policies that seek to provide DV counseling and treatment to MFM women.*

In Kenya, as in much of Sub-Saharan Africa (SSA), women are disproportionately affected by both HIV (UNAIDS, 2012) and domestic violence (Goo & Harlow, 2012; Jewkes, 2002; Kishor & Johnson, 2004; Koenig et al., 2003; Wanyoni & Lumumba, 2010). Among Kenyans aged 15 to 49 years, 8% of women compared with 4% of men report HIV infection (Kenya National Bureau of Statistics [KNBS] & ICF Macro, 2010), and higher prevalence of domestic violence among Kenyan women has been previously reported (Abuya, Onsomu, Moore, & Piper, 2012; Fonck, Leye, Kidula, Ndinya-Achola, & Temmerman, 2005; Goo & Harlow, 2012; Kishor & Johnson, 2004; Wanyoni & Lumumba, 2010). Despite the high prevalence of both DV and HIV among Kenyan women, the relationship between DV and HIV remains unclear. Although several investigators have observed an association between DV and HIV (Dude, 2011; Jewkes, Dunkle, Nduna, & Shai, 2010; Shi, Kouyoumdjian, & Dushoff, 2013; Silverman, Decker, Saggurti, Balaiah, & Raj, 2008), in the largest study on this topic—which incorporated data from 10 developing countries including Kenya—an association was not observed (Harling, Msisha, & Subramanian, 2010). All of these studies, however, are subject to important methodology and context limitations that may in part explain the discrepant findings. In the current study, we have addressed many of the limitations found in the existing literature in order to more accurately assess the relationship between DV and HIV infection among Kenyan women. An accurate understanding of the relationship between DV and HIV is paramount to the development of interventions to address these deeply rooted societal problems, which take a particularly heavy toll among women in Kenya and women throughout SSA.

Intimate partner violence (IPV), which includes DV, is the most common form of gender-based violence (García-Moreno, Jansen, Ellsberg, Heise, & Watts, 2006). It is defined as "the range of sexually, psychologically and physically coercive acts used against adult and adolescent women by current or former male intimate partners" (World Health Organization [WHO], 1997, p. 5). Experts estimate that in African countries, 25%–48% of women will suffer abuse at one point in their lives (Goo & Harlow, 2012; Jewkes, 2002; Kishor & Johnson, 2004; Koenig et al., 2003; Wanyoni & Lumumba, 2010). Its prevalence in Kenya is established (Abuya et al., 2012; Fonck et al., 2005; Goo & Harlow, 2012; Kishor & Johnson, 2004; Wanyoni & Lumumba, 2010), and Abuya and colleagues (2012) showed that physical (42%) and sexual (14%) violence toward Kenyan women fell in the middle range of multicountry estimates reported by the WHO, 14%–61% and 6%–59%, respectively (WHO, 2005). Emotional violence is also rampant (Abuya et al., 2012; Fonck et al., 2005; Goo & Harlow, 2012; Kimuna & Djamba, 2008).

Physical and sexual violence, including sexual assault within marriage, increase transmission of the virus as tears and lacerations to the vaginal canal enable its invasion of the vaginal epithelia (García-Moreno & Watts, 2000; Kishor & Johnson, 2004; van der Straten et al., 1998; Wittenberg, Joshi, Thomas, & McCloskey, 2007). Socially, the threat of IPV often impedes open communication regarding disease risk. Women refrain from discussing their husband's risky behaviors, such as having extramarital partners or frequenting sex workers (Karamagi, Tumwine, Tylleskar, & Heggenhougen, 2006; Lary, Maman, Katebalila, McCauley, & Mbwambo, 2004; Lasee & Becker, 1997), and avoid disclosing their own HIV serostatus in fear of accusations of infidelity, abandonment, discrimination, physical and emotional violence, and disruption of family relationships (Antelman et al. 2001; Gaillard et al., 2002; Medley, García-Moreno, McGill, & Maman, 2004).

Women reporting physical and emotional IPV also reported impaired emotional and social functioning, including depression, helplessness, resignation, and isolation from friends, family, and religious groups (Dietz et al., 1997; Wittenberg et al., 2007). Further, IPV has been shown to affect a woman's participation in household decision making, including decisions about her own health, for example, whether to seek skilled health care (Antelman et al., 2001; Dietz et al., 1997; Dunkle et al., 2004; Fonck et al., 2005; Gaillard et al., 2002; Goo & Harlow, 2012; Izugbara & Ngilangwa, 2010; Malhotra, Schuler, & Boender, 2002; Maman et al., 2002; Medley et al., 2004; WHO, 2005).

IPV is also associated with increased HIV risk in women because men who abuse their wives exhibit other risky behaviors, including drug abuse and alcohol misuse (Gielen, McDonnell, & O'Campo, 2002; Karamagi et al., 2006; Zablotska et al., 2009), multiple sexual partners (Martin et al., 1999; Onsomu et al., 2013), and lack of condom use (Gielen et al., 2002; Karamagi et al., 2006). Patriarchal cultural pressures that encourage men toward early sexual initiation and multiple sexual partners prior to marriage are also associated with increased incidence of infection (Abuya et al., 2012; Dunkle et al., 2006; Lary et al., 2004; Silverman et al., 2008). These factors are exacerbated by dominant and controlling men who manipulate their partners (Wang & Rowley, 2007; Wingood & DiClemente, 1998) and increase women's risk of contracting HIV (Decker et al., 2008; Dude, 2011; Silverman et al., 2008).

One of the nine priority areas in the UNAIDS Outcome Framework for 2009–2011 (2009) is to end violence against girls and women, especially because it increases their susceptibility to HIV infection (Andersson, Cockcroft, & Shea, 2008; Campbell et al., 2008; García-Moreno & Watts, 2000; Martin & Curtis, 2004; WHO, 2004). Although prevalence varies, many countries acknowledge the association between violence and HIV susceptibility among women. For instance, in eastern and southern Africa, IPV is associated with high risk of HIV infection (Abuya et al., 2012; Dunkle et al., 2004; Fonck et al., 2005; Jewkes, Levin, & Penn-Kekana, 2003; Jewkes et al., 2010; Karamagi et al., 2006; Kiarie et al., 2006; Lary et al. 2004; Maman et al., 2002; van der Straten et al., 1998).

Additionally, qualitative studies have highlighted the links among HIV/AIDS, gender inequities, and DV as an outcome of the patriarchal nature of African societies and notions of masculinity that emphasize male strength and toughness and perpetuate control of women (Coovadia, Jewkes, Barron, Sanders, & McIntyre, 2009; Go et al., 2003; Jewkes et al., 2010). Such norms have led some women to accept and tolerate male dominance to the extent of rationalizing IPV (Izugbara & Ngilangwa, 2010; Lawoko, 2008). For example, researchers found that traditional practices in some rural Kenyan communities could predispose women to higher risk of physical violence (Abuya et al., 2012). The prevalence of violence impedes women's ability to negotiate for safe sex, which often results in low condom use (Abuya et al., 2012; Andersson et al., 2008; Campbell et al., 2008; García-Moreno & Watts, 2000; Go et al., 2003; Karamagi et al., 2006; WHO, 2004).

Although research has shown that women are at greater risk of HIV infection, particularly in areas where HIV infection is high, prevention messages largely continue to focus on HIV testing, male condom use (Go et al., 2003), treatment of sexually transmitted diseases, and, most recently, male circumcision and antiretroviral treatment. Notably, interventions have not focused on gender-specific problems nor benefited vulnerable women (Christofides & Jewkes, 2010; Wawer et al., 2009).

From the foregoing arguments, research continues to show that gender-based violence, usually an outcome of male dominance, results in high-risk sexual behavior (Dunkle et al., 2004; Gilbert, El-Bassel, Schilling, Wada, & Bennet, 2000; Jewkes et al., 2003, 2006; Wingood & DiClemente, 1998; Zablotska et al., 2009). Women who experience violence in highly unequal relationships have greater chances of contracting HIV (Decker et al., 2008; Dude, 2011; Jewkes & Morrell, 2010; Karamagi et al., 2006; Silverman et al., 2008). Nonetheless, scholars examining HIV and IPV among women in 10 developing countries, including Kenya, found no association (Harling et al.,

2010). In the current study, we provide further evidence about the association between DV and HIV serostatus among married and formerly married (MFM) women in Kenya and improve on previous estimates by controlling for possible confounders.

METHODS

Data Source

Our cross-sectional study used a population-based national sample, the 2008/2009 Kenya Demographic and Health Survey (KDHS, 2008/09), with data collected between November 2008 and February 2009. This survey was the second to collect information on HIV serostatus, following the KDHS-2003 (Central Bureau of Statistics [Kenya], Ministry of Health [Kenya], and ORC Macro, 2004). Data were limited to a subsample of women aged 15–49 from a merged dataset that considered those who were married ($n = 5,041$) or formerly married ($n = 863$); of these women, 4,906 (83.1%) responded to questions about DV. Among these married and formerly married women, 2,669 of them agreed to be tested for HIV; among them, 442 did not respond to DV questions and were excluded from the final analyses. The total sample of 2,227 (83.4%) were tested for HIV and responded to DV questions, which allowed us to estimate the association between DV and HIV serostatus. Study data were weighted to account for a clustering effect to eliminate over- and underestimation in the standard errors (StataCorp, 2013).

Survey Measures

HIV serostatus. National Public Health Laboratory Services personnel were involved in the collection of dried blood spot (DBS) samples, voluntary counseling and testing, and laboratory testing for HIV. All positive samples and a random selection of negative samples (10%) were subjected to further testing at the HIV laboratory of the Kenya Medical Research Institute (KEMRI) using the same procedure. Further analysis by polymerase chain reaction of the deoxyribonucleic acid (DNA) in the same laboratory on 30 discrepant samples were conducted. See KNBS and ICF Macro (2010, pp. 9–10) for a complete description of the HIV procedures and testing. All DBS testing was done in early June 2009.

Domestic violence. Evaluation of DV among married and formerly married women was based on a modified Conflict Tactics Scale (CTS) used in the KDHS-2008/09, which has proven effective in measuring DV across cultures (Strauss, 1990, cited in KNBS & ICF Macro, 2010). Questions were asked to evaluate abuse and coded as no, "0," or yes, "1." Common factor analysis was used to group and identify patterns from the various questions while maintaining the needed information with minimal loss.

The factors that mostly explained/measured certain themes based on rotated factor loadings were retained and named based on the overall theme represented by their constituent items; these themes were named and used for analyses as the study exposures. Dichotomous variables generated from the retained factors explained most of the total variance (40%–62%) for each of the four themes identified: (a) physical violence (push you, shake you, or throw something at you?; slap you?; twist your arm or pull your hair?; punch you with his fist or with something that could hurt you?; kick you or drag you or beat you up?); (b) emotional violence (say or do something to humiliate you in front of others?; threaten to hurt or harm you or someone close to you?; insult you or make you feel bad about yourself?); (c) sexual violence (physically forced you to have sexual intercourse even when you did not want to?; force you to perform any sexual acts you did not want to?); and (d) violence with aggravated bodily harm (AGBH; try to choke you or burn you on purpose?; threaten to attack you with a knife, gun, or any other weapon?). A fifth theme was generated from all of the four variables and named "all forms of violence." All themes were coded as "0" if respondents indicated that they did not experience violence, and "1" if they did. Weights and correlations between each variable (factor loading) were determined at <0.3 (UCLA Institute for Digital Research and Education, n.d.).

Sociodemographic factors. The survey captured several partner, personal, social, and demographic characteristics, and since they could have an effect on or explain the association between DV and HIV serostatus, we controlled for them in the final logistic multivariable models. They include the following: (a) age, measured in 5-year increments, and ranging from 15 to 49 years, considered reproductive age; (b) risky sexual behavior, a variable generated from three questions: Were you given or did you receive money/gifts for sex in the past 12 months?; How many individuals have you had sex with other than your husband in the last 12 months?; and Was a condom used in the last intercourse?; (c) number of lifetime sexual partners; (d) whether husband consumes alcohol; (e) presence of an STD, a variable constructed from two questions: Have you had a genital sore/ulcer? and Genital discharge in the last 12 months?; (f) number of cowives, coded as no other cowife or two or more cowives; (g) education; (h) religion; (i) wealth index, a variable generated from the household's ownership of consumer goods, dwelling characteristics, drinking water source, and toilet facilities, among other socioeconomic characteristics (Gwatkin et al., 2000, cited in KNBS & ICF Macro, 2010); (j) residence; (k) age at first marriage; (l) occupation; (m) health insurance; and (n) perceived risk of acquiring HIV.

Data Analysis

The survey responses and HIV test result datasets were merged. All descriptive, bivariate, univariate, and multivariable data analyses were conducted using Stata/SE 13.1 with a "svyset" command, taking into consideration the weights, strata, cluster, and single unit to attain linearized standard errors. Hence, we accounted for nonindependence within the primary sampling unit and survey nonresponse. Bivariate analyses were used to estimate the prevalence of HIV serostatus. Univariate logistic regression analyses were used to estimate the association between the main outcome measure (HIV serostatus) and independent variables. Multivariate logistic regression analyses were conducted by including variables identified through the forward stepwise regression method and manual inclusion. Univariate (unadjusted) and multivariable (adjusted) analyses are reported using odds ratios (ORs) and 95% confidence intervals (CIs), with study significance set at a two tailed p value of $<.05$.

Institutional Review Board Approval

The current study involved secondary data analysis of the KDHS-2008/09. Administration of the survey involved multiple organizations, including the KNBS, the MEASURE Demographic and Health Survey (DHS) program at ICF Macro, the United States Agency for International Development (USAID), among others. For the HIV test, the blood specimen collection and analysis protocol was developed by the DHS program, with revisions completed by KEMRI and the Kenya National AIDS Control Council. It was reviewed and approved by KEMRI Scientific and Ethical Review Committee (KNBS & ICF Macro, 2010). Further human subject review and study oversight were granted by the Winston-Salem State University Institutional Review Board under exempt status.

RESULTS

Descriptive Statistics

The study included both MFM women aged 15–49 ($n = 2,227$). Overall, HIV prevalence among those who responded to DV questions was 10.67%, which differed between those who were currently married (7.03%), formerly married (34.19%), and both (MFM) women (10.67%). Prevalence of any DV was 44%, 42%, and 43% among these groups of women, respectively. Figure 1 reports the various forms of DV among MFM women, ranging from a low of 4% for married women experiencing violence with AGBH to a high of 32% for formerly married women experiencing physical violence. Overall, physical, emotional, sexual, and violence with AGBH were slightly higher among formerly married women with the exception of all forms of violence (see Table 1 and Figure 1).

TABLE 1 Study Population Characteristics, KDHS-2008/09

Study characteristics	Married		Formerly married		Married and formerly married	
	n	%	n	%	n	%
HIV serostatus ($n = 2,227$)						
Negative	1789	93	203	66	1992	89
Positive[§]	146	7	89	34	235	11
Physical violence ($n = 2,224$)						
No	1370	72	186	68	1556	71
Yes	563	28	105	32	668	29
Emotional violence ($n = 2,226$)						
No	1442	74	201	73	1643	73
Yes	493	26	90	27	583	27
Sexual violence ($n = 2,225$)						
No	1567	79	219	78	1786	79
Yes	366	21	73	22	439	21
Violence with AGBH[β] ($n = 2,224$)						
No	1861	96	253	88	2114	95
Yes	72	4	38	12	110	5
All forms of violence ($n = 2,227$)						
No	1106	56	153	58	1259	57
Yes	829	44	139	42	968	43
Risky sexual behavior ($n = 2,224$)						
No	1825	95	152	51	1977	89
Yes	107	5	140	49	247	11
Number of lifetime sexual partners ($n = 2,221$)						
One	901	43	61	22	962	40
Two	566	32	84	28	650	31
Three	279	16	75	27	354	17
Four or more	183	9	72	23	255	11
Husband consumes alcohol ($n = 2,224$)						
No	1290	65	134	42	1424	62
Yes	643	35	157	58	800	38
Sexually transmitted diseases ($n = 2,226$)						
No STDs	1799	94	267	92	2066	94
STDs present	135	6	25	8	160	6
Number of cowives ($n = 1,934$)						
No other wife	1645	88	—	—	1645	88
Two or more	289	12	—	—	289	12
Education ($n = 2,227$)						
Less than primary/none	348	11	48	11	396	11
Primary	1059	59	171	63	1230	60
Secondary	393	24	58	22	451	23
Higher/college/graduate	135	6	15	4	150	6
Age ($n = 2,227$)						
15–19	93	3	3	1	96	3
20–24	427	21	41	14	468	20
25–29	435	26	42	16	477	24
30–34	361	19	60	19	421	19
35–39	266	13	48	12	314	13

(continued on next page)

TABLE 1 Study Population Characteristics, KDHS-2008/09 *(continued)*

Study characteristics	Married		Formerly married		Married and formerly married	
	n	%	*n*	%	*n*	%
40–44	184	10	44	20	228	11
45–49	169	9	54	19	223	10
Religion (*n* = 2,226)						
Protestant	1140	66	171	67	1311	67
Roman Catholic	380	22	76	24	456	22
Muslim	343	8	37	7	380	8
Other religions	71	3	8	2	79	3
Wealth index (*n* = 2,227)						
Poorest	448	19	64	20	512	19
Poorer	311	17	59	19	370	17
Middle	317	17	49	18	366	18
Richer	362	20	45	18	407	20
Richest	497	26	75	25	572	26
Residence (*n* = 2,227)						
Urban	519	23	80	25	599	24
Rural	1416	77	212	75	1628	76
Age at first marriage (*n* = 2,227)						
≥25	196	9	31	15	227	10
20–24	562	31	82	27	644	30
15–19	973	50	146	47	1119	50
≤14	204	10	33	11	237	10
Occupation (*n* = 2,222)						
Not working	754	34	57	18	811	32
Teaching and professional	381	19	63	22	444	20
Agriculture-self employed	478	29	77	29	555	29
Sales	124	7	24	9	148	7
Other occupations	194	10	70	22	264	12
Health insurance (*n* = 2,226)						
No	1800	92	284	97	2084	92
Yes	134	8	8	3	142	8
Perceived risk of acquiring HIV (*n* = 2,214)						
No risk at all	159	8	26	7	185	8
Small risk	705	33	106	40	811	34
Moderate risk	725	41	93	31	818	40
Great risk	336	18	64	21	400	18

§Exact HIV prevalence: married women (7.03%), formerly married women (34.19%), and married and formerly married women (10.67%).
βAGBH: aggravated bodily harm.

Bivariate Analysis

Of married women who experienced physical violence, 11.9% tested positive for HIV compared with 5.8% ($F_{1, 378}$ = 14.24, $p < .001$) among those who did not experience physical violence. Also, 11.2% of married women who experienced sexual violence tested positive for HIV compared with 6.7% ($F_{1, 378}$ = 3.83, $p < .05$) among those who did not experience sexual

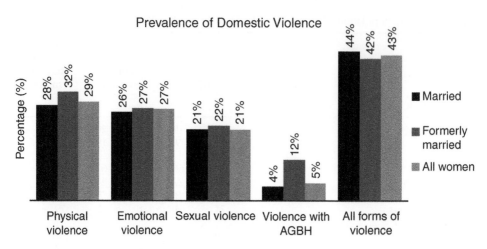

FIGURE 1 Percentage of domestic violence among married and formerly married women agreeing to be tested for HIV in Kenya, KDHS 2008/2009.
AGBH: aggravated bodily harm.

violence. Overall, 10.6% of married women who experienced all forms of violence tested positive for HIV compared with 5.2% ($F_{1, 378} = 6.22$, $p < .05$) among those who did not. For formerly married women, 20.5% who reported previous sexual violence tested positive for HIV compared with 33.8% ($F_{1, 190} = 5.01$, $p < .05$) of those who did not experience sexual violence. For married and formerly married women who experienced physical violence, 14.8% tested positive for HIV compared with 8.7% ($F_{1, 379} = 5.76$, $p < .05$) among those who did not (see Table 2).

Certain characteristics entered into the final model through stepwise forward multivariate analysis and the manual selection method were associated with HIV serostatus. The following were not associated; age at first marriage, husband's alcohol consumption, and education (selected by stepwise forward multivariate method), and health insurance status, wealth index, and age, which were selected manually and added back in the final model. These variables have been identified as relevant in previous studies of DV and HIV serostatus (Decker et al., 2008, 2009; Dude, 2011; Gielen et al., 2002; Jewkes et al., 2006, 2010; Maman et al., 2002; Shi et al., 2013; Silverman et al., 2008).

Association Between HIV Serostatus and Domestic Violence

Unadjusted results. Table 3 presents unadjusted (crude) odds ratios (ORs) in a univariate logistic regression model of the association between DV and HIV serostatus. Among married women, the OR for HIV infection was higher among those who experienced physical violence compared with those who did not 2.42 ($p < .001$). The ORs were also higher among married women who experienced sexual violence and all forms of violence compared with those who did not 1.66 ($p < .05$) and 1.83 ($p < .01$), respectively.

TABLE 2 Bivariate Analysis, Number, and Percentage of the Association Between HIV Serostatus and Domestic Violence, KDHS-2008/09

Characteristic	Negative (n)	Positive (n)	HIV Prevalence	p value
Married women				
Physical violence	n = 1,933			
No	1291	79	5.8	X^2 (n = 1933, df = 378) = 14.25***
Yes	496	67	11.9	
Emotional violence	n = 1,935			
No	1347	95	6.6	X^2 (n = 1935, df = 378) = 0.88^{NS}
Yes	442	51	10.3	
Sexual violence	n = 1,933			
No	1462	105	6.7	X^2 (n = 1933, df = 378) = 3.83*
Yes	325	41	11.2	
Violence with AGBH[β]	n = 1,933			
No	1724	137	7.4	X^2 (n = 1933, df = 378) = 1.53^{NS}
Yes	63	9	12.5	
All forms of violence	n = 1,935			
No	1048	58	5.2	X^2 (n = 1935, df = 378) = 6.22*
Yes	741	88	10.6	
Formerly married women				
Physical violence	n = 291			
No	130	56	30.1	X^2 (n = 291, df = 189) = 0.4^{NS}
Yes	73	32	30.5	
Emotional violence	n = 291			
No	138	63	31.3	X^2 (n = 291, df = 189) = 0.87^{NS}
Yes	65	25	27.7	
Sexual violence	n = 292			
No	145	74	33.8	X^2 (n = 292, df = 190) = 5.01*
Yes	58	15	20.5	
Violence with AGBH[β]	n = 291			
No	171	82	33.4	X^2 (n = 291, df = 189) = 1.92^{NS}
Yes	32	6	15.4	
All forms of violence	n = 292			
No	103	50	32.7	X^2 (n = 292, df = 190) = 1.97^{NS}
Yes	100	39	28.1	
Married and formerly married women				
Physical violence	n = 2,224			
No	1421	135	8.7	X^2 (n = 2224, df = 379) = 5.76*
Yes	569	99	14.8	
Emotional violence	n = 2,226			
No	1485	158	9.6	X^2 (n = 2226, df = 379) = 0.02^{NS}
Yes	507	76	13	
Sexual violence	n = 2,225			
No	1607	179	10	X^2 (n = 2225, df = 379) = 0.19^{NS}
Yes	383	56	12.8	
Violence with AGBH[β]	n = 2,224			
No	1895	219	10.4	X^2 (n = 2224, df = 379) = 1.04^{NS}
Yes	95	15	13.6	
All forms of violence	n = 2,227			
No	1151	108	8.6	X^2 (n = 2227, df = 379) = 0.68^{NS}
Yes	841	127	13.1	

*$p < .05$; **$p < .01$; ***$p < .001$; NS: not significant.
[β]AGBH: aggravated bodily harm.

TABLE 3 Unadjusted Odds Ratios and 95% Confidence Intervals of HIV Serostatus and Domestic Violence Among Married and Formerly Married Women in Kenya, in a Univariate Logistic Regression Model, KDHS-2008/09

HIV serostatus	Married women			Formerly married women		
	ORs	95% CI		ORs	95% CI	
Physical abuse	$n = 1{,}933$			$n = 291$		
No	1 Ref			1 Ref		
Yes	2.42***	1.51	3.87	0.78 NS	0.36	1.69
Emotional abuse	$n = 1{,}935$			$n = 291$		
No	1 Ref			1 Ref		
Yes	1.24 NS	0.79	1.95	0.69 NS	0.31	1.52
Sexual abuse	$n = 1{,}933$			$n = 292$		
No	1 Ref			1 Ref		
Yes	1.66*	0.99	2.77	0.42*	0.19	0.91
Violence with AGBH[β]	$n = 1{,}933$			$n = 291$		
No	1 Ref			1 Ref		
Yes	1.68 NS	0.73	3.88	0.46 NS	0.15	1.42
All forms of violence	$n = 1{,}935$			$n = 292$		
No	1 Ref			1 Ref		
Yes	1.83**	1.13	2.96	0.6 NS	0.29	1.24

*$p < .05$; **$p < .01$; ***$p < .001$; NS: not significant.
1 Ref: Reference Category | ORs: Odds Ratios | CIs: Confidence Intervals.
[β]AGBH: aggravated bodily harm.

Among formerly married women, the OR for HIV infection among those who experienced sexual violence compared with those who did not was 0.42 ($p < .05$).

Among married women, the OR for HIV infection among those with risky sexual behavior compared with those without was 0.25 ($p < .001$). Married women reporting two, three, and four or more lifetime sexual partners compared with those who reported only one lifetime sexual partner had increased ORs for HIV infection: 1.77 ($p < .05$), 1.73 ($p < .001$), and 1.48 ($p < .001$), respectively. Similarly, among married women, the OR for HIV infection among those whose husbands had two or more other wives compared with those who were the only wife was 2.8 ($p < .001$).

Among married women aged 20–24, 35–39, and 45–49 compared with those aged 15–19, the ORs for HIV infection were 0.28 ($p < .01$), 0.76 ($p < .05$), and 0.79 ($p < .01$), respectively. Among formerly married women between age groups 20–24 and 45–49 compared with those aged 15–19, the ORs for HIV infection were higher with more than 8.12 ($p < .001$). Among married Muslims, the OR for HIV infection compared with those affiliated with Protestant religions was 0.65 ($p < .05$). The OR for HIV infection was 0.39 ($p < .01$) among formerly married Muslims. Among married women, the OR for HIV infection among those who perceived themselves to have a small risk of acquiring HIV compared with those who perceived themselves to have no risk at all was 0.42 ($p < .05$).

Adjusted results. After controlling for sociodemographic, partner, and personal characteristics, statistically significant associations were observed between HIV serostatus and DV (see Table 4). Among married women, the OR for HIV infection was higher among those who experienced physical violence compared with those who did not 2.01 ($p < .05$). In modeling the association between physical violence and HIV serostatus among married women, other covariates that had statistically associations with HIV serostatus were risky sexual behaviors, number of lifetime sexual partners (three and four or more), number of cowives, age, religion (Muslim), and age at first marriage (≤ 14 years).

Of the married women in the study experiencing all forms of violence (44%), the OR for HIV infection among those with risky sexual behaviors compared with those without was 0.21 ($p < .001$). Among married women who experienced physical violence, the OR for HIV infection was higher among those who had two or more cowives compared with those without cowives was 2.6 ($p < .001$). Among married women experiencing various types of violence, those who indicated that they had previously had two, three, or four or more lifetime sexual partners had higher ORs for HIV infection ranging from 1.49 ($p < .01$) to 1.93 ($p < .05$) compared with those who reported only one lifetime sexual partner.

Among married women who experienced physical violence, the ORs for HIV infection among those aged 20–24 (21%) and 45–49 (10%) compared with those aged 15–19 was 0.18 ($p < .01$) and 0.68 ($p < .001$), respectively. Furthermore, among women experiencing physical violence, higher OR for HIV infection among those who were aged ≤ 14 (10%) at first marriage compared with those who were aged ≥ 25 was 1.72 ($p < .01$). Among women experiencing all forms of violence, the OR for HIV infection was 1.76 ($p < .001$). Among married Muslims (8%), the ORs for HIV infection among those experiencing various types of abuse compared with those affiliated with Protestant religions ranged between 0.52 and 0.56 ($p < .05$).

DISCUSSION

Researchers sought to evaluate the association between domestic violence and HIV serostatus among married and formerly married women in Kenya. This objective was motivated by contradictory findings in the literature on the association between IPV and HIV/AIDS in different contexts, including Kenya (Harling et al., 2010), and methodological issues (Shi et al., 2013) that demanded reexamination. Establishing the pathways by which violence may both be a marker for and directly facilitate HIV infection among women should inform prevention and treatment strategies (Abuya et al., 2012; Decker et al., 2008; Dunkle et al., 2004; Fonck et al., 2005; Goo & Harlow, 2012; Jewkes et al., 2003; Maman et al., 2002; Martin & Curtis, 2004; Silverman et al., 2008; van der Straten et al., 1998). Compared with other studies that examined the association between DV and HIV infection (Decker et al., 2008, 2009; Dude, 2011; Gielen et al., 2002; Jewkes et al., 2006, 2010; Maman et al.,

TABLE 4 Adjusted Odds Ratios and 95% Confidence Intervals of HIV Serostatus and Domestic Violence Among Married Women in Kenya, in a Multivariable Logistic Regression Model, KDHS-2008/09

HIV serostatus	Physical violence§ ORs	95% CI	Emotional violence§ ORs	95% CI	Sexual violence§ ORs	95% CI	Violence with AGBH$^{\beta}$,§ ORs	95% CI	All forms of violence§ ORs	95% CI
Domestic violence										
No	1 Ref		1 Ref		1 Ref		1 Ref		1 Ref	
Yes	2.01*	1.12, 3.6	0.93[NS]	0.55, 1.58	1.14[NS]	0.63, 2.07	1.15[NS]	0.41, 3.23	1.37[NS]	0.78, 2.4
Risky sexual behavior										
No	1 Ref		1 Ref		1 Ref		1 Ref		1 Ref	
Yes	0.2***	0.1, 0.41	0.21***	0.1, 0.42	0.21***	0.1, 0.42	0.21***	0.1, 0.42	0.21***	0.1, 0.43
Number of lifetime sexual partners										
One	1 Ref		1 Ref		1 Ref	1	1 Ref		1 Ref	
Two	1.86[NS]	0.99, 3.51	1.94*	1.04, 3.61	1.9*	3.61	1.93*	1.04, 3.59	1.87[NS]	0.99, 3.52
Three	1.56*	1.06, 2.28	1.64**	1.14, 2.35	1.62**	1.13, 2.34	1.63**	1.14, 2.35	1.59*	1.09, 2.31
Four or more	1.49**	1.13, 1.98	1.52**	1.16, 1.99	1.5**	1.14, 1.98	1.52**	1.16, 1.98	1.49**	1.13, 1.96
Number of cowives										
No other wife	1 Ref		1 Ref		1 Ref		1 Ref		1 Ref	
Two or more	2.6***	1.46, 4.61	2.68***	1.53, 4.69	2.68***	1.53, 4.69	2.67***	1.52, 4.69	2.67***	1.52, 4.68
Age										
15–19	1 Ref		1 Ref		1 Ref		1 Ref		1 Ref	
20–24	0.18**	0.06, 0.53	0.18**	0.06, 0.54	0.18**	0.06, 0.54	0.18**	0.06, 0.53	0.18**	0.06, 0.52
25–29	0.57*	0.35, 0.93	0.59*	0.37, 0.93	0.58*	0.37, 0.93	0.58*	0.37, 0.93	0.58*	0.36, 0.93
30–34	0.58**	0.4, 0.83	0.59**	0.41, 0.84	0.59**	0.41, 0.84	0.59**	0.41, 0.84	0.58**	0.41, 0.83
35–39	0.62***	0.47, 0.83	0.63***	0.48, 0.83	0.63***	0.48, 0.83	0.63***	0.48, 0.83	0.63***	0.48, 0.83
40–44	0.7*	0.54, 0.89	0.7*	0.55, 0.89	0.7*	0.55, 0.88	0.7**	0.55, 0.88	0.69**	0.54, 0.88
45–49	0.68***	0.55, 0.86	0.69***	0.55, 0.86	0.69***	0.55, 0.86	0.69***	0.55, 0.86	0.68***	0.55, 0.85

	OR	CI	CI	OR	CI	CI	OR	CI	CI	OR	CI	CI
Religion												
Protestant	1 Ref			1 Ref			1 Ref			1 Ref		
Roman Catholic	0.73[NS]	0.39	1.37	0.73[NS]	0.39	1.36	0.73[NS]	0.39	1.36	0.72[NS]	0.39	1.35
Muslim	0.56*	0.34	0.91	0.52*	0.32	0.86	0.52*	0.32	0.87	0.53*	0.32	0.87
Other religions	0.7[NS]	0.37	1.34	0.7[NS]	0.38	1.28	0.69[NS]	0.37	1.28	0.69[NS]	0.37	1.29
Age at first marriage												
≥25	1 Ref			1 Ref			1 Ref			1 Ref		
20–24	1.6[NS]	0.6	4.28	1.71[NS]	0.62	4.68	1.67[NS]	0.61	4.56	1.61[NS]	0.59	4.4
15–19	1.09[NS]	0.63	1.87	1.18[NS]	0.68	2.06	1.16[NS]	0.67	2.04	1.13[NS]	0.65	1.96
≤14	1.72**	1.13	2.61	1.81**	1.17	2.82	1.81**	1.16	2.77	1.76**	1.15	2.69

$n = 1{,}927$; *$p < .05$; **$p < .01$; ***$p < .001$; NS: not significant.

1 Ref: Reference Category | ORs: Odds Ratios | CIs: Confidence Intervals.

§Other variables controlled for but were nonsignificant: husband alcohol consumption, sexually transmitted diseases, education, wealth index, residence, occupation, health insurance, and perceived risk of acquiring HIV.

βAGBH: aggravated bodily harm.

Note: Formerly married women did not respond to the question, does your husband/partner have other wives or does he live with other women as if married?

2002; Shi et al., 2013; Silverman et al., 2008; van der Straten et al., 1998), our study controlled for most of the identified confounders.

Overall, we found HIV prevalence among those who responded to DV questions to be 10.67%; this was higher than the 8% reported for women aged 15–49 by the KDHS 2008/2009 (KNBS & ICF Macro, 2010). The prevalence of DV was 44%, 42%, and 43% among married and formerly married women and women who have been both, respectively, which confirms the findings of Abuya and colleagues (2012), Fonck and colleagues (2005), Goo and Harlow (2012), Kishor and Johnson (2004), and Wanyoni and Lumumba (2010), who established the continued prevalence of IPV in Kenya. The finding that 42% of formerly married women have experience DV is consistent with a study by Abuya and colleagues (2012) that established the prevalence of physical violence at 42% based on the 2003 KDHS. Given that our study used the 2008/2009 KDHS, we see no significant change in the prevalence of physical violence against formerly married women in Kenya. It falls within the middle range of the 14%–61% reported in a 2005 WHO multicountry study on women's health and DV.

We found that married women who experienced physical violence had 2.01 ($p < .05$) times the odds of testing positive for HIV compared with those who did not experience physical violence. This finding corroborates the work of scholars in the last decade who have reported associations between partner violence and high risk of HIV infection in eastern and southern Africa (Abuya et al., 2012; Dunkle et al., 2004; Fonck et al., 2005; Jewkes et al., 2003, 2010; Karamagi et al., 2006; Kiarie et al., 2006; Lary et al., 2004; Maman et al., 2002; van der Straten et al., 1998). The need to implement the UNAIDS Outcome Framework for 2009–2011 priority to end violence against girls and women, therefore, is urgent (UNAIDS, 2009). Emotional violence, sexual violence, violence with AGBH, and all forms of violence were not observed to have any significant association with HIV serostatus. Except for emotional violence, however, they had higher ORs of HIV infection compared with those who did not experience any DV. Another explanation for lack of significance for other forms of DV can be due to the small sample size as observed from the CIs.

Aside from DV, other factors that increased the likelihood of testing positive for HIV among married women included number of lifetime sexual partners, number of cowives, and age at first marriage. These factors, including risky sexual behaviors and age, have been associated with increased risk of infection, not only among women, but also among men, who then spread the disease to their female partners (Martin et al., 1999). Our study found that married women aged 20–49 who experienced physical violence, however, had less risk (OR: 0.18 to 0.7) of testing positive for HIV compared with their counterparts aged 15–19. With regard to age at first marriage, the study found that women who were aged ≤14 when first married and experienced physical violence had 1.72 ($p < .01$) times the odds of testing positive for HIV compared with those aged ≥25. Overall, these findings implicate marriage as a risk factor for contracting HIV and age at first marriage with contracting the virus later in life.

The patriarchal nature of African society is known to support a notion of masculinity that perpetuates control of women by their male partners (Coovadia et al., 2009). In many African societies, including Kenya, women are expected to accept and to tolerate male dominance to the extent of rationalizing severe forms, such as domestic violence (Izugbara & Ngilangwa, 2010; Lawoko, 2008). Furthermore, age differences in sexual partnerships have long been associated with increased risk of intergenerational HIV transmission (Gregson et al., 2002), especially between older men and younger women (Longfield, Glick, Waithaka, & Berman, 2004), in part because older men have had time to acquire sexually transmitted infections from other partners (Kelly et al., 2003). Younger women are also likely to be economically dependent on their often older partners and unlikely to leave a sexually risky or abusive relationship (Luke, 2003). Younger wives experiencing DV are unlikely to ask their husbands about their HIV status and other previous or current sexual partners, leaving them more vulnerable to infection (Sa & Larsen, 2007).

Our study may be limited by the survey on which it is based. Since our measurements of the variables are restricted to one time point, we could not assess the relationship between DV and HIV serostatus over time. Our findings are also limited to Kenya and cannot be generalized to other SSA countries. While the instrument was found to be sensitive to cultural differences and effective in measuring DV (Strauss, 1990, cited in KNBS & ICF Macro, 2010), self-response might have led to underreporting. Because our data were limited to women who responded to DV questions and agreed to be tested for HIV, a large percentage of women who responded to DV questions were not considered in the final analyses. This raises questions about differences between women who experienced DV and tested for HIV versus those who experienced DV and were not tested for HIV.

Cultural expectations and norms in the context of most African countries, including Kenya, could have led some respondents to think that some forms of violence are acceptable and not "actual domestic violence." Furthermore, the survey did not capture a timeline for violence, which could have caused recall bias, leading to nondifferential misclassification of the exposure (DV) and possibly biasing the findings toward the null (Birkett, 1992; Dosemeci, Wacholder, & Lubin, 1990). These married and formerly married women would probably identify most of these forms as DV and respond appropriately, however, reducing the possibility of nondifferential misclassification. Potential recall bias by HIV serostatus could have been possible among women who were aware of being HIV positive at the time of the survey. These women, especially those who were formerly married, may have been more likely to report a history of violence than women who had not tested HIV positive previously. This could explain the high HIV prevalence rates for various types of DV among formerly married women that ranged between 15.4% and 30.5%.

Overall, our findings have significant policy implications for women's health outcomes in Kenya. They call for increasing the level of awareness, protection, and subsequent empowerment of women. Articles 3, 7, and10 (Domestic Violence and Sexual Violence) of the Sexual Offenses Act (No. 3 of 2006, rev. 2007) address domestic violence (Kenya Law Reports and the Government of Kenya, 2009). The adoption of effective and concrete measures to combat domestic and sexual violence against women, sensitization of society as a whole on these issues, prosecution of perpetrators, and provision of assistance and protection to victims are some of the measures proposed.

The importance of women's protection and empowerment is premised on consistent findings from prior studies and the current study, which show that violence, particularly physical abuse, makes women susceptible to HIV infection and other STDs (Abuya et al., 2012; Decker et al., 2008; Dunkle et al., 2004; Fonck et al., 2005; Jewkes et al., 2003; Maman et al., 2002; Martin & Curtis, 2004; Silverman et al., 2008; van der Straten et al., 1998). Our study argues strongly for the immediate implementation of the proposals in the Sexual Offences Act of 2006.

In Kenya, services for victims of gender-based violence have been provided mainly by nonstate actors. The Kenyan government should be more involved and develop nationwide emergency shelters to provide accommodation, medical care, and counseling services for victims of gender-based violence (Federation of Women Lawyers [FIDA], 2011). They are essential because many women are economically and emotionally dependent on their abusers (FIDA, 2011; Luke, 2003). Our study supports this notion and reiterates the need to implement the UNAIDS (2009) critical priority to end violence against girls and women, especially to protect young women from early marriage, which we found increases their risk for testing positive for HIV later in life compared with those who married when they were aged ≥ 25. One plausible explanation is that such young women are more likely to be economically dependent on their older partners, which prevents them from leaving what are often sexually risky and abusive relationships.

Additionally, both men and women in marital relationships should be sensitized about ways to protect themselves against HIV infection. In particular, younger women who experience domestic violence and are afraid to ask their husbands about their previous or current sexual partners and HIV status are more vulnerable to infection (Sa & Larsen, 2007). Also, economic empowerment and microfinancing programs for women in countries like Kenya will go a long way toward making women less dependent on men and more able to make informed choices when faced with circumstances that threaten their sexual and personal health.

This study adds to the body of literature associating IPV and HIV serostatus by critically examining numerous risk factors. Women responding to questions about IPV were categorized as married and formerly married to provide finer distinction on life status and a more nuanced analysis; however, for formerly married women, the sample ($n = 292$) was not sufficient to allow multiple logistic regression analysis. A major innovation of our study was the examination of different components of DV (physical, emotional, sexual, violence with AGBH, and all forms of violence) which could contribute to the literature on IPV. Our study did associate physical violence and HIV serostatus among married women. Because of the high prevalence of HIV (all forms of violence) among formerly married women (28.1%), which could be explained by the fact that their husbands might have died from HIV, prospective studies should be conducted to identify the silent factors of DV that were not captured by the national survey among this vulnerable group. Such study findings can be used to develop interventions targeting formerly married women. This high HIV prevalence for various DVs—physical (30.5%), emotional (27.7%), sexual (20.5%), violence with AGBH (15.4%), and all forms of violence (28.1%)—have never been reported before.

By virtue of their life status, formerly married women who are HIV positive may experience triple jeopardy: the disease, alienation, and stigma. Emotionally, these women need support to achieve better health outcomes. Studies show that women who report IPV also report impaired emotional and social functioning, including depression, helplessness, resignation, and isolation from friends, family, and religious groups (Dietz et al., 1997; Wittenberg et al., 2007). Broad community-based initiatives to deal with the underlying gender norms and social attitudes about HIV/AIDS and DV against women must accompany individually focused initiatives to create a safer and more comfortable environment for women. Given the prevalence of HIV among married and formerly married women experiencing IPV, initiatives that support them toward healthy lifestyles should be encouraged through policies that enable tailored counseling and medication services.

Only an end to violence against women can promote their physical, social, and emotional integrity. Curbing IPV will enable them to make optimal decisions about their life and health, including safeguards against STDs including HIV, so their contributions to society can flourish.

FUNDING

This study was supported by the UNC Center for AIDS Research, an NIH funded program (P30 A150410), Ronald I. Swanstrom, PhD, Principal Investigator.

REFERENCES

Abuya, B. A., Onsomu, E. O., Moore, D., & Piper, C. N. (2012). Association between education and domestic violence among women being offered an HIV test in urban and rural areas in Kenya. *Journal of Interpersonal Violence, 27*, 2022–2038.

Andersson, N., Cockcroft, A., & Shea, B. (2008). Gender-based violence and HIV: Relevance for HIV prevention in hyperendemic countries of southern Africa. *AIDS, 22*(Suppl. 4), S73–86.

Antelman, G., Smith Fawzi, M. C., Kaaya, S., Mbwambo, J., Msamanga, G. I., Hunter, D. J., Fawzi, W. W. (2001). Predictors of HIV-1 serostatus disclosure: A prospective study among HIV-infected pregnant women in Dar es Salaam, Tanzania. *AIDS, 15*, 1865–1874.

Birkett, N. J. (1992). Effect of nondifferential misclassification on estimates of odds ratios with multiple levels of exposure. *American Journal of Epidemiology, 136*, 356–362.

Campbell, J. C., Baty, M. L., Ghandour, R. M., Stockman, J. K., Francisco, L., & Wagman, J. (2008). The intersection of intimate partner violence against women and HIV/AIDS: A review. *International Journal of Injury Control and Safety Promotion, 15*, 221–231.

Central Bureau of Statistics [Kenya], Ministry of Health [Kenya], and ORC Macro. (2004). *Kenya demographic and health survey 2003.* Calverton, MD: Author.

Christofides, N., & Jewkes, R. (2010). Acceptability of universal screening for intimate partner violence in voluntary HIV testing and counseling services in South Africa and service implications. *AIDS Care, 22*, 279–285.

Coovadia, H., Jewkes, R., Barron, P., Sanders, D., & McIntyre, D. (2009). The health and health system of South Africa: Historical roots of current public health challenges. *Lancet, 374*(9692), 817–834.

Decker, M. R., Miller, E., Kapur, N. A., Gupta, J., Raj, A., & Silverman, J. G. (2008). Intimate partner violence and sexually transmitted disease symptoms in a national sample of married Bangladeshi women. *International Journal of Gynaecology and Obstetrics, 100*(1), 18–23.

Decker, M. R., Seage, G. R. III, Hemenway, D., Raj, A., Saggurti, N., Balaiah, D., & Silverman, J. G. (2009). Intimate partner violence functions as both a risk marker and risk factor for women's HIV infection: Findings from Indian husband–wife dyads. *Journal of Acquired Immune Deficiency Syndromes, 51*, 593–600.

Dietz, P. M., Gazmararian, J. A., Goodwin, M. M., Bruce, F. C., Johnson, C. H., & Rochat, R. W. (1997). Delayed entry into prenatal care: Effect of physical violence. *Obstetrics and Gynecology, 90*, 221–224.

Dosemeci, M., Wacholder, S., & Lubin, J. H. (1990). Does nondifferential misclassification of exposure always bias a true effect toward the null value? *American Journal of Epidemiology, 132*, 746–748.

Dude, A. M. (2011). Spousal intimate partner violence is associated with HIV and other STIs among married Rwandan women. *AIDS and Behavior, 15*(1), 142–152.

Dunkle, K. L., Jewkes, R. K., Brown, H. C., Gray, G. E., McIntyre, J. A., & Harlow S. D. (2004). Gender-based violence, relationship power, and risk of HIV infection in women attending antenatal clinics in South Africa. *Lancet, 363*(9419), 1415–1421.

Dunkle, K. L., Jewkes, R. K., Nduna, M., Levin, J., Jama, N., Khuzwayo, N., … Duvvury, N. (2006). Perpetration of partner violence and HIV risk behavior among young men in the rural Eastern Cape, South Africa. *AIDS, 20*, 2107–2114.

Federation of Women Lawyer's Kenya (FIDA). (2011). *Assessment of the implementation of the previous concluding observations on Kenya (CCPR/CO/83/KEN) at the time of the review of the Third Periodic Report.* Nairobi, Kenya: Author.

Fonck, K., Leye, E., Kidula, N., Ndinya-Achola, J., & Temmerman, M. (2005). Increased risk of HIV in women experiencing physical partner violence in Nairobi, Kenya. *AIDS and Behavior, 9,* 335–339.

Gaillard, P., Melis, R., Mwanyumba, F., Claeys, P., Muigai, E., Mandaliya, K., . . . Temmerman, M. (2002). Vulnerability of women in an African setting: Lessons for mother-to-child HIV transmission prevention programmes. *AIDS, 16,* 937–939.

García-Moreno, C., Jansen, H. A., Ellsberg, M., Heise, L, & Watts, C. H. (2006). Prevalence of intimate partner violence: Findings from the WHO multi-country study on women's health and domestic violence. *Lancet, 368*(9543), 1260–1269.

García-Moreno, C., & Watts, C. (2000). Violence against women: Its importance for HIV/AIDS. *AIDS, 14*(Suppl. 3), S253–265.

Gielen, A. C., McDonnell, K. A., & O'Campo, P. J. (2002). Intimate partner violence, HIV status, and sexual risk reduction. *AIDS and Behavior, 6,* 107–116.

Gilbert, L., El-Bassel, N., Schilling, R. F., Wada, T., & Bennet, B. (2000). Partner violence and sexual HIV risk behaviors among women in methadone treatment. *AIDS and Behavior, 4,* 261–269.

Go, V. F., Sethulakshmi, C. J., Bentley, M. E., Sivaram, S., Srikrishnan, A. K., Solomon, S., & Celentano, D. D. (2003). When HIV-prevention messages and gender norms clash: The impact of domestic violence on women's HIV risk in slums of Chennai, India. *AIDS and Behavior, 7,* 263–271.

Goo, L., &. Harlow, S. D. (2012). Intimate partner violence affects skilled attendance at most recent delivery among women in Kenya. *Maternal and Child Health Journal, 16,* 1131–1137.

Gregson, S., Nyamukapa, C. A., Garnett, G. P., Mason, P. R., Zhuwau, T., Carael, M., . . . Anderson, R. M. (2002). Sexual mixing patterns and sex-differentials in teenage exposure to HIV infection in rural Zimbabwe. *Lancet, 359*(9321), 1896–1903.

Harling, G., Msisha, W., & Subramanian, S. V. (2010). No association between HIV and intimate partner violence among women in 10 developing countries. *PLoS ONE, 5*(12), e14257. doi:10.1371/journal.pone.0014257

Izugbara, C. O., & Ngilangwa, D. P. (2010). Women, poverty and adverse maternal outcomes in Nairobi, Kenya. *BioMed Central Womens Health, 10,* 33. doi:10.1186/1472-6874-10-33

Jewkes, R. (2002). Intimate partner violence: Causes and prevention. *Lancet, 359*(9315), 1423–1429.

Jewkes, R., Dunkle, K., Nduna, M., Levin, J., Jama, N., Khuzwayo, N., . . . Duvvury, N. (2006). Factors associated with HIV sero-status in young rural South African women: Connections between intimate partner violence and HIV. *International Journal of Epidemiology, 35,* 1461–1468.

Jewkes, R. K., Dunkle, K., Nduna, M., & Shai, N. (2010). Intimate partner violence, relationship power inequity, and incidence of HIV infection in young women in South Africa: A cohort study. *Lancet, 376*(9734), 41–48.

Jewkes, R. K., Levin, J. B., & Penn-Kekana, L.A. (2003). Gender inequalities, intimate partner violence and HIV preventive practices: Findings of a South African cross-sectional study. *Social Science & Medicine, 56,* 125–134.

Jewkes, R., & Morrell, R. (2010). Gender and sexuality: Emerging perspectives from the heterosexual epidemic in South Africa and implications for HIV risk and prevention. *Journal of the International AIDS Society*, *13*, 6. doi:10.1186/1758-2652-13-6

Karamagi, C. A., Tumwine, J. K., Tylleskar, T., & Heggenhougen, K., (2006). Intimate partner violence against women in eastern Uganda: Implications for HIV prevention. *BMC Public Health*, *6*, 284. doi:10.1186/1471-2458-6-284

Kelly, R. J., Gray, R. H., Sewankambo, N. K., Serwadda, D., Wabwire-Mangen, F., Lutalo, T., & Wawer, M. J. (2003). Age differences in sexual partners and risk of HIV-1 infection in rural Uganda. *Journal of the Acquired Immune Deficiency Syndrome*, *32*, 446–451.

Kenya Law Reports and the Government of Kenya. (2009). *The Sexual Offences Act (Number 3 of 2006)*. Nairobi, Kenya: The National Council for Law Reporting with the Authority of the Attorney General. Retrieved from http://www.kenyalaw.org/family/statutes/download.php?file=Sexual%20Offences%20Act.pdf

Kenya National Bureau of Statistics (KNBS) & ICF Macro. 2010. *Kenya demographic and health survey 2008–09*. Calverton, MD: Author.

Kiarie, J. N., Farquhar, C., Richardson, B. A., Kabura, M. N., John, F. N., Nduati, R. W., & John-Stewart, G. C. (2006). Domestic violence and prevention of mother-to-child transmission of HIV-1. *AIDS*, *20*, 1763–1769.

Kimuna, S. R., &. Djamba, Y. K. (2008). Gender based violence: Correlates of physical and sexual wife abuse in Kenya. *Journal of Family Violence*, *23*, 333–342.

Kishor, S., & Johnson, K. (2004). *Profiling domestic violence—A multi-country study*. Calverton, MD: ORC Macro.

Koenig, M. A., Lutalo, T., Zhao, F., Nalugoda, F., Wabwire-Mangen, F., Kiwanuka, N., ... Gray, R. (2003). Intimate partner violence in rural Uganda: Evidence from a community-based study. *Bulletin of World Health Organization*, *81*(1), 53–60.

Lary, H., Maman, S., Katebalila, M., McCauley, A., & Mbwambo, J. (2004). Exploring the association between HIV and violence: Young people's experiences with infidelity, violence and forced sex in Dar es Salaam, Tanzania. *International Family Planning Perspectives*, *30*, 200–206.

Lasee, A., & Becker, S. (1997). Husband-wife communication about family planning and contraceptive use in Kenya. *International Family Planning Perspectives*, *23*, 15–20.

Lawoko, S. (2008). Predictors of attitudes toward intimate partner violence: A comparative study of men in Zambia and Kenya. *Journal of Interpersonal Violence*, *23*, 1056–1074.

Longfield, K., Glick, A., Waithaka, M., & Berman, J. (2004). Relationships between older men and younger women: Implications for STIs/HIV in Kenya. *Studies in Family Planning*, *35*, 125–134.

Luke, N. (2003). Age and economic asymmetries in the sexual relationships of adolescent girls in sub-Saharan Africa. *Studies in Family Planning*, *34*, 67–86.

Malhotra, A., Schuler, S. R., & Boender, C. (2002). *Measuring women's empowerment as a variable in international development*. Washington, DC: World Bank, Gender and Development Group.

Maman, S., Mbwambo, J. K., Hogan, N. M., Kilonzo, G. P., Campbell, J. C., Weiss, E., & Sweat, M. D. (2002). HIV-positive women report more lifetime partner violence: Findings from a voluntary counseling and testing clinic in Dar es Salaam, Tanzania. *American Journal of Public Health, 92,* 1331–1337.

Martin, S. L., & Curtis, S. (2004). Gender-based violence and HIV/AIDS: Recognizing links and acting on evidence. *Lancet, 363*(9419), 1410–1411.

Martin, S. L., Kilgallen, B., Tsui, A. O., Maitra, K., Singh, K. K., & Kupper, L. L. (1999). Sexual behaviors and reproductive health outcomes: Associations with wife abuse in India. *Journal of the American Medical Association, 282,* 1967–1972.

Medley, A., García-Moreno, C., McGill, S., & Maman, S. (2004). Rates, barriers and outcomes of HIV serostatus disclosure among women in developing countries: Implications for prevention of mother-to-child transmission programmes. *Bulletin of the World Health Organization, 82,* 299–307.

Onsomu, E. O., Kimani, J. K., Abuya, B. A., Arif, A. A., Moore, D., Duren-Winfield, V., & Harwell, G. (2013). Delaying sexual debut as a strategy for reducing HIV epidemic in Kenya. *African Journal of Reproductive Health, 17*(2), 46–57.

Sa, Z., & Larsen, U. (2007). Gender inequality increases women's risk of HIV infection in Moshi, Tanzania. *Journal of Biosocial Science, 40,* 505–525.

Shi, C.-F., Kouyoumdjian, F. G., & Dushoff, J. (2013). Intimate partner violence is associated with HIV infection in women in Kenya: A cross-sectional analysis. *BMC Public Health, 13,* 512. doi:10.1186/1471-2458-13-512

Silverman, J. G., Decker, M. R., Saggurti, N., Balaiah, D., & Raj, A. (2008). Intimate partner violence and HIV infection among married Indian women. *Journal of the American Medical Association, 300,* 703–710.

StataCorp. (2013). *Stata statistical software: Release 13.* College Station, TX: Author.

UCLA Institute for Digital Research and Education. (n.d.). *Stata annotated output: Factor analysis.* Retrieved from http://www.ats.ucla.edu/stat/stata/output/fa_output.htm

UNAIDS. (2009). *Joint action for results: UNAIDS outcome framework, 2009–2011.* UN document UNAIDS/09.13E/JC1713E. Retrieved from http://www.unaids.org/en/media/unaids/contentassets/dataimport/pub/basedocument/2010/jc1713_joint_action_en.pdf

UNAIDS. (2012). *Regional fact sheet 2012: Sub-Saharan Africa.* Retrieved from http://www.unaids.org/en/media/unaids/contentassets/documents/epidemiology/2012/gr2012/2012_FS_regional_ssa_en.pdf

van der Straten, A., King, R., Grinstead, O., Vittinghoff, E., Serufilira, A., & Allen, S. (1998). Sexual coercion, physical violence, and HIV infection among women in steady relationships in Kigali, Rwanda. *AIDS and Behavior, 2*(1), 61–73.

Wang, S. H., & Rowley, W. (2007). *Rape: How women, the community and the health sector respond.* Geneva, Switzerland: Sexual Violence Research Initiative and World Health Organization. Retrieved from http://www.svri.org/rape.pdf

Wanyoni, M., & Lumumba, V. (2010). *Gender-based violence. Kenya demographic and health survey 2008–09.* Calverton, MD: KNBS and ICF Macro.

Wawer, M. J., Makumbi, F., Kigozi, G., Serwadda, D., Watya, S., Nalugoda, F., . . . Gray, R. H. (2009). Circumcision in HIV-infected men and its effect on HIV transmission to female partners in Rakai, Uganda: A randomised controlled trial. *Lancet, 374*(9685), 229–237.

Wingood, G. M., & DiClemente, R. J. (1998). Rape among African American women: Sexual, psychological, and social correlates predisposing survivors to risk of STD/HIV. *Journal of Women's Health*, 7(1), 77–84.

Wittenberg, E., Joshi, M., Thomas, K. A., & McCloskey, L. A. (2007). Measuring the effect of intimate partner violence on health-related quality of life: A qualitative focus group study. *Health and Quality of Life Outcomes*, 5, 67. doi:10.1186/1477-7525-5-67

World Health Organization (WHO). (1997). *Violence against women: A priority health issue*. WHO/FRH/WHD/97.8. Geneva, Switzerland: Author.

World Health Organization (WHO). (2004). *Violence against women and HIV/AIDS: Critical intersections (Intimate Partner Violence and HIV/AIDS)*. Geneva, Switzerland: Author.

World Health Organization (WHO). (2005). *Multi-country study on women's health and intimate partner violence against women: Summary report of initial results on prevalence, health outcomes and women's responses*. Geneva, Switzerland: Author.

Zablotska, I. B., Gray R. H., Koenig, M. A., Serwadda, D., Nalugoda, F., Kigozi, G., . . . Wawer, M. (2009). Alcohol use, intimate partner violence, sexual coercion and HIV among women aged 15–24 in Rakai, Uganda. *AIDS and Behavior*, *13*, 225–233.

Risk for Family Rejection and Associated Mental Health Outcomes Among Conflict-Affected Adult Women Living in Rural Eastern Democratic Republic of the Congo

ANJALEE KOHLI

Johns Hopkins University School of Nursing, Baltimore, Maryland, USA

NANCY A. PERRIN

Center for Health Research, Portland, Oregon, USA

REMY MITIMA MPANANO

Programme d'Appui aux Initiatives Economiques (PAIDEK), Bukavu, Democratic Republic of the Congo

LUKE C. MULLANY

Johns Hopkins Bloomberg School of Public Health, Baltimore, Maryland, USA

CLOVIS MITIMA MURHULA, ARSÈNE KAJABIKA BINKURHORHWA, ALFRED BACIKENGI MIRINDI, JEAN HERI BANYWESIZE, NADINE MWINJA BUFOLE, and ERIC MPANANO NTWALI

Pigs for Peace, Bukavu, Democratic Republic of the Congo

NANCY GLASS

Johns Hopkins University School of Nursing; and Johns Hopkins Center for Global Health, Baltimore, Maryland, USA

Stigma due to sexual violence includes family rejection, a complex outcome including economic, behavioral, and physical components. We explored the relationship among conflict-related trauma, family rejection, and mental health in adult women living in rural eastern Democratic Republic of the Congo, who participate in a livestock-based microfinance program, Pigs for Peace. Exposure to multiple and different types of conflict-related trauma, including sexual assault, was associated with increased likelihood of family rejection, which in turn was associated with poorer mental health outcomes. Design of appropriate and effective interventions will require understanding family relationships and exposure to different types of trauma in postconflict environments.

The authors focus on the health of women who have experienced on-going conflict, violence against women, and limited access to social services including health care and economic opportunity. We apply concepts of stigma to better the understanding of factors that influence mental health outcomes amongst women who have experienced trauma. In Africa and worldwide, conflict and violence are a key concern. A better understanding of how outcomes due to war-related violence influence health is essential to improve interventions in these settings. To learn more about these issues, we conducted a study in the Democratic Republic of Congo (DRC).

Since 1996, civilian populations living in eastern DRC have endured ongoing war and violence resulting in disruption of economic opportunities and destruction of basic health and social services (Alberti et al., 2010; Coghlan et al., 2007; Réseau des Femmes pour un Développement Associatif, Réseau des Femmes pour la Défense des Droits et la Paix, & International Alert, 2005). Women living in North and South Kivu provinces and Ituri District reported high exposure to physical (17.2%), movement (7.8%), and property (23.6%) rights violations including sexual violence (39.7%) between 1994 and 2010 (Johnson et al., 2010). These findings are consistent with other studies where researchers attempted to quantify conflict and nonconflict-related sexual violence in eastern DRC (Steiner et al., 2009; Wakabi, 2008). Several scholars have documented that exposure to war-related violence including surviving rape or sexual assault, lacking basic necessities (e.g., food, water), lacking medical care when ill, and being in a combat situation are risk factors for mental illness (Betancourt, Brennan, Rubin-Smith, Fitzmaurice, & Gilman, 2010; Kubiak, 2005; Miller et al., 2002; Roberts, Damundu, Lomoro, & Sondorp, 2010; Roberts, Ocaka, Browne, Oyok, & Sondorp, 2008).

Individual-level consequences of sexual violence include poor health, stigma, rejection, and fear of rejection. Women survivors of sexual violence accessing health services at Panzi Hospital (in Bukavu) or one of two rural nongovernmental organizations (NGOs) in eastern DRC reported abandonment by their husband (29%) and communities (6%) after the assault (Kelly, Betancourt, Mukwege, Lipton, & Vanrooyen, 2011). Similar estimates of rejection have been reported in studies with participants in NGO programs (Steiner et al., 2009) and with community members (Vinck, Pham, Baldo, & Shigekane, 2008). Such stigma and rejection arises from family and community beliefs that women were voluntary participants in the assault; the trauma and humiliation associated with public, witnessed rape; cultural beliefs that sex, whether or not voluntary, means that a woman is married to her partner/aggressor; fear of return of the aggressor; family and community pressure to reject survivors; cultural beliefs that women should represent purity; and pregnancy due to rape (Harvard Humanitarian Initiative, 2009; Kohli et al., 2012; Réseau des Femmes pour un Développement Associatif et al., 2005; Sideris, 2003).

Female survivors of sexual assault and their male partners living in Walungu Territory, South Kivu province, described family rejection as complex and multifaceted, including, for example, forced removal from the family home, loss or limited financial support by family, children of the survivor (even those not born from rape) being rejected by the family, lack of communication and affection, limited assistance or involvement in household activities, reduced or absence of sexual activity, and loss of property (Kohli et al., 2012). Community members described difficulties that all villagers faced due to their exposure to different types of conflict-related trauma, and they expressed a need to understand and address the multiple risk factors and consequences of those varied exposures on both family relationships and individual outcomes.

Theoretical Consideration on Violence and Stigma

A brief introduction into moral stigma may provide an understanding of how family rejection is related to exposure to multiple types of trauma and mental health outcomes. Stigma is a process involving the use of labels and stereotypes, separation of individuals from a group, and discrimination against labeled individuals. Stigma and the associated outcomes result from an interaction between individual behavior and characteristics and social and cultural norms, morals, and beliefs (Link & Phelan, 2001). Yang and colleagues (Yang & Kleinman, 2008; Yang et al., 2007, p. 1528) propose a cultural understanding of stigma, where stigma is "embedded in the moral life of sufferers." In this context, moral is defined as that which is most important in the daily life and interaction of ordinary people. Thus, communities employ stigma as a means of protecting the larger group and preserving social and cultural norms, meanings, and values (Kleinman & Hall-Clifford, 2009; Yang et al., 2007).

Corrigan and Miller (2004) explain that family members may be stigmatized because of their choice to continue to interact with the marginalized individual. This places great social pressure on families to reject stigmatized persons, even if the individual members express a desire to practice acceptance. In the DRC, male partners of survivors of sexual assault have described the difficulty they face in accepting their wife/female partner for reasons that include the family and peer pressure they face to remarry a woman who has not been raped (Kohli et al., 2012). In the DRC, people develop and define their identity as a part of a larger social whole, favoring the well-being of the group over individual needs (Menkiti, 1984). Experiences of family rejection in the DRC may fall within the realm of moral stigma whereby individuals grow and live in a family and social unit, and threats to the moral character of society and family are considered dangerous to the character and cohesion of the group. As a result, decisions to reject family members may be related to experiences where individuals are held responsible or blamed for their trauma; for example, sexual violence. There may be other conflict-related traumatic exposures that similarly result in a stigmatizing experience within the family and community leading to negative health outcomes.

Research Aims

In response to community requests to understand the relationship between traumatic experiences and stigma within family relationships, we explored the relationship among conflict-related trauma, family relationships, and mental health amongst female participants in the baseline data collection of an impact evaluation of a Congolese-led livestock microfinance program, Pigs for Peace (PFP). PFP is a collaborative project between Programme d'Appui aux Initiatives Economiques, a Congolese microfinance organization, and the Johns Hopkins University School of Nursing (Glass, Ramazani, Tosha, Mpanano, & Cinyabuguma, 2012) that was designed to address the social, health, and economic effects of conflict and poverty on families and communities. Members of PFP receive a loan in the form of a 2- to 4-month-old female pig. The PFP model uses pigs as a loan because animals are an important source of economic well-being in these rural villages and there are no cultural taboos or gender-based responsibilities for raising or selling pigs. Each member cares for his or her pig with support from trained Congolese PFP Research and Microfinance agents. When the pig gives birth, members repay their pig loan in the form of two female piglets, which are then used to provide new pig loans in the same village. Consistent with prior research on family relationships, we hypothesized that (a) family rejection would be associated with a past experience of conflict-related traumas; and (b) an experience of family rejection would more strongly predict poorer mental health outcomes than experiences of conflict-related trauma including sexual assault. Last, the relationship between specific circumstances of sexual assault and family rejection is examined.

METHODS

Study Design

In 2011, a National Institutes of Health/National Institute of Minority Health and Health Disparities-funded randomized community trial was initiated to evaluate the effectiveness of PFP on health, economic, and community-level outcomes. Ten rural villages of Walungu Territory, South Kivu Province, were selected for participation in PFP based on the following: (a) feasibility of delivering an intervention over a wide geographic area; (b) commitment to the intervention and study by traditional chiefs and administrators; and (c) findings from village-level assessments.

Study Sample

Adults, aged 16 years and older, were eligible for the study if they expressed a commitment to and understanding of microfinance principles (e.g., repayment of loans), were permanent residents of the village, and were responsible individuals in the household (e.g., married 16 year old, 16 year old responsible for younger siblings because of death of parent). Participation was limited to one member (male or female) of a household. Following a participatory village meeting, eligible and interested community members attended a second meeting where each individual was randomly assigned, through a village lottery, to intervention and delayed control group.

Data Collection

Baseline data collection took place after randomization but prior to initiation of the intervention. Translation and back translation of the questionnaire from English to French was conducted as well as translation to local languages—Swahili and Mashi. The questionnaire was pilot tested before finalizing it and use of the tablet for interviews. To address logistical challenges of conducting research (e.g., limited infrastructure), trained interviewers (male and female) collected baseline data in two phases of five villages each: between May and June 2012 and August and September 2012. A few participants were not available (e.g., participant hospitalized) during the baseline data collection period; therefore, the final baseline interview was completed in November 2012.

The Institutional Review Board (IRB) of the Johns Hopkins Medical Institute approved this study. As there is no local IRB in South Kivu province, a committee of respected Congolese educators at the Universite Catholique at Bukavu reviewed and approved this study, including risks and benefits to participants. Pilot and study interviews were initiated only after receiving oral, voluntary, and informed consent. All data recorded through the tablet-based program were backed-up and uploaded to a password-protected server managed by the study team. Participant names were centrally removed from the dataset and stored in a separate file. As interviews were conducted during the day when members would be earning their daily income, compensation (~U.S.$1.50) for the time (~90 minutes) spent away from work was provided. All interviews took place in a private setting of the respondent's choice, most often their home.

Study Questionnaire

Participants reported their current age category (e.g., 15–19 years, 20–24 years). Age was included in the model as a continuous variable with values between 0 and 4 where the reference group was 15–19 years and persons over 60 years were coded as four.

Exposure to trauma. Participants were asked about their exposure to 18 different conflict-related traumatic events over the past 10 years, a time period when rural villagers experienced conflict-related violence using an adapted version of the Harvard Trauma Questionnaire (HTQ; Mollica, McDonald, Massagli, & Silove, 2004). Exposure to conflict-related trauma was examined in two ways: as a single continuous variable (experience of 1–18 different events) and as multiple binary variables indicating exposure to one or more events within categories of traumatic events. These categories were defined through a slight adaptation of those proposed by Mollica and colleagues (Mollica, Henderson, & Tor, 2002) and include the following: (a) material deprivation (three events: lack of food or water, lack of shelter, and ill health without access to medical care); (b) warlike conditions (one event: combat situation); (c) bodily injury (four events: torture or witnessed torture, serious injury, rape or sexual assault, other type of sexual humiliation); (d) coercion (six events: imprisonment, brainwashing, lost or kidnapped, being close to death, forced isolation, forced separation from family members); and (e) violence to others (four events: unnatural death of family member or friend, murder of family member or friend, murder of stranger, witness rape or sexual abuse).

Sexual assault. Female participants who reported any type of sexual assault or kidnapping in the past 10 years were asked when they were assaulted. As not all would have been raped (e.g., sexual humiliation, verbal abuse), only those reporting rape were asked a series of follow-up questions about the assault(s).

Family rejection. Questions on family rejection were developed through qualitative work with survivors of sexual violence (Kohli et al., 2012). Participants reported whether they ever experienced rejection (financial, emotional, or physical) by family members (spouse/male partner, parents, or in-laws). In the first iteration of the family rejection section (i.e., surveys implemented between May and June 2012), all those participants reporting sexual assault provided information on their experience of family rejection. In July 2012, this module on family rejection was revised and expanded to include all participants (i.e., not limited to those reporting sexual assault only). This revision was done in response to participants noting that trauma-related factors, other than sexual assault, can be linked to family rejection.

Mental health. A 16-item version of the HTQ was used to understand the frequency of experiencing post-traumatic stress symptoms in the prior week (Mollica et al. 2004). The 15-item Hopkins Symptom Checklist (HSCL) was used to understand the frequency of experiencing depression-related symptoms in the prior 4 weeks (Mollica et al., 2004). Both the HSCL and HTQ have been validated for use in other conflict settings and in East Africa (Bass, Ryder, Lammers, Mukaba, & Bolton, 2008; Roberts et al., 2008; Sabin, Lopes Cardozo, Nackerud, Kaiser, & Varese, 2003). An average individual symptom score was calculated for post-traumatic stress disorder (PTSD) and depression where the symptom frequency "not at all" was scored as 1 and "extremely" as 4. Where individual-level missing data on the frequency of experiencing symptoms were small for a syndrome (<25% missing data for total symptoms), the individual's average symptom score was the average of the available items. Individuals who were missing data for >25% of items within a scale were not included in the analysis.

Data Analysis

Female participants in the baseline interview who responded to questions on family rejection and had experienced at least one traumatic event in the past 10 years were included in this analysis. To test our first hypothesis that family rejection would be associated with a past experience of more violent conflict-related traumas, we used bivariate logistic regression. Each category of trauma was tested as a predictor of ever being rejected by family. Multiple linear regression was used to test the second hypothesis that experience of family rejection would more strongly predict poorer mental health outcomes than experiences of conflict-related trauma including sexual assault. For each dependent variable (PTSD, depression), we estimated seven multivariable linear regression models to test the relative importance of exposure to the different trauma categories and family rejection in predicting mental health. Each model included a different trauma category (e.g., number of different trauma exposures, material deprivation, bodily injury, rape, or sexual assault). Age was included as a covariate in all multiple linear regression models. Within this sample size, we were able to detect with 80% power small to moderate associations in the analysis for both hypotheses. In exploratory analyses amongst the subset of women who reported ever experiencing rape ($N = 51$), we used Pearson's chi-square test to examine bivariate relationships between specific experiences of assault and family rejection. All statistical analyses were formed using STATA version 11.2 (Stata Corporation, College Park, Texas, USA).

RESULTS

This analysis includes 315 women in 10 villages who experienced at least one conflict-related traumatic event and provided information on family

TABLE 1 Descriptive Statistics of Female Participants in Pigs for Peace Who Experienced at Least One Conflict-Related Trauma in the Past 10 Years

Item	Frequency	Percent
Village (N = 315)		
Karhagala	33	10.48
Kamisimbi	46	14.60
Cagombe	2	0.63
Cahi	55	17.46
Lurhala	4	1.27
Kahembari	52	16.51
Irhaga	76	24.13
Karherwa	6	1.90
Cize	12	3.81
Izege	29	9.21
Current age group (N = 315)		
16–19 years	6	1.90
20–24 years	46	14.60
25–34 years	89	28.25
35–44 years	71	22.54
45–60 years	93	29.52
> 60 years	10	3.17
Current marital status (N = 314)		
Married	218	69.43
Widowed	72	22.93
Separated/divorced/abandoned	19	6.05
Never married	5	1.59
Symptoms of PTSD (N = 308)*		
Mean score (95% confidence interval)	2.22 (2.14, 2.30)	
Standard deviation of mean score	0.71	
Possible range of average symptom score	(1–4)	
Symptoms of depression (N = 314)*		
Mean score (95% confidence interval)	1.85 (1.80, 1.91)	
Standard deviation of mean score	0.50	
Possible range of average symptom score	(1–4)	

*PTSD and Depression were scored according to the standards laid out in the instrument. 16 different symptoms were used to understand symptoms of PTSD and 15 symptoms for depression.

rejection. Owing to the previously described revisions to the family rejection section, the majority of participants (262) were from Phase II villages. Most participants were married (69.43%) and between 45 and 60 years (29.52%; Table 1). Average PTSD and depression scores were available for a total of 308 (97.78%) and 314 (99.68%) females, respectively, out of the 315 total women included in this analysis. The average post-traumatic stress symptom score was 2.22 (95% CI = 2.14, 2.30) and the mean depression score was 1.85 (95% CI = 1.80, 1.91).

The average number of different traumatic experiences was 4.64 (95% CI = 4.15, 5.14) (Table 2). In the past 10 years, respondents reported experiencing material deprivation (87.94%), warlike conditions (52.70%), and rape or sexual assault (15.56%). Of the 315 women who experienced at least one conflict-related trauma, 60 (19.05%) reported being rejected by at least

TABLE 2 Frequency of Experiencing Individual and Grouped Traumatic Events Amongst Female Participants Who Experienced at Least One Conflict-Related Traumatic Event (N = 315)

Item	Frequency	Percent
Average number of traumatic events (range: 1–18)	4.64 (4.15, 5.14)	
Material deprivation trauma	277	87.94
Ill health without access to medical care	224	71.11
Lack of food or water	212	67.30
Lack of shelter	78	24.76
Warlike condition (combat trauma)	166	52.70
Coercion	149	47.30
Forced separation from family members	99	31.43
Being close to death	76	24.13
Brainwashing	55	17.46
Forced isolation	47	14.92
Lost or kidnapped	38	12.06
Imprisonment	34	10.79
Violence to others	111	35.24
Unnatural death of family or friend	81	25.71
Murder of family or friend	70	22.22
Witness rape or sexual abuse	47	14.92
Murder of stranger	25	7.94
Bodily injury	105	33.33
Serious injury	69	21.90
Tortured or witnessed torture	61	19.37
Rape or sexual assault	49	15.56
Other types of sexual humiliation	32	10.16

one family member (husband/male partner, parents, in-laws; see Table 3). Women who experienced more types of traumatic events (OR = 1.09; 95% CI = 1.03, 1.15), violence to others (OR = 1.97; 95% CI = 1.12, 3.49), coercion (OR = 2.24; 95% CI = 1.25, 4.00), and bodily injury trauma (OR = 2.61; 95% CI = 1.47, 4.64) were significantly more likely to be rejected by family members in bivariate logistic regression (Table 4).

Association of Trauma and Family Rejection With Mental Health

In all seven multivariate linear regression models between trauma, family rejection, and PTSD, family rejection was significantly associated with

TABLE 3 Frequency of Family Rejection Amongst Women That Reported Experience of at Least One Conflict-Related Trauma (N = 315)

Item	Frequency	Percent
Ever experienced family rejection (husband, parents, in-laws)	60	19.05
Ever rejected by husband/male partner	44	13.97
Ever rejected by parents and/or in-laws	27	8.57

TABLE 4 Bivariate Logistic Regression Between Experience of at Least One Traumatic Event in the Past 10 Years and Family Rejection ($N = 315$)

Item	Ever experienced family rejection		
	No. (%) who never experienced family rejection*	Odds Ratio	95% Confidence interval
Number of different traumatic events (1–18 events)		1.09	1.03, 1.15
Material deprivation trauma	54 (19.49%)	1.29	0.51, 3.24
Warlike conditions trauma	35 (21.08%)	1.33	0.75, 2.34
Violence to others trauma	29 (26.13%)	1.97	1.12, 3.49
Coercion trauma	38 (25.50%)	2.24	1.25, 4.00
Bodily injury trauma	31 (29.52%)	2.61	1.47, 4.64

*Comparison of number and percent of participants rejected by family who experienced specific traumatic events compared with those who did not experience the traumatic event.

post-traumatic stress symptoms (Table 5). Material deprivation was not significantly related to PTSD symptoms. Experience of rape or sexual assault in the past 10 years was more strongly related to increased symptoms of PTSD than family rejection (as evidenced by the standardized β). Family rejection was significantly related to having symptoms of depression in all seven multiple linear regression models (Table 6). Family rejection showed a stronger association with depression-related symptoms than the experience of increased number of different traumatic events, coercion, violence to others, and rape/sexual assault. Neither the experience of material deprivation nor warlike conditions were significantly related to symptoms of depression.

Experience of Sexual Assault

Fifty-one women in the 10 villages reported rape (Table 7). Amongst this subset, 16 (31.37%) reported ever experiencing family rejection, consistent with previous studies in eastern DRC, with most reporting rejection by their husband. About one-third of women reported that member(s) of an armed combatant group sexually assaulted them more than once. The most recent sexual assault was frequently witnessed by others (52.94%), involved more than one perpetrator (60.88%), and took place in the forest (45.10%) or the woman's home (43.14%). Bivariate analysis showed that repeated rape, witness of rape by others, having multiple perpetrators (i.e., gang rape), or having a child due to sexual assault were significantly associated with family rejection (Table 8).

TABLE 5 Multivariate Linear Regression of Severity of PTSD Symptoms, Experience of at Least One Traumatic Event and Family Rejection ($N = 308$)

Model	B	Standard error	β	p value	Adjusted R^2
Model 1					
No. of different traumatic events (1–18 events)	0.07	0.01	0.43	.000	
Family rejection	0.39	0.09	0.22	.000	0.276
Age in years	0.09	0.03	0.15	.003	
Model 2					
Material deprivation trauma	0.14	0.12	0.06	.243	
Family rejection	0.51	0.10	0.28	.000	0.101
Age in years	0.09	0.03	0.15	.005	
Model 3					
Warlike conditions	0.30	0.08	0.21	.000	
Family rejection	0.49	0.10	0.27	.000	0.141
Age in years	0.09	0.03	0.15	.005	
Model 4					
Coercion	0.45	0.07	0.31	.000	
Family rejection	0.43	0.09	0.24	.000	0.194
Age in years	0.08	0.03	0.14	.008	
Model 5					
Violence to others	0.46	0.08	0.31	.000	
Family rejection	0.44	0.09	0.25	.000	0.193
Age in years	0.09	0.03	0.15	.004	
Model 6					
Bodily injury	0.63	0.07	0.42	.000	
Family rejection	0.37	0.09	0.21	.000	0.269
Age in years	0.09	0.03	0.14	.004	
Model 7					
Rape or sexual assault	0.72	0.10	0.35	.000	
Family rejection	0.43	0.09	0.23	.000	0.228
Age in years	0.10	0.03	0.17	.000	

DISCUSSION

This cross-sectional analysis of trauma-related predictors and mental health outcomes of experience of family rejection amongst conflict-affected adult women living in rural eastern DRC provides evidence of the importance of family relationships to mental health. Female participants reported high exposure to traumatic events. Almost one in five women reported an experience of family rejection (19.05%). While qualitative studies and this data point to the importance of sexual assault in family rejection (Kelly et al., 2011; Kohli et al., 2012; Steiner et al., 2009), community members in Walungu Territory presented the importance of all types of trauma experiences to changes in family and community relationships. We quantified the importance of trauma exposures, by category, to family rejection and found that exposure to more events, violence to others, coercion and bodily trauma were significantly associated with family rejection.

TABLE 6 Multivariate Linear Regression of Severity of Depression Symptoms, Experience of at Least One Traumatic Event and Family Rejection ($N = 308$)

Model	B	Standard error	β	p value	Adjusted R^2
Model 1					
No. of different traumatic events (1–18 events)	0.02	0.01	0.22	.000	
Family rejection	0.44	0.07	0.34	.000	0.214
Age in years	0.07	0.02	0.17	.001	
Model 2					
Material deprivation trauma	0.09	0.08	0.06	.254	
Family rejection	0.49	0.07	0.38	.000	0.171
Age in years	0.07	0.02	0.17	.001	
Model 3					
Warlike conditions	0.06	0.05	0.06	.226	
Family rejection	0.48	0.07	0.37	.000	0.171
Age in years	0.08	0.02	0.17	.001	
Model 4					
Coercion	0.12	0.05	0.12	.021	
Family rejection	0.46	0.07	0.36	.000	0.182
Age in years	0.07	0.02	0.17	.001	
Model 5					
Violence to others	0.14	0.05	0.14	.009	
Family rejection	0.47	0.07	0.36	.000	0.186
Age in years	0.07	0.02	0.17	.001	
Model 6					
Bodily injury	0.34	0.05	0.32	.000	
Family rejection	0.41	0.06	0.32	.000	0.266
Age in years	0.07	0.02	0.16	.001	
Model 7					
Rape or sexual assault	0.41	0.07	0.29	.000	
Family rejection	0.46	0.02	0.34	.000	0.256
Age in years	0.08	0.06	0.18	.000	

A focused analysis of sexual assault and family rejection provided detailed information on factors associated with the assault that could result in family rejection. For example, women reporting that there were people, other than the perpetrators, who witnessed the assault (e.g., family, friends) or more than one perpetrator were more likely to have an experience of family rejection. Women who were raped multiple times by armed groups and who became pregnant as a result of the assault were also more likely to report family rejection. These situational risk factors for family rejection of survivors of sexual assault are supported by qualitative research (Kelly et al., 2011; Kohli et al., 2012; Réseau des Femmes pour un Développement Associatif et al., 2005). In the framework of moral stigma, it is not surprising that the more public experiences of rape (e.g., witnessed assault, gang rape, multiple rapes) were associated with rejection. These types of rape experiences are difficult to hide from other family members and the larger community. With each of the categories of trauma (e.g., warlike conditions, coercion, violence

TABLE 7 Descriptive Statistics of Female Participants Who Reported Having Ever Been Sexually Assaulted

Item	Frequency	Percent
Number of women reporting sexually assault, ever ($N = 701$)	51	7.27
Report being rejected by any family member ($N = 51$)	16	31.37
Report being rejected by husband ($N = 33$)	13	39.39
Report being rejected by parents ($N = 36$)	4	11.11
Report being rejected by in-laws ($N = 29$)	6	20.69
Report being rejected by children ($N = 47$)	1	2.13
Number of times assaulted sexually		
One time	34	66.67
Two times	5	9.80
Three times	8	15.69
Four or more times	4	7.84
Most recent sexual assault was witnessed ($N = 51$)	27	52.94
Witnessed by husband	4	7.84
Witnessed by parents	2	3.92
Witnessed by children	9	17.65
Witnessed by other family members	9	17.65
Witnessed by friends	7	13.73
Ever abducted by perpetrators of sexual assault ($N = 51$)	43	84.31
Number of different perpetrators in most recent sexual assault		
One person	20	39.22
Two people	7	13.73
Three people	11	21.57
Four people	5	9.80
Five people	5	9.80
Six or more people	3	5.88
Place of most recent sexual assault		
Forest	23	45.10
Home	22	43.14
Other (in field, on route, market, etc.)	6	11.76
Family possessions were taken during most recent sexual assault ($N = 51$)	38	74.51
Animals were taken	27	52.94
Money was taken	15	29.41
Business materials	13	25.49
House	1	1.96
Agricultural products	13	25.49
Other	17	33.33
Had a child from sexual assault ($N = 51$)	12	23.53
Sought medical care after most recent sexual assault ($N = 51$)	33	64.71
3 days or less	11	33.33
4–7 days after assault	5	15.15
More than 1 week, but less than 6 months after assault	12	36.36
Between 6 months to 1 year after assault	3	9.09
One year or more after the assault	2	6.06

to others, bodily injury), there is the possibility to blame the survivor for her experience and to interpret it as a threat to the moral attitudes that guide social interaction and family relationships. Family rejection, related to any type of trauma exposure, may be an act to preserve sociocultural morals and

TABLE 8 Experience of Ever Being Rejected by a Family Member Amongst Women Who Were Sexually Assaulted

Item	No. and percent ever rejected by a family member ($N = 51$)	Chi square	p value
Number of times raped			
Once	8 (23.53%)	4.41	.036
More than once	9 (52.94%)		
Most recent sexual assault was witnessed			
Yes	15 (55.56%)	12.75	<.0001
No	2 (8.33%)		
Ever abducted by perpetrators of sexual assault			
Yes	14 (32.56%)	0.07	.785
No	3 (37.50%)		
Number of perpetrators in most recent sexual assault			
One	2 (10.0%)	8.06	.005
More than one	15 (48.39%)		
Location of most recent sexual assault			
Home	10 (43.48%)	1.94	.164
Away from home (e.g., forest, field, market, etc.)	7 (25%)		
Possessions were stolen during most recent sexual assault			
Yes	13 (34.21%)	0.05	.820
No	4 (30.77%)		
Had a child as a result of sexual assault			
Yes	8 (66.67%)	7.85	.005
No	9 (23.08%)		
Sought medical care after most recent sexual assault			
Yes	12 (36.36%)	0.39	.534
No	5 (27.78%)		

protect the family and community, albeit at the expense of certain vulnerable individuals.

The association between family rejection and increased symptoms of depression and PTSD regardless of the trauma exposure is consistent with other research on the importance of social conditions in producing individual outcomes apart from, or in addition to, exposure to conflict-related trauma (Amone-P'olak et al., 2013; Miller, Omidian, Rasmussen, Yaqubi, & Daudzai, 2008; Miller & Rasmussen, 2010; Sideris, 2003). Women who have experienced violence in war have referred to the social impact of the violence as overwhelming and debilitating, affecting their access to resources and support (Mukamana & Brysiewicz, 2008; Sideris, 2003). While individual trauma experiences, including sexual assault/rape, were generally more strongly related to PTSD, family rejection consistently predicted symptoms of depression. In a study focused on the mental health effects of political violence in Nepal, Kohrt similarly reports that conflict-related violence predicted PTSD, but social factors, such as socioeconomic factors, more strongly predicted depression (Kohrt & Hruschka, 2010; Kohrt et al., 2012). Material deprivation was not significantly associated with family rejection or increased symptoms of PTSD or depression. Because material deprivation was widespread in families and the larger community, it may not be associated with an assumption of culpability, and individuals may not experience the stigma and mental health outcomes associated with other types of trauma.

Results from this study demonstrate the importance of relationships to mental health outcomes in eastern DRC, and likely other conflict-affected countries (Farhood, 2004; Igreja, Kleijn, & Richters, 2006). Individual experiences of different categories of trauma (conflict and nonconflict related) remain important. Their long-term significance may be understood, in part, however, through how the trauma affects social relationships. Broadening the lens of interventions from addressing individual needs to include family and community relationships may present an opportunity to address the multilevel outcomes of conflict in an appropriate and culturally acceptable manner. Partnering with local organizations to understand, design, and adapt interventions for rural communities is critical. For example, in the DRC, local communities emphasize the importance of building on community resources to provide mediation to resolve family conflict. Support to enhance family mediation interventions (Kohli et al., 2012) or adaptation of promising group psychotherapy approaches (Bass et al., 2013) to address family relationships may reduce some of the negative outcomes associated with trauma. Survivors of trauma frequently describe the economic impact of conflict on individuals and families. Economic interventions that prioritize the needs of the family and larger community, perhaps through inclusion of awareness or counseling, may also reduce some of the negative outcomes of conflict while contributing toward improved outcomes.

There are several limitations to this study. First, as a 10-year history of trauma experience(s) and cumulative experience of family rejection was assessed, conclusions on causality are precluded. Longitudinal data on family rejection, trauma exposure, and mental health would provide insight into causality and change over time and whether family rejection mediates all or part of the relationship between trauma and mental health. Second, the measure of family rejection was developed based on qualitative research in these communities, but it did not involve the use of a validated scale which might more accurately measure the different manifestations of family rejection.

CONCLUSION

The experience of multiple and different types of trauma in conflict settings affects family relationships and may lead to rejection of survivors of trauma including those who have experienced sexual assault. Exposure to conflict-related violence and family rejection both had independent, significant relationships with poor mental health. In the future, researchers should explore whether family rejection mediates the relationship between trauma and mental health outcomes. Further, exploration of how family rejection affects access to social services including health care and economic opportunity is important given that survivors in other studies have described the multidimensional aspects of family rejection. Intervention design should be guided by an understanding of family dynamics and must address trauma experiences more broadly rather than offering an exclusive focus on one type of trauma at the expense of other trauma exposures associated with poor health outcomes.

ACKNOWLEDGMENTS

The authors of this study are grateful to all the participants in the Pigs for Peace program who provided detailed information on their lives during and after experiences of violence.

FUNDING

This study was conducted as part of the National Institutes of Health (NIH)/National Institute of Minority Health and Health Disparities (NIMHD)-funded randomized trial of a livestock-based microfinance intervention. Additional support was provided from the Health Systems Program Award for Doctoral Student Research, the Student Grant Award from the Center for Public Health and Human Rights, and the Goodermote Humanitarian Award Scholarship from the Center for Refugees and Disaster Response at the Johns Hopkins School of Public Health.

REFERENCES

Alberti, K. P., Grellety, E., Lin, Y. C., Polonsky, J., Coppens, K., Encinas, L., ... Mondonge, V. (2010). Violence against civilians and access to health care in North Kivu, Democratic Republic of Congo: Three cross-sectional surveys. *Conflict and Health*, 4, 17. doi:10.1186/1752-1505-4-17

Amone-P'olak, K., Jones, P. B., Abbott, R., Meiser-Stedman, R., Ovuga, E., & Croudace, T. J. (2013). Cohort profile: Mental health following extreme trauma in a northern Ugandan cohort of ar-ffected youth study (The WAYS Study). *Springerplus*, *2*(1), 300. doi:10.1186/2193-1801-2-300

Bass, J. K., Annan, J., McIvor Murray, S., Kaysen, D., Griffiths, S., Cetinoglu, T., . . . Bolton, P. A. (2013). Controlled trial of psychotherapy for Congolese survivors of sexual violence. *New England Journal of Medicine*, *368*, 2182–2191. doi:10.1056/NEJMoa1211853

Bass, J. K., Ryder, R. W., Lammers, M. C., Mukaba, T. N., & Bolton, P. A. (2008). Post-partum depression in Kinshasa, Democratic Republic of Congo: Validation of a concept using a mixed-methods cross-cultural approach. *Tropical Medicine & International Health*, *13*, 1534–1542. doi:10.1111/j.1365-3156.2008. 02160.x

Betancourt, T. S., Brennan, R. T., Rubin-Smith, J., Fitzmaurice, G. M., & Gilman, S. E. (2010). Sierra Leone's former child soldiers: A longitudinal study of risk, protective factors, and mental health. *Journal of the American Academy of Child & Adolescent Psychiatry*, *49*, 606–615. doi:10.1016/j.jaac.2010.03.008

Coghlan, B., Ngoy, P., Mulumba, F., Hardy, C., Bemo, V. N., Stewart, T., . . . Brennan, R. (2007). *Mortality in the Democratic Republic of Congo: An ongoing crisis (2006–2007)*. Melbourne, Australia: International Rescue Committee, Burnet Institute.

Corrigan, P. W., & Miller, F. E. (2004). Shame, blame, and contamination: A review of the impact of mental illness stigma on family members. *Journal of Mental Health*, *13*, 537–548.

Farhood, L. F. (2004). The impact of high and low stress on the health of Lebanese families. *Research and Theory for Nursing Practice*, *18*, 197–212.

Glass, N., Ramazani, P., Tosha, M., Mpanano, M., & Cinyabuguma, M. (2012). A Congolese-US participatory action research partnership to rebuild the lives of rape survivors and their families in eastern Democratic Republic of Congo. *Global Public Health*, *7*, 184–195. doi:10.1080/17441692.2011 .594449

Harvard Humanitarian Initiative. (2009). *Characterizing sexual violence in the Democratic Republic of the Congo: Profiles of violence, community response and implications for the protection of women*. New York, NY: Harvard Humanitarian Initiative, Open Society Institute.

Igreja, V., Kleijn, W., & Richters, A. (2006). When the war was over, little changed: Women's posttraumatic suffering after the war in Mozambique. *Journal of Nervous and Mental Disease*, *194*, 502–509. doi:10.1097/01.nmd. 0000228505.36302.a3

Johnson, K., Scott, J., Rughita, B., Kisielewski, M., Asher, J., Ong, R., & Lawry, L. (2010). Association of sexual violence and human rights violations with physical and mental health in territories of the Eastern Democratic Republic of the Congo. *Journal of the American Medical Association*, *304*, 553–562. doi:10.1001/jama.2010.1086

Kelly, J. T., Betancourt, T. S., Mukwege, D., Lipton, R., & Vanrooyen, M. J. (2011). Experiences of female survivors of sexual violence in eastern Democratic Republic of the Congo: A mixed-methods study. *Conflict and Health*, *5*, 25. doi:10.1186/1752-1505-5-25

Kleinman, A., & Hall-Clifford, R. (2009). Stigma: A social, cultural and moral process. *Journal of Epidemiology and Community Health*, *63*, 418–419.

Kohli, A., Tosha, M., Ramazani, P., Safari, O., Bachunguye, R., Zahiga, I., ... Glass, N. (2012). Family and community rejection and a Congolese led mediation intervention to reintegrate rejected survivors of sexual violence in Eastern Democratic Republic of Congo. *Health Care for Women International, 34,* 736–756. doi:10.1080/07399332.2012.721418

Kohrt, B. A., & Hruschka, D. J. (2010). Nepali concepts of psychological trauma: The role of idioms of distress, ethnopsychology and ethnophysiology in alleviating suffering and preventing stigma. *Culture, Medicine, and Psychiatry, 34,* 322–352. doi:10.1007/s11013-010-9170-2

Kohrt, B. A., Hruschka, D. J., Worthman, C. M., Kunz, R. D., Baldwin, J. L., Upadhaya, N., ... Nepal, M. K. (2012). Political violence and mental health in Nepal: Prospective study. *British Journal of Psychiatry, 201,* 268–275. doi:10.1192/bjp.bp.111.096222

Kubiak, S. P. (2005). Trauma and cumulative adversity in women of a disadvantaged social location. *American Journal of Orthopsychiatry, 75,* 451–465. doi:10.1037/0002-9432.75.4.451

Link, B. G., & Phelan, J. C. (2001). Conceptualizing stigma. *Annual Review of Psychology, 27,* 363–385.

Menkiti, I. A. (1984). Person and community in African traditional thought. In R. A. Wright (Ed.), *African philosophy: An introduction* (3rd ed.). Lanham, MD: University Press of America.

Miller, K. E., Omidian, P., Rasmussen, A., Yaqubi, A., & Daudzai, H. (2008). Daily stressors, war experiences, and mental health in Afghanistan. *Transcultural Psychiatry, 45,* 611–638. doi:10.1177/1363461508100785

Miller, K. E., & Rasmussen, A. (2010). War exposure, daily stressors, and mental health in conflict and post-conflict settings: Bridging the divide between trauma-focused and psychosocial frameworks. *Social Science & Medicine, 70*(1), 7–16. doi:10.1016/j.socscimed.2009.09.029

Miller, K. E., Weine, S. M., Ramic, A., Brkic, N., Bjedic, Z. D., Smajkic, A., ... Worthington, G. (2002). The relative contribution of war experiences and exile-related stressors to levels of psychological distress among Bosnian refugees. *Journal of Traumatic Stress, 15,* 377–387. doi:10.1023/A:1020181124118

Mollica, R. F., Henderson, D. C., & Tor, S. (2002). Psychiatric effects of traumatic brain injury events in Cambodian survivors of mass violence. *British Journal of Psychiatry, 181,* 339–347.

Mollica, R. F., McDonald, L. S., Massagli, M. P., & Silove, D. M. (2004). *Measuring trauma, measuring torture: Instructions and guidance on the utilization of the Harvard Program in Refugee Trauma's Versions of The Hopkins Symptom Checklist-25 (HSCL-25) and The Harvard Trauma Questionnaire.* Cambridge, UK: Harvard Program in Refugee Trauma.

Mukamana, D., & Brysiewicz, P. (2008). The lived experience of genocide rape survivors in Rwanda. *Journal of Nursing Scholarship, 40,* 379–384. doi:10.1111/j.1547-5069.2008.00253.x

Réseau des Femmes pour un Développement Associatif, Réseau des Femmes pour la Défense des Droits et la Paix, & International Alert. (2005). *Women's bodies as a battleground: Sexual violence against women and girls during the war in the Democratic Republic of Congo, South Kivu (1996–2003).* London, UK: International Alert.

Roberts, B., Damundu, E. Y., Lomoro, O., & Sondorp, E. (2010). The influence of demographic characteristics, living conditions, and trauma exposure on the overall health of a conflict-affected population in Southern Sudan. *BMC Public Health, 10*, 518. doi:10.1186/1471-2458-10-518

Roberts, B., Ocaka, K. F., Browne, J., Oyok, T., & Sondorp, E. (2008). Factors associated with post-traumatic stress disorder and depression amongst internally displaced persons in northern Uganda. *BMC Psychiatry, 8*, 38. doi:10.1186/1471-244X-8-38

Sabin, M., Lopes Cardozo, B., Nackerud, L., Kaiser, R., & Varese, L. (2003). Factors associated with poor mental health among Guatemalan refugees living in Mexico 20 years after civil conflict. *Jouranl of the American Medical Association, 290*, 635–642. doi:10.1001/jama.290.5.635

Sideris, T. (2003). War, gender and culture: Mozambican women refugees. *Social Science & Medicine, 56*, 713–724.

Steiner, B., Benner, M. T., Sondorp, E., Schmitz, K. P., Mesmer, U., & Rosenberger, S. (2009). Sexual violence in the protracted conflict of DRC programming for rape survivors in South Kivu. *Conflict and Health, 3*, 3. doi:10.1186/1752-1505-3-3

Vinck, P., Pham, P., Baldo, S., & Shigekane, R. (2008). *Living with fear: A population-based survey on attitudes about peace, justice and social reconstruction in Eastern Democratic Republic of Congo.* Berkeley, CA: Human Rights Center at University of California Berkeley, Payson Center for International Development, and International Center for Transitional Justice.

Wakabi, W. (2008). Sexual violence increasing in Democratic Republic of Congo. *Lancet, 371*(9606), 15–16. doi:10.1016/S0140-6736(08)60051-3

Yang, L. H., & Kleinman, A. (2008). "Face" and the embodiment of stigma in China: The cases of schizophrenia and AIDS. *Social Science & Medicine, 67*, 398–408. doi:10.1016/j.socscimed.2008.03.011

Yang, L. H., Kleinman, A., Link, B. G., Phelan, J. C., Lee, S., & Good, B. (2007). Culture and stigma: Adding moral experience to stigma theory. *Social Science & Medicine, 64*, 1524–1535. doi:10.1016/j.socscimed.2006.11.013

Intimate Partner Violence and the Utilization of Maternal Health Care Services in Nigeria

DOROTHY NGOZI ONONOKPONO

Department of Sociology and Anthropology, University of Uyo, Uyo, Nigeria

EZINWANNE CHRISTIANA AZFREDRICK

Department of Guidance and Counselling, University of Ibadan, Ibadan, Nigeria

Our aim in this study is to examine the association between women's lifetime experiences of physical, sexual, and emotional intimate partner violence (IPV) and the use of maternal health care services. We used data from the 2008 Nigeria Demographic and Health Survey. Analysis was based on responses from 17,476 women (for antenatal care [ANC]) and 17,412 (for delivery assisted by a skilled health provider) who had had deliveries in the 5 years preceding the survey. We found an overall IPV prevalence rate of 33.4%. Physical IPV was associated with low use of ANC. Emotionally abused women were less likely to use delivery assistance from skilled health care providers. Based on our findings, we suggest the importance of designing interventions to address the health care needs of women who have experienced violence from their partners.

Intimate partner violence (IPV) is one of the most common forms of violence perpetrated against women by current or former husband or intimate partner (Krug, Mercy, Dahlberg, & Zwi, 2002). In sub-Saharan Africa, the prevalence of IPV ranges between 20% and 70% (Devries et al., 2013; Jewkes, Levin, & Penn-Kekana, 2002). The use of maternal health care services, however, remains poor. We examined the relationship between IPV and the use of maternal health care services in Nigeria. Understanding the relationship has the potential to provide a policy tool for designing interventions to address women's health care needs in Africa.

Substantial progress has been made globally to reduce maternal mortality. Nigeria, however, is still in the list of countries that contribute the highest rates of maternal mortality in sub-Saharan Africa. In 2012, the maternal mortality ratio (MMR) in Nigeria was 630 per 100,000 live births (World Bank, 2013), contributing to about 10% of the global maternal deaths annually (Babalola & Fatusi, 2009). The poor maternal health outcome in the country has been linked to inadequate or nonuse of maternal health care services such as antenatal care (ANC) and delivery care (Doctor, 2011; Osubor, Fatusi, & Chiwuzie, 2006). ANC and delivery assisted by a skilled health provider have been widely recognized as important factors contributing to the reduction of maternal mortality. The use of these maternal health care services (ANC and assisted deliveries by a skilled health provider), however, remains low in Nigeria. According to the 2008 Nigeria Demographic and Health Survey (NDHS) report, about 58% of women in Nigeria received skilled ANC; fewer than half received the four ANC visits recommended by the World Health Organization (WHO), while only 39% of deliveries were assisted by a skilled health provider (National Population Commission [NPC] & ICF Macro, 2009).

Several studies indicate that low use of ANC and delivery assisted by a skilled health provider is associated with increased risk of poor pregnancy outcomes (Jasinski, 2004; Koenig & Ahmed, 2006). Adamu (2011) found that the utilization of maternal health care service varied across the regions of Nigeria, and that education and family wealth index were strongly related to service utilization in all the regions. Although researchers have identified socioeconomic and demographic factors associated with the use of ANC and delivery care (Bullock, Bloom, Davis, Kilburn, & Curry, 2006; Ononokpono & Odimegwu, 2014; Rai, Singh, Singh, & Kumar, 2014), the role that IPV plays in the utilization of ANC and delivery assistance from a skilled health provider has received less attention. Nigeria is a culturally diverse country with institutionalized gender roles and structural power imbalances between women and men. The social inequalities can increase the risk of IPV, which consequently may constrain women from having access to maternal health care. Thus a better understanding of the relationship between IPV and the use of maternal health care services is important especially in highly patriarchal societies such as Africa and particularly Nigeria, where culture and societal norms allow men to make decisions on the issue of women's reproductive health (Isiugo-Abanihe, 2003; Odimegwu et al., 2005).

Intimate partner violence (IPV) is the most common form of violence against women and consists of a range of physical, sexual, and emotional acts perpetrated against women by a current or former husband or intimate partner (Krug et al., 2002; Rahman, Nakamura, Seino, & Kizuki, 2012). Globally, the estimate of lifetime IPV prevalence ranged between 10% and 70% (Rahman, Nakamura, Seino, & Kizuki, 2013, while in sub-Saharan Africa the prevalence of IPV is between 20% and 70% (Ellsberg, Caldera, Herrera,

Winkvist, & Kullgren, 1999; Jewkes et al, 2002; WHO, 2013). Researchers in Nigeria found an IPV prevalence rate ranging between 17% and 34% (Antai, 2011; Osuora, Omolo, Kamweya, Harder, & Mutai, 2012). The huge range of IPV prevalence estimates is assumed to be related to the acceptance of IPV as a justifiable punishment and societal norm in many parts of Africa (Osuora et al., 2012).

Adverse health outcomes have been linked to IPV (Campbell, 2002; Sharps, Laughon, & Giangrande, 2007). Studies in developing countries revealed that women's experience of physical violence was significantly associated with low use of contraception, unwanted pregnancy, and repeat pregnancy (Scribano, Stevens, & Kaizar, 2013; Stephenson, Koenig, Acharya, & Roy, 2008). Further, Sarkar (2008) found that IPV significantly increased the risk for low birth weight infants, preterm delivery, and neonatal death. In a study in Seattle, researchers showed that women reporting any IPV during pregnancy were twice as likely as unexposed women to experience an antenatal hospitalization (Lipsky, Caetano, Field, & Larkin, 2006). Rahman and colleagues (2012) found that maternal experience of physical IPV was associated with low use of sufficient ANC and assisted deliveries from a skilled provider. Studies in Kenya showed that IPV was related to polygamy, parity, and receipt of skilled attendance during parturition (Makayoto, Omolo, Kamweya, Harder, & Mutai, 2013; Goo & Harlow, 2012). Furthermore, Emenike and colleagues (2008) found a significant association between physical/emotional/sexual abuse of women and negative reproductive health outcomes such as terminated pregnancies and infant mortality. In Nigeria, women's exposure to IPV was associated with low use of contraception, miscarriages, induced abortion, and child mortality (Okenwa, Lawoko, & Jansson, 2011; Osuora et al., 2012). Antai (2011) found a strong association between IPV and traumatic physical consequences.

In several publications researchers have established the association between IPV and adverse women's reproductive and maternal health outcomes. Most focused on the linkage between IPV and various health consequences such as low contraceptive use, unwanted pregnancies, miscarriages, sexually transmitted diseases (STDs), low birth weight, and neonatal and child mortality (Chibber & Krishnan, 2011; Silverman, Gupta, Decker, Kapur, & Raj, 2007; Stephenson, Koenig, & Ahmed, 2006). Rahman and colleagues (2012) argued that most studies have been conducted in developed countries and are clinic-based studies. Further, several studies have focused on the relationship between physical and sexual IPV and health outcomes (Heidi, Ruchira, & Naved, 2008; Rahman et al., 2012), and little is known about the association between emotional (psychological) violence and the utilization of maternal health care services. Therefore, examining the role of emotional IPV would make an important contribution to studies on IPV and the use of maternal health care services.

Researchers who examined the association between IPV and ANC have measured ANC using single indicators such as type of provider, content of ANC, and frequency of ANC visits (for example, Rahman et al., 2012). Some argued the adequacy of ANC to a large extent is shaped by the way in which utilization is measured (Kotelchuck, 1994). The ANC Adequacy Utilization Index, which takes into consideration both the utilization of ANC and the timing of ANC initiation, is considered more appropriate because it offers a more accurate and comprehensive measure of ANC utilization (Kotelchuck, 1994). To the best of our knowledge, studies that have examined the association between IPV and ANC utilization have rarely used the ANC Adequacy Utilization Index to measure antenatal care utilization. For a better understanding of the relationship between IPV and ANC, there is need for a more appropriate measurement of ANC utilization. Our aim in this study is to examine the association between physical, sexual, and emotional violence and the utilization of adequate ANC and delivery assisted by a skilled health care provider. We hypothesize that emotional IPV is associated with a lower likelihood of the use of maternal health care services.

METHODS

We drew data from a cross-sectional survey, the 2008 NDHS. The survey provided information on population and health indicators at the national and state levels. Nigeria is made up of 36 states and a Federal Capital Territory (FCT, Abuja). All the states and the FCT of Abuja were selected to be in the sample. Each state is subdivided into Local Government Areas (LGAs). Each LGA is divided into census enumeration areas (EAs). The primary sampling units (PSUs) were derived from a sampling frame created for the 2006 Nigerian census. The PSU or cluster was selected from the lists of EAs. A stratified, two-stage cluster design was adopted to select a sample of 888 primary sampling units: 286 urban and 602 rural areas. A weighted probability sample of 36,800 households was selected in the survey. A listing of households and mapping was done and on the average a total of 41 households were selected in each cluster. A minimum of 950 interviews were completed for each state, and a total of 33,385 women aged 15–49 were selected, yielding a response rate of 96.5% (NPC & ICF, 2009). Of the 33,385 women, 19,389 were surveyed with the Demographic and Health Survey (DHS) IPV module. Out of the 19,389 women, 1,361 women who did not have their last delivery in the 5 years before the survey were excluded, while 18,028 women who had had deliveries in the 5 years preceding the survey were included in our study. For ANC and delivery assisted by a skilled health care provider, 552 and 616 missing cases, respectively, were excluded. This is because the percentages were small (less than 1%). The final sample included 17,476 women for ANC and 17,412 women for delivery assistance from a skilled health care provider.

Variables

Antenatal care (ANC) utilization and delivery assisted by a skilled health care provider are the outcome variables. We assessed ANC utilization through the ANC Adequacy Utilization Index, which is based on duration of pregnancy at first ANC visit and number of ANC visits (Trinh, Dibley, & Byles, 2006). The WHO recommended at least four ANC visits during pregnancy for women without complications and a minimum of one visit within the first 4 months of gestation. Antenatal care (ANC) adequacy was assessed using the "at least four ANC visits" and "initiation of first visit within 4 months" criteria. Details about the construction of the ANC Adequacy Utilization Index have been described elsewhere (Trinh et al 2006). Although the ANC Adequacy Utilization Index proposed by Trinh and colleagues classified use of antenatal care as either sufficient, intermediate, insufficient, missing; in our study we classified the use of ANC as adequate or inadequate. The "adequate" category in our study corresponds to the sufficient and intermediate categories of the ANC Adequacy Utilization Index, while the "inadequate" category corresponds to the insufficient category. A woman is classified as having adequate utilization of ANC if she had four or more visits and the initial visit within the first 4 months of pregnancy, and by the fifth or sixth month. Antenatal care (ANC) utilization is classified as inadequate if a woman attends fewer than the four recommended visits and initiates the first visit in 7 months or later, or she had no ANC. The adequate category was coded 1 and inadequate 0. Delivery assisted by a skilled health provider is a binary variable and was constructed from the combined responses to the question whether the respondent was assisted by a health professional (doctor, nurse/midwife, and auxiliary nurse) during delivery. Responses to these questions were grouped into two categories and coded 1 if a woman was assisted by a doctor, nurse/midwife/auxiliary nurse during delivery and 0 if not.

IPV is the main explanatory variable and is measured as experience of violence by women perpetrated by their current or former husband or intimate partner since age 15. It is defined as a lifetime experience of IPV. The variable is measured using the modified Conflict Tactics Scale (CTS) approach as embodied in the DHS domestic violence module. This approach guarantees a high level of reliability and constructive validity (Straus, Hamby, Boney-McCoy, & Sugarman, 1996). Three types of IPV were considered in our study: physical, sexual, and emotional violence. Physical IPV was assessed through seven items. Each woman was asked whether her husband or partner perpetrated the following acts against her: (a) pushing, shaking, or throwing something at her; (b) slapping; (c) twisting of her arm or pulling her hair; (d) punching her with his fist or with something that could hurt her; (e) kicking dragging, or beating; (f) trying to choke or burn her on purpose; or (g) threatening or attacking her with a knife, gun, or any other weapon. Women could respond "yes" or "no" to each item. A "yes" response to one or more items (a) to (g) above constitutes evidence of physical violence (NPC & ICF Macro, 2009). Sexual violence was measured through the question of whether the respondent's husband or partner had ever physically forced her to have sexual intercourse with him even when she did not want to. A binary variable was created to assess whether a woman had ever experienced emotional violence. In the 2008 NDHS, respondents were asked whether the husband or partner said or did something to humiliate her in front of others, threatened to hurt or harm her or someone close to her, or insulted her or made her feel bad about herself.

Other covariates that have been theoretically and empirically proven to be significantly associated with IPV were included in our analyses (Bates, Schuler, Islam, & Islam, 2004; Uthman, Lawoko, & Moradi, 2009). Maternal age was categorized as follows: 15–24, 25–34, and 35–49 years of age. The educational attainment of the woman and the partner was classified as follows: no education, primary, or secondary or higher. Employment status is categorized as working or not working. A woman's decision-making autonomy was defined as decision making regarding her own health and was determined by whether a woman made decisions alone or jointly with her husband or partner, including if the husband alone or others made decisions for her health care. In previous studies (Ononokpono, Odimegwu, Adedini, & Imasiku, 2013), mass media exposure has been found to be strongly associated with maternal health outcomes. This variable was grouped into three categories: newspaper, radio, and television. A dichotomous variable was created for each media exposure category.

Parity was classified as 1, 2–3, or 4+. The NDHS wealth index is measured as a standardized composite variable made up of quintiles. This was determined through principal component analysis (from factor analysis) and was based on household assets (e.g., type of flooring, water supply, electricity, radio, television, refrigerator, and type of vehicle). The index was constructed by assigning a factor score to each of the household assets. Each household was assigned a score for each asset, and individuals were then ranked according to the total score of the household in which they live (NPC & ICF Macro, 2009). The household wealth index of the sample was then categorized into five quintiles. Each quintile represented a relative measure of a household's socioeconomic status (Rutstein & Johnson, 2004).

Household size was defined as total number of household members and categorized as follows: < = 4, 5–6, 7+. Type of place of residence was categorized as urban or rural. Region was defined as any one of the geopolitical zones with administrative boundaries categorized as North Central, North East, North West, South East, South South, and South West.

Statistical Analyses

Descriptive statistics were used to describe the sociodemographic characteristics of the respondents, IPV, and the utilization of maternal health care service indicators. For bivariate analysis, frequencies and cross tabulations were used to identify the distributions of the outcome variables by selected background characteristics. The chi-square test of association was used to test the statistical significance of the differences in the perpetration of IPV. Sample weights provided in the DHS data were applied for the univariate and bivariate analyses to adjust for nonresponse and oversampling of some areas. For all analyses, the Stata 11.1 software package was used. The level of significance was set at $p < .05$. At the multivariate level, logistic regression was employed. The outcome measures are dichotomous variables and as such binary logistic regression models were used to assess the relationship between IPV and the maternal health care outcomes. This makes it possible to estimate the odds of the use of adequate ANC and delivery assisted by a skilled health care provider. A total of four models were estimated (two models for each outcome variable). Model 1 contained each of the IPV variables (physical, sexual, and emotional violence) and the outcome variable. This enabled the assessment of the association between each of the IPV variables and the maternal health care indicators. Model 2 contained the IPV variables while controlling for other covariates. This is to enable a simultaneous examination of these variables and to assess whether the IPV variables were significantly associated with the use of maternal health care services after controlling for other covariates. The multicollinearity of the variables was checked by examining the variance inflation factors (VIFs) of the independent variables, which was approximately 2. The strength of the associations between the dependent variables and independent variables was estimated using the odds ratio (ORs) and 95% confidence intervals.

Ethical Considerations

Our study comprised analyses of existing survey data with all identifier information removed. The conduct of the survey was approved by both the Ethics Committee of the Opinion Research Corporation Macro International Incorporated (ORC Macro Inc.), at Calverton in the USA and the National Ethics Committee in the Federal of Ministry of Health in Nigeria. Written and signed informed consent was obtained from all the participants before participation in the survey, and information was collected anonymously and confidentially (NPC & ICF Macro, 2009, p. 528).

RESULTS

Sociodemographic Profile of the Respondents

In Table 1 we display results to show almost half (47%) of the women were between the ages of 25 and 34 years. About 45.4% of the sample population had no formal education. Over two-thirds of the women (66%) were employed.

Of the total sample, 7.4% were exposed to reading a newspaper, 50.4% listened to the radio, and 22.4% reported that they watched television regularly. Regarding autonomy, 58.1% reported that their husbands or partners make decisions regarding health care. The household wealth index showed that 45.3% of the sample population were in the poor wealth quintile category. The majority of the women (69.8%) resided in the rural areas. The highest proportion of the women resided in South East. Fewer than half (48.8%) of the women had adequate ANC, while fewer (40.8%) had delivery assistance from a skilled health provider. With respect to IPV experience, 13.9% of the sample population reported that they had experienced physical IPV, 4% had experienced sexual IPV, and 15.5% indicated that they had experienced emotional IPV.

The bivariate relationship showed that there was a high correlation among those living in the rural areas and the different measures of IPV (physical, sexual, and emotional) and respondents who reported that their husband and others make decisions regarding their health care. The proportion of physical, sexual, and emotional IPV was higher for women aged 25–34 years. Respondents with higher education had a higher proportion of physical and sexual IPV, while emotional IPV was more frequent among women with no education. Women who had no access to any media reported more experiences of all three forms of IPV than those who had access to mass media. There was also a high prevalence of all three forms of IPV among women who are working than those who are not working. Women with parity of one had lower experience of any form of IPV than women with parity above two. It is also worthwhile to mention that the lowest level of IPV experience was observed in households where women alone make decisions. Experience of physical IPV was higher for women who belong to the rich wealth quintile than their counterparts in poor households. Women residing in large households (seven or more household members) had a higher proportion of sexual and emotional IPV experience. Reports of all three forms of IPV were significantly higher among women residing in the South West.

Table 2 shows that women who reported ever experiencing physical IPV were as likely to use adequate ANC compared with those who had no experience of physical IPV. Emotional IPV was associated with low use of adequate ANC (OR = 0.76; 95% CI = 0.69–0.81). The association between physical IPV and utilization of delivery assistance by a skilled health care

TABLE 1 Descriptive Statistics for Sociodemographic Characteristics of Women and Distribution According to Different Forms of IPV, 2008 Nigeria Demographic and Health Survey (DHS)

Characteristics	All women n (%)	Physical IPV%	Sexual IPV%	Emotional IPV%
Maternal age				
15–24	4,528 (26.0)	23.3**	28.3	25.6
25–34	8,239 (47.0)	52.6	50.1	48.4
35–49	4,709 (27.0)	24.1	21.6	26.0
Maternal education				
No education	7,926 (45.4)	28.0***	30.6***	43.8**
Primary	3,989 (22.8)	33.4	33.2	26.4
Secondary/higher	5,561 (31.8)	38.6	36.2	29.8
Partner's education				
No education	6,450 (38.5)	23.3***	24.0***	34.4**
Primary	3,624 (21.5)	27.5	32.5	25.6
Secondary/higher	6,774 (40.0)	49.2	43.5	40.0
Employment status				
Not working	5,905 (34.0)	26.4***	29.1*	30.5**
Working	11,450 (66.0)	73.6	70.9	69.5
Woman's autonomy				
(decision making on own health)				
Husband alone/others	9,582 (58.1)	46.2***	51.0	57.4**
Husband /wife	5,456 (38.1)	38.8	37.6	31.1
Wife alone	1,443 (8.8)	15.0	11.4	11.5
Parity				
1	3,506 (23.9)	19.5**	18.8**	19.2***
2–3	6,455 (44.1)	48.0	45.0	48.0
4+	4,663 (32.0)	32.5	36.2	32.8
Media access				
Newspaper				
No	16,058 (92.6)	94.5**	95.77**	95.2***
Yes	1,281 (7.4)	5.5	4.234	4.8
Radio				
No	8,637 (49.6)	53.7***	52.45	55.88***
Yes	8,769 (50.4)	46.3	47.55	44.12
Television				
No	11,813 (77.6)	76.5	80.4*	82.9***
Yes	3,414 (22.4)	23.5	19.6	17.1
Household wealth index				
Poor	7,920 (45.3)	36.6***	37.4***	45.8***
Middle	3,317 (19.0)	23.3	27.3	23.0
Rich	6,238 (35.7)	40.1	35.3	31.2
Household size				
< = 4	5,016 (28.7)	32.9*	31.9***	30.9***
5–6	5,083 (29.1)	35.7	31.0	32.8
7+	7,376 (42.2)	31.4	37.1	36.3
Place of residence				
Urban	5,279 (30.2)	29.4	25.9*	25.2***
Rural	12,196 (69.8)	70.6	74.1	74.8
Region				
North Central	3,049 (17.5)	18.0***	6.7***	7.8***
North East	2,507 (14.4)	19.0	11.6	18.4
North West	2,733 (14.6)	13.0	23.1	16.0
South East	5,302 (30.3)	12.6	13.0	27.8

(Continued on next page)

TABLE 1 Descriptive Statistics for Sociodemographic Characteristics of Women and Distribution According to Different Forms of IPV, 2008 Nigeria DHS Demographic and Health Survey (DHS) *(Continued)*

Characteristics	All women n (%)	Physical IPV%	Sexual IPV%	Emotional IPV%
South South	1,595 (9.1)	11.4	12.9	13.3
South West	2,290 (13.1)	27.0	32.7	16.7
ANC adequacy				
Inadequate	8,951 (51.2)	47.2	51.6	54.2***
Adequate	8,525 (48.8)	52.8	48.4	45.8
Delivery assistance				
Unskilled health provider	10,300 (59.2)	51.2***	58.6	60.8**
Skilled health provider	7,113 (40.8)	48.8	41.4	39.2
IPV prevalence		13.9	4.0	15.5

Note: IPV = intimate partner violence; ANC (antenatal care) adequacy is measured as making four or more ANC visits and an initial visit in the first 4 months of pregnancy; skilled health providers include doctors, nurses/midwives, and auxiliary nurses.
Significance level $*p < .05; **p < .01; ***p < .001$.

provider was statistically significant. Women who reported that they had been emotionally abused were less likely to use delivery assistance from a skilled health care provider (OR = 0.77; 95% CI = 0.70–0.86).

The association between physical IPV and the use of adequate ANC remained statistically significant after controlling for other covariates in Model 2 (AOR = 0.72; 95% CI = 0.61–0.85). Maternal age, maternal and partners' education, employment status, parity, household wealth index, media access (reading newspaper and listening to radio), rural residence, and region of residence were significantly associated with both use of adequate ANC and delivery assistance from a skilled health care provider. Women who made decisions jointly with their husbands or partners were significantly more likely to use adequate ANC compared with women whose husbands or partners made decisions alone.

DISCUSSION

We found an overall IPV prevalence rate of 33.4%. This finding is consistent with the lifetime prevalence of IPV in sub-Saharan Africa and Nigeria (Jewkes et al., 2002; Osuora et al., 2012). The high prevalence of IPV found in this study could suggest the patriarchal ideology in traditional societies such as Nigeria where gender roles are being skewed to justify violence against women who are assigned an inferior role to men (Antai, 2011). We also identified significant associations between IPV and the utilization of maternal health care services in Nigeria. The finding that women who reported they have ever experienced physical or emotional IPV were significantly less likely to use adequate ANC and delivery assisted by a skilled health

TABLE 2 Logistic Regression Odds Ratio for the Association Between Different Forms of IPV and the Use of Maternal Health Care Services, 2008 Nigeria Demographic and Health Survey (DHS)

Characteristics	Adequate ANC		Delivery assistance (skilled health provider)	
	Model 1 odds ratio (95% CI)	Model 2 adjusted odds ratio (95% CI)	Model 1 odds ratio	Model 2 adjusted odds ratio (95% CI)
Physical IPV				
No	1.00	1.00	1.00	1.00
Yes	1.18 (1.06–1.31)**	0.72 (0.61–0.85)***	1.37 (1.23–1.53)***	0.92 (0.77–1.10)
Sexual IPV				
No	1.00	1.00	1.00	1.00
Yes	0.99 (0.81–1.20)	1.00 (0.76–1.33)	0.93 (0.75–1.12)	0.98 (0.72–1.33)
Emotional IPV				
No	1.00	1.00	1.00	1.00
Yes	0.76 (0.69–0.81)***	0.99 (0.85–1.15)	0.77 (0.70–0.86)***	1.02 (0.86–1.21)
Maternal age				
15–24		1.00		1.00
25–34		1.35 (1.17–1.55)***		1.23 (1.05–1.45)*
35–49		1.27 (1.05–1.53)*		1.45 (1.16–1.80)***
Maternal education				
No education		1.00		1.00
Primary		1.54 (1.33–1.79)***		1.43 (1.20–1.69)***
Secondary/higher		2.14 (1.79–2.55)***		2.89 (1.39–3.50)***
Husband/partner´s education				
No education		1.00		1.00
Primary		1.71 (1.47–1.98)***		1.46 (1.22–1.75)***
Secondary/higher		2.02 (1.74–2.36)***		1.81 (1.51–2.17)***
Employment status				
Not working		1.00		1.00
Working		1.19 (1.07–1.34)***		1.24 (1.09–1.42)***
Woman's autonomy[a] (decision making)				
Husband alone/others		1.00		1.00
Husband /wife		1.32 (1.18–1.49)***		1.10 (0.96–1.25)
Wife alone		1.13 (0.92–1.40)		0.96 (0.77–1.21)

(Continued on next page)

TABLE 2 Logistic Regression Odds Ratio for the Association Between Different Forms of IPV and the Use of Maternal Health Care Services, 2008 Nigeria Demographic and Health Survey (DHS) (*Continued*)

Characteristics	Adequate ANC		Delivery assistance (skilled health provider)	
	Model 1 odds ratio (95% CI)	Model 2 adjusted odds ratio (95% CI)	Model 1 odds ratio	Model 2 adjusted odds ratio (95% CI)
Parity				
1		1.00		1.00
2–3		0.81 (0.70–0.94)**		0.66 (0.56–0.79)***
4+		0.72 (0.59–0.89)***		0.59 (0.46–0.75)***
Media access				
Newspaper				
No		1.00		1.00
Yes		1.84 (1.36–2.48)***		2.07 (1.53–2.80)***
Radio				
No		1.00		1.00
Yes		1.53 (1.36–1.71)***		1.32 (1.16–1.51)***
Television				
No		1.00		1.00
Yes		1.02 (0.84–1.23)		1.15 (0.95–1.40)
Household wealth index				
Poor		1.00		1.00
Middle		2.02 (1.77–2.31)***		1.91 (1.64–2.22)***
Rich		2.89 (2.40–3.47)***		3.87 (3.18–4.71)***
Household size				
<= 4		1.00		1.00
5–6		1.06 (0.92–1.22)		1.04 (0.88–1.21)
7+		1.00 (0.86–1.17)		1.01 (0.85–1.21)
Place of residence				
Urban		1.00		1.00
Rural		0.69 (0.60–0.79)***		0.62 (0.53–0.72)***
Region				
North Central		1.00		1.00
North East		3.31 (2.62–4.17)***		2.54 (2.02–3.20)***
North West		1.44 (1.19–1.75)***		1.19 (0.97–1.45)*
South East		1.16 (0.94–1.42)		0.59 (0.47–0.73)***
South South		0.55 (0.45–0.67)***		0.27 (0.22–0.34)***
South West		1.87 (1.47–2.38)***		3.02 (2.34–3.90)***
Log-likelihood	−9287.5136	−4482.5054	−8898.3313	−3577.1492
Pseudo R2	0.0016	0.3059	0.0023	0.4118

aWoman's autonomy is defined as decision making on a woman's own health care.

Note: IPV = intimate partner violence; ANC = antenatal care (adequate or inadequate).

Significance level *$p < .05$; **$p < .01$; ***$p < .001$.

care provider confirms the hypothesis of this study. The explanation to the significant association between emotional IPV and the maternal health care indicators is that emotional violence could affect a woman's emotional and physical health; and this in turn may lead to lack of incentive to pursue appropriate maternal health care (Rahman et al., 2012). This suggests the need for interventions such as counselling and trauma management for emotionally abused women by health care providers. Surprisingly, the relationship between sexual IPV and the use of the two maternal health care indicators was not statistically significant. Our finding that maternal age, higher education, employment status, belonging to the rich wealth quintile, and having access to media (reading newspaper and listening to radio) were significantly associated with the use of maternal health care services is consistent with studies elsewhere (Ciceklioglu, Soyer, & Öcek, 2005; Gayawan, 2013).

The higher proportion of the use of maternal health care services found among women with higher education, women from the rich wealth quintile, and women who were employed could reflect higher socioeconomic status and supports the notion that women who are better off are more likely to access health care services than disadvantaged women (Doctor, 2011). This finding suggests the need for programs to empower disadvantaged women socially and economically, especially through employment to secure means of livelihood and thus enhance their ability to utilize maternal health care services and challenge the acceptance of IPV. Higher parity was associated with low use of adequate ANC and deliveries assisted by a skilled health care provider, and this could be linked to better maternity experiences (Gabrysch & Campbell, 2009). Consistent with previous studies, the low use of maternal health care services found in our study was more likely among the disadvantaged women.

Our study, however, has some limitations. First, the cross-sectional design of the study does not permit a cause–effect relation of the independent variables to the dependent variable. Second, IPV is often associated with stigmatization (Rahman et al., 2012); therefore, the possibility of underreporting of IPV in our study should be taken into consideration. Third, the 2008 NDHS was collected retrospectively. This may be associated with recall bias, however, given that the events took place 5 years following the survey. Fourth, it is unclear whether the IPV acts preceded the use of maternal health care use, and this may raise some methodological questions. Finally, the study assessed lifetime IPV and the use of maternal health care services rather than IPV within the last 12 months. These limitations notwithstanding, our study has its strengths. First, it is a large population-based study with national coverage, and findings could be easily generalized across the whole country and other developing countries. Second, we make an important contribution to existing studies regarding the relationship between emotional (psychological) IPV and the use of maternal health care services.

CONCLUSION

Based on strong associations between IPV and the use of maternal health care services found in our study, we suggest the importance of designing an intervention to address the health care needs of women who have experienced violence from their husbands or partners. Interventions to reduce the risk of IPV should be considered a public health priority. Further, in highly patriarchal societies such as Nigeria where gender norms are indifferent to IPV, there is a need to educate men on IPV prevention and maternal health care service programs. Health care providers should create a social environment that enables women report their experience of IPV with less difficulty. To encourage the use of maternal health care services in the face of IPV, women should be empowered educationally and economically. Programs to increase women's education may help reduce their dependence in matters relating to their health care needs. Interventions to reduce household poverty and unemployment may enhance women's economic status and even reduce IPV. The government should use effective media such as radio and television to create awareness regarding IPV and maternal health care services. Further research is needed to understand possible pathways through which IPV influences the use of maternal health care.

ACKNOWLEDGMENTS

The authors are grateful to Measure DHS and ICF International for the 2008 Nigeria DHS data used in this study.

REFERENCES

Adamu, H. S. (2011). *Utilization of maternal health care services in Nigeria: An analysis of regional differences in the patterns and determinants of maternal health care use.* (Published thesis). University of Liverpool, Liverpool, UK.

Antai, D. (2011). Traumatic physical health consequences of intimate partner violence against women: What is the role of community factors? *BMC Women's Health, 11,* 56.

Babalola, S., & Fatusi, A. (2009). Determinants of use of maternal health services in Nigeria—Looking beyond individual and household factors. *BMC Pregnancy and Childbirth, 9*(43). doi:10.1186/1471-2393-9-43.

Bates, L. M., Schuler, S. R., Islam, F., & Islam, M. K. (2004). Socioeconomic factors and processes associated with domestic violence in rural Bangladesh. *International Family Planning Perspective, 30,* 190–199.

Bullock, L., Bloom, T., Davis, J., Kilburn, E., & Curry, M. A. (2006). Abuse disclosure in privately and Medicaid-funded pregnant women. *Journal of Midwifery & Women's Health, 51*(5), 361–369.

Campbell, J. C. (2002). Health consequences of intimate partner violence. *Lancet, 359*(9314), 1331–1336.

Chibber, K. S., & Krishnan, S. (2011). Confronting intimate partner violence: A global health priority. *Mount Sinai Journal of Medicine: A Journal of Translational and Personalized Medicine, 78*(3), 449–457.

Devries, K. M., Mak, J. Y. T., García-Moreno, C., Petzold, M., Child, J. C., Falder, G., ... Watts, C. H. (2013). The global prevalence of intimate partner violence against women. *Science, 340*, 1527–1528.

Ciceklioglu, M., Soyer, M. T., & Öcek, Z. A. (2005). Factors associated with the utilization and content of prenatal care in a western urban district of Turkey. *International Journal for Quality in Health Care, 17*(6), 533–539.

Doctor, H. V. (2011). Intergenerational differences in antenatal care and supervised deliveries in Nigeria. *Health & Place, 17*, 480–489.

Ellsberg, M., Caldera, T., Herrera, A., Winkvist, A., & Kullgren, G. (1999). Domestic violence and emotional distress among Nicaraguan women: Results from a population-based study. *American Psychologist, 54*(1), 30–36.

Emenike, E., Lawoko, S., & Dalal, K. (2008). Intimate partner violence and reproductive health of women in Kenya. *International Nurse Review, 55*(1), 97–102.

Gabrysch, S., & Campbell, O. M. R. (2009). Still too far to walk: Literature review on the determinants of delivery service use. *BMC Pregnancy and Childbirth, 9*, 34.

Gayawan, E. (2013). A poison regression model to examine spatial patterns in antenatal care utilization in Nigeria. *Population, Space and Place, 20*(5). doi:10.1002/psp.1775

Goo, L., & Harlow, S. D. (2012). Intimate partner violence affects skilled attendance at most recent delivery among women in Kenya. *Maternal and Child Health Journal, 16*(5), 1131–1137.

Heidi, B., Ruchira, J., & Naved T. (2008). A call for a public health response. *Journal of Health Population and Nutrition, 26*, 366–377.

Isiugo-Abanihe, U. C. (2003). *Male role and responsibility in fertility and reproductive health in Nigeria*. Ibadan, Nigeria: The Centre for Population Activities and Education for Development (CEPAED).

Jasinski, J. L. (2004). Pregnancy and domestic violence: A review of the literature. *Trauma Violence Abuse, 5*, 47–64.

Jewkes, R., Levin, J., & Penn-Kekana, L. (2002). Risk factors for domestic violence: From a South African cross-sectional study. *Social Science & Medicine, 55*(9), 1603–1617.

Koenig, S. A., & Ahmed, S. (2006). Domestic violence and symptoms of gynecologic morbidity among women in North India. *International Family Planning Perspective, 32*, 201–220.

Kotelchuck, M. (1994). An evaluation of the Kessner adequacy of prenatal care index and a proposed adequacy of prenatal care utilization index. *American Journal of Public Health, 84*(9), 1414–1420.

Krug, E. G., Mercy, J. A., Dahlberg, L. L., & Zwi, A. B. (2002). *The world report on violence and health.* Geneva, Switzerland: World Health Organization (WHO).

Lipsky, S., Caetano, R., Field, C. A., & Larkin, G. L. (2006). The role of intimate partner violence, race, and ethnicity in help-seeking behaviors. *Ethnicity and Health, 11*(1), 81–100.

Makayoto, L. A., Omolo, J., Kamweya, A. S., Harder, V. S., & Mutai, J. (2013). Prevalence and associated factors of intimate partner violence among pregnant women attending Kisumu District Hospital, Kenya. *Maternal and Child Health Journal, 17*(3), 441–447.

National Population Commission (NPC) [Nigeria] & ICF Macro. (2009). *Nigeria Demographic and Health Survey 2008.* Abuja, Nigeria: National Population Commission and ICF Macro.

Odimegwu, C., Adewuyi, A., Odebiyi, T., Aina, B., Adesina, Y., Olatubara, O., & Eniola, F. (2005). Men's role in emergency obstetric care in Osun State of Nigeria. *African Journal of Reproductive Health, 9*(3), 59–71.

Okenwa, L., Lawoko, S., & Jansson, B. (2011). Contraception, reproductive health and pregnancy outcomes among women exposed to intimate partner violence in Nigeria. *European Journal of Contraception and Reproductive Health Care, 16*(1), 18–25.

Ononokpono, D. N., & Odimegwu, C. O. (2014). Determinants of maternal health care utilization in Nigeria: A multilevel approach. *Pan African Medical Journal, 17*(Suppl. 1), 2.

Ononokpono, D. N., Odimegwu, C. O., Imasiku, E., & Adedini, S. (2013). Contextual determinants of maternal health care service utilization in Nigeria. *Women & Health, 53*(7), 647–668.

Osubor, K., Fatusi, A., & Chiwuzie, J. (2006). Maternal health-seeking behavior and associated factors in a rural Nigerian community. *Maternal and Child Health Journal, 10*(2), 159–169. doi:10.1007/s10995-005-0037-z

Osuora, D., Antai, D., Ezeudu, C., & Chukwujekwu, E. (2012). Effect of maternal exposure to intimate partner violence on under-five mortality in Nigeria. *Niger Journal of Paediatrics, 39*(3), 97–104.

Rahman, M., Nakamura, K., Seino, K., & Kizuki, M. (2012). Intimate partner violence and use of reproductive health services among married women: Evidence from a national Bangladeshi sample. *BMC Public Health, 12*(1), 913.

Rahman, M., Nakamura, K., Seino, K., & Kizuki, M. (2013). Does gender inequity increase the risk of intimate partner violence among women? Evidence from a national Bangladeshi sample. *PLoS ONE, 9*(2), e91448. doi:10.1371/journal.pone.009144

Rai, R. K., Singh, P. K., Singh, L., & Kumar, C. (2014). Individual characteristics and use of maternal and child health services by adolescent mothers in Niger. *Maternal and Child Health Journal, 18*(3), 592–603.

Rutstein, S. O., & Johnson, K. (2004). *The DHS Wealth Index. DHS comparative report.* Calverton, MD: ORC Macro.

Sarkar, N. N. (2008). The impact of intimate partner violence on women's reproductive health and pregnancy outcome. *Journal of Obstetrics and Gynaecology, 28*(3), 266–271.

Scribano, P. V., Stevens, J., & Kaizar, E. (2013). The effects of intimate partner violence before, during, and after pregnancy in nurse visited first time mothers. *Maternal and Child Health Journal, 17*(2), 307–318.

Sharps, P. W., Laughon, K., & Giangrande, S. K. (2007). Intimate partner violence and the childbearing year: Maternal and infant health consequences. *Trauma Violence Abuse, 8*(2), 105–116.

Silverman, J. G., Gupta, J., Decker, M. R., Kapur, N., & Raj, A. (2007). Intimate partner violence and unwanted pregnancy, miscarriage, induced abortion, and stillbirth among a national sample of Bangladeshi women. *British Journal of Gynaecology, 114*, 1246–1252.

Stephenson, R., Koenig, M. A., Acharya, R., & Roy, T. K. (2008). Domestic violence, contraceptive use, and unwanted pregnancy in rural India. *Studies in Family Planning, 39*(3), 177–186.

Stephenson, R., Koenig, M. A., & Ahmed, S. (2006). Domestic violence and contraceptive adoption in Uttar Pradesh, India. *Studies in Family Planning, 37*(2), 75–86.

Straus, M., Hamby, S., Boney-McCoy, S., & Sugarman, D. (1996). The revised Conflict Tactics Scales (CTS2): Development and preliminary psychometric data. *Journal of Family Issues, 17*, 283–316.

Trinh, L. T. T., Dibley, M. J., & Byles, J. (2006). Antenatal care adequacy in three provinces of Vietnam: Long An, Ben Tre, and Quang Ngai. *Public Health Reports, 121*, 468–475.

Uthman, O. A., Lawoko, S., & Moradi, T. (2009). Factors associated with attitudes towards intimate partner violence against women: A comparative analysis of 17 sub-Saharan countries. *BMC International Health and Human Rights, 9*(14), 1–15.

World Bank. (2013). *Trends in maternal mortality: 1990-2010. Estimates developed by WHO, UNICEF, UNFPA and The World Bank.* Retrieved from http://data.worldbank.org/indicator/SH.STA.MMRT

World Health Organization (WHO). (2013). *Violence against women: A global health problem of epidemic proportions.* Geneva, Switzerland: Author.

Relationship Difficulties Postrape: Being a Male Intimate Partner of a Female Rape Victim in Cape Town, South Africa

EVALINA VAN WIJK

Department of Psychiatric Nursing, Western Cape College of Nursing, Cape Peninsula University of Technology (CPUT), Cape Town, South Africa

TRACIE C. HARRISON

School of Nursing, The University of Texas at Austin, Austin, Texas, USA

In a longitudinal phenomenological study, the lived experience of being a male intimate partner (MIP) of a female rape victim in Cape Town, South Africa, is presented. Nine men participated in four face-to-face, semistructured interviews. The authors describe changes in communication and sexual intimacy postrape and how these changes spiralled into a dysfunctional relationship. Participants were interested in interventions for both partners and particularly for education to improve their communication and sexual relationships postrape. Researchers need to reconsider existing policies related to training programs to develop interventions that can address the needs of couples postrape and, ultimately, enhance their recovery.

Rape is an international problem. In a report published in September 2013, the United Nations found that one in four of the men surveyed in six South Asian countries had committed rape at some point in their lives (Karim, 2013). The frequency of rape in these countries is similar to other areas where research of this kind has been conducted, including South Africa (Karim, 2013).

The authors of this article add to the existing body of research by examining the lived experience of MIPs of female rape victims with emphasis on how the rape of their female partners has affected their relationship postrape. We found that in the case of the men, the rape was perceived as a crisis that adversely affected their communication and levels of intimacy with their partners. Because rape is a worldwide problem, we believe that the findings of this study are applicable not only to South Africa, but also internationally. Although the focus of this work is on the intimate male partner of women, we believe that further studies are needed to explore the impact of rape on partners of any gender or sexual orientation. The findings may be used by health care professionals to prepare and institute interventions to address the challenges and needs of both the primary victim and her partner at health facilities that serve rape victims in order to promote healing. Campaigners (or advocates) may also have a basis for expanding the impact of rape to intimate partners of the victims. International policymakers may also come together to discuss the crisis for couples postrape and to decide how best to support healing communities.

BACKGROUND

In South Africa, with its violent and oppressive history, the prevalence of rape is soaring (Dartnall & Jewkes, 2013; Meel, 2005). A total of 68,332 cases were reported to the South African Police Services during the period 2009/10, with the reported rape crime ratio of 100 per 100,000 of the population (South African Police Service, 2012). Most rapes occurred at the victim's home, and in 90% of cases the victims knew their attackers (Meel, 2005). Current South African statistics do not reflect the extent of sexual assault on women due to under reporting (Jacobson, 2009).

After reviewing literature in the field of sexual violence, it becomes clear that rape is a very traumatic experience for the female victims and for their partners (Banyard, Moynihan, Walsh, Cohn, & Ward, 2010; Remer, 2007). The effects of rape extend beyond the impact on the victim, and the authors therefore classify and discuss those effects as either primary or secondary. Although MIPs are classified as secondary victims, their experience is not downplayed; indeed, although they were not the direct recipient of the sexual assault trauma, they bear a serious burden (Remer, 2007; Remer & Ferguson, 1995).

Postrape, MIPs have been found to display some of the same symptoms that are found in primary rape victims (PRVs), including fearfulness, rage, and depression (Smith, 2005). It has also been documented that MIPs often experience a reluctance to talk about the rape with the PRV, display a constant fear for their safety as a couple, report recurrent thoughts about what could have been done to prevent the rape, and experience avoidance and arousal symptoms consistent with a post-traumatic stress disorder

(PTSD) diagnosis, such as avoiding the place where the rape took place and feeling hyperaroused to the point of being unable to sleep (Christiansen, Bak, & Elklit, 2012; McNair, 2010; Ullman, Townsend, Filipas, & Starzynski, 2007).

Consistent with PTSD, it is well documented that many PRVs feel angry, irritable, and have an increased level of arousal that manifests itself in feeling jumpy, agitated, jittery, and shaky; being easily startled; having trouble concentrating; and experiencing disorganized sleep patterns (Ahrens & Campbell, 2000; Christiansen et al., 2012; Duma, 2006; McNair, 2010; Smith, 2005). Often, MIPs are aggravated by this behavior and feel unhappy and frustrated with the way their partners have dealt with the rape. Barcus's case study (1997) of a therapy group for MIPs found that men felt isolated, confused, angry, powerless, and frustrated when living with their intimate partners' emotional reactions, which ranged from expressing grief and depression to exhibiting withdrawal, anxiety, phobias, fear, insomnia, and nightmares re-experiencing the trauma; crying; losing interest in people and past activities; lashing out at the MIP; and showing other emotional symptoms that manifest as changes in personality (Haansbaek, 2006a).

Ahrens and Campbell (2000) used victimization perspective theory (Janoff-Bulman & Frieze, 1983) to explain how secondary rape victims (SRV) try to help the PRV to cope with the psychological changes that follow rape. According to this theory, MIPs often do not understand how and why their female partners cope in the way they do with the rape. Male intimate partners (MIPs) believe that because they are raised to be strong and not allowed to cry in front of others, they should ignore their own emotions while remaining supportive of their female partners' needs (van Wijk, 2011). In the face of ineffective efforts to care for their partner, the MIP would often feel helpless and frustrated, which would strain his ability to cope with the rape and his relationship with the PRV (Ahrens & Campbell, 2000).

There are multiple ways in which the aftermath of rape can be studied in order to provide caregivers with the best tools to foster a couple's psychological healing after rape. Almost all of this work has been done by researchers aiming to improve the psychological adjustment of the PRV (Kilpatrick et al., 2003; Martin, Young, Billings, & Bross, 2007). Most international and South African researchers focus on the rape victim's experience of how the event affected the couple's relationship (Campbell & Wasco, 2005; Van den Berg & Pretorius, 1999). Other researchers have documented that the MIP is seldom assessed to establish how the rape event disrupted the couple's interpersonal and sexual relationship (Ahrens & Campbell, 2000; Campbell & Wasco, 2005; Daane, 2005; Duma, Mekwa, & Denny, 2007b; Smith, 2005).

Researchers have documented that rape can have a long-term psychological impact on the relationship of couples (Conner, 2006; Connop & Petrak, 2004, Jones, Schultz, & van Wijk, 2001; Smith, 2005). Various writers

(Janoff-Bulman & Frieze, 1983; Davis, Taylor, & Bench, 1995: Kilpatrick, Saunders, Veronen, Best, & Von, 1987) have indicated that postrape, couples face many challenges. These include, for example, blame for the primary victim's rape, fear of unwanted pregnancy, disenchantment with the criminal justice system, and overwhelming demands from the medical system. Due to the profound psychological effects of these challenges, there is a strong possibility that both partners may develop PTSD.

The psychological impact of the rape may culminate and manifest itself in how the couple resumes their sexual relationship. Because of the range of stressors the PRV experiences after an assault, consensual romantic sexual relationships can be placed under heavy strain, ultimately making sex a reminder of the rape. Overall, the effects of the rape on the couple's sexual functioning are multifaceted (Christiansen et al., 2012; Holmstrom & Burgess, 1979; White & Rollins, 1981). It may take time for the PRV to disassociate the sexual assault from consensual sex. Sexual encounters may trigger painful flashbacks. Although some survivors may not wish to be sexually active for a period of time, they may still have the need and desire for physical comfort and closeness. Male intimate partners (MIPs) may mistakenly think the PRV needs distance; the PRV misreads the MIP's distance as blaming and rejection. Most PRVs withdraw from sexual relationships and intimacy because they feel contaminated or ruined as a result of the assault. An individual reaction of this type is usually related to specific cultural definitions and stigmas assigned to being raped (Foa, Hembree, Riggs, Rauch, & Franklin, 2007).

Researchers have demonstrated that the tense and uncomfortable atmosphere between the couple and purposeful avoidance of each other may result in future difficulties with intimacy (Foa et al., 2007). While some couples find it helpful to stop having sex for a period of time while they work through the tragedy, some intimate partners may pressure their male partners into sex to ensure that the rape does not interfere with their sex life (Orzek, 1983). The result is an ongoing, unpleasant argument between the PRV and her MIP; this cycle demonstrates the way the rape disrupts the relationship (Foa et al., 2007). It is clear from the literature that interventions are needed to support the couple.

Despite the high number of negative consequences that a rape can have on a couple's relationship, Ahrens and Campbell (2000) and Haansbaek (2006a) found that the participants in their studies became closer and more intimate after the assault. This is consistent with the findings of Janoff-Bulman and Frieze (1983), who emphasize that if both the PRV and MIP are included from the beginning in support services offered to the rape victim, then the MIP will have a better understanding of his reactions and feelings, which will enable him to cope better with his reactions and feelings toward the rape. This in turn means the MIP will be better able to understand and support the victim. These authors make pragmatic suggestions that social support, especially the support of family, lovers, or friends, is a crucial aspect in the adjustment of the rape victim after rape.

In summary, there is minimal information available on how rape affects individuals close to the PRV, particularly her intimate partner. In South Africa, where the incidence of rape is high (Jacobson, 2009), little is known about the form of relational support that women receive after being raped, and how that support, or lack of support, contributes to healing after rape. It is possible that the rape of a woman could become a normative event in countries where the occurrence is inordinate. If researchers do not take the time to understand how the MIPs perceive this event, there will be no insights into the extent to which women are forced to return to homes where their rape is perceived by their partner as insignificant, stigmatizing, or upsetting. The rape should also be explored from the perspective of the MIP because, in this way, a clear identification of experiences may be made. Our current lack of understanding and knowledge restricts service providers and is a challenge to researchers who should provide a scientific basis for intervention strategies to combat the effect of sexual assault. The researchers conducted the study described in this article in an attempt to shed some light on this lack of understanding.

As far as could be ascertained, the first author of this article is the first person in South Africa to involve the participating intimate partners over an extended period. From a mental health perspective, 6 months is the minimum period required to study the delayed effects of rape and the victim's coping and adaptive strategies (or lack thereof). Hence, the victim's intimate partner must be followed for the same period of time while he responds to her postrape reactions. The primary aim of the researchers in conducting this study was to explore, analyze, and interpret the meaning that MIPs of female rape victims attach to their lived experience.

The research question that guided the researchers was the following: What are the lived experiences of intimate partners of female rape victims during the 6 months following the rape?

METHODOLOGY

A longitudinal, hermeneutic phenomenological approach was used to examine the phenomena of interest, after approval from the local institutional review board. While phenomenologists concentrate on the lived experiences of individuals within their life-world, eliciting commonalities and shared meanings, researchers using the hermeneutic interpretive theory of Paul Ricoeur focus on the interpretation of language and the meanings of individuals' experiences (Byrne, 1998; Creswell, 2004). Furthermore, hermeneutic phenomenology allows researchers to describe and to interpret the phenomenon while uncovering the lived experience in the text (Creswell, 2004). Ricoeur's analytical process shows the way that interpretation proceeds through multiple stages of understanding, where the interpreter seeks to understand what is expressed and unexpressed within the text (Ricoeur, 1976; Speziale & Carpenter, 2003).

The principal investigator designed the study to focus on the interpretation of language, and Ricoeur's work guided our approach to understanding the multiethnic world of the male in South Africa (Creswell, 2012; Lindseth & Norberg, 2004). First, the men's experiences were read and interpreted, bearing in mind the ethnic beliefs prevailing in the social environment from which the men originated. Next, the initial coding remained true to their words within their experiences as individuals, not as a group. At that stage, commonalities were found only if both the grammatical words and the ethnic meaning indicated an overlap; this was verified through several iterations based on the multiple interviews. Each MIP was interviewed four times over a period of 6 months. The multiple interviews provided a stronger base from which to interpret and understand their meaning, as change in the men's experience was always rooted in a description of prior meaning. The final themes, describing the essence of their experiences, represented how the men as a group experienced the impact of rape. By using a hermeneutic philosophical perspective we were able to draw from contextual meaning before finalizing that understanding.

Due to the therapeutic recommendation of involving the MIP in treatment immediately after the partner's rape (Janoff-Bulman & Frieze, 1983), the researchers chose to begin this investigation immediately after reporting the incident; the researchers followed the MIPs for a minimum of 6 months afterward. That period of 6 months allowed the MIP to explore his own lived experience as an MIP (Molloy, Woodfield, & Bacon, 2002) while he responded to the victim's adjustment to the event.

Ethical Considerations

Ethical approval was obtained from the Human Research Ethics Committee of the Faculty of Health Sciences, University of Cape Town, and from the recruitment site management. The researchers conducted the study in accordance with the principles of the Declaration of Helsinki (World Medical Association, October 2008). Provision was made for referral to counsellors in the case of those participants who either verbalized or displayed distress as a result of the interviews. All the participants' partners had been assaulted in or near their homes and thus participants were provided with other options for the interviews, as an interview in their homes might cause distress for the MIP and might be a safety issue for the interviewers. Participants were interviewed at a mutually agreed upon time and at a safe, comfortable venue. A thorough review of the ethical considerations was published with the pilot data (van Wijk & Harrison, 2013).

A reflective journal enabled the primary researcher to record perceptions, emotions, thoughts, and ideas related to the interviews. The principal investigator (first author) adhered to the principle of reflexivity by disclosing personal feelings, background, perceptions, preconceptions, biases, assumptions, and her role in the study (Guba & Lincoln, 1989; Patton, 2002).

Credibility was achieved through prolonged engagement with the phenomenon of interest and careful attention to the philosophically based design of the study.

Setting

Participants were recruited from a specialized center for the comprehensive treatment and support of victims of rape and sexual assault mostly living in low socioeconomic areas of Cape Town, South Africa. These participants were living in low-income housing or in informal settlements within 20 miles of the geographical area of the recruitment site. The center provided services for people from the surrounding areas, which comprised formal and informal housing settlements. The men were interviewed at times arranged by mutual agreement between the primary researcher and the participants.

Recruitment and Retention

Procedures for ethically accessing MIPs postrape were piloted to ensure feasibility (van Wijk & Harrison, 2013). This process was begun by contacting the attending medical and nursing staff who identified female rape victims who were in an intimate relationship with a partner of any gender; this identification was done either directly after the rape or at their 72-hour follow-up visit. The staff members were requested to inform victims gently of the nature of the study and to ask, without any pressure, whether they would meet with the researcher. Although 217 rape victims attended the selected facility during the time period, fewer than half learned of the study. The nurses at the facility reported they were either too busy or too short staffed, or they had forgotten about the study. From the 112 who were informed of the study, 44 chose not to participate or were hesitant to inform their partners. The 68 MIPs who were interested in the study were given the printed research information as well as the researcher's contact details to take to their partners.

A total of 68 MIPs contacted the primary researcher with an interest in participating in the study. After contact was initiated, the researcher met the potential participants. The nature of the study and the requirements for participation were explained. Of the 68 potential MIPs, 26 agreed to participate. In order to retain the sample, two contact numbers were recorded for each participant so that regular telephone contact could be maintained to remind participants of upcoming interviews. Seventeen participants completed the first two interviews, and nine participants successfully completed all four interviews scheduled. This analysis is based on data from the nine participants who completed the full study. Although all nine were positive about their involvement in the study, three participants related independently that speaking about their experiences appeared, at times, to elicit unanticipated negative feelings. They preferred, nevertheless, to continue to participate in the study. None of the participants needed or required referral for treatment related to these feelings. They also said that compensation for expenses incurred for taking part was not the reason for their involvement. Numerous attempts by the first author to contact those who did not appear for their follow-up interviews were unsuccessful, despite reimbursement. Analysis of the data of the recruits who did not complete all four interviews did not occur because those recruits did not satisfy the objectives of the longitudinal design. There are some possible explanations for their withdrawal: for example, they could have lost interest in the study, lost the researcher's contact details, or no longer wished to contribute to the knowledge base.

Sampling

Using purposeful sampling, we considered for the study all MIPs of victims who received treatment for rape at the previously mentioned center in Cape Town, South Africa, during the study period, if they met the inclusion criteria. The participants met those criteria if they were in an intimate relationship with a female rape victim before and immediately after the rape (as revealed by the rape victim to the nursing staff), were older than 18 years, were able to communicate in one of the three main languages spoken in the region, that is, isiXhosa, English, or Afrikaans, and, voluntarily contacted the researcher telephonically within 14 days of learning of the study to indicate willingness and availability to participate in the study for a period of 6 months. Partners of male rape victims were excluded from the study because of the specific issues relating to male rape; this would require a separate study from the perspective of an investigator applying a hermeneutic phenomenological approach.

Participants

Of the nine MIPs, six spoke English and three spoke isiXhosa. Demographic information obtained from each participant is detailed in Table 1. All nine cases of rape had been reported to the police. In all but one instance, persons

TABLE 1 Demographic Profile of Nine Male Intimate Partners

ID	Age	Education	Marriage status	Employment	Children
1	39	Five years of schooling	Married 5 years	Employed at a factory manufacturing building materials	2 children (ages 2 and 5)
2	38	Standard 8	Partner with girlfriend for 5 years	Grade 1 level security guard	Partner pregnant with twins
3	43	Standard 10	Married for 11 years	Waiter in a local restaurant	3 children (ages 2, 7, and 9)
4	37	Completed secondary school	Married for 9 years	Degree in civil engineering— temporary employment	4 children (ages 1, 5, 8, and 13)
5	33	Standard 8	Partner with girlfriend for 7 years	Panel beater	Partner 6 months pregnant; 1 child (age 4 years)
6	25	Postsecondary education— art and drama	Partner with girlfriend for 1 year	Unemployed	None
7	54	Standard 7	Married for 19 years	Truck driver at a beer factory	4 children
8	42	Postsecondary education— business administration	Married for 15 years	Manager of guest house	2 children (ages 11 and 13)
9	41	Standard 8	Partner with girlfriend for 14 months	Clothing industry	2 children (ages 9 and 11)

unknown to the victims or to the MIP were reported to have committed the crime. In the one instance, a neighbor was reported to have raped the MIP's wife. Six of the participants were South African, and the other three were either economic migrants or refugees from Central Africa.

Data Collection

The first author collected audio-taped data between August 2008 and August 2009. She conducted four face-to-face, in-depth interviews within a 6-month period with each participant. At each interview the research question had a specific focus as detailed in Table 2. Probes, active listening, and reflective comments were used to encourage the participants to elaborate on their feelings, as well as on positive and negative emotions and experiences. At the end of each interview session, key issues were summarized and discussed by the first author and the participant in English or through an isiXhosa

TABLE 2 Interview Guide

Interview	Timing of interview	Primary question	Probes
1	Within 14 days of the rape of partner	Your partner was raped on [date]. Have you experienced any changes between you and your partner since the incident?	I also would like you to tell me how you are dealing with these experiences.
2	End of the first month	Have you experienced any changes between you and your partner since the incident?	I also would like you to tell me how you are dealing with these experiences. Since your partner was raped, how are the communication and intimate relationship between you and your partner?
3	End of the third month	Have you experienced any changes between you and your partner since the incident?	I also would like you to tell me how you are dealing with these experiences. Since your partner was raped, how are the communication and intimate relationship between you and your partner?
4	End of 6 months: Final reflective interview	It is now 6 months since your partner was raped. Last time you said [depending on responses from previous interview session]. Today, I would like us to talk about how you are feeling now.	It is now 6 months since your partner was raped. Last time you said [depending on responses from previous interview session]. Today, I would like us to talk about how is the relationship now between you and your partner?

interpreter. These discussions were documented in field notes and were later incorporated into the analysis described below. The audio-taped data were transcribed verbatim and stored in a secure location after all data were deidentified to protect the confidentiality of participants. After the study, all contact information was destroyed.

Translation

A pilot study was conducted with two participants who met the criteria for inclusion in the study (van Wijk & Harrison, 2013). The pilot study enabled the primary researcher to modify the interview questions and ensure that the meaning in each of the languages was understood (Kim, 2011). As the first author was fluent in two of the three local languages, the pilot also highlighted the need for an isiXhosa-speaking interpreter to facilitate the recruitment process and expand data collection. The interpreter was trained in study procedures in order to ensure accurate understanding for final interpretations. Interviews were interpreted and translated into English during data collection, and then the verbatim transcriptions were checked and back-checked for accuracy by two bilingual translators. Preliminary data analysis of an interview transcript was done prior to the next interview with each participant in order to provide the foundation for the next interview.

Data Analysis

The data analysis methods of Colaizzi (1978) and the within-case and across-case approach of Ayres, Kavanaugh, and Knafl (2003) were used to analyze and interpret the transcribed data and the field notes. This time-sequenced approach to hermeneutic phenomenology and the lived experience is consistent with the work by Harrison and Stuifbergen (2005), which built on the reinterpretation of the past over time. In that respect, time unified and solidified the phenomenon for analysis. In this study, the authors build on that ability to understand a phenomenon with time and in doing so, analyze meaning as it unfolds repeatedly. For our MIPs, past experiences were brought into consciousness, while present time did not exist in conscious thought until it had passed and was given a reinterpretation; the result was a new discussion of past and present. Because what the MIPs "experience as present always contains memory of what has just been present" (Dilthey, 1985, p. 150), the potential for us to understand change in meaning was always present with each interview.

As a first step in the analysis, the transcribed and translated data were read through several times in chronological order. Next, significant statements relating to the MIP's perception of the couple's experience were identified. The meaning of each statement was labeled and organized into clusters. Those significant concepts that emerged were given a label that formed the basis of the categorization scheme. A Microsoft Word file was opened to create a conceptual file for each category. Thereafter, the researchers reduced the text with similar concepts into more manageable components for the purposes of retrieval and review. This process allowed the researchers to view the impact on the couple over time. Finally, a descriptive theme was created that captured the changes perceived in each couple's relationship over time.

The interpretation of the data involved reflecting, repeatedly, on what the researchers read in the transcribed text, with the aim of ensuring a comprehensive understanding of the findings. Dilthey (1985) wrote that hermeneutic understanding occurred within the mind-constructed world.

That world was an interaction of the lived experience, the insight into the mind, the understanding of other people, and the understanding of the historical community. Dilthey recognized that part of "understanding was irrational because life is irrational" (1985, p. 162). There are limits to the application of logic in understanding the lived experience. Hence, within our interpretation of the MIPs' words in this study, it was not our goal to justify or make their experiences seem logical, acceptable, or permissible; instead, our goal was to present their world to the reader. In doing this, as was the case for Ricoeur (1983), the objective of our interpretation was to produce an emotional relationship with the text that generated a new interpretation from the reader of this report.

FINDINGS

Over time, the MIPs discussed the evolution of their feelings toward their partners. This evolution allowed the researchers to witness as the MIPs struggled with how the rape impacted the foundation for their connection to their partners. Although the interpersonal struggles of the men will be published elsewhere, the researchers, in the following section, provide insight into the minds of the men as they discussed their relationship with the women in their lives after they were raped. The following themes best relate how these discussions were interpreted. They include the following: fear of infection; the sex act; given a blind eye; and connecting with her emotions.

Fear of Infection

All participants, at the initial interview session, stated that before the rape they had a good relationship with their partners. What was before and the reality of what existed now was evident in their statements. During the initial interview sessions the fear of contracting an infection and, more specifically, human immunodeficiency virus (HIV), was clearly evident. The MIPs voiced their fears, their struggles with sexual restraint, and their desires for interfamilial safety. For instance, one participant acknowledged that he could be directly, physically injured due to the rape of his wife by an attacker. He said, "What now if my partner has been infected? You know, it's going to affect me for the rest of my life." Another participant acknowledged that the impact could have a long-standing impact on his health, the health of his children, and the health of his wife:

> They pulled her blood, and in that time that she was waiting for the blood results, I told her that we can't have sex because I was very scared that she will get the HIV and also me. I was thinking of our two children, that their mother can die, and then my wife is dead.

The realization that an infection of their wives through rape could affect them and their families affected multiple aspects of the men's lives, including their sexual activities. A participant stated, "So the thought of HIV really affects my sex life; in fact, I have no sex life on the moment." This remained a large part of their focus a month after the rape. One participant struggled with the idea of using a condom as if this represented a barrier to intimacy and a reminder of the rape. He stated, "Our sex life is bad because I don't want to use a condom any longer, but I still have a fear to get AIDS."

As time progressed, the fear of infection remained, regardless of the level of desire for sexual intimacy and their fondness for their wives. The MIPs' reports did, however, move from descriptions of fears and responses directly voiced from the perspective of the men, to reports echoing the perspective of the united couple. This trend is clear in the statement of one participant, who told of how the use of a condom became a new normal for their sexual relationship. He stated, "We're still using protection because I know she is my partner, and she knew the same. We didn't use protection before, and although the blood results were negative, we rather want to be safe."

This was not to infer that the men gradually reached a level of acceptance in their relationships. It was quite the contrary; there were relationship challenges due to fears of infection that seemed to never abate. As one participant explained, his fears of infection coupled with his wife's response to the possibility of infection caused friction within their sex lives and on-going relationship:

> We try to understand each other, and at the moment, our sex life is slowly becoming a little bit better, but I am still a bit scared because she did tell me last time that she must still go back for her blood results to see if she is infected with the sickness or not. She didn't go and fetch it up till now. And this causes sometimes friction between us.

The MIPs' movement from voicing an individual fear to voicing a couple's needs was the most indicative of their perception that they were in the experience together. The desire to protect the self, but to also remain committed to the relationship, demonstrated the MIPs' commitment to more than just their own wants and needs. This was clear when a participant who had been initially upset by using a condom stated after months had passed, "If I just think of that, I am so bitter and angry. In that time, I felt very distant from her because I have to use a condom, but I was thinking if it is the best for me and for her, then I will do so."

The Sex Act

In this theme, the researchers examine the men's views of the sex act as a performance of their interpersonal bond and how that bond was, or was not, restored. If the MIPs could go beyond the pain felt due to the rape of their partners, then they resumed an active sex life as soon after the rape as permissible. For the MIPs, the relationship with their partners encompassed an inflexible need that connected the physical and emotional aspects of their bodies.

Regardless of the state of their relationship at the time of the interviews, the MIPs all voiced a need for sexual activity. The participants believed that sex not only enhanced their relationships, but it was also a defining aspect. The sex act was a means to fulfilling a masculine sense of self, regardless of their fears of infection. This was evident when an MIP stated, "Because the thing that hurts me the most is that she disrespects my sexual needs. It's very disturbing to me to not have sex with my wife. It's very, very disturbing." This was in contrast to a participant who reported that he and his partner had a mutual understanding of their sexual needs, which had always helped him cope with life's circumstances:

> Although I am afraid of getting HIV, we use a condom for our own protection, but nothing have [sic] changed between me and her; there is no difference in our sex life after the rape. Both of us think of each other and show that we have a need for sex. As it was all the time of our life together.

The men also voiced a need for sex as a means to assert their masculine role and status within the relationship. A need for sex as a means of asserting masculinity was evident when an MIP stated, "Since my wife was raped, both of us have a desire for sex, and although I used a condom, I just tell her, 'I am your husband,' and we hug and kiss each other, and both of us enjoy it." The MIP was clear that sex was a part of his role within their relationship, and within that role sex either was, or should be, pleasurable. This view of sex was expressed by another participant:

> Even if I refrain myself from embarrassing her about sex sometimes, I do ask. And then after lots of begging from my side, we have sex. But she just do it but doesn't feel or enjoy anything. This is not how I know my wife.

The nature of the sex act subsequently became a symbol for the condition of their relationship after the rape. As a participant stated, "I want that our sex life must get stronger, and our communication with each other must be the same as before the rape took place." Without the sex act, the relationship and the man would suffer. This was clear when a participant stated, "I crave doing sex, things that I have before. In fact, there is now nothing between us, which I cannot accepted [sic] any longer."

During interview sessions 3 months after the rape, two participants indicated that although they understood that their partners did not desire sex due to their feelings surrounding the rape, they hoped that their partners would understand the MIPs' physical and emotional needs, demonstrated through the sex act. They believed that such an understanding would eventually lead their partners to desire sexual intercourse again. The participants added that as men they need the same physical contact and intimacy as before the rape, which require her emotional commitment to the act. The rape had not affected the meaning of the sex act from the MIPs' perspective. The MIPs still needed the same sexual acts, but they perceived that their partners had changed, as one man related:

> When it comes to the point where I ask her for sex, she get very cross, and then I say to her, "I am tired of those excuses to avoid having sex." That's why I say those problems will be for a long time, if not permanent with us, you know; it's for a long time. I can't go on any longer; I cannot see that I can have sex with my wife ever again after someone else put his penis into her. I just sleep without touching her, and sometimes I sleep in another room. It's changed the foundation of my marriage permanently. But my faith as a Christian is what still keeps me with her.

"Given a Blind Eye"

While some participants initially described an understanding of their partner's avoidance of sex and her negative emotions, most participants grew increasingly frustrated with time as they lost sight of the bonds they shared before the rape. What they thought was a temporary crisis continued, as if the event had permanently blinded their partner to their needs. In this theme, the researchers identify and describe a lonely, isolated sentiment: A connection no longer existed for a recipient. It was this severing of linkages that prevented most MIPs from connecting to their partners; however, in some cases, it was what allowed the couple to move past the rape.

Those participants with minimal sexual interactions with their partners after the rape expressed that if they did have sex, it was repulsive. They spoke openly of how their partners' negative remarks and lethargic attitude toward sex disappointed and frightened them. An MIP stated, "After the rape, her personality changed. She is cold and does not want to be touched; if I talk to her about it, she gets angry and ignores me. It makes me so frustrated to get on without sex." Another participant explained how his partner's negative attitude toward sex and her fear of being touched concerned him in terms of their future. He said, "For 2 weeks we have not done sex because my girlfriend is afraid to be touched and just give me a blind eye. I can take anything but that." For these men, being given a blind eye meant more than being denied sex. It meant that their needs were not seen and not acknowledged.

Two participants specified that their lack of sexual activity and their partners' unwillingness to restore their lives were troubling. Those two participants described continuous frustrations and obstructions that affected their feelings toward their partners. This was clear in the excerpt below:

> From a few days ago, she don't want anything to do with our sexual life; she has so many excuses and said she is too scared for it. Sex let her think of the day she was raped. Although I try to understand that the incident is still fresh in her mind, I don't know how I can explain to her that she must accept and forget about the rape. I mean, I try so hard to make peace with it. Why can she also not try to do the same?

It was as if the men were no longer recognized by their partners as the men they were before the rape. They sensed they could choose between being gone or being wrong, "because nothing that I am doing seems right in her eyes." Another participant explained how his partner's negative attitude toward their life together as a couple affected his feelings of being understood as a man with emotional and physical needs within their marriage. On one day he shared what he had told her:

> "Although you are not feeling for sex, do you not understand my needs?" ... The way she treated me makes me so agitated and sexually frustrated. But the consequences of the rape are the cause of the problems between us. She is associating sex with violence. So, there's no kissing. There's no more hugging. You know, if she sleep [sic] this side, I look that side. That it is not well, and it cause tension between us.

While some participants described a decline in the quality of their relationships, and some entertained the thought of taking lovers, there were others who saw how to be fully present for their partners. Indeed, as one MIP suggested, these men learned to give the rapist a blind eye. The MIP stated, "We both forget the rape now, so, ja, there are no bad things between me and my woman." This required a conscious effort to keep the rapist out of their marriage through the heartfelt adage, "Every time when we are down, I hold her while telling her that we're not making him part of our life."

Connecting With Her Emotions

There are times when people in intimate relationships are able to communicate their thoughts and desires without saying a word. Years of conflict and subsequent resolution have typically built up a good interpersonal understanding, which means that, often, little needs to be said in words. Thus, men and women do not need to speak to their partners in order to be understood; the partner could be fully aware and responsive to the other's feelings without sharing as much as a whisper. The severity and uniqueness of rape in the lives of couples, however, demands that words be spoken. Clarity was not found in the silent assumptions of the MIPs as to the needs of the rape victims.

Because a disturbance in communication between the MIPs and their partners was evident months after the rape, some participants admitted that they preferred to avoid conversations with their partners about the rape for fear of evoking unpleasant feelings between them. As one MIP stated, "When I start talking to her about how the rape affected both our lives and marriage, the one moment, she start to cry, the other moment, she is so agitated and accuse me that I don't care about how she is feeling and that I don't know what she is going through." Due to the MIPs' perceptions of their partners' emotions, they were unsure of how to approach their partners and of what to say. Silence was often the solution. Initially they feared that talking about the rape could worsen their relationship, as illustrated in the following excerpt:

> My communication with my wife regarding this issue, I think we don't talk about it. I think it is my fault; I am just safeguarding her for her own interest because I wouldn't want her to reflect on the issue again. But on the other hand, it is more harmful for our relationship, and if we want to both get over it, we will have to talk about it, but I think also we are both scared of how and what to say to each other.

The MIPs attempted to go about their lives struggling to hide their feelings while trying not to trigger the expression of their partners' feelings. An MIP noted how he danced around her emotions; he stated, "I rather keep quiet because I am not sure how she will react. I rather struggle on my own, which is no good for me." One participant reported that although a slight improvement in communication between him and his partner was apparent, he preferred to omit the event from their conversations, fearing that the topic might evoke feelings in both of them, as he disclosed:

> Although my girlfriend is in the Eastern Cape with her parents to help her with the babies, we communicate each day. But we don't even go so far as to discuss the rape because it's going to be like now. I am afraid I will go back to that thing where I wasn't feeling well, but sometimes we can tell each other how we are feeling. It was not like this till 2 months ago.

Ultimately, the decision to avoid discussing their feelings left the MIPs isolated. One participant specified that his partner's behavior was irritating him.

He believed that together with his alcohol problem, which began after the rape, their lack of communication was preventing them from progressing with their lives together:

> Because she was pregnant and not feeling so good, we never had time to talk about the rape so we leave the issue of the rape out of our conversations. I also don't know her feelings yet. So both of us are not okay; and my heavy drinking since the rape added stress in our relationship, which caused so much conflict between us and because of all these, both of us are not moving on with our lives.

As time continued passing, 24 weeks after the rape, the MIPs spoke of an improvement in their communication with their partners. They began to know their partners again. They were no longer "strangers." The women they knew before the rape and the connection that made them partners reemerged. As a participant stated, "I love her very much, she's my wife. In the beginning, as I told you, she felt like a stranger to me, but now, I'm start talking to her about the rape, and she talks to me. I tell her, 'Don't worry.'" The renewal of the relationship through understanding also gave the couple permission to forgive and forget. This was voiced by a participant who had struggled greatly with his own fears postrape:

> Like I said earlier on, if she is not okay, I just tell her to like forget what happened to her, and forgive, and just try to get on with her life. And, also, because we talk now, how we feel after he [sic] rape. We support each other. I think me and she's coping quite well.

Although communication did not fully improve for all of the couples, it was clear that communication had been altered by the rape, and that once it improved, the MIPs were more satisfied with the whole of their relationships.

DISCUSSION

The goal of the researchers was to conduct a study providing insights into the mind-constructed world of rape victims in South Africa, as described by MIPs. The study has limitations; for example, the small sample size with multiple drop-outs and refusals may have skewed the results toward those participating MIPs who may have experienced the event in way that differed from the others who left the study. Furthermore, these men might have had a connection to their partners that differed from those MIPs who refused to participate, leaving the reader with a biased view of how men perceive their partner's rape. For these reasons, the results should be considered with some degree of caution. Regardless, a strong point of this study was the longitudinal design, which allowed the researchers to follow these MIPs as their life worlds were interpreted and reinterpreted over 6 months. This design prevented the researchers from drawing quick conclusions, yielding to the temptation of interpreting the MIP experience based upon momentary or one-time descriptions, or both possibilities.

Furthermore, the philosophical perspective driving the researchers was carefully integrated into the analysis, allowing the researchers to understand how changes in meaning were interpreted with time. The men spoke openly about the changing meaning the rape had for their lives. The connections they had with their partners were broken or damaged and although they felt their partners' pain they also felt their own needs. Logic and rational decision making might have demanded a different response from the men as they deciphered what the rape meant for them and their futures. Instead, the MIPs spoke of how their partners' objective bodies were given new meaning either by her or by the MIP based upon the rape performed by a stranger.

As mental health and women's health researchers and advocates, we do not suggest that the MIPs' needs equal or surpass those of the rape victim. It is important we understand the MIPs' experience, however, in order to bests prepare the rape victim for the environment to which she will return postrape. Health care providers should also offer the couple the best opportunity for long-term adjustment. In this effort, while we are not generalizing to the larger population, we did build on previous findings and we added to the literature in four ways. First, the MIP's initial reaction may not be his main focus over time; second, the MIP may put his partners needs above his own; third, the MIP may be able to overcome his resentments directed at the rapist by "turning a blind eye" to the assailant; and, finally, intimacy, communication, and sexual acts may have enduring significance in the MIP's mind-constructed world.

Van Manen (1990), who approached the life world in terms of the lived space and time, characterized relationships as fragmented, communication as tentative, and intimacy as erratic unless renegotiated. Consistent with this phenomenological understanding of relationships in time and space, the rape of a partner set off a sequence of events that changed how the MIPs perceived the nature of their relationships with the primary victims. For instance, the interpretation of the use of a condom moved from being perceived as a loss of pleasure to a protective sacrifice for both the MIP and his partner. The meanings were not static and the past was reinterpreted. Beckham and Beckham (2004) reported that after the rape, a couple's belief in a safe and secure environment is shattered. The lack of safety within the relationship was not a prominent theme throughout this study. This may be due to the frequency of rape in South Africa. It is most likely due to the type of analysis performed here, however, which focused primarily on the phenomenon over time. Threatened safety may be more fixed in space and time at the beginning of their experiences with less reinterpretation than is intimacy and the act of sex. The consequences of the rape, which were reported as lost intimacy and sexual contact, have been found to become part of psychological identity after rape (Christiansen et al., 2012; Remer & Ferguson, 1995).

Secondary victims experience trauma symptoms similar to those of the primary victims and survivors (Morrison, Quadara, & Boyd, 2007; Remer, 2001). Secondary victims often receive recognition, not because they are also traumatized, but rather because of the need for their attention by the primary victim during his or her healing process. The actions and reactions of secondary victims can affect the recovery process of the primary victims (Duma, 2006; Morrison et al., 2007; Remer, 2001). The experiences of the MIPs after the rape of their spouse shed light on their struggles as reactions to the rape, unique from the direct effects experienced by his partner. For instance, the MIP who began drinking after his pregnant wife was raped reported that his actions compounded the detrimental effects the rape had on his partner, his relationship, and on his health. The MIPs' ability to cope postrape deserves attention due to the MIPs' potential to assist their partners' healing, but it also deserves attention due to the profound impact the rape may have on their mental and physical health.

In this study, the MIPs experienced sexual rejection from their partners. This rejection threatened their masculinity and their role within the relationship. In accordance with the results of Smith (2005) and Smith and Kelly (2001), the MIPs reported that, although they had secure positive relationships with their partners before the rape, the rape left them psychologically traumatized and confused about how to show their support for their partner and how to deal with the possible health damaging consequences of rape. They struggled with supporting their partner and maintaining their past sense of self. In contrast to the findings of Holmstrom and Burgess (1979), who found that most of the respondents in their study blamed their partner, the female victim, for the rape, none of the MIPs in our study discussed these feelings. In the process of comforting their partners, over time the MIPs preferred to put their own needs and feelings aside for their partners. It is unclear how long the MIPs may be able to maintain this position.

Various writers such as Christiansen and colleagues (2012), Smith and Kelly (2001), and Rudd (2003) found that most of the respondents in their studies had experienced problems in their relationship with the rape victim. Their findings are in accordance with prior studies. This emphasizes, further, the view that rape is a devastating experience and a shared crisis for couples, which is consistent with the view of the MIPs in this study. For example, relationship problems of a communicative nature were particularly common.

Intimacy, particularly sexual intimacy, is for many couples an intensely private space, in which there is a sense of knowing and being known.

The violation of one partner creates disequilibrium, a loss of that which is known and precious, and the fear of entering a space that is no longer safe and even sacred. Because the normal sexual style of the couple becomes disrupted after a rape, most of the MIPs reported a fear of infection and a loss of what was pleasurable and customary in the past.

The outcome of this study has implications for policymakers, nurse-training providers, and health care professionals who provide support services for female rape victims. The MIPs in this study repeatedly stressed the need for information and integrated counselling for couples. Despite the plea for support postrape, there was limited support in South Africa for couples (Duma et al., 2007b; Duma, Mekwa, & Denny, 2007a; Rudd, 2003; Van den Berg & Pretorius, 1999).

The scope of the study was limited to the experience of the nine participants who dedicated hours of their lives to improving our understanding of the essence of being an MIP of a rape victim. The transferability of the finding is accentuated by the researchers' careful attention to the methodological procedures for analysis, by the inclusion of multiple researchers' insights, and by the systematic in-depth data collection and analysis.

CONCLUSION

The authors of this article reported on the lived experiences of male intimate partners (MIPs) postrape in South Africa. The study was conducted by applying a hermeneutic phenomenological design using longitudinal interviews with nine men over a 6-month period. It is our conclusion that the prospective design allowed us to capture changes in meaning, which were subtle but clearly evident as the men moved from a focus on individual needs to the needs of the couple. Despite a limited sample size and multiple drop-outs, the findings highlighted how future research should consider the experience of the MIP in the couples' healing postrape.

FUNDING

The authors disclosed receipt of the following financial support for the research, authorship, and or publication of this article: the research was partially funded by an African Doctoral Dissertation Research Fellowship award offered by the African Population and Health Research Centre (APHRC) in partnership with the International Development Research Centre (IDRC) and also partially funded by a bursary from Margaret McNamara Research Foundation.

REFERENCES

Ahrens, C. E., & Campbell, R. (2000). Assisting rape victims as they recover from rape. *Journal of Interpersonal Violence, 15*(9), 959–986.

Ayres, L., Kavanaugh, K., & Knafl, K. A. (2003). Within-case and across-case approaches to qualitative data analysis, *Qualitative Health Research, 13*(6), 871–883.

Banyard, V. L., Moynihan, M. M., Walsh, W. A., Cohn, E. S., & Ward, S. (2010). Friends of survivors: The community impact of unwanted sexual experiences. *Journal of Interpersonal Violence, 25*(2), 242–256.

Barcus, R. (1997). Partners of survivors of abuse: A men's therapy group. *Psychotherapy, 34*(3), 316–323.

Beckham, E., & Beckham, C. (2004). *Coping with trauma and post traumatic stress disorder.* Retrieved from http://www.drbeckham.com/handouts/CHAP11_COPING_WITH_PTSD.pdf

Byrne, M. (1998). *Hermeneutics 101.* Retrieved from http://www.coe.uga.edu/quig/byrne.html

Campbell, R., & Wasco, S. (2005). Understanding rape and sexual assault: 20 years of progress and future directions. *Journal of Interpersonal Violence, 20*(1), 127–131.

Christiansen, D., Bak, R., & Elklit, A. (2012). Secondary victims of rape. *Violence and Victims, 27*(2), 246–262.

Colaizzi, P. (1978). Psychological research as the phenomenologist views it. In R. Valle & M. King (Eds.), *Existential-Phenomenological Alternatives for Psychology* (pp. 48–71). New York, NY: Oxford University Press.

Conner, M. G. (2006). *Coping and surviving violent and traumatic events.* Retrieved from http://www.tsunamisupportnetwork.org.uk/sa_index.asp?id = 42631

Connop, V., & Petrak, J. (2004). The impact of sexual assault on heterosexual couples. *Sexual & Relationship Therapy, 19*(1), 29–38.

Creswell, J. W. (2004). *Five qualitative approaches to inquiry.* Retrieved from http://209.85.129.104/search?q = cache:qEkrlejaA8EJ:www.sagepub.com/upm-data/1342

Creswell, J. W. (2012). *Qualitative inquiry and research design. Choosing among the five traditions* (3rd ed.). Thousand Oaks, CA: Sage.

Daane, D. M. (2005). The ripple effects: Secondary sexual assault survivors. In F. P. Reddington & B. W. Kreisel (Eds.), *Sexual assault: The victims, the perpetrators and the criminal justice system* (pp. 48–71). Durham, NC: Carolina Academic Press.

Dartnall, E., & Jewkes, R. (2013). Sexual violence against women: The scope of the problem. Best practice and research. *Clinical Obstetrics & Gynaecology, 27*(1), 3–13.

Davis, R. C., Taylor, B., & Bench, S. (1995). Impact of sexual and non sexual assault on secondary victims. *Violence and Victims, 10*(1), 73–84.

Dilthey, W. (1985). Draft for a critique of historical reason. In K. Mueller-Vollmer (Ed.), *The Hermeneutic Reader* (pp. 148–164). New York, NY: Continuum.

Duma, S. (2007). *Women's journey of recovery from sexual assault trauma.* Retrieved from http://www.curationis.org.za/index.php/curationis/article/download/1111/1046

Duma, S., Mekwa, J., & Denny, L. (2007a). Women's journey of recovery from sexual assault trauma: A grounded theory. Part 1. *Curationis, 30*(3), 4–11.

Duma, S., Mekwa, J., & Denny, L. (2007b). Women's journey of recovery from sexual assault trauma: A grounded theory. Part 2. *Curationis, 30*(4), 12–20.

Foa, E. B., Hembree, E. A., Riggs, D., Rauch, S., & Franklin, M. (2007). *Common reactions after trauma.* Retrieved from http://www.fthood.healthandperformance solutions.net/.../Common%20Reactions%2

Guba, E. G., & Lincoln, Y. (1989). *Fourth generation evaluation.* Newbury Park, CA: Sage.

Haansbaek, T. (2006). Partner to a rape victim: How is he doing? *Journal of Sex Research, 43*(1), 2–37.

Harrison, T., & Stuifbergen, A. (2005). A hermeneutic phenomenological study of women aging with childhood onset disability. *Health Care for Women International, 26,* 731–747.

Holmstrom, L., & Burgess, A. (1979). Rape: The husband's and boyfriend's initial reactions. *JSTOR: Family Coordinator, 28*(3), 321–330.

Jacobson, C. (2009). *Rape linked to manhood in South Africa.* Retrieved from http://www.chicagodefender.com/article-5462-rape-linked-to-manhood-in-south-afric a.html

Janoff-Bulman, R., & Frieze, I. H. (1983). A theoretical perspective for understanding reactions to victimization. *Journal of Social Issues, 39,* 1–17.

Jones, P. M., Schultz, H., & van Wijk, T. (2001). *Trauma in Southern Africa: Understanding emotional trauma and aiding recovery.* Retrieved from http://www. saps.gov.za/statistics/reports/farmattacks/_pdf/part17.pdf

Karim, A. (2013). *Rape culture is a worldwide problem and these organizations are solving it.* Retrieved from http://www.policymic.com/articles/64525/rape-culture-is-a-worldwide-problem-and-these-organizatizations-are-solving-it

Kilpatrick, D. G., Ruggiero, K. J., Acierno, R., Saunders, B. E., Resnick, H. S., & Best, C. L. (2003). Violence and risk of PTSD, major depression, substance abuse/dependence, and comorbidity: Results from the National Survey of Adolescents. *Journal of Consulting and Clinical Psychology, 71,* 692–700.

Kilpatrick, D. G., Saunders, B. E., Veronen, L. J., Best, C. L. & Von, J. M. 1987. Criminal victimisation: Lifetime prevalence, reporting to police, and psychological impact. *Crime and Delinquency, 33*(4), 479–489.

Kim, Y. (2011). The pilot study in qualitative inquiry. *Qualitative Social Work, 10*(2), 190–206.

Lindseth, A., & Norberg, A. (2004). A phenomenological hermeneutical method for researching lived experience. *Scandinavian Journal of Caring Sciences, 18*(2), 145–153.

Martin, S. L., Young, S. K., Billings, D. L., & Bross, C. C. (2007). Health care-based interventions for women who have experienced sexual violence: A review of the literature. *Trauma, Violence and Abuse, 8,* 3–18.

McNair, R. (2010). *Coping with rape: A husband's journey.* Retrieved from http://www.womensweb.ca/violence/rape/husband.php

Meel, B. L. (2005). Incidence of HIV infection at the time of incident reporting, in victims of sexual assault, between 2000 and 2004, in Transkei, Eastern Cape, South Africa. *African Health Sciences, 5*(3), 207–212.

Molloy, D., Woodfield, K., & Bacon, J. (2002). *Longitudinal qualitative research approaches in evaluation studies, Working Paper No. 7.* London, England: Her Majesty's Stationery Office (HMSO).

Morrison, Z., Quadara, A., & Boyd, C. (2007). Ripple effects of sexual assault. *Australian Institute of Family Studies, 7,* 1–3. Retrieved from http://aifs.gov.au/acssa/pubs/issue/i7html

Orzek, A. M. (1983). Sexual assault: The female victim, her male partner, and their relationship. *The Personnel and Guidance Journal, 62*(3), 143–146.

Patton, M. Q. (2002). *Qualitative research & evaluation methods* (2nd ed.). Thousand Oaks, CA: Sage.

Remer, R. (2001). *Secondary victims of trauma: Secondary survivors.* Retrieved from http://www.uky.edu/~rremer/secondarysur/SOCIASEC.doc

Remer, R. (2007). *Secondary victims of trauma: Secondary survivors.* Retrieved from http://www.uky.edu/~rremer/secondarysur/SOCIASEC.doc

Remer, R., & Ferguson, R. A. (1995). Becoming a secondary survivor of sexual assault. *Journal of Counselling & Development, 73*(4), 407–413.

Ricoeur, P. (1976). *Interpretation theory: Discourse and the surplus of meaning.* Fort Worth, TX: Texas Christian Press.

Ricoeur, P. (1983). *Time and narrative.* (K. McLaughlin & D. Pellauer, Trans.). Chicago, IL: University of Chicago Press.

Rudd, L. (2003). *The effects of rape on the social functioning of the family.* Retrieved from http://www.ujdigispace.uj.ac.za:8080/dspace/bitstream/.../ThesissubmissionChps123.pdf

Smith, M. E. (2005). Female sexual assault: The impact on the male significant other. *Issues in Mental Health Nursing, 26*(2), 149–167.

Smith, M. E., & Kelly, L. M. (2001). The journey of recovery after a rape experience. *Issues in Mental Health Nursing, 22*(4), 337–352.

South African Police Service. (2012). *Crime Statistics: April 2011–March 2012.* Retrieved from http://www.saps.gov.za/statistics/reports/crimestats/2012/crime_stats.htm

Speziale, H. J., & Carpenter, D. J. (2003). *Qualitative research in nursing. Advancing the humanistic imperative* (3rd ed.). Philadelphia, PA: Lippincott Williams & Wilkins.

Ullman, S. E., Townsend, S. M., Filipas, H. H., & Starzynski, L. L. (2007). Structural models of the relations of assault severity, social support, avoidance coping, self-blame, and PTSD among sexual assault survivors. *Psychology of Women Quarterly, 31*(1), 23–37.

Van den Berg, D., & Pretorius, R. (1999). The impact of stranger rape on the significant other. *Acta Criminologica, 13*(3), 92–104.

Van Manen, M. (1990). *Researching lived experience.* London, Ontario: State University of New York Press.

van Wijk, E. (2011). *The lived experience of male intimate partners of female rape victims in Cape Town, South Africa.* Retrieved from http://www.research2011.uct.ac.za

van Wijk, E., & Harrison, T. (2013). *Managing ethical problems in qualitative research involving vulnerable populations, using a pilot study.* Retrieved from http://ejournals.library.ualberta.ca/index.php/IJQM/article/view/18806 January 2014

White, P. N., & Rollins, J. C. (1981). Rape: Family crisis. *Family Relations*, *30*(1), 103–109.

World Medical Association. (2008, October). *Declaration of Helsinki: Ethical principles for medical research involving human subjects.* Paper presented at the 59th General Assembly, Seoul, South Korea.

The Place of Birth in Kafa Zone, Ethiopia

RUTH JACKSON

Alfred Deakin Research Institute, Deakin University, Geelong, Victoria, Australia

In this qualitative study, I used an ethnographic approach to provide an understanding about the place of birth in rural and semi-urban Kafa Zone, Ethiopia. I interviewed women about birth at home and asked what would happen if there were serious problems and a woman was taken to a health facility. The development of health services aimed at reducing maternal mortality implies that the place of birth must change from home to health facility, but the distance from international policy to its implementation is vast and the pathway is not a direct, linear route.

Childbirth is a process personal, collective, physical, symbolic, significant in countless ways. It is also a sometimes precarious deliverer of life and death. —Lukere, 2002, p. 201

Of all the health statistics monitored by the World Health Organization (WHO), maternal mortality has the highest discrepancy between developing and developed countries (WHO, United Nations International Children's Emergency Fund [UNICEF], United Nations Population Fund [UNFPA], & The World Bank, 2012). Maternal mortality levels in many developing countries are similar to those of the more developed regions of the world at the late nineteenth century (De Brouwere et al., 1998; Loudon, 1992). The reduction of maternal mortality by three quarters by 2015 was endorsed as a major international development goal at the Millennium Summit in 2000 (United Nations, 2000), but data to monitor the progress of the Millennium Development Goals (MDGs) shows that sub-Saharan Africa has the lowest level of maternal mortality ratio (MMR) decline. Although there has been international consensus about the need to prioritize maternal mortality as a health issue, there has not always been consensus about how to do this. This issue needs further attention as distance to health services is a common barrier for women in remote locations in developing countries such as Ethiopia.

In the key medical literature, many researchers take for granted that high rates of maternal mortality and disability will be reduced through the transfer of modern health service interventions. For example, the health center intrapartum-care strategy means that all women should have access to skilled birth attendants, referral for emergency obstetric care (EmOC), and other strategies that complement those targeted at the intrapartum period including antenatal (ANC) and postpartum care, family planning, safe abortion, and treatment for preexisting ill health particularly those causing indirect death such as infections, chronic disease, or malaria (Campbell & Graham, 2006; see also The Partnership for Maternal, Newborn & Child Health, 2010). A skilled attendant is an accredited health professional—such as a midwife, doctor, or nurse—who has been educated and trained to proficiency in the skills needed to manage normal (uncomplicated) pregnancies, childbirth and the immediate postnatal period, and in the identification, management, and referral of complications in women and newborns (WHO, 2004). Other researchers argue for a more comprehensive perspective to understand the problems of maternal mortality and include, for example, "the macrostructural—i.e. the social, cultural, economic and political—determinants of health" (Gil-González et al., 2006, p. 904) as service availability alone is not enough to increase utilization and reduce maternal mortality (Barker et al., 2007; Jackson, 2013).

Ethiopia is committed to achieving the MDGs as a framework for measuring progress toward sustainable development and eliminating poverty—one of the aims of Ethiopia's *Reproductive Health Strategy* is to "ensure its place in the national development agenda" (Ministry of Health [MOH], 2006a, p. 7). The MDG 5 aims to reduce by three-quarters, between 1990 and 2015, the MMR. The MMR measures the number of maternal deaths during a given time period per 100,000 live births during the same time period (WHO et al., 2012). A case in point is Ethiopia with an MMR of 350 maternal deaths per 100,000 live births in 2010 and a lifetime risk of maternal death of one in 67 (WHO et al., 2012). Hogan and colleagues (2010) estimate, however, that the MMR in Ethiopia was 590 per 100,000 live births and the 2011 Ethiopian Demographic and Health Survey (DHS) MMR estimate was 676 maternal deaths per 100,000 live births for the 7-year period preceding the survey (Central Statistical Authority [CSA] & ICF International, 2012).

Many strategic objectives in Health Sector Development Program IV 2010/11–2014/15 emphasize maternal and newborn care (MOH, 2010), but the targets for reducing the MMR and increasing the proportion of births attended by a skilled birth attendant are unlikely to be met by 2015 (Koblinsky et al., 2010). Only 10% of women give birth with the assistance of a trained or skilled health professional, and 28% of birthing women are supported by a traditional birth attendant (TBA). The majority of births are attended by a relative or some other person (57%), and 4% of women give birth without any type of assistance at all (CSA & ICF International, 2012). The most important barriers to accessing health services during pregnancy and birth are lack of transportation, lack of money, and distance to a health facility (CSA & ICF International, 2012).

I conducted a qualitative study to examine the place of "normal" birth in rural and semiurban southwest Ethiopia and also considered what it means for women if they are transferred to a health facility when there is a problem during childbirth. In this article, I also examine the importance of the mother–daughter relationship and decision making because these factors impact on the reason normal birth takes place at home. My article is drawn from a larger study from 2007, where reproductive health, in particular MDG 5, provided an entry point to study Ethiopia's development agenda (Jackson, 2010).

METHOD

My research was not an anthropological account of childbirth but an ethnographic approach to juxtapose women's experiences of birth at home with that in a health facility to explore the sociocultural processes that influence women's choices affecting ANC and childbirth. During the fieldwork I focused on the relationships women form and the work they do in and around their households because I wanted to contextualize how childbirth fits into their world. Maternal mortality is the antithesis of birth as a life-giving process; it can also reveal the complexity of the issues and the diverse social, cultural, economic, and environmental settings for changes in maternal health to take place (Boddy, 1998). The intention was that women and their pattern of living can "methodologically, be used as a window onto the society of which they are a part" (Poluha, 2004, p. 16). I used participant observation to describe the research setting and semistructured interviewing to collect data about women's experiences about giving birth in rural Ethiopia. As the majority of Ethiopia's population live in rural areas, lack of transportation and distance to a health facility are cited as major problems for 71% and 66% of women, respectively (CSA & ICF International, 2012).

Study Site

The studied area was in and around Bonga town, located in the Ghimbo district (*woreda*) and the northern part of Decha *woreda*. Kafa Zone covers an area of 11,114 square km, dominated by steep hills, gorges, and streams with large areas of natural forest that are the habitat of wild Ethiopian coffee and has been described as one of the "biodiversity hotspots" of the world

(Schmitt, 2006). Most people are engaged in agriculture, with the average land holding per family between 1.25 and 2.0 hectares (Schmitt, 2006). The total population in 2007 was 880,251, with 92.3% living in rural areas (CSA, 2007).

Participants

The selection of women was based on snowballing techniques after I was introduced to women through my interpreter and her family. I interviewed 22 women in their homes and one woman who was an inpatient at Chiri Health Center (CHC; funded by Lalmba, a small U.S.-based nongovernmental organization [NGO]). Of these women, five of them had had one pregnancy and eight of the women had had over seven pregnancies. One woman had been pregnant 14 times. With women's permission, I also sat in during ANC examinations at Bonga Hospital and at Deckia Clinic and CHC. At CHC, I interviewed 17 women waiting for ANC. I specifically asked people to refer me to Manjo women they knew, and I subsequently interviewed five Manjo women. Five to 10% of the total population of Kafa Zone are Manjo—the largest minority class facing prejudice and discrimination—who survive by making charcoal and carrying it or firewood to sell in towns (Gezahegn Petros, 2003).

In the larger study, interview data from key personnel in government, NGOs, one UN agency, and 16 health institutions (including Bonga Hospital, health centers and health posts) examined the processes through which skilled health workers provide ANC, intrapartum care, and EmOC. In this article, however, I focus mainly on the views of the women interviewed and the location of birth.

Data Collection and Analysis

Ethical clearance was sought from and approved by Deakin University Human Ethics Committee. The Ethiopian MOH also provided formal letters of introduction. Informed consent was requested from all participants either orally or in writing. I gave all participants pseudonyms to provide confidentiality and presented interview data in such a way that would make it difficult to identify individual responses.

All interviews were recorded on a voice recorder. A female interpreter was present at most interviews and later transcribed audio recordings verbatim. I was assisted by a male interpreter at CHC and with interviews with two Manjo women in their homes. This interpreter also checked interview data that were unclear or needed further clarification. For example, we discussed the meanings of proverbs at great length because they could be interpreted in more than one way.

Analysis of interview data followed a process of data reduction, data display, and conclusion drawing/verification occurring concurrently: as interview data were transcribed, the data were organized around key themes (Miles & Huberman, 1994). I used the participants' words and thematic analysis guided by the Three-Delays framework developed by Thaddeus and Maine (1994). The themes of mobility and accessibility to health facilities were commonly described by participants. Travel distances and transportation reflect the themes of accessibility found in Phase II of the Three Delays. The benefit of doing participant observation meant I could see how long it took and how much energy was required to travel to the health facilities from remote regions of Kafa Zone.

RESULTS

Where Does Birth Take Place?

Rural Ethiopian woman live and work in a setting of loosely collected family households embedded in domestic agriculture and industry. Production, reproduction, and consumption are oriented to the household unit of husband, wife, and their children. Work takes place in and around the household with tasks allocated by age and gender (Pankhurst, 1992; Poluha, 1988).

The women I interviewed live a gendered existence performing most household tasks such as food preparation; washing clothes; going to the mill planting and weeding vegetables, root crops, and spices around the home; threshing; pounding; and assisting with animal production tasks including milking, butter churning, and cheese making. Ploughing the fields, sowing the seed, harvesting, processing, storing and marketing of coffee, producing cereal and legumes, and performing animal husbandry and bee keeping are men's work because these are the crops that are more likely to generate cash income (Abiyu Million et al., 2002; Holden & Tewodros Tefera, 2008). Men are not supposed to be involved in household activity with the exception of occasionally collecting firewood, and there are cultural beliefs that a man busying himself with household activities will be seen as "becoming a female" and not capable of running his household properly (Abiyu Million et al., 2002).

Based on my observations with women in their homes and while walking with or passing women on the road and visiting health facilities, it was common to see women walking together on the road. Manjo women carried heavy bags of charcoal or firewood for sale in Bonga, and older women walked together on their saints' day to the Orthodox Church on the hilltop with their crosses. Women carried baskets of food to a neighbor who had had a baby or lost a relative through death, or they hauled large bundles of vegetables or grain on their way to the market on Tuesday or Saturday. Many women walked 1 to 2 hours each way in mountainous terrain to go to the market or the mill. Going to the market, however, was not just about obtaining cash money. Women welcomed the opportunity to get out of the house and socialize with other women and to talk on the way and at the market. Stopping at a favorite *tej* (wine made from honey and the local *gesho* plant) or *tella* (mild alcoholic drink made from maize or barley) house (*bet*) on the way home is a social occasion as women gather together to gossip and catch up with all the news with friends and neighbors before the long walk home. Women also walked to the health post, health center, or hospital to have their children immunized, for Depo-Provera injections, and for ANC.

Childbirth generally takes place in the privacy of the home, a round thatched hut or *tukul*, although in some parts of Kafa Zone a separate hut is built in the compound for menstruating and birthing women. Generally local communities in Ethiopia "perceive that the resources and knowledge necessary for a healthy pregnancy" are "available within the community": this includes advising women not to travel long distances or to expose themselves to the sun during pregnancy (MOH, 2006b) or "to be exposed to cold while going to or staying in the health facility, [or] to expose one's body to others as they believe to get desired assistance while at home" (Mirgissa Kaba, 2000, p. 24).

Going to a health facility. In Kafa Zone, in 2007, there were three doctors, five health officers, and 150 nurses with certificates or diplomas including 11 midwives, one laboratory technologist, nine laboratory technicians, and 360 Health Extension Workers, with another 223 in training. Neighborhoods (kebeles) can be a long way from the *woreda* center where the referral health center is located, so inaccessibility is a problem for many people, especially in the rainy season. Many of the woredas are a long way (up to 4-days walk away) from Bonga Hospital, which is the only facility with an operating theater. Moreover, the shortage of vehicles for transportation was obvious as all buses and Isuzu trucks on the road were always overcrowded and had to turn potential passengers away.

In practice, the referral system creates many delays, and women often arrive at the health facility needing emergency treatment. If women are referred to health centers and midwives and nurses are unable to remove a retained placenta or assist with obstructed labor, they must refer the woman to Bonga Hospital, which could be another day's travel away. One midwife stated that he referred women with uterine rupture, malpresentation or very high blood pressure immediately to Bonga Hospital, but if a woman needed a blood transfusion she would need to go immediately to Jimma Hospital, 3 to 4 hours by road from Bonga. In essence, women who were referred to Bonga Hospital were described as "lucky" by one doctor because there was so much going against a woman receiving emergency treatment. All the women in remote Deckia talked about the possibility of dying on the way to Bonga. One woman explained: "Other women, when they carry them to Bonga or Chiri on the stretcher, she gets tired and passed away on the way.

Many mothers died from childbirth related problems. Other lucky women are survived by God's help."

Many health workers said that if people recognize there is a problem during birth, they do not understand how serious it is but instead they just "hope" that things will get better and that the baby will come soon. There is also a cultural taboo about staying in the dark and about avoiding cold air or blowing wind known as *birrd*. If birth is at night, it means waiting until the morning: "For one girl the placenta is stuck. We couldn't go to the hospital because it was night. God helped me (Addisalem)." No one travelled at night, even staff from CHC, which had the resources and vehicles, as it was deemed too dangerous to be on the road at night.

Meseret's baby died on the way from remote Agaro Bushi to CHC. Meseret was around 25 to 27 years old, and had had five pregnancies: three children, two stillborn. All of her other babies were born at home with the help of her husband and mother-in-law. She had walked to Chiri 2 weeks earlier for ANC after referral for swollen ankles and breech presentation at Deckia Clinic. She said she planned to give birth at Chiri this time, but she went home to wait until the baby was due. Meseret's labor started in the night, 9 days early. After some time had passed, her husband started to organize the neighbors to carry her. He said this took about 3 hours. Making a stretcher took around 30 minutes. He then had to borrow money from her cousins. This took about 30 minutes. Then the journey from Agaro Bushi to Chiri took about 8 hours over mountainous terrain. Around 20 men helped to carry Meseret on the stretcher. Along the way, she was in terrible, agonizing pain, tied to the stretcher. She told me she cried the whole way. Half way to Chiri, they knew the baby had died. The baby was removed at CHC and later the health officer told me that she had been in labor for at least 2 days. Although the baby's body had been delivered, the head was stuck. What Meseret did not tell me was that only the day before her labor started, her neighbor's child had been washed out of his father's arms trying to cross the river on the way to Chiri for medical care. She was afraid of crossing the river. This is why they delayed. This happened in the middle of the rainy season.

Why Do Women Give Birth At Home?

Giving birth marks a milestone in the mother–daughter relationship, and some Ethiopian women return to their mother's home or village to give birth so they are surrounded by other women providing care (Mendlinger & Cwikel, 2006). As most women move near their patrilineal kin at marriage, however, for those women who have moved far from their mother's home, the importance of a good relationship with ones neighbors and the community becomes evident during birth. This relationship is reflected in the proverb: "A close neighbor is much better than a faraway relative" (Knutsson, 2004, p. 103).

Most of the women in this study gave birth at home with the assistance of their neighbor, mother, mother in-law, husband, or sister. In addition to close neighbors or family members, many women called on God and Mary (*Maryam*) during their labor to help them deal with the pain. Only two of the four women who gave birth in a hospital or health center had planned to do so. During labor at home, the main role for the birth assistant is to hold the woman tightly on the shoulders from behind so she feels supported and to massage her abdomen with *kibbi* (butter) or hair food (Vaseline). Almost all the women reported that someone had massaged their abdomen during labor, which is a common practice to deal with pain and speed up labor. When I demonstrated with my fingers and asked if the massage was gentle or with pressure, all the women said the massage had been gentle. By contrast, health practitioners who were asked about abdominal massage said that it is one of the main causes for stillbirth, uterine rupture, bleeding, and even death.

Several women said that birth should be kept secret, and others stated that it was best not to have too many people around as it might bring bad luck. I asked this question knowing how common it was for women to be invited to visit each other, to drink coffee, and to enjoy sitting around, talking, and gossiping. For Abaynesh, "Everyone should not know a woman is in labor except the intimate friend. We don't want others around until she delivers the child. That's why we keep it a secret but nothing bad happens." Hirut from Wushwush related the following:

> This one time—it is different. What happens is she is having labor pains and if they [other family members] are asked, "Where is your mother?" and they want to say she has a headache or even she is not around. That time they make a secret, anything that is not a labor pain connection.... Too many people are not good for the baby. They pray for Our Lady and they are waiting and Maryam helps them. They do not tell to anyone else.

Wolete from Deckia also said, "They keep it silent until they give birth; they don't tell anyone."

On the other hand, Wubealem related another tradition:

> When a woman is giving birth, the husband must leave the house and wait outside. He should be invited in [afterward] to visit his wife if she delivered normally. But if the pain continues, he is told to take her to the health center. Everyone knows when she is in labor—passers-by can bring bad luck.

Sara was one of the women I interviewed from rural Sheyka; about 2-hours walk from Bonga town. Her house was far from other houses, and Sara expressed how isolated she felt at birth. She was not only far from her own family, especially her mother, but she felt she had no close friends or neighbors to call on to support her, only her husband who assisted by massaging her abdomen and holding her shoulders during the labor. Sara expressed her sorrow about being "alone" during birth by saying that no one was there to watch over her, even when she felt she was at "death's door."

None of the women interviewed gave birth totally "alone," but several women said that they did not want others, with the exception of the close neighbor or friend, to know that they were in labor. Yet other women stated that birth is an event that involves social interaction with close family members and neighbors, and religious interaction with God and Maryam through prayer. Whatever happens, the role of female relatives and neighbors is to support the birthing woman. For those women with no family or neighbors close by, there is a sense of being "alone."

The mother–daughter relationship. Although it is important for women to bear children, especially sons, to carry on their father's name, the importance of having a daughter is also an important theme in the women's lives because it is daughters who can buy a dress, plait their mother's hair with *kibbi* or hair food (Vaseline), make coffee, clean the house for her mother, and so on—all little things that show that they care. All the women interviewed had children or grandchildren with them during the day. For those women who had babies or toddlers, the child was breastfed on demand. Older children assisted with the daily chores by collecting water and firewood, helping out in the garden or the fields, or running errands to the local shop or neighbor. Typically, girls spent a lot of time with their mothers; older daughters assisted their mother during labor and birth.

Almaz lived in her son's house and had no regular income. She has had 12 pregnancies, but only three of her children are alive. Her daughters are too poor to assist her and her son who is a teacher a long way away occasionally sends a small amount of money. Almaz still grieved for her daughter who had died the previous year and commented that there was no one to help her out as her clothes were falling to pieces: "Since Azeb's mother has died, who will give me a new dress?" Almaz's life is bound up with that of her two surviving daughters and numerous grandchildren who depend on her for guidance and stability because the future looks bleak for all of them with no regular income.

Amina was my next-door neighbor in *Kebele* Three in Bonga. Amina lived with her three grandsons, only one who had a regular income as he worked for a tailor in town. I often invited her over for coffee, and on one occasion we talked about how well her middle grandson had played the role of someone who was "down and out" in a recent play. Relating this story, however, had an unexpected effect. She held back the tears and then gave in and wept as she told us how worried she was about her grandsons' future. Since her daughter died, she had become even more concerned for them because there was no one else to care for them. This meant also that there was no one to care for her. From these and other conversations with women, I felt that although women must bear sons to do the heavy work on the farm, it is daughters whom women grieved for the most.

Decision making. Building good relationships with neighbors and the community is a critical role for women (Abiyu Million et al., 2002). Although women are not expected to go to meetings at the church or kebele because they are normally represented by their husband, women are expected to provide food and drink for the men. There is an expectation that women's ability to work and perform all the tasks expected of a woman is synonymous with a broad understanding of women's health: on the one hand, Ethiopian women define their health as a disease-free state, and on the other hand, they emphasize that being healthy is a social obligation. It is not just that the unhealthy woman is regarded as a failure; she is unable to perform the tasks expected of women (Yemane Berhane, Gossaye, Emmelin, & Högberg, 2001). A common way women build relationships is by sharing in the coffee ceremony. Preparing coffee is an activity that is central to Ethiopian culture and one that enables the building of good relationships with neighbors and the community.

Marriage is viewed as universal in Ethiopia and is the principal indicator of a woman's exposure to pregnancy. It takes place relatively early: the median age of first marriage for women aged 25–49 is 16.5 years (CSA & ICF International, 2012). All the women I interviewed were married or had been married. Only two women were not living with their husband. One was Abebech from the outskirts of Bonga town whose husband had left her for another woman. Abebech was a single mother with seven children. The other woman was Birke, who had been forced to leave her husband after the birth (and death) of her last child, which left her with chronic health problems. In many countries including Ethiopia, women do not decide to seek medical health care on their own, nor would they have money to pay for their treatment. This decision is made by their husband or other senior members of their family, including the mother and mother-in-law, often after traditional means in the village have been tried first.

Decision making about accessing health care is dependent on a number of factors including availability of money or assets that can be sold, rented, or used for getting a loan and the willingness of people to lend money. Sometimes, the community or the funeral association (the traditional get together to support one another in case of funerals or other emergency situations known an *iddir*) is mobilized to help with financial costs and human power to carry the woman to the health facility (Endale Workalemahu, 2003). If there is no *iddir*, the husband relies on relatives and neighbors. In my interviews, *all* the women and *all* health practitioners and staff from NGOs confirmed that the husband was the decisionmaker about whether a woman would be taken to biomedical health care. With only one exception, all the women and health workers I interviewed talked about the difficulties for women around the financial cost of treatment. Some women stated that those women who were poor and could not afford medicine or to go to the hospital might die.

Two examples serve to show how women have little power to make decisions around fertility and pregnancy. During an interview at Bonga Hospital, I was told how "clever" women go the market via the hospital for a Depo-Provera injection. Women carry their foodstuffs and tell their husbands they are going to the market, but they stop on the way to seek "urgent" attention at the hospital so their husband will not find out where they have been.

Second, while observing ANC at Deckia Clinic, a pregnant woman came in exhibiting such extreme discomfort that she could hardly walk. The nurse thought it was likely that she had a urinary tract infection, but her argumentative husband who had accompanied her did all the talking and refused to pay for the treatment. He demanded that the nurse massage his wife's stomach "to take away the pain." The nurse refused, and they left without treatment.

CONCLUSION

Substantial effort has been made in Ethiopia and other developing countries to bring health facilities closer to where people live in rural and semiurban areas. The findings from this study contribute to a growing body of literature that shows that while many women in developing countries access ANC, family planning, and child vaccination, there is a need to consider the sociocultural environment and the barriers that prevent women accessing health services during pregnancy and childbirth.

Why do women in Ethiopia give birth at home? Is it just because it is taken for granted to do so? The short answer is probably yes because the alternative appears to be restricted to "abnormal" births, an alternative that involves imagining the worst outcome for the woman. Researchers who focus on cultural beliefs around childbirth in developing countries suggest that women birthing at home are expected to be stoic (e.g., Bedford et al., 2013; Sargent, 1990). My findings show that when stoicism is combined with the normalization of prolonged labor at home, it means calling on God or Maryam to assist and just "hoping the baby will come." When childbirth is at home, the importance of close relationships with neighbors, family members, and local communities is manifested as these people support the birthing women, sometimes in secret, other times more openly.

Since Thaddeus and Maine (1994) developed the Three-Delays model, researchers report that distance is a common barrier for women and their families to access health facilities in developing countries. This was also the case in this study as participants described how the distance to a health facility was a barrier because they felt they would "die on the way." I believe that in Kafa Zone it is taken for granted that most people's lives are to some extent slowed to a walking pace because that is often the only way to travel both short and long distances. If walking is seen only as a mode of transportation to collect water and firewood, to go to the market, a neighbor's house, or to the church or health facility, however, this does not fully describe the act of walking. Women did not describe walking as "work" or "going to work," although I would argue that is what they are doing when they are carrying heavy loads. Women welcome the opportunity to get out of the house. Observing and listening to them as they barter and buy what they can afford at the marketplace, while queuing up at the "grind house" or commenting on the quality of the butter to braid their hair, there is no doubt that women can argue and negotiate to achieve better outcomes for themselves. Women come up with innovative ways to get family planning on the way to the market. They stop on the way home to socialize and gossip over a drink with other women. They find ways to cope with the loss of mothers and daughters by walking to a friend's house to share food and drink coffee together. If they are concerned about their pregnancy, they walk long distances to attend ANC.

I concur that people walk to health facilities, but during childbirth it appears to be a last resort because "normative health behavior" is characterized by a "wait-and-see" attitude to see if things improve on their own (Kloos et al., 1987). Abaynesh's husband described to me how they watched and waited for 2 days before they carried his friend's wife to the hospital. What happens when a woman's husband, her relatives, and neighbors decide to take a woman to a health facility? I observed how local communities come together to provide transportation to EmOC health services as women are carried on a stretcher for many hours or even days to a health facility.

By and large, my findings corroborate the work of other researchers including the Ethiopian DHS, which shows that women are not considered part of the decision-making process about health-seeking behavior. Decisions to travel to a health facility are primarily made by a woman's husband, close relatives, and neighbors. In doing so, the decision-making process generally involves people who have no training about when to refer women to skilled health personnel. Thus it is argued that the influence of husbands is not "trivial" because women who are married to men who approve of health care are more likely to use it (Belay Biratu & Lindstrom, 2006). Women in this study, however, did find ways to access some health services without their husband's permission. Cost is also a significant factor in the decision-making process.

Many researchers who focus on the discrepancy between maternal mortality levels in developing and developed countries and the lack of progress toward reaching MDG 5 suggest that increasing the proportion of deliveries with skilled attendance will itself reduce maternal mortality and disability. The findings in this research add to the literature by providing additional understanding about how the sociocultural cultural dimensions of childbirth need to be considered. The alternative is that we would only have a partial explanation of the dangers and problems that women, along with their husbands, mothers, mothers-in-law, and neighbors face. From a distance, it appears straightforward to employ skilled birth attendants and to refer a woman to health facilities if there are problems during a difficult birth in developing countries. In places such as Kafa Zone, however, "roads" are in mountainous terrain. In the rainy season, it is slippery and muddy and sometimes there are rivers that are impossible to cross. For women being carried on a stretcher, the topography and lack of transportation also contribute to the delays, and many women do die on the way. Future research using ethnographic methods could explore whether women's fears that they will die "on the way" to a health facility contribute to delays in seeking maternal health care services.

REFERENCES

Note: All Ethiopian names are entered, as is traditional practice, in alphabetical order of the author's first name followed by the father's name.

Abiyu Million, Wondwosen Terefe, Shiferaw G. M., Wubit Bekele, Elfenesh Wondiumu, Wudenesh Adelo, & Groenendijk, N. (2002). The economic contribution of women, decision-making processes in the family and gender related behavior in the Kafa Zone. (Unpublished report). Bonga, Ethiopia: FEDCMD/SUPAK.

Barker, C. E., Bird, C. E., Pradhan, A., & Shakya, G. (2007). Support to the Safe Motherhood Programme in Nepal: An integrated approach. *Reproductive Health Matters, 15*(30), 81–90.

Bedford, J., Gandhi, M., Admassu, M., & Girma, A. (2013). "A normal delivery takes place at home": A qualitative study of the location of childbirth in rural Ethiopia. *Maternal and Child Health Journal, 17*(2), 230–239.

Belay Biratu & Lindstrom, D. P. (2006). The influence of husbands' approval on women's use of prenatal care: Results from Yirgalem and Jimma towns, south west Ethiopia. *Ethiopian Journal of Health Development, 20*(2), 84–92.

Boddy, J. (1998). Remembering Amal: On birth and the British in northern Sudan. In M. Lock & P. A. Kaufert (Eds.), *Pragmatic women and body politics* (pp. 28–57). Cambridge, England: Cambridge University Press.

Campbell, O. M. R., & Graham, W. J. (2006). Strategies for reducing maternal mortality: Getting on with what works. *The Lancet, 368*(9543), 1284–1299.

Central Statistical Authority (CSA). (2007). *2007 population and housing census.* Retrieved from http://www.csa.gov.et/pdf/Cen2007_firstdraft.pdf

Central Statistical Authority (CSA) & ICF International. (2012). *Ethiopia demographic and health survey 2011*. Addis Ababa, Ethiopia: Author.

De Brouwere, V., Tonglet, R., & Van Lerberghe, W. (1998). Strategies for reducing maternal mortality in developing countries: What can we learn from the history of the industrialized West? *Tropical Medicine and International Health, 3*(10), 771–782.

Endale Workalemahu. (2003). Assessment on health care seeking behaviour West Hararghe Zone. (Unpublished report). Addis Ababa, Ethiopia: CARE International Ethiopia.

Gezahegn Petros. (2003). Kafa. In D. Freeman & A. Pankhurst (Eds.), *Peripheral people: The excluded minorities of Ethiopia* (pp. 80–96). London, England: Hurst & Co.

Gil-González, D., Carrasco-Portiño, M., & Ruiz, M. T. (2006). Knowledge gaps in scientific literature on maternal mortality: A systematic review. *Bulletin of the World Health Organization, 84*(11), 903–909.

Hogan, M. C., Foreman, K. J., Naghavi, M., Ahn, S. Y., Wang, M., Makela, ... Murray, C. J. L. (2010). Maternal mortality for 181 countries, 1980–2008: A systematic analysis of progress towards Millennium Development Goal 5. *The Lancet, 375*(9726), 1609–1623.

Holden, S., & Tewodros Tefera. (2008). *From being property of men to becoming equal owners? Early impacts of land registration and certification on women in Southern Ethiopia*. Retrieved from http://www.statkart.no/filestore/Eiendomsdivisjonen/PropertyCentre/Pdf/EarlyImpactsonWomenFinalReport2007sh.pdf

Jackson, R. (2010). *(Un)safe routes: Maternal mortality and Ethiopia's development agenda*. (Unpublished doctoral dissertation). Deakin University, Geelong, Australia.

Jackson, R. (2013). "Waiting-to-see" if the baby will come: Findings from a qualitative study in Kafa Zone, Ethiopia. *Ethiopian Journal of Health Development, 27*(2), 118–123.

Kloos, H., Alemayehu Etea, Assefa Degefa, Hundessa Aga, Berhanu Solomon, Kabede Abera, Abebe Abegaz, & Geta Belemo. (1987). Illness and health behaviour in Addis Ababa and rural Central Ethiopia. *Social Science and Medicine, 25*(9), 1003–1019.

Knutsson, A. (2004). *"To the best of your knowledge and for the good of your neighbour": A study of traditional birth attendants in Addis Ababa, Ethiopia*. (Doctoral dissertation). Acta Universitatis Gothoburgensis, Göteborg, Sweden.

Koblinsky, M., Tain, F., Asheber Gaym, Ali Karim, Carnell, M., & Solomon Tesfaye. (2010). Responding to the maternal health care challenge: The Ethiopian Health Extension Program. *Ethiopian Journal of Health Development, 1*(24), 105–109.

Loudon, I. (1992). *Death in childbirth: An international study of maternal care and maternal mortality, 1800–1960*. Oxford, England: Clarendon.

Lukere, V. (2002). Conclusion: Wider reflections and a survey of literature. In V. Lukere & M. Jolly (Eds.), *Birthing in the Pacific: Beyond tradition and modernity?* (pp. 178–202). Honolulu, Hawaii: University of Hawaii Press.

Mendlinger, S., & Cwikel, J. (2006). Health behaviors over the life cycle among mothers and daughters from Ethiopia. *Nashim: A Journal of Jewish Women's Studies and Gender Issues, 12*, 57–94.

Miles, M., & Huberman, A. (1994). *Qualitative data analysis: An expanded source-book* (2nd ed.). Thousand Oaks, CA: Sage.

Ministry of Health (MOH). (2006a). *National reproductive health strategy 2006–2015*. Addis Ababa, Ethiopia: Family Health Department.

Ministry of Health (MOH). (2006b). *Report on safe motherhood community-based survey, Ethiopia*. Addis Ababa, Ethiopia: Family Health Department.

Ministry of Health (MOH). (2010). *Health Sector Development Program IV 2010/11–2014/15*. Retrieved from http://phe-ethiopia.org/admin/uploads/attachment-721-HSDP%20IV%20Final%20Draft%2011Octoberr%202010.pdf

Mirgissa Kaba. (2000). A qualitative study on health seeking behavior and community based health care potentials in Kafa-Sheka Zone, SNNPR. (Unpublished report). Jimma, Ethiopia: Jimma University.

Pankhurst, H. (1992). *Gender, development and identity: An Ethiopian study*. London, England: Zed Books.

The Partnership for Maternal, Newborn & Child Health. (2010). *Consensus for maternal, newborn and child health*. Retrieved from http://www.who.int/pmnch/topics/maternal/consensus_12_09.pdf

Poluha, E. (1988). The producers cooperative as an option for women: A case study from Ethiopia. In H. G. B. Hedlund (Ed.), *Cooperatives revisited* (pp. 139–152). Uppsala, Sweden: Nordic Africa Institute.

Poluha, E. (2004). *The power of continuity: Ethiopia through the eyes of its children*. Uppsala, Sweden: Nordic Africa Institute.

Sargent, C. F. (1990). The politics of birth: Cultural dimensions of pain, virtue, and control among the Bariba of Benin. In W. P. Handwerker (Ed.), *Births and power: Social change and the politics of reproduction* (pp. 69–79). Boulder, CO: Westview.

Schmitt, C. B. (2006). *Montane rainforest with wild coffea arabica in the Bonga region (SW Ethiopia): Plant diversity, wild coffee management and implications for conservation*. (Doctoral dissertation). Center for Development Research, University of Bonn, Bonn, Germany.

Thaddeus, S., & Maine, D. (1994). Too far to walk: Maternal mortality in context. *Social Science and Medicine, 38*(8), 1091–1110.

United Nations. (2000). *Resolution adopted by the General Assembly, United Nations Millennium Declaration (A/RES/55/2)*. Retrived from http://www.un.org/millennium/declaration/ares552e.pdf

World Health Organization (WHO). (2004). *Making pregnancy safer: The critical role of the skilled attendant: A joint statement by WHO, ICM and FIGO*. Geneva, Switzerland: Author. Retrieved from http://whqlibdoc.who.int/publications/2004/9241591692.pdf

World Health Organization (WHO), United Nations International Children's Emergency Fund (UNICEF), United Nations Population Fund (UNFPA), & The World Bank. (2012). *Trends in maternal mortality: 1990 to 2010 WHO, UNICEF, UNFPA, & The World Bank estimates*. Retrieved from http://whqlibdoc.who.int/publications/2012/9789241503631_eng.pdf

Yemane Berhane, Gossaye, Y., Emmelin, M., & Högberg, U. (2001). Women's health in a rural setting in societal transition in Ethiopia. *Social Science and Medicine, 53*(11), 1525–1539.

Women's Health in Women's Hands: A Pilot Study Assessing the Feasibility of Providing Women With Medications to Reduce Postpartum Hemorrhage and Sepsis in Rural Tanzania

GAIL C. WEBBER

Department of Family Medicine, University of Ottawa, Ottawa, Ontario, Canada

BWIRE CHIRANGI

Shirati District Hospital, Shirati, Tanzania

In rural Africa, deaths from childbirth are common and access to health care facilities with skilled providers is very limited. Leading causes of death for women are bleeding and infection. In this pilot study, we establish the feasibility of distributing oral medications to women in rural Tanzania to self-administer after delivery to reduce bleeding and infection. Of the 642 women provided with medications, 90% of the women took them appropriately, while the remaining 10% did not require them. We conclude that is it feasible to distribute oral medications to rural women to self-administer after delivery.

Context of Maternal Mortality in Africa

Death from childbirth is one of the largest challenges facing African women today, particularly in rural communities. The United Nations' fifth Millennium Development Goal addressed this concern with the aim to improve maternal health and reduce by two-thirds by 2015 the enormously high numbers of women dying while giving birth (United Nations, 2013). Although, several African countries have made some progress toward this goal, there are still many thousands of women dying as a result of childbirth annually. In 2010, an estimated 164,800 women lost their lives while giving birth in Africa—56% of the number of women dying globally of childbirth (African Union Commission, Economic Commission for Africa, African Development Bank Group, & United Nations Development Program, 2013). In Tanzania, with a maternal mortality ratio of 454 per 100,000 (National Bureau of Statistics Tanzania & ICF Macro Tanzania, 2011), this reality equates to one woman dying in childbirth almost hourly (Ministry of Finance and Economic Affairs, Republic of Tanzania, 2009).

Two of the largest causes of maternal mortality are bleeding and infection, causing 25% and 15% of maternal deaths globally, respectively (Sullivan & Hirst, 2011). In Africa, 34% of maternal deaths are attributed to hemorrhage (Haeri & Dildy, 2012). Women who deliver outside of a health care institution are most at risk, as they do not have access to life-saving medications or skilled attendants. More than 50% of women delivering in sub-Saharan Africa lack a skilled birth attendant at their delivery, and there is evidence that this concerning statistic is unlikely to change soon (Crowe, Utley, Costello, & Pagel, 2012). In addition to increasing access to health care services for rural women, strategies are urgently needed to provide women with alternative methods to reduce their risks at the time of delivery that are not dependent on the presence of skilled health care workers.

Postpartum Hemorrhage

Saving mothers' lives from the risks of childbirth does not always involve costly interventions. The recommendations for the period immediately after delivery of the baby, referred to as the third stage of labor, are to provide injectable uterotonic medications such as oxytocin or ergometrine to prevent bleeding. Unfortunately, for women delivering in the villages or on the way to a facility, this is not possible as these medications require refrigeration and a skilled provider to administer them. Six hundred micrograms of oral misoprostol has been shown to be an effective alternative to injectable uterotonics in low-resource settings (Gülmezoglu, Forna, Villar, & Hofmeyr, 2011; Sheldon, Blum, Durocher, & Winikoff, 2012). The World Health Organization (WHO) and the International Federation of Gynecology and Obstetrics (FIGO) have both endorsed the use of misoprostol for the prevention of postpartum hemorrhage (PPH) in settings where oxytocin in not available, although only when administered by a skilled or lay health care provider (FIGO Safe Motherhood and Newborn Committee, 2012; WHO, 2012a). The United Nations Commission on Life-Saving Commodities for Women and Children has listed misoprostol for the prevention and treatment of PPH as one of 13 key commodities to reduce deaths of women and children (Every Women Every Child, 2012).

Community distribution of misoprostol for PPH prevention through various providers has been demonstrated to be effective in India (Derman et al., 2006), Afghanistan (Sanghvi et al., 2010), Nepal (Rajbhandari et al., 2010), Bangladesh (Nasreen, Nahar, Al Mamun, Afsana, & Byass, 2011), and Pakistan (Mir Wajid, & Gull, 2012), as well as several other countries in Africa and Asia (Smith, Gubin, Holston, Fullerton, & Prata, 2013). In Tanzania, there have been two studies of misoprostol for PPH prevention. In the first (Prata, Mbaruki, Grossman, Holston, & Hsieh, 2009), misoprostol was successfully distributed through traditional birth attendants (TBAs). Unfortunately, this is no longer feasible as the Tanzanian government has officially restricted the work of TBAs, and while women still attend these caregivers, it is unlikely that TBAs would be permitted to engage in misoprostol distribution. In the second study, the intervention entailed dispensary nurses delivering misoprostol at the antenatal visits after 32 weeks gestation (Ifakara Health Institute, Venture Strategies Innovations, Bixby Center for Population, Health and Sustainability, Population Services International [PSI]/Tanzania, 2011); however, the researchers found that many women did not receive the medications because they did not attend antenatal care during the latter weeks of their pregnancy. The WHO has recognized that task shifting needs to occur in maternal and child health in order to optimize care, but, they have stopped short of promoting misoprostol distribution to pregnant women for self-administration to prevent PPH (WHO, 2012b).

Puerperal Sepsis

In addition to PPH, puerperal sepsis, or life-threatening infection associated with childbirth, is another major cause of death for mothers. Puerperal sepsis has been estimated to contribute to 75,000 deaths per year, mostly in developing countries (Hussein & Fortney, 2004). It has been proposed that the provision of antibiotics to prevent life-threatening sepsis and oral misoprostol to prevent postpartum bleeding could augment facility strengthening in Africa to reduce deaths from childbirth by one-third (Pagel et al., 2009). There is evidence that prophylactic antibiotic use prevents sepsis in elective and nonelective caesarian sections and in women at high risk of sepsis (van Dillen, Zwart, Schutte & van Roosmalen, 2010). In a study of prophylactic antibiotics at delivery in HIV-positive women, researchers have also documented a reduction in postpartum infections (Sebitloane, Moodley, & Esterhuizen, 2008), although a study of HIV infected and noninfected women was unable to demonstrate a positive effect of prophylactic antibiotics given during the antenatal and intrapartum periods to women in urban health care facilities in Malawi, Tanzania, and Zambia (Aboud et al., 2009).

Purpose and Objectives

In order to address the problem of maternal mortality for rural women living in Rorya District, Tanzania, we conducted a 6-month study in 2012. The purpose of this research was to assess the feasibility of misoprostol and erythromycin distribution to rural Tanzanian women to prevent PPH and puerperal sepsis. Our objectives were to demonstrate that the community provision of these medications was both acceptable to the community and safe for the women, in preparation for a later scale-up to the larger Mara Region.

METHODS

Research Design

This research used a mixed method design composed of both quantitative and qualitative methods. After receiving the study medications, the women were surveyed by the research assistants about their demographic information and the facts of their delivery experience (quantitative results). The results of the survey are the focus of this article. In addition, interviews were conducted with women, traditional birth attendants, and dispensary nurses; these results are reported elsewhere (Webber & Chirangi, n.d.).

Research Setting

Rorya District is bordered by Lake Victoria to the west, Serengeti National Park to the east, and the Kenyan border to the north. Mara Region has one of the highest nonfacility birth rates in Tanzania, with more than 60% of women delivering in their villages where no skilled attendants are available (Ministry of Finance and Economic Affairs, Republic of Tanzania, 2009). We chose to conduct the study in the villages serviced by 12 rural dispensaries in Rorya that were located farthest from the district hospital.

Ethics and Data Collection

Ethical approval for the study was obtained from the Ottawa Hospital Research Ethics Board in Canada and the National Institute of Medical Research in Tanzania, which is responsible for ethical approval of all medical research in Tanzania.

In this study, research assistants and dispensary nurses distributed misoprostol and erythromycin to rural women for self-administration after delivery (i.e., the women could take the medication themselves or designate a family member or TBA to administer it to them). We used a misoprostol dose of 600 micrograms because this is the recommended dose for prevention of

PPH (WHO, 2011). We included 500 mg of erythromycin, an antibiotic that is used to treat Group A streptococcus, historically a common cause of puerperal sepsis (Hussein & Fortney, 2004). It is important to note that in order to maximize distribution, we provided these medications to women during their pregnancy for self-administration after delivery and we attempted to include all willing women in the catchment area, not just those who attended antenatal clinics for prenatal care, unlike some previous studies (Smith et al., 2013).

From February to July 2012, the research assistants visited the study villages and with the assistance of local health workers, they met with women who were currently pregnant and due to deliver before August. In addition to distributing the medications directly from the research assistants, the dispensary nurses were provided with the study medications and were instructed how to enroll women in the study. The research assistants and dispensary nurses explained the study to the women in the local language of Swahili or Luo, and they provided an information letter in Swahili to the women. The women were asked to sign a consent form indicating their agreement to participate in the study. The consent form was read to women who lacked the literacy skills to read it themselves. Women who consented to be part of the study were provided with a small bag containing three tablets of misoprostol (200 micrograms each) and two tablets of erythromycin (250 mg each). The women were instructed to store the medication in a safe location, to take it with them wherever they chose to deliver, and to swallow the medications immediately after the birth of the infant and not before. The women were also warned about the possible side effects of the medications, particularly shivering and an upset stomach. We sought ethics permission from the Canadian ethics committee to include only women 18 years and older; hence younger women are not represented in this report.

After the women delivered, the research assistants returned to survey them about their birth experience. The research assistants collected demographic information on the women (including age, parity, and distance living from the hospital and dispensary), in addition to details about the delivery (location, attendance at delivery, whether study medications were taken, whether the woman would consider taking the study medications in future deliveries, side effects, and the health of the baby).

Analysis and Validity

All data were entered into an Excel spreadsheet by the principal investigator or a research assistant, and 20% of the data entries were double-entered for accuracy. All errors were corrected. The data were then analyzed using SPSS for descriptive statistics.

RESULTS

A total of 642 women were surveyed after they used the study medications. The results of the survey are provided in Table 1.

Demographic Information

The mothers' ages ranged from 18 to 47, with a median age of 26. The women's parity also had a wide spread, from 1 to 14 with a median parity of fou children. The median distance from the hospital for the women was 34 km, although the farthest was 90 km. The median distance from the dispensary was 4 km, while the range extended from 0.25 km to 57 km.

Experience of Delivery

Most of the women surveyed delivered in their own home (47.9%) or the TBA's home (21.1%). A further 3.4% delivered en route to a health facility. Thus 72.4% of this cohort of women delivered outside of a health care facility. The remainder of the women delivered in a variety of health care

TABLE 1 Survey Results ($n = 642$)

Survey item	Results
Age of mothers (years; $n = 642$)	Range 18–47 (median 26)
Parity of mothers ($n = 642$)	Range 1–14 (median 4)
Distance from hospital (km; $n = 642$)	Range 2–90 (median 34)
Distance from dispensary (km; $n = 640$)	Range 0.25–57 (median 4)
Place of delivery ($n = 641$)	Home: 307 (47.9%)
	TBA's home: 135 (21.1%)
	Dispensary: 83 (12.9%)
	Hospital: 79 (12.3%)
	On the way: 22 (3.4%)
	Health center: 12 (1.9%)
	Pharmacy: 3 (0.5%)
Attendance at delivery ($n = 642$)	TBA: 244 (38.0%)
	Family/neighbors only: 195 (30.4%)
	Dispensary nurses: 97 (15.1%)
	Hospital staff: 78 (12.1%)
	Alone: 22 (3.4%)
	Others: 6 (0.9%)
Number who took study medications ($n = 642$)	Yes: 578 (90.0%)
	No: 64 (10.0%)*
	*All received injection at institution.
Number who would take study medications again in future pregnancies ($n = 642$)	Yes: 640 (99.7%)
	No: 2 (0.3%)*
	*One wanted tubal ligation, one had not used meds.

facilities: dispensary (12.9%), hospital (12.3%), health center (1.9%), and local pharmacy (0.5%).

More than two-thirds of the women were not attended by a skilled health care provider for their delivery. About one-third was either alone (3.4%), or only with family or neighbors (30.4%), or with others (0.9%). More than one-third (38%) were attended by a TBA. The remaining women had the skilled attendance of a dispensary nurse (15.1%) or hospital staff (12.1%).

When asked about whether they took the study medications, 90% of the women stated they did. The remaining 10% who did not take the medications all received an injectable medication at a health care institution, and thus they did not require the study medications. Of note, some of the women who delivered in an institution where injectable medication was available still insisted on using the study medication, despite the instructions of the health care staff to accept the injectable medication. All the women except for two, including those who had not used the medication, stated they would take them in a future pregnancy. Of the two who declined, one had not used the medications, and the second did not intend to have more children.

The women were asked if they sought medical attention for bleeding ($n = 641$). The vast majority (99.4%) stated they did not. Of the four women who admitted to requiring further attention for bleeding, two women had bleeding after using the misoprostol. One of these women got assistance from a health care provider and received injectable medication, while the other received local medications. The other two women who bled had received injectable medications first, and subsequently they decided to take the study medications.

When asked if they sought medical attention for infection, 636 of the 642 women surveyed (99.1%) stated that they did not. The six women who did seek medical attention for infection just reported on side effects. One of the six had not received misoprostol. Of the five women who had used the misoprostol, three reported abdominal pain, while one each reported palpitations and lack of energy. Two women stated that they subsequently used traditional medicine.

The women were also asked if the baby was born healthy ($n = 641$). For 631 women (98.4%), they agreed that the baby was healthy. For the remaining 10 women (1.6%), the responses follow: death of baby for seven (from prematurity, cord around neck, convulsions), spontaneous abortion (one), prematurity at 7 months (one), and no reason given (one).

DISCUSSION

About half of the women surveyed lived more than 30 km from the hospital and more than 4 km from the dispensary, and most had no access to transportation. A total of 72.4% of this cohort delivered outside of a health care facility. This percentage is higher than the average for the region (Ministry of Finance and Economic Affairs, Republic of Tanzania, 2009). Such a statistic is not surprising, however, as we chose to conduct this project in the most rural dispensaries in the district. There are many barriers to women in this region reaching a facility for delivery, including geographic distances, lack of affordable transportation, and insufficient time to undertake the trip before delivery.

An earlier study also documented multiple barriers facing Tanzanian women seeking a facility delivery (Women's Dignity and CARE International in Tanzania, 2008). In this study, women noted that in addition to distance and cost of delivery at a health care facility, the negative attitudes of health care providers and the lack of qualified staff and supplies were other barriers to seeking a health care facility for childbirth. Despite the existence of multiple barriers, Mbaruku and colleagues have demonstrated that many Tanzanian women would prefer a facility birth over birthing with a TBA if they had the choice because they are aware of the need for a skilled birth attendant to ensure a safe delivery (Mbaruku, Msambichaka, Galea, Rockers, & Kruk, 2009).

Only about a quarter of women in our cohort were attended by a trained health care provider, and a third of the women delivered without even the presence of a TBA. Interventions to help these women will be most effective if they can be easily administered by the women themselves or by those who are with her at the time of delivery. While the challenges for women to attend health care facilities for delivery are significant, the women who participated in our study were very positive about the availability of oral medications for them to take. All the women who took the study medications would use them again. Indeed, almost all of the women who did not take them would also use them in another pregnancy, as the word had spread about how effective the medications were. In future studies, more education about available drugs and their effectiveness is needed as some of the participating women chose to use misoprostol even when the superior medication oxytocin was available at a health care facility. Community distribution of misoprostol will help ensure that women have access to a uterotonic drug at the time of delivery for prevention of PPH, as the lower-level health care facilities (e.g., dispensaries) often do not have oxytocin in stock (Plotkin, Tibaijuka, Makene, Currie, & Lacoste, 2010).

There is not enough evidence to warrant including an oral antibiotic for sepsis prevention currently, and this will be abandoned in future research. Instead, in our scale-up project we intend to provide rural women with 600 micrograms of misoprostol in combination with a birth kit. How to effectively deliver these kits containing misoprostol to the most women has yet to be determined (Smith et al., 2013) and will be a focus of future research.

Limitations

There were several limitations to the research. It was not feasible to randomize the population; therefore, a convenience sample of women was used. Unfortunately, we were unable to include the TBAs in the distribution of the misoprostol as current government policy has prohibited them from practicing (although many still service the rural population). We did not record the number of women who declined to participate and the reasons for this; however, the participating dispensary nurses could only recall one woman who actively declined taking the study medications. Future research should capture this data, including which family members are making the decision for women to access care. We relied on self-report of the women about using the medication, which could elicit some bias. In addition, we did not confirm the timing of when the medication was taken; this oversight will be addressed in the scale-up study. Finally, in the future we will seek ethics approval to include younger women in the study (obtaining parental consent for their participation), as it is not uncommon for women aged 14 to 17 to become pregnant in this region, and excluding them from access to this important intervention because of age would be unethical.

Conclusions

Investment in maternal health is a human right, and results in improved health for the whole family as mothers are the main caregivers for children. It also makes economic sense, for every dollar spent on maternal health has the potential to multiply twentyfold in economic benefits (The Partnership for Maternal, Newborn and Child Health, 2013). Like thousands of women living in rural Africa, many women in rural Tanzania lack the resources and time to access health care providers at the time of their deliveries. Until there is sufficient resources to construct and staff health care facilities in the most rural areas of the country, there is a role for provision of oral medications for home deliveries. Women are both willing and able to safely take oral medications provided to them in pregnancy at the time of their deliveries, even when delivering at home with a TBA, family member, or alone. Through this study we conclude that it is feasible to distribute misoprostol to women for self-administration for PPH prevention, and in fact this is confirmed by a recent review of the literature (Smith et al., 2013). Qualitative data from interviews with participating women, TBAs, and dispensary nurses demonstrate that this program is very acceptable to women, their health care providers, and their communities (Webber & Chirangi, n.d.). As noted earlier, the benefits of misoprostol in preventing PPH are well established (Derman et al., 2006; Guülmezoglu et al., 2011; Sheldon, Blum, Durocher, & Winikoff, 2012) and it is now recommended that misoprostol be provided at all deliveries where access to injectable uterotonic medications is limited (FIGO, 2012; WHO,

2012a). While the WHO has not yet endorsed the distribution of misoprostol for self-administration for PPH prevention (WHO, 2012a, 2012b), we would argue that there is an imperative to undertake larger studies demonstrating the safety and effectiveness of this. Hundreds of thousands of women could be saved by access to this inexpensive medication: the time for further research is now.

ACKNOWLEDGMENTS

The authors thank the research coordinator Philegona Oloko and the research team members for their dedication to the project; the dispensary nurses, TBAs, and home-based care workers for their collaboration; and our advisory committee, particularly Mark Walker. We also appreciate the support of the Tanzanian Ministry of Health and Social Welfare, Rorya District Medical Officer, Mara Regional Medical Officer, the National Institute of Medical Research, and the project funders Grand Challenges Canada. We especially thank the women who participated in the project. We sincerely hope this research can make a difference for Tanzanian women in the future.

FUNDING

This project was funded by Grand Challenges Canada.

REFERENCES

Aboud, S., Msamanga, G., Read, J. S., Wang, L., Mfalila, C., Sharma, U., ... Fawzi, W.W. (2009). Effect of prenatal and perinatal antibiotics on maternal health in Malawi, Tanzania, and Zambia. *International Journal of Gynecology and Obstetrics, 107*, 202–207.

African Union Commission, Economic Commission for Africa, African Development Bank Group, & United Nations Development Program. (2013). *Executive summary MDG report 2013: Assessing progress in Africa toward the Millennium Development Goals* [Report]. Retrieved from http://www.undp.org/content/dam/undp/library/MDG/english/MDG%20Regional%20Reports/Africa/MDG%20report%202013%20summary_EN.pdf

Crowe, S., Utley, M., Costello, A., & Pagel, C. (2012). How many births in sub-Saharan Africa and South Asia will not be attended by a skilled birth attendant between 2011 and 2015? *BioMed Central Pregnancy and Childbirth, 12*, 4. doi:10.1186/1471-2393-12-4

Derman, R. J., Kodkany, B. S., Goudar, S. S., Geller, S. E., Naik, V. A., Bellad, M. B., Moss, N. (2006). Oral misoprostol in preventing postpartum haemorrhage in resource-poor communities: A randomised controlled trial. *The Lancet, 368*, 1248–1253.

Every Women Every Child. (2012). *UN Commission on life-saving commodities for women and children: Commissioners' report.* Retrieved from http://www.everywomaneverychild.org/images/UN_Commission_Report_September_2012_Final.pdf

FIGO Safe Motherhood and Newborn Committee. (2012). Prevention and treatment of postpartum hemorrhage in low-resource settings. *International Journal of Gynecology and Obstetrics, 117,* 108–118.

Guülmezoglu, A., Forna, F., Villar, J., & Hofmeyr, G. J. (2011). Prostaglandins for preventing postpartum haemorrhage. *Cochrane Database of Systematic Reviews, Issue 3.*

Haeri, S., & Dildy, G. A. (2012). Maternal mortality from hemorrhage. *Seminars in Perinatology, 36,* 48–55.

Hussein, J., & Fortney, J. A. (2004). Puerperal sepsis and maternal mortality: What role can new technologies play? *International Journal of Gynecology and Obstetrics, 85*(Suppl. 1), S52–S61.

Ifakara Health Institute, Venture Strategies Innovations, Bixby Center for Population, Health and Sustainability, Population Services International (PSI)/Tanzania. (2011). *Prevention of postpartum hemorrhage at home births: Misoprostol distribution during antenatal visits final report.* Ifakara, Tanzania: Authors.

Mbaruku, G., Msambichaka, B., Galea, S., Rockers, P. C., & Kruk, M. E. (2009). Dissatisfaction with traditional birth attendants in rural Tanzania. *International Journal of Gynecology and Obstetrics, 107,* 8–11.

Ministry of Finance and Economic Affairs, Republic of Tanzania. (2009). *Poverty and human development report 2009.* Retrieved from http://www.povertymonitoring.go.tz/WhatisNew/PHDR%202009%20text.pdf

Mir, A. M., Wajid, A., & Gull, S. (2012). Helping rural women in Pakistan to prevent postpartum hemorrhage: A quasi experimental study. *BioMed Central Pregnancy and Childbirth, 12,* 120. doi:10.1186/1471-2393-12-120

Nasreen, H., Nahar, S., Al Mamun, M., Afsana, K., & Byass, P. (2011). Oral misoprostol for preventing postpartum haemorrhage in home births in rural Bangladesh: How effective is it? *Global Health Action, 4.* doi:10.3402/gha.v4i0.7017

National Bureau of Statistics Tanzania & ICF Macro Tanzania. (2011). *Demographic and health survey 2010.* [Report]. Retrieved from http://www.measuredhs.com/pubs/pdf/FR243/FR243[24June2011].pdf

Pagel, C., Lewycka, S., Colbourn, T., Mwansamba, C. M., Mefuid, T., Chiudzu, G., . . . Costello, A.M.L. (2009). Estimation of potential effects of improved community-based drug provision, to augment health-facility strengthening, on maternal mortality due to post-partum haemorrhage and sepsis in sub-Saharan Africa: An equity-effectiveness model. *The Lancet, 374,* 1441–1448.

The Partnership for Maternal, Newborn and Child Health. (2013). *Economic case for investment in RMNCH.* [Report]. Retrieved from http://www.who.int/pmnch/topics/part_publications/ks24_re_20130403_low.pdf

Plotkin, M., Tibaijuka, G., Makene, C. L., Currie, S., & Lacoste, M. (2010). Quality of care for prevention and management of common maternal and newborn complications: A study of 12 regions in Tanzania. *Report 2: Findings on Labour, Delivery and Newborn Care.* [Report]. Retrieved from http://www.mchip.net/sites/default/files/mchipfiles/Tanzania_%20QoC_StudyReport_FINAL_0.pdf

Prata, N., Mbaruki, G., Grossman, A. A., Holston, M., & Hsieh, K. (2009). Community-based availability of Misoprostol: Is it safe? *African Journal of Reproductive Health, 13*, 117–128.

Rajbhandari, S., Hodgins, S., Sanghvi, H., McPherson, R., Pradhan, Y. V., & Baqui, A. H. (2010). Expanding uterotonic protection following childbirth through community-based distribution of misoprostol: Operations research study in Nepal. *International Journal of Gynecology and Obstetrics, 108*, 282–288.

Sanghvi, H., Ansari, N., Prata, N.J.V., Gibson, H., Ehsan, A. T., & Smith, J. M. (2010). Prevention of postpartum hemorrhage at home birth in Afghanistan. *International Journal of Gynecology and Obstetrics, 108*, 276–281.

Sebitloane, H. M., Moodley, J., & Esterhuizen, T. M. (2008). Prophylactic antibiotics for the prevention of postpartum infectious morbidity in women infected with human immunodeficiency virus: A randomized controlled trial. *American Journal of Obstetrics and Gynecology, 198*, 189.e1–189.e6.

Sheldon, W. R., Blum, J., Durocher, J., & Winikoff, B. (2012). Misoprostol for the prevention and treatment of postpartum hemorrhage. *Expert Opinions in Investigative Drugs, 21*, 235–250.

Smith, J. M., Gubin, R., Holston, M. M., Fullerton, J., & Prata, N. (2013). Misoprostol for postpartum hemorrhage prevention at home birth: An integrative review of global implementation experience to date. *BioMed Central Pregnancy and Childbirth, 13*, 44. doi:10.1186/1471-2393-13-44

Sullivan, T., & Hirst, J. (2011). Reducing Maternal Mortality: A review of progress and evidence-based strategies to achieve Millennium Development Goal 5. *Health Care for Women International, 32*, 901–916.

United Nations. (2013). *The Millennium Development Goals 2013.* [Report]. Retrieved from http://www.un.org/millenniumgoals/pdf/report-2013/mdg-report-2013-english.pdf

van Dillen, J., Zwart, J., Schutte, J., & van Roosmalen, J. (2010). Maternal sepsis: Epidemiology, etiology and outcome. *Current Opinion in Infectious Diseases, 23*, 249–254.

Webber, G & Chirangi, B. (n.d.). "Please do not forget us"—Views of women, nurses, and traditional birth attendants on community distribution of medications to prevent postpartum hemorrhage and sepsis: A qualitative pilot study in rural Tanzania. Unpublished manuscript.

Women's Dignity and CARE International in Tanzania. (2008). *"We have no choice": Facility-based childbirth: The perception and experiences of Tanzanian women, health workers, and traditional birth attendants* [Report]. Retrieved from http://www.policyforum-tz.org/files/childbirth.pdf

World Health Organization (WHO). (2011). *The selection and use of essential medicines: Report of the WHO Expert Committee, 2011 (including the 17th WHO Model List of Essential Medicines and the 3rd WHO Model List of Essential Medicines for Children)* [Report]. Retrieved from http://whqlibdoc.who.int/trs/WHO_TRS_965_eng.pdf

World Health Organization (WHO). (2012a). *WHO recommendations for the prevention and treatment of postpartum haemorrhage* [Report]. Retrieved from http://

www.who.int/reproductivehealth/publications/maternal_perinatal_health/9789
241548502/en/

World Health Organization (WHO). (2012b). *Optimizing health worker roles to improve access to key maternal and newborn health interventions through task shifting: Optimize MNH* [Report]. Retrieved from http://apps.who.int/iris/bitstream/10665/77764/1/9789241504843_eng.pdf

What Are the Factors That Interplay From Normal Pregnancy to Near Miss Maternal Morbidity in a Nigerian Tertiary Health Care Facility?

IKEOLA A. ADEOYE

Department of Epidemiology and Medical Statistics, College of Medicine, University of Ibadan, Ibadan, Nigeria

OMOTADE O. IJAROTIMI

Department of Obstetrics, Gynaecology and Perinatology, College of Health Sciences, Obafemi Awolowo University, Ile-Ife, Nigeria

ADESEGUN O. FATUSI

Department of Community Health, College of Health Sciences, Obafemi Awolowo University, Ile-Ife, Nigeria

Researchers in Nigeria examined the epidemiological charac-teristics and factors associated with maternal outcomes using a mixed method approach: a prospective case control study design involving 375 pregnant women who received maternal care from a tertiary facility and in-depth interviews reporting the experience of near-miss survivors. A generalized ordered logit model was used to generate the estimates of partial proportional odds ratios (and 95% confidence intervals) across categories of the outcome variable. Factors strongly associated with maternal morbidity were late refer-ral of women, presence of complications at booking antenatal visits, low birth weight, and severe birth asphyxia. The nearmiss women were further characterized, and a low proportion (25%) had organ dysfunction or failure. The challenge of such diagnoses in resource-constrained settings raises questions about the appropriateness of using organ dysfunction criteria in developing countries.

BACKGROUND

Maternal health issues in Nigeria are of global concern as the country records the second highest number of annual maternal deaths in the world after India: Nigeria contributes 14% of the total global maternal deaths figure of 287,000), while India contributes 19% (World Health Organization [WHO], 2012). Improving maternal health is one of the eight Millennium Development Goals (MDGs) with the target of reducing maternal mortality ratio by three-quarters between 1990 and 2015. According to the WHO, considerable progress has been made toward the reduction of maternal mortality over the last two decades although the challenge still persists (WHO, 2012). Unfortunately, for each maternal death that occurs, another 20 women are likely to suffer serious health sequellae (Chowdhury, Ahmed, Kalim, & Koblinsky, 2009). As many as 15 million women are estimated to be affected by maternal morbidities worldwide (Koblinsky, Chowdhury, Moran, & Ronsmans, 2012). Hence, while maternal mortality has been described as the "tip of the iceberg," maternal morbidity constitutes the "base" but has not received adequate attention (Fortney & Smith, 1996; Hardee, Gay, & Blanc, 2012). As such, maternal morbidity and disability and their consequences have recently been described as the "neglected agenda in maternal health" (Koblinsky et al., 2012, p. 124).

Maternal morbidity refers to the health problems that women encounter during pregnancy, delivery, or in the postpartum period. Unlike maternal mortality, which is a singular and distinct event, however, maternal morbidity is often more complex, resulting from many conditions of varying duration and severity. The lack of a uniform, standardized, and reproducible definition of maternal morbidity as well as the difficulty associated with ascertaining and measuring maternal morbidity has been a major challenge in research (Firoz et al., 2013; Say, Souza, & Pattinson, 2009). As in the case of maternal mortality, developing countries disproportionately bear the burden of maternal morbidity. Maternal health occurs along a spectrum, with the two extremes as normal health and death, and maternal morbidity exists within these extremes. Across the spectrum of maternal health, pregnancy and childbirth can move from normal pregnancy to being complicated (acute maternal morbidity) and to becoming life threatening, otherwise referred to as "near-miss" cases (WHO, 2004).

A near miss is defined as a woman who nearly died but survived a complication that occurred during pregnancy, childbirth, or within 42 days of termination of pregnancy. Three different approaches have generally been reported in literature for identifying near misses: (a) disease-specific criteria; (b) intervention criteria such as emergency hysterectomy to control hemorrhage; and (c) organ system based criteria which is based on the dysfunction or failure of a major organ such as the occurrence of pulmonary edema or disseminated intravascular coagulopathy, which are markers of cardiac and coagulation systems, respectively (Mantel, Buchmann, Rees, & Pattinson, 1998; Souza, Cecatti, Hardy, Serruya, & Amaral, 2007). In addition to near-miss events being useful in assessing the quality of services, it has a special advantage in that the woman who survived a life-threatening condition is able to recount her experience: such narratives can contribute to a deeper understanding of the social factors that are associated with maternal morbidity (WHO, 2012). Studies reporting the experiences of the survivors of near miss events, however, are very few (Souza, Cecatti, Parpinelli, Krupa, & Osis, 2009; Tuncalp, Huldin, Kwame, & Adamu, 2012).

Nigeria is making progress toward the achievement of MDG 5: from an estimated 1,100 maternal deaths per 100,000 in 1990, the country's maternal mortality ratio reduced to 820 maternal deaths per 100,000 in 2005, and to 630 per 100,000 in 2010 (WHO, 2012). Maternal mortality remains a substantial challenge in the country, with about 40,000 maternal deaths recorded annually. Besides, many important maternal health indices with implications for maternal and newborn outcomes are still poor, and they suggest that the level of maternal morbidity may be quite high. For instance, while 58.9% of mothers received antenatal care services from skilled service providers, only 38.9% had skilled attendance during delivery (National Population Commission [NPC] & ICF Macro, 2009). Social and community factors, in addition to health facility factors, have been strongly implicated in maternal health outcomes in Nigeria (Babalola & Fatusi, 2009; Wall, 1998) and many other low- and middle-income countries (Gabrysch & Campbell, 2009; Thaddeus & Maine, 1994). Overall, maternal morbidity has been inadequately researched in Nigeria, and there is a need to determine its current pattern as well as to investigate associated factors.

In this study, we investigated the spectrum of maternal events from uncomplicated pregnancy (normal) to complicated (acute maternal morbidity) and life-threatening cases (near misses) by examining their characteristics and the associated factors in the Ife-Ijesa zone of Osun State, southwest Nigeria. We also explored some factors associated with the occurrence of severe maternal morbidities through the lens of near-miss cases by reviewing their narratives. Finally, we examined and characterized women who had experienced organ dysfunction or organ failures among women with life-threatening complications.

METHODS

This study provides a further analysis of a prospective case control study that was carried out at the Obafemi Awolowo University Teaching Hospitals Complex (OAUTHC), Ile-Ife, southwest Nigeria from July 2006 to June

2007. The study was carried out simultaneously at two maternity hospitals under OAUTHC, which are situated in two separate local government areas (LGAs) of Osun State (Wesley Guild Hospital, Ilesa in Ilesa East LGA, and Ife Hospital Unit in Ife Central LGA). The study participants were pregnant women who sought maternal care at the hospitals during the antenatal (third trimester) or intrapartum period or within 42 days after delivery. Four un-matched controls were selected for every near-miss event. The details of the methodology (namely, study setting, population, sample size, and se-lection) have been described in an earlier publication (Adeoye, Onayade, & Fatusi, 2013). Here, we present fresh perspectives from the quantitative data and also include findings from qualitative aspects of the study based on a collection of narratives from near-miss survivors and subsequent narrative analysis (Hancock, Windridge, & Ockleford, 2007). The qualitative findings were used to put the quantitative data into a social context.

Trained research assistants carried out a narrative interview with each of the 75 women who had experienced a near miss. The interview started with a "generative narrative question" whereby each woman was requested to relate her experience of the near-miss event and the associated events/factors. This was then followed by relevant questions from the data collector, drawing from a study guide, to gain better perspectives of the associated social and community factors. Where necessary, the information from the interview of the affected woman was supplemented with information from another adult, usually a woman and a close relative who was caring for the woman at the time of the near-miss event. The initial theme was based on the content of the interview guide. The interviews, on the whole, provided an opportunity to obtain a verbatim account of the pregnancy and the delivery experience as well as information on related maternal health issues including the use of birth preparedness plans, knowledge of warning signs, types of delays encountered, male involvement, access to funds, and perception of the quality of care. The interviews were performed by the bedside when patients became clinically stable enough to respond to the questions. The responses were documented in writing and not recorded because some of the study participants were not comfortable with the use of a tape recorder and did not give consent to that effect. The narrative analysis was carried out manually. The study protocol was approved by the Ethics and Research Committee of the hospital.

Operational Variable Definitions

Dependent variable. Dependent variables included maternal outcome categorized into three groups: normal pregnancy, acute maternal morbidities, and near misses:

- *Normal pregnancy* describes a pregnant woman who had spontaneous vertex delivery of a live infant, without any obstetric complication and did not require any health intervention like caesarian section, induction of labor, and manual removal of placenta to facilitate or complete the birth process.

- *Acute maternal morbidities:* Women who had non-life-threatening complication in current pregnancy, during delivery, and puerperium that could adversely affect maternal and perinatal outcomes as well as those that required any health intervention like caesarian section, induction of labor, or manual removal of placenta to facilitate or complete the birth process. This category also included women who have had complications in their previous pregnancies that influenced obstetric management in the current pregnancy.

- *Near misses* were based on the disease-specific criteria described by Filippi and colleagues (2005): (a) hemorrhage (leading to shock, emergency hysterectomy, coagulation defects, and/or blood transfusion of 2 or more liters of blood); (b) hypertensive disorders in pregnancy—eclampsia and severe preeclampsia with clinical or laboratory indication for termination of pregnancy to save the woman's life; (c) dystocia—uterine rupture and impending rupture, such as prolonged obstructed labor with previous caesarian section; (d) infection—septicemia from any cause; and (e) severe anemia (hemoglobin <6 g/dl).

Independent variables. Independent variables included sociodemographics (maternal age, maternal education, marital status), obstetric (parity, gestational age at delivery, antenatal care attendance, complications noted during booking visit, referral status, fetal presentation during labor), and perinatal characteristics (low birth weight, birth asphyxia, stillbirth).

Statistical Analysis

Statistical analysis for the quantitative aspect was performed using STATA version 12. The differences in the proportion of women with normal pregnancy, acute maternal morbidities, and near misses with specific characteristics were compared using a chi-square test at a 5% level of statistical significance. Multivariate analysis was done using a generalized ordered logit model with maternal event—normal pregnancy, acute maternal morbidity, and near miss—as the outcome. This was used to generate the estimates of partial proportional odds ratios across the categories of the outcome variable: (a) any maternal morbidity (acute maternal morbidity and near misses) versus normal pregnancy and (b) near misses versus other pregnancy outcomes (acute maternal morbidity and normal pregnancy). The generalized ordered logit model works well in situations where the proportionality or parallel slopes assumption of ordinal logistic regression is violated (Williams, 2005). This assumption was assessed during the preliminary analysis using the omodel test. The test showed a violation of the proportionality assumption of odds across response categories ($\chi^2 = 80.42, p < .001$): hence, ordinal logistic regression could not be used for the analysis. The "gologit2" command was used in STATA to fit the generalized ordered logit model. The partial proportional odds ratios and 95% confidence intervals are reported.

RESULTS

Sociodemographic, Maternal, and Perinatal Characteristics

A total of 375 parturient women were analyzed in this study, consisting of 130 women with normal pregnancy (34.7%), 170 women with acute maternal morbidities (45.3%), and 75 women with near misses (20.0%). There was no significant difference between the mean age of the groups ($p = .554$): 29.5 (±5) years for women who had normal pregnancy (NP), 30.0 (±5) for those with acute maternal morbidity (AMM) and 28.6n (±6) for those with near misses (NM). As Table 1 shows, there were significant differences between the three groups of women with respect to maternal education ($p = .044$) and marital status ($p < .001$) but not with parity ($p = .685$).

The three groups of women differ significantly with respect to the maternal experiences at delivery ($p < .001$ in each case): gestational age at delivery, proportion with complications noted during booking visit, proportion referred to tertiary facility, and proportion with emergency caesarean section. For each variable, the proportion was highest among women with near miss and lowest among those with normal pregnancy. Similarly, the three groups of women differed significantly ($p < .001$) with respect to the following perinatal outcomes: low birth weight, birth asphyxia, and stillbirth rate, with the near-miss group recording the highest proportion for each of these negative outcomes.

Maternal/Fetal Conditions Among Acute Maternal Morbidities

Figure 1 shows the rate of occurrence of various complications experienced by the women who had acute maternal morbidities. Prolonged labor was the most common cause of maternal morbidity, accounting for about a third (32.4%) of all the morbidities. The other leading causes were abnormal presentation (14.6%), fetal distress (11.6%), and hemorrhage (11.0%).

Specific Clinical, Laboratory, and Health Care Features of Near Misses

Table 2 shows the specific clinical, laboratory and health care features of near misses. Of the 75 women who had near-miss events, 61 (81.0%) had developed their complications prior to their arrival at the hospital, while 14 (19%) developed life-threatening complications while on admission at the tertiary health facility. The major causes of near-miss events were severe hemorrhage

TABLE 1 A Comparison of Sociodemographic, Obstetric, and Perinatal Characteristics in Women With Normal Pregnancies, Acute Maternal Morbidity, and Near Miss Events

	Spectrum of maternal health			
Characteristics	Normal pregnancy (n = 130)	Acute maternal morbidity (n = 170)	Near misses (n = 75)	p value
Maternal age (years)				
<35 years	102(78.5)	127(74.7)	53(77.3)	.554
≥35 years	28(21.5)	43(25.3)	17(22.7)	
Maternal education				
≤Secondary	76(58.5)	76(44.7)	42(56.0)	.044
≥Postsecondary	54(41.5)	94(55.3)	33(44.0)	
Marital status				
Married	123(94.6)	151(88.8)	55(73.3)	<.001
Not married	7(5.4)	19(11.2)	20(26.7)	
Parity				
Primipara	55(42.3)	67(39.4)	35(46.7)	.685
2nd–3rd deliveries	50(38.5)	75(44.1)	30(40.0)	
>3 deliveries	25(19.2)	28(16.5)	10(13.3)	
Gestational age at delivery				
<38 weeks	14(10.8)	26(15.8)	26(35.6)	<.001
≥38 weeks	116(89.2)	139(84.2)	47(64.8)	
Antenatal care				
OAUTHC	101(77.7)	119(70.0)	21(28.0)	<.001
Not OAUTHC	29(22.3)	51(30.0)	54(72.0)	
Complications noted during booking visit				
Yes	13(10.0)	35(20.6)	23(30.7)	<.001
No	117(90.0)	124(79.4)	52(69.3)	
Referred				
Yes	21(16.1)	44(25.9)	28(37.3)	<.001
No	109(83.9)	126(74.1)	47(62.7)	
Cephalic presentation				
Yes	130(100.0)	136(80.5)	71(96.0)	<.001
No	0(0.00)	33(19.5)	3(4.0)	
Emergency and caesarean section				
Yes	0(0.0)	97(57.4)	41(57.7)	<.001
No	123(100.0)	72(42.6)	30(42.3)	
Low birth weight				
Yes	14(12.0)	24(14.5)	28(44.4)	<.001
No	103(88.5)	141(85.5)	35(55.6)	
Birth asphyxia				
Yes	3(2.6)	13(8.70)	10(22.2)	<.001
No	113(97.4)	137(91.3)	35(77.8)	
Stillbirth				
Yes	0(0.00)	12(7.45)	17(27.0)	<.001
No	117(100.0)	149(92.7)	46(73.0)	

(41.3%), hypertensive disorders of pregnancy (37.3%), prolonged obstructed labor (18.6%), severe septicemia (14.6%), and severe anemia (13.3%). Severe hemorrhage was mostly secondary to retained placenta and uterine atony and was associated with hypovolemic shock in the majority of women who experienced severe hemorrhage (77.4%). The estimated mean blood loss

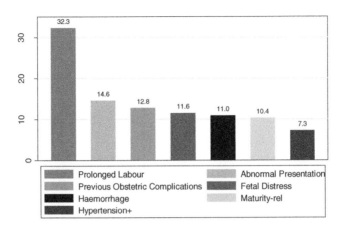

FIGURE 1 Distribution of acute maternal morbidities by specific causes.

was 1.21 (±0.76 liters). Emergency hysterectomies were performed in four women, consisting of two who had ruptured uterus, one woman with morbidly adherent placenta, and another with uncontrolled hemorrhage. Among women who had pregnancy-induced hypertension (PIH), the mean systolic and mean diastolic blood pressures were 194.3 (±23.3) and 126.3 (±23.8), respectively. The associated clinical features were severe headache (24.0%), hypochondria pain (18.6%), and convulsions (12.0%). The electrolytes evaluated included serum sodium [132 ± 5.3], serum potassium [132 ± 5.3], and serum urea [5.7 ± 3.2] levels. Chorioamnionitis and wound infections were causes of septicemia in 27.2% and 73.3% of cases, respectively. The mean body temperature measured was 39.0 ± 0.6 degrees Celsius.

Nineteen of the near misses (25.0%) had identifiable organ dysfunction. Acute pulmonary edema (10.6%) was the most common cause of organ dysfunction followed by acute renal failure (8.0%), intractable uterine atony warranting hysterectomy (5.3%), and disseminated intravascular dissemination (1.3%) (see Figure 2).

Multivariate Analysis

In Table 3 we display the result of the generalized ordered logit estimates that are expressed as partial proportional odds ratios (POR) with their 95% confidence intervals. In the first set of comparisons, women who had any form of maternal morbidity (acute morbidity or near misses) were assessed against those who had normal pregnancies. The following were the significant risk factors for maternal morbidity: the presence of complications during booking visit [POR = 2.94; 95% CI = 1.53 – 5.63]; referral to the tertiary facility [POR = 3.84; 95% CI = 1.1 – 13.26]; and, severe asphyxia [POR = 3.14; 95% CI = 1.36 – 8.52].

Second, women who had life-threatening complications were compared with other maternal outcomes (acute maternal morbidity or normal

TABLE 2 Specific Clinical, Laboratory, Health Care Features of Near Misses

Types of near miss	Frequency (%) ($n = 75$)	Mean (+*SD* or IOR)
Severe hemorrhage	31(41.3%)	
Specific causes		
Retained placenta	11/31(35.5%)	
Uterine atony	9/31(29.0%)	
Antepartum hemorrhage	11/31(35.5%)	
Mean blood loss (mL)		1208.2 ± 760
Hypovolemia shock	24/31(77.4%)	
Emergency hysterectomy	4/31(12.9%)	
Hypertensive disorders of pregnancy	28(37.3%)	
Mean systolic blood pressure		194.3 ± 23.3
Mean diastolic blood pressure		126.3 ± 23.8
+ Convulsion	9/28(32.1%)	
Associated features		
Severe headache	18/28(64.3%)	
Hypochondria pain	14/28(50.0%)	
Pulmonary Edema	5/28(17.9%)	
Electrolytes		
Mean sodium		132 ± 5.3
Mean potassium		3.65 ± 0.6
Mean urea		5.7 ± 3.2
Prolonged obstructed labor	14/75(18.6%)	
Mean duration of labor		36.93 ± 20.1
Comorbidities	8/14(57.1%)	
Severe septicemia	11/75(14.6%)	
Causes		
Chorioamnionitis	3/11(27.2%)	
Wound infection	8/11(72.3%)	
Mean temperature		39.0 ± 0.6
Specimen for culture	5/11(45.5%)	
Severe anemia	10/75(13.3%)	
Median PCV		13.5(IQR 12–15)
Median pints of blood transfusion		4(IQR 3–6)
Proportion with organ dysfunction	19/75(25.0%)	

pregnancy). The presence of complications during booking visit [POR = 2.94; 95% CI = 1.53 –5.63], referral to the tertiary facility [POR = 3.84; 95% CI = 1.1 – 13.26], and, severe asphyxia [POR = 3.14; 95% CI = 1.36–8.52] remained significant factors. In addition, having a low birth weight baby was also a significant factor associated with the near-misses experience [POR = 3.31; 95% CI = 1.43 – 7.63].

Qualitative Data Findings

We present illustrative narratives from our study to highlight the interplay of these factors within our study context based on the classical three-delay model of Thaddeus and Maine (1994), as well as the four-pronged classification of Gabrysch and Campbell (2009) on factors associated with adverse

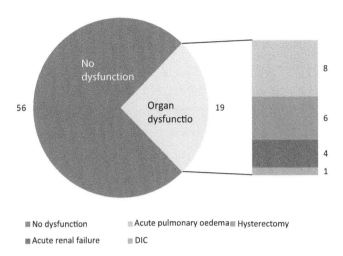

FIGURE 2 Percentage distribution of women with near miss by presence and type of organ dysfunction.

maternal outcomes: (a) sociocultural factors, (b) perceived benefit or need of skilled attendance, (c) economic accessibility, and (d) physical accessibility.

Delay in presenting at the health facility. Some women had been experiencing serious pregnancy-related problems (warning signs in pregnancy) but underestimated their significance and did not respond appropriately due to poor maternal health knowledge. Thus there was a delay in accessing and obtaining appropriate health care:

> I was having headache for over more than a week and I used Panadol (a pain reliever). Later on the headache became very serious and I began to have swollen feet and poor vision. It was then I went to the comprehensive health center at Iloko Ijesa where I had registered for antenatal care. The nurses told me my blood pressure was very high so they referred me here. *(30 year old secondary school teacher with imminent eclampsia)*

> I started passing fluid from my private part (vagina) about 10 days ago. At that time my baby was still moving. I went to the maternity center in my area. There I was told to go home that there was no problem. But the fluid never stopped coming. After a week, the baby movement stopped. One of my relatives advised me to go to the teaching hospital. *(27 year-old unbooked para 3, i.e., woman that has had her third birth, who had a macerated stillbirth and anemia complicated by septicemia. She also had gram negative septicemia shock.)*

> I had been feeling weak and dizzy for some time now, but I thought it was because I was pregnant. My husband and I decided to travel home to be cared for by my Mum in Ilesa. When we arrived home, she insisted I had to come to the hospital. Here I was told I have anemia. *(26-year-old primigravida from Abuja, who had severe anemia secondary to*

TABLE 3 Odds Ratios of Ordered Logistic Regression on Normal Pregnancies, Acute Maternal Morbidity, and Near Misses

Item	(Acute maternal morbidity and near misses) versus normal pregnancy		Near misses versus (acute maternal morbidity and normal pregnancy)	
	Odds ratio	95% Confidence interval	Odds Ratio	95% Confidence interval
Age				
<35 years (RC)				
≥35 years	0.90	0.49–1.62	0.90	0.49–1.62
Maternal education				
≤Secondary school (RC)				
Postsecondary	2.00	1.2–3.34	0.89	0.43–1.87
Marital status				
Not married (RC)				
Married	0.52	0.24–1.44	0.52	0.24–1.44
ParityPrimipara				
2–3 deliveries	1.03	0.72–1.46	1.03	0.72–1.46
≥3 deliveries				
Antenatal attendance				
OAUTHC	1.08	0.33–3.49	1.08	0.33–3.49
No (RC)				
Complications noted at booking				
No	2.94	1.53–5.63	2.94	1.53–5.63
Yes				
Referred				
No				
Yes	3.84	1.11–13.26	3.84	1.11–13.26
Gestational age at delivery				
<38 weeks				
≥38 weeks	0.52	0.25–1.08	0.52	0.25–1.08
Low birth weight				
Yes	1.14	0.54–2.44	3.31	1.43–7.63
No				
Severe asphyxia				
Yes	3.14	1.36–8.52	3.14	1.36–8.52
No				

HIV/AIDS. She was unaware of her HIV status until she got to the hospital. Her husband also tested HIV positive.)

Perceived benefit or need of skilled attendance and economic accessibility. These are factors that influence the perception of how a facility delivery with skilled attendance would benefit the mother and newborn, how "big" the personal need for such care is, or both. These factors affect the decision to seek care from skilled attendants and health facilities. The narratives obtained in our study showed that some categories of women opted for care from unskilled attendants largely because they do not see the value of skilled attendants and facilities largely based on their experience in previous pregnancies. Poor financial status also interplays in this decision-making process as illustrated by the following narrative:

> My two previous deliveries were without any problem. I had always received care from the mission home. However in this pregnancy, I started bleeding since the pregnancy was about 6 months. When the bleeding became very frequent, the church birth attendant asked me to do an ultrasound scan. She told me to go to the hospital but I refused because I had no money. I also believed that I was going to be fine because God is in control. As the day of delivery drew near, the bleeding became very heavy and unfortunately my husband had gone to the farm. I did not know when I got here. I was told my relatives and neighbors brought me here. (*34-year-old unbooked para 3 who had disseminated intravascular coagulopathy following severe antepartum, intrapartum, and postpartum hemorrhages secondary to placenta previa. She received 10 pints of blood.*)

Physical accessibility to emergency obstetric facilities and health system factors. The narratives from our women show two categories with respect to accessibility to emergency obstetric facilities and health system factors: (a) seeking care from health facilities that lack obstetrics emergency care capacities, largely because the accessibility to emergency obstetric care facilities is more challenging; and (b) inability to receive appropriate care from health facilities with emergency obstetric care capacities due to poor quality of care or broader health systems factor such as industrial action by health workers:

> I delivered a dead baby at home. Thereafter, the placenta did not come out, so I went to a private hospital close by where the placenta was removed. Few days after I was discharged, I started bleeding heavily, so I reported back to the same hospital, but I was referred to Wesley Guild Hospital because the bleeding was just too much. (*35-year-old unbooked grand multiparous (para 6) woman with severe hemorrhage from retained placenta following stillbirth*)

> I had a stillbirth in my last delivery, but I believed that all would be well this time. After I had delivered my baby at home, the placenta wouldn't come out and I also started bleeding. I was taken to a private clinic, but they refused to take me into the facility because of the seriousness of the bleeding. My husband was told to take me to Wesley Guild Hospital. (*Near miss with postpartum hemorrhage secondary to retained placenta*)

> The man that impregnated her lives close to us; we did not realize she was pregnant for quite some time. Although he did not deny the pregnancy, he has not provided funds for her care. When she fell into labor, we took her to the primary health center here (in our community) where she was in labor for 3 days without progress. Then, she was referred to LAUTECH Teaching Hospital (which is not far from us). Unfortunately when we got

there, there was a strike. So we had to come here. (*Mother of a 20-year-old primigravida with prolonged obstructed labor with septicemia*)

On Sunday afternoon I had a sharp pain in my stomach. At that time, my baby was still moving. I was told that I was bleeding inside because of placenta separation. Eventually, I was taken to the theater, by which time my baby had stopped kicking. (*Booked but unmarried primigravida who had ruptured uterus that was mistaken for concealed abruption placenta. She had uterine repair instead of hysterectomy because of her low parity.*)

DISCUSSION

Maternal morbidity has been aptly described as a neglected agenda in women's health as it has received scant attention in comparison with maternal mortality, though it occurs at a much higher level (Koblinsky et al., 2012). Although Nigeria, which has the second highest burden of annual maternal deaths in the world (WHO, 2012), is expected to have very high rates of maternal morbidity, scant research attention has been given to this issue. Our study examined the pattern in maternal health spectrum from normal pregnancy, to acute maternal morbidity, to near misses in a Nigerian tertiary health care facility and explored associated factors.

The most important factor associated with maternal morbidity (both acute maternal morbidity and near misses) found in our study was the referral status of women. Women who were referred from another facility to the tertiary care center had a fourfold risk (OR = 3.84) of experiencing maternal morbidity compared with women who were not referred. One probable reason for this was that referrals were mostly late, which usually resulted from delay in seeking care from the primary (referring) center. Referrals to a tertiary facility, in most cases, inadvertently meant that severe complications had already set in or were imminent. Several narratives from near-miss cases strongly suggest that the act of first approaching lower-level centers (which lack emergency obstetric care capacity) during obstetrics emergencies inadvertently lengthened the referral process. Specifically, four-fifths (81%) of the near misses were in serious condition upon arrival at the hospital. This is similar to the findings of Filippi and colleagues (2005) in their study on near misses in three African countries were most of the women (83%) were already in critical condition upon arrival at the hospital.

Evidently, strengthening the referral system in Nigeria will reduce maternal morbidity and mortality, but this needs to be complemented with efforts to overcome critical demand- and supply-side barriers to produce optimal results. Fournier and colleagues (2009) have shown, in a quasiexperimental study of maternal mortality in six rural health districts in Mali that the risk of maternal death could be reduced with appropriate constellation of services or intervention. The risk of maternal death in that study was reduced by half (OR = 0.48) following health system improvement that involved basic and comprehensive emergency obstetric care, transportation, and a community financing scheme. The approach used in Mali showed that it is not just a question of improving the link between facilities, but that other ancillary factors, particularly finance and transportation issues, must be addressed especially in the context of low-resourced communities. For instance, lack of funds was one of the factors that did not allow some of the women in our study to take the advantage of the referral provided to them. Therefore, "active referral" rather than a passive referral of women needs to be vigorously promoted. Active referrals involve proactive participation and support of the referring facility and personnel in ensuring that the referred individuals access emergency care. The issue of absence of skilled attendants at birth is also implicated in maternal morbidity occurrence in this study because a number of our women indicated in their narratives that they used the services of traditional or faith-based birth attendants. This is an area of significant concern in the maternal health effort because the last Nigeria Demographic and Health Survey reported that more than a third of pregnant women in Nigeria still deliver outside an orthodox health facility or without the presence of skilled attendants (NPC & ICF Macro, 2009).

Identifying maternal-related complication in a woman during her first antenatal (booking) visit was also strongly associated with maternal morbidity. There was a threefold odds (OR = 2.94) of having maternal morbidity among this category of women compared with those in whom no complication was observed at their booking visit. Although obstetric complications are often unpredictable, which makes the use of the risk approach in antenatal care ineffective, our findings strongly suggest that complications during the first antenatal visit might be a risk marker. Thus, women who present with complications at first antenatal booking visit may require more intensive surveillance. Significant attention, therefore, must also be paid to counseling for possible referral, having a birth preparedness plan, regular education, and close clinical monitoring during each antenatal visit.

Low birth weight (OR = 3.31) and severe birth asphyxia (OR = 3.14) were also strongly associated with maternal morbidity, especially with near misses. This finding supports the point that the health of the mother and her child are intricately linked. Low birth weight may be a consequence of preterm delivery and could be also be an indicator of poor fetomaternal nutrition. Poor fetomaternal nutrition may result from poor nutritional status and inadequate nutritional intake during pregnancy. In addition, heavy placenta parasitemia from severe malaria infection is an important cause of low birth weight in malaria holoendemic areas like Nigeria. Low birth weight, a major determinant of mortality, morbidity, and disability in neonates, infancy, and childhood, could have a long-term impact on health outcomes in adult life (United Nations Children's Fund (UNICEF) & WHO, 2004). Specifically, having low birth weight can program the infant for future disease in adult life (Balci, Acikel, & Akdemir, 2010).

Furthermore, we found prolonged obstructed labor occurring in almost a fifth of women with acute maternal morbidities. Cephalopelvic disproportion, which may result from poorly developed pelvic bones of mothers, could account for most cases of prolonged labor. An inadequate pelvis is usually a sequellae of prolonged undernutrition in the mother from her childhood or adolescent years. Poor childhood nutrition and early pregnancy, both of which have fairly high rates in Nigeria, are associated with cephalopelvic disproportion. Thus, improving nutrition in childhood and adolescence, preventing early marriage and pregnancy, and reducing fertility rates may all contribute toward the reduction of maternal morbidity in our study population.

Finally, the proportion of near-miss cases with organ dysfunction or failure of a major organ system was 25%. This is comparable with the findings of Thomas van den Akker and coworkers in Malawi where only 22% of the near miss events were discovered using the organ systemic dysfunction criteria (van den Akker, Beltman, Leyten, Mwagomba, & Meguid, 2013). Near misses with organ failure, for example renal or cardiopulmonary failures, comprise the most severe forms of maternal morbidity because they faced the highest risk of death but only survived because of the quality maternal care they had received. The WHO Working Group on Maternal Mortality and Morbidity classification has proposed that the organ system dysfunction criteria might be the most promising approach compared with the disease-specific criteria (which has been widely used in developing countries) or intervention-based approach. The strong appeal of the organ dysfunction approach includes its sensitivity in capturing true near-miss events as well as its suitability for comparison across different setting. Its use may be challenging in low-income settings, however, because of the shortage of sophisticated equipment and skills required to diagnose organ dysfunction or failures (Pattison & Hall, 2003).

Not unexpectedly, our findings show that the organ failure criteria are likely to document only a subset of women with life-threatening complications: as such, this results in an underestimation of the true burden of near misses. A recent systematic review on the prevalence of maternal near misses revealed that prevalence of near misses was much lower when the identification criteria was based on organ failures or dysfunction (Tuncalp, Hindin, Souza, Chou, & Say, 2012). Furthermore, for better surveillance and timely interventions in women with life-threatening complications, concentration on those who meet the disease-specific criteria may be better than those with organ failures who have a comparatively lower likelihood of survival. Besides, the time of progression to organ failure and death may move very fast along the maternal health spectrum. Therefore, the disease-based approach might be the most suitable in low-resource settings that bear disproportionately higher burdens of maternal ill-health and mortality. The position of the WHO Working Group in its preference for an organ-system dysfunction approach may require further research, particularly in elucidating factors that affect the time of progression to fatal or near-fatal outcomes in pregnancy and childbirth.

CONCLUSIONS

Overall, the findings from our study highlight some factors that are associated with the spectrum of maternal morbidity in a Nigerian environment. Many of these factors, interestingly, are modifiable, thus providing some directions for possible evidence-based interventions. Health systems strengthening (HSS) is an important interventional approach for improving accessibility to and quality of maternal service delivery. HSS should address factors associated with improved availability as well as geographical and financial accessibility to essential obstetrics facilities, as well as the strengthening of the referral system. Individual and household targeted interventions are also important, particularly health education for women to improve maternal health seeking behavior and the use of a birth preparedness plan. As we have indicated earlier, maternal morbidity has not received adequate research attention. Thus, this study opens a window of opportunity for better understanding of maternal morbidity challenges, its patterns, and associated factors. More studies are needed, particularly in low- and middle-income countries to improve the understanding of the factors at play in maternal morbidity and serve as platforms for effective program design and implementation.

The low proportion of the near-miss cases that had organ dysfunction in our study and the challenge of such diagnosis in a resource-constrained environment raise questions about the appropriateness of using organ dysfunction criteria in low- and middle-income countries. We advocate, instead, that a disease-based approach appears more feasible and practicable for most developing countries to identify and address the challenge of severe maternal morbidities. This issue deserves more research and consensus building between maternal health researchers and experts. In addition, we share the perspective of Van der Akker and colleagues (2013) that "by only monitoring near-miss cases and mortality, we underestimate the impact on women who will live with non-life threatening, yet serious maternal morbidities" (p. 1–5).

ACKNOWLEDGMENTS

We acknowledge the role of physicians and nurses in the Department of Obstetrics and Gynaecology, OAUTHC, in facilitating the study. A. Jegede of the Department of Sociology, University of Ibadan, Ibadan, and Olanrewaju Afolabi of the Medical Research Council, The Gambia, critiqued the initial drafts of the manuscript and gave useful input.

REFERENCES

Adeoye, I. A., Onayade, A. A., & Fatusi, A. O. (2013). Incidence, determinants and perinatal outcomes of near miss maternal morbidity in Ile-Ife Nigeria: A prospective case control study. *BMC Pregnancy and Childbirth, 13*, 93. doi:10.1186/1471–2393–13–93

Babalola, S., & Fatusi, A. (2009). Determinants of use of maternal health services in Nigeria—Looking beyond individual and household factors. *BMC Pregnancy Childbirth, 9*, 43. doi:10.1186/1471–2393–9–43

Balci, M. M., Acikel, S., & Akdemir, R. (2010). Low birth weight and increased cardiovascular risk: Fetal programming. *International Journal of Cardiology, 24*, 110–111.

Chowdhury, M. E., Ahmed, A., Kalim, N., & Koblinsky, M. (2009). Causes of maternal mortality decline in Matlab, Bangladesh. *Journal of Health, Population and Nutrition, 27*, 108–123.

Filippi, V., Ronsmans, C., Gandaho, T., Graham, W., Alihonou, E., & Santos, P. (2003). Women's reports of severe near miss obstetric complications in Benin. *Studies in Family Planning, 31*, 309–324.

Filippi, V., Ronsmans, C., Gohou, V., Goufodji, S., Lardi, M., Amina, S., . . . de Brouwere, V. (2005). Maternity wards or emergency obstetric rooms? Incidence of near miss events in African hospitals. *Acta Obstetricia et Gynacologica Scandinavica, 84*, 11–16.

Firoz, T., Chou, D., von Dadelszen, P., Agrawal, P., Vanderkruik, R., Tunçalp, O., . . . Say, L. (2013). Measuring maternal health: Focus on maternal morbidity. *Bulletin of the World Health Organization, 91*, 794–796.

Fortney, J. A., & Smith, J. B. (1996). *The base of the iceberg: Prevalence and perceptions of maternal morbidity in four developing countries.* The Maternal Morbidity Network. Research Triangle Park, NC: Family Health International. Retrieved from http://pdf.usaid.gov/pdf_docs/Pnacg698.pdf

Fournier, P., Dumont, A., Tourigny, C., Dunkley, G., & Dramé, S. (2009). Improved access to comprehensive emergency obstetric care and its effect on institutional maternal mortality in rural Mali. *Bulletin of the World Health Organzation, 87*, 30–38. doi:10.2471/BLT.07.047076

Gabrysch, S., & Campbell, O. M. (2009). Still too far to walk: Literature review of the determinants of delivery service use. *BMC Pregnancy Childbirth, 11*(9), 34. doi:10.1186/1471–2393–9–34

Hardee, K., Gay, J., & Blanc, A. K. (2012). Maternal morbidity: Neglected dimension of safe motherhood in the developing world. *Global Public Health, 7*, 603–617. doi: 10.1080/17441692.2012.668919

Hancock, B., Windridge, K., & Ockleford, E. (2007). *An introduction to qualitative research.* Nottingham, UK: The NIHR Research Design Service for Yorkshire & the Humber.

Koblinsky, M., Chowdhury, M. E., Moran, A., & Ronsmans, C. (2012). Maternal morbidity and disability and their consequences: Neglected agenda in maternal health. *Journal of Health, Population and Nutrition, 30*, 124–130.

Mantel, G. D., Buchmann, E., Rees, H., & Pattinson, R. C. (1998). Severe acute maternal morbidity: A pilot study of a definition for a near miss. *British Journal of Obstetrics and Gynaecology, 105*, 985–990.

National Population Commission (NPC) & ICF Macro. (2009). *Nigeria demographic and health survey, 2008*. Abuja, Nigeria: Author. Retrieved from http://population.gov.ng/index.php/110-publications/recent-publications/195-ndhs-2008

Pattison, R. C. & Hall, M. (2003). Near misses: A useful adjunct to maternal death enquires. *British Medical Bulletin, 67*, 231–243.

Say, L., Souza, J. P., & Pattinson, R. C. (2009). WHO working group on Maternal Mortality and Morbidity classifications. Maternal near miss—Towards a standard tool for monitoring quality of maternal health care. *Best Practice and Research: Clinical Obstetrics and Gynaecology, 23*, 287–296.

Souza, J., Cecatti, J. G., Hardy, E. F., Serruya, S. J., & Amaral, E. (2007). Appropriate criteria for identification of near miss maternal morbidity in tertiary care facilities: A cross sectional study. *BMC Pregnancy and Childbirth, 7*, 20.

Souza, J. P., Cecatti, J. G., Parpinelli, M. A., Krupa, F., & Osis, M. J. (2009). An emerging maternal Near Miss Syndrome: Narratives of women who almost died during childbirth and Pregnancy. *Birth, 36*, 149–158.

Thaddeus, S., & Maine, D. (1994). Too far to walk: Maternal mortality in context. *Social Science and Medicine, 38*, 1091–1110.

Tuncalp, O., Huldin, M., Kwame, A., & Adanu, R. (2012). Listening to women's voices: The quality of care of women experiencing severe maternal morbidity, in Accra, Ghana. *PloS ONE, 7*(8), e44536. doi:10.1371/journal.pone.0044536

Tuncalp, O., Huldin, M., Souza, J., Chou, D., & Say, L. (2012). The prevalence of maternal near miss: A systematic review. *British Journal of Obstetrics and Gynaecology, 119*, 653–661.

United Nations Children's Fund (UNICEF) & World Health Organization (WHO). (2004). *Low birth weight: Country, regional and global estimates*. New York, NY: UNICEF. Retrieved from http://www.childinfo.org/files/low_birthweight_from_EY.pdf

Van den Akker, T., Beltman, J., Leyten, J., Mwagomba, B., & Meguid, T. (2013). The WHO maternal near miss approach: Consequences at Malawian District level. *PLoS ONE, 8*, e54805. doi:10.1371/journal.pone.0054805

Wall, L. L. (1998). Dead mothers and injured wives: The social context of maternal morbidity and mortality among the Hausa of Northern Nigeria. *Studies in Family Planning, 29*, 341–359.

William, R. (2005) Generalized ordered logit/partial proportional odds model for ordinal dependent variables. *Stata Journal, 6*(1), 58–82.

World Health Organization (WHO). (2004). *Beyond the numbers: Reviewing maternal deaths and complications to make pregnancy safer*. Geneva, Switzerland: Author. Retrieved from http://whqlibdoc.who.int/publications/2004/9241591838.pdf

World Health Organization (WHO). (2012). *Trends in maternal mortality: 1990 to 2010. WHO, UNICEF, UNFPA, and the World Bank estimates*. Geneva, Switzerland: Author. Retrieved from https://www.unfpa.org/webdav/site/global/shared/documents/publications/2012/Trends_in_maternal_mortality_A4–1.pdf

Comparison Between an Independent Midwifery Program and a District Hospital in Rural Tanzania: Observations Regarding the Treatment of Female Patients

KATHLEEN MILLER

Department of Pediatrics, University of Wisconsin, Madison, Wisconsin, USA

MICHAEL McLOUGHLIN

Des Moines Internal Medicine Residency, University of Iowa, Des Moines, Iowa, USA

Tanzania faces a significant shortage of physicians. In light of this, nurse–midwives have been critical in reducing maternal mortality in Tanzania in recent years. Despite the importance of both entities in providing health care to women in Tanzania, there have been few studies addressing the cultural competency of each entity. We shadowed and assisted both an independent nurse–midwife as well as physicians and nurse–midwives at a large district hospital in rural Tanzania. In this article we describe our observations regarding the treatment of female patients within the culture of an independent midwifery practice and at a large district hospital.

Maternal mortality ratio (MMR) measures the risk of death during pregnancy or shortly after delivery, and it is considered a measure of the safety of childbirth (World Health Organization [WHO], 2005). Tanzania, located in East Africa, has a high MMR, with most recent estimates placing its MMR at 449/100,000 (Hogan et al., 2010). It has been well documented that the majority of deaths and disabilities due to childbirth are avoidable, which is demonstrated by the disparity between MMR in developed versus developing nations (Maclean, 2010; Mrisho et al., 2007). One of the most consistent methods of decreasing maternal mortality is to provide professional care during and after labor (Kruk, Paczkowski, Mbaruku, de Pinho, & Galca, 2009; Mrisho et al., 2007; Nyamtema et al., 2008; Sarker et al., 2010; WHO,

2005). Lawn and colleagues (cited in Mrisho et al., 2007) also noted that professional care also lessens the risk of death for the infant, as over 50% of neonatal deaths occur after home birth without skilled care attendance. Tanzania has a low percentage of births attended by skilled health professionals: 50% of women deliver at home, and only 51% have a skilled health professional assisting while giving birth (National Bureau of Statistics, 2011). Health infrastructure in Tanzania is relatively developed, however, with 90% of the population living within 10 km of a health facility providing antenatal and delivery care (Peter, 2003; Prytherch et al., 2007). Additionally, while Tanzania has a very high percentage of antenatal care (96%), its MMR is still distressingly high (National Bureau of Statistics, 2011).

In part, the lack of assistance of skilled health professionals is due to a workforce shortage. There is a severe shortage of health care professionals in Tanzania, especially physicians (Lowell et al., 2006; Nyamtema et al., 2008). Only an estimated 32% of the recommended skilled health care workforce is available (Nyamtema et al., 2008). There are approximately 1,600 physicians in the nation, who are primarily concentrated in urban areas (Lowell et al., 2006), for a population of 43 million people (National Bureau of Statistics, 2011). There are, however, an estimated 15,000 nurse–midwives in the nation (Lowell).

Nurse–midwives have been increasingly utilized in Tanzania to bridge the gaps in maternal care. It has been well documented that nurse–midwives can play a substantial role in lessening maternal mortality, especially when utilized in association with larger referral centers (Mrisho et al., 2007; WHO, 2005). The WHO states that nurse–midwives can decrease maternal mortality to below 200 per 100,000, even when large hospitals are not readily available (2005). Eighty percent of antenatal care in Tanzania is provided by nurses and nurse–midwives (National Bureau of Statistics, 2011). Thus, nurse–midwives can play an important role in Tanzania in reducing health care disparities and providing care to women. Physicians, while in short supply, are necessary for the provision of higher levels of care, in particular cesarean sections, when complications occur.

Given the importance of both physicians and midwives in the reduction of maternal mortality, we also wondered about the cultural sensitivity of each entity. In order to improve maternal health, we must have an in-depth understanding of barriers to care. While factors such as cost, distance to hospitals, predisposing medical conditions (anemia, HIV, malnutrition, etc.) have all been described, there has been very little research documenting health care providers' cultural and ethical treatment of women in the developing world. In certain cases, discriminatory treatment of women may constitute a barrier to care. This basic subject is of utmost importance as we seek to improve maternal health. The primary question we sought to answer is whether there is a difference in the treatment of female patients—rom the perspectives of human rights, ethics, and cultural sensitivity—by practitioners in a public government hospital versus a local midwife. Here, we will describe our experiences working with both an independent midwife and physicians employed at a government facility. Our conclusions are the result of our own qualitative observations as well as an in-depth review of pertinent literature.

METHODS

The first author spent 2 consecutive weeks shadowing and assisting a licensed midwife in rural Tanzania, followed by 5 consecutive weeks at a rural district hospital in Tanzania. The second author spent 8 consecutive weeks at the same district hospital. Both authors were medical students participating in a global health elective during medical school. Conversations with providers were conducted in English. Conversations with patients were either conducted in English or with the use of bilingual health care employees who served as interpreters. Out of respect for the privacy of the physicians and midwife, we will not refer to either location by name, but rather we describe the demographics of each location below.

Project Sites

Maternity home.   The maternity home where the first author spent 2 weeks is located in a small village approximately 20 minutes outside of Moshi, Tanzania. It is directed by a licensed RN and midwife from the area who is fluent in Swahili, English, and the local dialect. The midwife employs two additional part-time employees at the maternity home—one with a 2-year nursing degree and the other a young student hoping to train to become a nurse. The maternity home is an independently operated business without government funding. It is located in a complex of buildings, with a small patient reception area, room for wound dressing and injections, a delivery room, and a room with two patient beds. In addition to attending to births at the maternity home, the midwife also provides prenatal care, HIV/AIDS screenings, treatment for common infectious diseases such as malaria and certain sexually transmitted infections, contraception, wound care, chronic disease management, and minor surgical procedures.

District hospital.   The district hospital where we participated in our global health elective is located 2 hours outside of Moshi, Tanzania, in a town of 20,000. The district itself is home to over 200,000 residents spread out over a large geographical area. The hospital has seven full-time physicians, several clinical officers who work in outpatient clinics, two operating theaters, and over half a dozen outpatient clinics. None of the physicians are female; however, it is relevant to note that there are four female nurse–midwives employed at the hospital. There are four hospital wards: a female, male, pediatric, and maternity ward. The labor and maternity ward is the busiest in the hospital. There are 20 beds each for prepartum and postpartum; the prepartum side of the ward often has two or even three women per bed.

RESULTS

Observations From the Maternity Home

The maternity home is located in a relatively traditional village, and it is in close proximity to many of the patients. Because the midwife lives within the village, her patients are able to come to the maternity home whenever their labor begins, even if that means coming in the middle of the night. In this way, she is able to provide services that even the large district hospitals cannot because of her geographical accessibility. She also performed frequent home visits, allowing her to provide care for women who were bedridden or busy caring for other children. The midwife also speaks the local dialect, which allows her to communicate with rural women who may not speak Kiswahili.

When patients arrived for care and the midwife was not immediately available, they frequently had to wait for her return; sometimes, this was up to several hours. However, I (the first author) never saw patients express annoyance with the long wait. Rather, patients seemed very content to wait until the midwife was available, and they expressed a great deal of faith in the quality of her care. She performed pelvic exams only after explaining the process to her patients and was gentle, and her patients did not appear distressed by the exams. She was also very conscientious of the privacy of her patients, and she would carefully cover her patients' waists and legs once she had finished her exam.

While she was very proficient with basic prenatal care and deliveries, she openly acknowledged her lack of surgical skills and ability to intervene in complicated deliveries. I (the first author) did not personally witness any referrals of women with high-risk pregnancies to the local district hospital. Additionally, a lack of resources was a considerable constraint. She was unable to provide anesthesia to women during delivery, and she had a very limited supply of medications for routine antenatal care. She frequently reused examination gloves or performed cervical exams during labor with nonsterile gloves.

District Hospital

The district hospital is able to provide care to women with complicated pregnancies and deliveries. Cesarean sections, epidurals, and other surgical interventions are readily available, as are a wide variety of medications. The physicians we worked with were skilled surgeons and clinically proficient. There is sufficient room for several dozen women to be hospitalized simultaneously, and multiple operating theaters. Additionally, there is a pediatric ward available in the event that neonatal resuscitation or hospitalization is required.

As with the maternity home, patients at the district hospital also faced long waits for appointments and care. Patients frequently traveled from long distances, and it was commonplace for high-risk pregnant patients to arrive up to a month prior to delivery and remain in the hospital until they delivered. While physicians were available during the mornings and early afternoons, however, they were usually unavailable in the late afternoons, evenings, and overnight, leaving the deliveries that took place during these hours to the overnight nursing staff.

Despite the availability of tertiary care, we (both authors) were distressed by the treatment of female patients. It was not unusual for physicians to make a patient bleed unnecessarily from a rough pelvic exam or slap a patient who cried out during an exam. In one instance, a woman was forcibly held down while a pelvic exam was performed against her will. Women were left completely undressed on the exam table during labor, and there was very little concern for privacy. Prior to cesarean sections, pregnant women were routinely instructed to lay naked on the operating table, where they would shiver until they were finally anesthetized for the procedure. Women who cried out during labor were often slapped. Patients frequently appeared fearful, and one patient expressed to us that many women are afraid of the district hospital because they have heard that women will be operated on without permission. Patient education regarding the necessity of surgical procedures was minimal.

There was also a general disregard for women's physical ailments. Chronic abdominal and pelvic pain were frequent complaints among the patients. If no immediate cause was found and antibiotics failed to resolve the problem, the women were often labeled "neurotic" or "depressed." For example, a teenage girl who had been in a car accident complained of pelvic pain for over a week before the treating physician ordered an X ray. Her pelvis was shattered, but the physician had insisted for days that the girl was simply traumatized and that the shock of the accident needed to wear off. Despite substantial evidence that she may have suffered a fracture, her complaints were minimized and ignored.

We note that a minority of physicians was extremely gentle, sensitive, and responsive to their patients' needs. The vast majority of the seven physicians, however, participated in the distressing treatment of patients described above. Of note, the four female nurse–midwives at the hospital also treated patients in a manner similar to that of the physicians.

DISCUSSION

Attitudes of Providers

There is literature suggesting that women in Tanzania tend to have positive impressions of nurse–midwives and negative impressions of physicians and staff at larger hospitals (Mrisho et al., 2007). This is consistent with our observations between two work sites: patients at the independent maternity home seemed content with the midwife's' services and comfortable with their relationship with her, while patients at the district hospital expressed discomfort with the care they were receiving. First-level care (that is, care provided by a midwife) takes place in "an area where a woman is comfortable with her surroundings, and where the fear and pain that go with giving birth are managed positively" (WHO, 2005, p. 71). In contrast, care provided by the physician takes place at an unfamiliar and often intimidating district hospital.

The independent nurse–midwife, while not equipped to provide care for complicated pregnancies or deliveries, was able to offer culturally sensitive care to the women she treated. This was not the case at the hospital, where we felt the care was all too frequently inhumane. Women who overcame all other barriers—such as geographical distance, lack of money, transportation, or support from their partners—frequently found themselves at the mercy of a discriminatory system.

Interestingly, the nurse–midwives who were employed at the District Hospital also participated in what we found to be disturbing treatment of female patients. The fact that this was not true of the independent nurse–midwife suggests that the difference in the cultural competency or empathy of providers may not be dependent on whether they are nurse–midwives or physicians, but also on the climate of the institution in which they are practicing. One theory is that the maternity home had a smaller volume of patients, which may have allowed the independent midwife to spend more time with her patients and avoid the burnout that may come with working at a larger institution. Additionally, perhaps the smaller community allowed the independent nurse–midwife to see her patients as fellow community members, rather than strangers who were sometimes from different tribes than the nurse–midwives practicing in the hospital. This is an area that requires further study, as we observed dramatically different treatment of patients by providers with similar levels training.

Kruk and colleagues noted that type of provider—be it midwife or physician—was less important to women than the provider's attitude and performance (2009). Mrisho and colleagues came to a similar conclusion regarding health care at hospitals in Tanzania:

> Poor staff attitude was perceived [by patients] to exist in most health facilities; including abusive language, denying women service, lacking compassion and refusing to assist properly. . . . In his observational study in Tanzania, the author was dissatisfied with the child birth experience, as women in labour lay in bed in complete isolation, in pain, without support. (2007, p. 869)

Perhaps one of the most notable (and common) experiences was that of women who were about to undergo a cesarean section. As described in the Results section, these women were left naked on the operating table while the surgical team prepared. At times, this took up to 1 hour. Physicians, nurses, and students entered and left the room frequently. These patients were clearly terrified, cold, and humiliated. What was most striking about this situation was that it would have been so easy to remedy: it would take only a single sheet to cover the patient and reinstate her dignity. We can only hypothesize that the hospital staff were so used to the daily occurrence of cesarean sections that they were unaware or unsympathetic to the distress it caused each patient.

Physical Exams and Patient Education

Other literature has reported that Masai women may perceive vaginal exams as painful or dehumanizing (Magoma, Requejo, Campbell, Cousens, & Filippi, 2010); in our observations, vaginal exams were performed more frequently by physicians than by the independent nurse–midwife, and with fewer explanations of their necessity. This may be due to the higher-risk nature of patients at the district hospital, however, who may require more frequent exams. Sarker and colleagues noted that in their study in Tanzania, the reason for clinical exams was often not explained to the patients (2010). Magoma and associates also reported that Masai and Watemi women fear they may endure unnecessary cesarean sections when delivering in health units, as cesarean sections are sometimes performed without explanation to the mother (2010). This, as well, was consistent with our observations: very little education was provided to patients regarding their care. This added to patients' anxiety and fears that surgery would ensue without their knowledge or permission.

Privacy

The independent nurse–midwife was also able to provide a higher level of privacy than the district hospital, in part because the district hospitals treated a greater number of patients. Even with a large patient volume, however, certain low-cost policies could lead to greater privacy for female patients: providing patients waiting for exams or surgeries with a sheet, for example. Lack of privacy has been cited as a reason why women may choose to give birth outside of a health care facility (Mrisho et al., 2007), making this an important concern.

Availability of Services

Additionally, the nurse–midwife was available to her patients at all hours of the day and night, in a geographically accessible location. Transportation has frequently been cited as a reason women fail to deliver in a medical setting (Kruk et al., 2009; Magoma et al., 2010; Mrisho et al., 2007). Other studies have found that district hospitals are often functional only in the morning, and are "virtually inactive the rest of the day and all the night" (Nyamtema et al., 2008). This was also consistent with our experience, as physicians seldom attended births that took place after 3 PM. Occasionally, doctors would come in after hours to perform emergency cesarean sections, but there was rarely a sense of urgency in performing the procedures; such attitudes have been associated with poor outcomes (Nyamtema et al., 2008).

The Role of Nurse–Midwives and Physicians Within the Community

The majority of nurse–midwives are female, allowing them to overcome certain gender differences that may prevent effective communication between female patients and male physicians. Many of the nurse–midwives we encountered in Tanzania, including the nurse–midwife observed at the maternity home, were from the area in which they worked and shared a common background with their patients. The physicians and midwives at the district hospital were assigned to that location by the government, and several expressed their discontent in living in that particular area. Many are serving in areas outside of the region of their tribes, which may lead to cultural discrepancies and miscommunication.

A Note on Cultural Relativism

As previously discussed, physicians in Tanzania face an overwhelming workload, and they are constantly assaulted with a barrage of life-threatening scenarios that they must deal with on a daily basis. To a certain extent, many of the attitudes that we found frustrating may stem from such frequent exposure to heartbreak: empathy comes at a high price in low-resourced nations. For these reasons, we find ourselves conflicted: it is difficult to fault the staff at the hospital when they deal with structural inequities on a daily basis. We also wished to defend the women who were treated so poorly in our presence, however. As outsiders, it is not our goal to pass judgment or criticize a culture that we are familiar with only in passing. It is easy to argue that we, as two medical students who were outsiders in the community, are not well placed to make rash conclusions regarding cultural competency. Nevertheless, we believe that there are certain human rights that transcend culture. In our opinion, this includes the right to medical care without discrimination or abuse. Even within our limited understanding of the culture, it was obvious that both of these were commonplace during our time at the district hospital in Tanzania. For that reason, we have chosen to explore this topic more thoroughly and describe the differences in the treatment of patients by an independent midwife and providers at a governmental hospital.

LIMITATIONS

This article did not seek to identify differences in the technical quality of care between midwives and physicians, nor did it attempt to quantify outcomes according to training level of the provider. The numbers of this study are limited, as only one independent nurse–midwife and only a small number of providers at the district hospital were observed. It is an observational study only, from the perspectives of outsiders to the community who do not speak the local dialects. Our findings are consistent, however, with literature published regarding the cultural competence of providers in Tanzania. While we understand the limitations of our study, we believe our observations make a contribution to the literature. They indicate a need for further research to determine the role of cultural competency of providers, as well as unethical treatment of women, as potential barriers to care.

CONCLUSIONS: WORKING TOWARD A BETTER FUTURE

Medical decisions are often based on cultural considerations. Without a health care environment that feels safe, women are unlikely to seek out care unless it is an emergency. This means that fewer women will seek pre-natal care, more women will wait until they are in labor or their labor fails to progress, and women are unlikely to treat chronic conditions until they become debilitating. In order to decrease maternal mortality, the medical care that is offered *must* be culturally sensitive and respectful if we are to expect women to utilize it. In our opinion, working toward this goal requires an increase in the cultural sensitivity within the context of large public hospitals.

This is not an easy task. High rates of burnout are inevitable because of the lack of resources and overwhelming burden of disease and poverty. Perhaps a start would be emphasizing the role of physicians and hospital staff in providing humans rights to their patients: if the daily task of coming to work could be reframed as a compassionate and heroic act, providers might be able to find purpose in an incredibly difficult area of work. Increasing the availability of ethical conferences and education would also be an appropriate step, as would be the inclusion of ethical coursework during medical education. Such campaigns are useless, however, if they are not coupled with attempts to improve the overall standing of women within society and do not address sexism within health care delivery.

Creating an atmosphere in which women are respected and listened to is essential if women are to feel safe in the health care environment. If we are to work toward reducing maternal mortality, promotion of women's right to respectful, ethical, and culturally competent health care is of utmost importance.

REFERENCES

Hogan, M. C., Foreman, K. J., Naghavi, M., Ahn, S. Y., Wang, M., Makela, S. M., . . . Murray, C. J. (2010). Maternal mortality for 181 countries, 1980–2008: A systematic analysis of progress towards Millennium Development Goal 5. *Lancet, 375*, 1609–1623. doi:10.1016/S0140-6736(10)60518-1

Kruk, M. E., Paczkowski, M., Mbaruku, G., de Pinho, H., & Galca, S. (2009). Women's preferences for place of delivery in rural Tanzania: A population-based discrete choice experiment. *American Journal of Public Health, 99*(9), 1666–1672. doi:10.2105/AJPH.2008.146209

Lowell, B., Rita, G., Salim, R., Ari, S., Elya, T., & Iain, W. (2006). *Investing in Tanzanian Human Resources for Health: An HRH report for the TOUCH Foundation, Inc.* Retrieved from http://www.touchfoundation. org/uploads/assets/documents/mckinsey_report_july_2006_5nYbVVVS.pdf

Maclean, G. D. (2010). An evaluation of the Africa Midwives Research Network. *Midwifery, 26*(6), e1–e8. doi:10.1016/j.midw.2009.04.004

Magoma, M., Requejo, J., Campbell, O., Cousens, S., & Filippi, V. (2010). High ANC coverage and low skilled attendance in a rural Tanzanian district: A case for implementing a birth plan intervention. *BMC Pregnancy and Childbirth, 10*(13). doi:10.1186/1471-2393-10-13

Mrisho, M., Schellenberg, J. A., Mushi, A. K., Obris, B., Mshinda, H., Tanner, M., & Schellenberg, D. (2007). Factors affecting home delivery in rural Tanzania. *Tropical Medicine and International Health, 12*(7), 862–872. doi:10.1111/j.1365-3156.2007.01855.x

National Bureau of Statistics, United Republic of Tanzania. (2011). *Tanzania 2010 Demographic and Health Survey.* Retrieved from http://www.measuredhs. com/pubs/pdf/FR243/FR243[24June2011].pdf

Nyamtema, A. S., Urassa, D. P., Massawe, S., Massawe, A., Lindmark, G., & Van Roosmalen, J. (2008). Staffing needs for quality perinatal care in Tanzania. *African Journal of Reproductive Health, 12*(3), 113–124. Retrieved from http://www.ncbi.nlm.nih.gov/pubmed/19435016

Peter, P. (2003). Major factors that impact on women's health in Tanzania: The way forward. *Health Care for Women International, 24*(8), 712–722.

Prytherch, H., Massawe, S., Kuelker, R., Hunger, C., Mtatifikolo. F., & Jahn, A. (2007). The unmet need for emergency obstetric care in Tanga Region, Tanzania. *BMC Pregnancy and Childbirth, 7*(16). doi:10.1186/1471-2393-7-16

Sarker, M., Schmid, G., Larsson, E., Kirenga, S., de Allegri, M., Lekule, I., & Müller, O. (2010). Quality of antenatal care in rural southern Tanzania: A reality check. *BMC Research Notes, 3*, 209. doi:10.1186/1756-0500-3-209

World Health Organization (WHO). (2005). *The World Health report 2005: Make every mother and child count.* Retrieved from http://www.who.int/whr/2005/ whr2005_en.pdf

Food Beliefs and Practices During Pregnancy in Ghana: Implications for Maternal Health Interventions

AMA DE-GRAFT AIKINS

Regional Institute for Population Studies, University of Ghana, Legon, Ghana

Ghanaian women's food beliefs and practices during pregnancy and the scope for developing more effective maternal health interventions were explored in this study. Thirty-five multiethnic Ghanaian women between the ages of 29 and 75 were interviewed about pregnancy food beliefs and practices. I show that, based on the data analysis, their knowledge about food was drawn from lifeworlds (family and friends), educational settings, health professionals, mass media, and body-self knowledge (unique pregnancy experiences). Core lay ideas converged with expert knowledge on maternal health nutrition. Multiple external factors (e.g., economics, cultural representations of motherhood) and internal factors (e.g., the unpredictable demands of the pregnant body) influenced pregnancy food practices. I suggest and discuss a need for culturally situated multilevel interventions.

Ghanaian women of childbearing age experience problems with nutrition. Poor women experience undernutrition; wealthier women experience overnutrition. These problems have implications for maternal and child health. Maternal nutrition interventions in Ghana are informed by a common assumption that lay nutrition knowledge is "incorrect" and expert nutrition knowledge is "correct." By pitting "good" expert knowledge against "faulty" lay knowledge, researchers and health practitioners fail to incorporate the complex range of beliefs, knowledge, and practices that shapes women's pregnancy experiences and food practices. In this study I apply the concepts of medical logic and social logic: (a) to examine the content, sources, and functions of women's beliefs about pregnancy foods; (b) to identify food practices during pregnancy and their mediating factors; and (c) to examine the implications for developing more appropriate dietary interventions for pregnant women. Interviews with 35 women of different ethnicities and socioeconomic status suggested that successful maternal interventions will have to consider the following: (a) pregnant women draw on multiple and often-conflicting sources of information; (b) lay and expert knowledge converge on core ideas of maternal health and antenatal nutrition; and (c) the pregnant body is a significant mediator of pregnancy food practices.

Ghanaian women of childbearing age from poor rural and urban communities experience food and micronutrient insecurities (Grant & Lartey, 2006; Ghana Statistical Service [GSS], Noguchi Memorial Institute for Medical Research [NMIMR], & ORC Macro, 2004, 2009). These insecurities increase their risk of disease and premature death. In Ghana iron-deficiency anemia is a major threat to maternal health, contributing to low birth weight and poor health and cognitive outcomes for babies, as well as increasing morbidity risks for mothers. At least 9% of Ghanaian women are chronically malnourished: high mortality rates are reported among women from the northern belt of Ghana and of low education. The prevalence of anemia among Ghanaian women is higher than the prevalence in other West African countries, including Benin, Guinea, Sierra Leone, and Senegal (GSS et al., 2009).

Women with higher income and education in urban settings experience overnutrition. This group of women has access to a wider diversity of local and foreign foods, report increased intake of fat-rich and sugar-rich diets, and are more likely to be overweight or obese (Biritwum, Gyapong, & Mensah, 2005; Dake, Tawiah, & Badasu, 2010; GSS et al., 2009; Levine et al., 1999). Thirty percent of Ghanaian women are reported to be overweight or obese: the Greater Accra Region—where this study was conducted—has the highest percentage (45%) of this group. Overweight and obese women are more likely to experience pregnancy-induced diabetes and hypertension, which undermine their physical and psychological well-being during pregnancy and increase their chance of delivering overweight babies, who—current knowledge suggests—may go on to develop obesity and diabetes as adults. Pregnancy-induced hypertension is a leading cause of maternal death in Ghana (Kumi-Aboagye, 2008; Lassey & Wilson, 1998).

There have been two broad responses to the dual challenge of undernutrition and overnutrition among Ghanaian women of childbearing age. At the national level, nutritionists and food researchers have developed micronutrient supplementation and local food fortification projects as well as public health education strategies on malnutrition and overnutrition (Owusu, Adom, Opoku, Afoakwah, & Ankrah, 2006; Quarshie, Amoaful, & Armah, 2006). At the community level, micronutrient supplementation has become central to maternal health and antenatal care. At (public) antenatal clinics across the country pregnant women receive generic micronutrient supplements such as folic acid, multivitamins, and b-complex vitamins free of charge. For women who face pregnancy risks such as preeclampsia, hypertension, and diabetes, diet restrictions are advocated alongside micronutrient supplementation. Restrictions focus largely on reducing salt, fat, and sugar intake and necessitate restructuring everyday food practices. It is important to note that maternal health care in Ghana is generally poor especially at district and community health facilities, and many health facilities lack nutritionists and dieticians (GSS et al., 2009; Initiative for Maternal Mortality Programme Assessment [IMMPACT], 2007). Reports suggest that pregnant women using district and community health facilities may not necessarily have access to expert knowledge on maternal nutrition. Current interventions have had mixed success. At the community level, women have not fully adopted the practice of taking daily micronutrient supplements although they understand the benefits of these supplements to their reproductive health. Similarly, compliance with antenatal micronutrient supplement intake (such as vitamin A and iron) and dietary advice across the country is reportedly low (GSS et al., 2009). Local experts advocate for the development of more effective nutrition interventions (Addo, Marquis, & Lartey, 2006; Quarshie et al., 2006).

In this article I report a qualitative study that examines pregnancy food beliefs and practices in Ghana. This study is a subset of a broader study reported elsewhere that focused on the role of culture in pregnancy and breastfeeding dietary practices (de-Graft Aikins, 2011). The study is based on the premise that nutrition interventions may not be successful because they fail to incorporate women's perspectives on food and nutrition and their daily food and nutrition practices. This approach is informed by a tendency to pit "good" expert knowledge against "faulty" lay knowledge. I had four aims: (a) to document the content, sources, and functions of women's beliefs about pregnancy foods; (b) to identify food practices during pregnancy and their mediating factors; (c) to examine the extent to which these representations and practices corresponded to or deviated from expert knowledge; and (d) to identify practical and effective dietary interventions for pregnant Ghanaian women.

CONCEPTUAL FRAMEWORK

Maternal nutrition interventions in Africa are informed by a common assumption that lay nutrition knowledge is "incorrect" and expert nutrition knowledge is "correct" (Appoh & Krekling, 2004; Gittelson & Vastine, 2003). Writing within the Ghanaian context—on maternal nutrition knowledge in the Volta Region—Lily Appoh and Sturla Krekling, state that "whereas nutritional knowledge obtained from formal education and community health services to a large extent may be relied on to be the right one, the same cannot be said of knowledge about nutrition obtained through friends and families that may be related to the culture, tradition and beliefs in the community" (2004, p. 1). The popular, but conceptually limiting, knowledge–attitude–behavior (KAB) model of health promotion posits that knowledge changes attitudes, which in turn change behavior (Joffe, 1996). Maternal health experts often draw explicitly or implicitly on the KAB model and assume that providing "good" expert nutrition knowledge to women who desire healthy pregnancies and babies enhances their ability to achieve healthy status and therefore should ensure adherence with nutrition interventions. Yet interventions have had mixed success.

The conceptual framework for this study was informed by the concepts of "social logic" and "medical logic." "Social logic" and "medical logic" were coined within the health psychology field to distinguish between the knowledge drawn on by people with illness and their caregivers to manage their condition and the knowledge drawn on by their health care providers (Herzlich & Pierret, 1987; Nettleton, 1995). "Medical logic" is drawn from the disease-centred approach to illness and focuses on a restricted repertoire of practical routines aimed at addressing the physiological dimension of the illness. "Social logic" draws from intersubjective experiences of the individual with illness and focuses on a broader repertoire of practical routines aimed at addressing the physiological as well as social dimensions of living with illness. Social logic will include what Appoh and Krekling refer to as "knowledge ... obtained through friends and families which may be related to the culture, tradition and beliefs in the community" (2004, p. 1). Researchers argue that the everyday knowledge and skill drawn from "social logic" confer expertise to the chronically ill and their caregivers that encapsulates and transcends the expertise of their health care providers; this expertise has to be brought to the fore (and legitimized) in trying to understand processes of medical and self-care. These observations are true for experiences of chronic diseases such as diabetes and cancer in Ghana (Clegg-Lamptey & Hodasi, 2007; de-Graft Aikns, 2003; de-Graft Aikins et al., 2014).

When applying this broad argument to maternal health, two corresponding scenarios can be developed. Expert knowledge on maternal nutrition, hereafter "medical nutrition logic," can be described as highly technical knowledge based on nutritional science and obstetrics that focuses on a restricted repertoire of practical nutrition management routines aimed at addressing the physical and physiological dimensions of pregnancy. On the other hand, lay knowledge on maternal nutrition, hereafter "social nutrition logic," draws on physiological, physical, as well as intersubjective and sociocultural dimensions of pregnancy experiences and as such instructs a broader repertoire of practical food and nutrition practices. Social nutrition logic essentially captures what pregnant women know, think, feel, and do about food during their pregnancies. This goes beyond the medical space and encompasses the social, cultural, and structural dimensions of everyday life.

TABLE 1 Participant Profiles

Participant information	No. of participants
Age	
21–40	13
41–60	14
61–80	8
>80	
Ethnicity	
Akan	13
Dagao	3
Ewe	2
Ga	5
Hausa	3
Education	
None	1
Primary	2
Secondary	7
Tertiary (polytechnic, vocational training) University	5
Occupation	
Professional (law, management, academic)	5
Professional (nursing, teaching, secretarial, support services)	5
Trader (market, store)	6
Retired (but working—consulting, running kindergarten, etc.)	3
Retired (no work)	1
Other (e.g., traditional leader)	6

METHODS

Thirty-five women of different ethnicities (Akan, Dagao, Ewe, Ga, and Hausa) and age groups (29 to 75) were recruited for the study. The study was exploratory, and the broader focus was on the role of culture in pregnancy and breastfeeding experiences. Therefore, I aimed to maximize diversity across ethnic identity and age in order to explore cultural differences (via ethnic difference) as well as the changes in the role of culture over time (via intergenerational experience). In Table 1 I present the profile of the study women. With the exception of one, all informants were educated. Educational status ranged from primary-level education to obtaining a postgraduate university degree. Occupations ranged from small-scale trading to white-collar professions. Some retired women continued to work. The number of children women had ranged between one (for the youngest informants) and four. The youngest age at first birth was 20 (for a woman in her late forties); the oldest age for first birth was 36 (a woman lactating at the time of the study).

After gathering demographic information (age, education, occupation[s], number and ages of children, ethnicity), the women were asked questions about the following:

(1) recommended and prohibited pregnancy foods, including sources of knowledge and functions of the foods;

(2) foods consumed during their own pregnancies and the factors mediating food practices; and

(3) their general health and well-being during pregnancy.

All the women generated their pregnancy food list using a free-recall approach. Question (1) produced a general pregnancy food list, and question (2) generated a participant-specific pregnancy food list. As interviews progressed and perspectives approached "meaning saturation" (the "stopping criterion" for qualitative research: the point at which no additional variety of meaning is gained from data collection (Gaskell, 2000), items on the cumulative pregnancy food list were used as memory prompts (for example, "I spoke to some women who said snails were good for pregnancy, what is your opinion on that?"). A key limitation of this open-ended approach with a cohort of women who were required to remember their pregnancy experiences dating back a number of years or decades was that certain details of everyday pregnancy experience such as food portions, quantity of herbs used in cooking, and frequency of food intake were lost. This kind of detailed information is best gathered by direct observation or the use of food diaries and would necessitate studying pregnant and lactating women over extended periods of pregnancy and breastfeeding (Messer, 1989). I interviewed the women along with two research assistants in English and the local languages: Asante-Twi, Fante-Twi, Ga, and Dagari. The interviews were conducted between October 2006 and April 2008. Notes were taken for all interviews; some women were interviewed more than once. Note-taking was preferred because it created a more relaxed interviewing setting, especially for opportunistic interviews. For some interviews, note-taking was the only practical option, for example, with market women interviewed during work. Using the operationalised notion of "social nutrition logic" analysis focused on content, sources, functions, and legitimation of food knowledge.

RESULTS

Results are presented in two parts. In Part 1 I focus on women's knowledge of recommended and prohibited foods for pregnancy. In Part 2 I focus on food practices during women's pregnancies. Cross-cutting themes include women's relationship with food during their pregnancies and the extent to which social nutrition logic structures everyday food practices and enhances or undermines compliance to expert nutrition interventions.

Part 1: Social Nutrition Logic: Contents, Sources, Functions, and Legitimation of Pregnancy Food Beliefs

Contents of social nutrition logic. The women generated a wide range of recommended foods and food supplements for pregnancy. The majority

of foods were indigenous to Ghanaian diets generally (e.g., green leafy vegetables, legumes, meat and fish, fruits). These indigenous foods are termed
traditional foods and supplements: their indigenous status allows identification of continuities and change in culturally mediated food consumption patterns. The list also included foreign foods such as beverages (tea,
Milo, Ovaltine, Horlicks), dairy products (milk, yogurt), and biscuits (diges-
tives, cream crackers). The contents of the food list, including incorporation
of foreign foods, was similar across different age groups. That is to say
pregnancy diets had not changed much across three generations (between
women in their late sixties, forties, and twenties). The majority of indigenous foods discussed cut across ethnic groups. Two notable, but expected,
differences occurred in terms of relative food availability (e.g., more fish in
southern Ghana, more meat in the northern Ghana) and mode of food preparation (e.g., preference for fermented maize/millet dough-based staples in
some ethnic groups and nonfermented maize/millet dough-based staples in

TABLE 2 Recommended Food and Food Supplements for Pregnancy

Raw foods	Cooked foods	Dry/processed foods
Fruits: bananas, oranges, pawpaw (papaya), pineapples, watermelon	Beans stew (with palm oil) [eaten with boiled white rice]	Beverages: tea, Milo, cocoa
Vegetables: carrots, cabbage, lettuce, "salads"	Bread (white, brown)	Biscuits: cream crackers, digestive
Honey	Fish: fried *keta school boys* (anchovies), smoked mackerel [with fresh pepper sauce, kenkey[ii]]	Fluids: soya milk, juices
Supplements: *kwawu nsua/nsaman troba* [i] (blended with water)	*Nkontomire* stew (made with palm oil) [with boiled sweet cassava[iii], or plantain, or yam]	Supplements: blood tonics; b-complex vitamins, biscuits (dry) folic acid, lucozade, multivitamins, pregnacare
	Palm-nut soup [with fufu[iv], banku[ii], rice]	
	Soups (other)—light (tomato & garden eggs); nkontonmire vegetable[v]	
	Snails (in soups)	
	Stews (other): garden eggs, Tuo Zaafi[v] [with vegetable soup]	
	Supplements: *alefi*[v]; *kwawu nsua/nsaman troba* (added to soups and stews); prekese	

Ethnic differences: [i]mentioned only by Akan women; [ii]made from fermented corn dough—common to
southern women (Akan, Ga); [iii]common to Nzema and Krobo communities; [iii]usually pounded plantain
and cassava, mentioned only by southern women; [v]mentioned only by northern women.

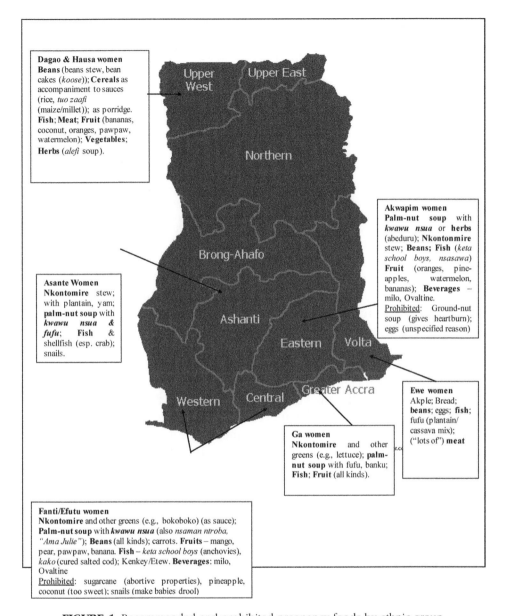

Dagao & Hausa women
Beans (beans stew, bean cakes (*koose*)); **Cereals** as accompaniment to sauces (rice, *tuo zaafi* (maize/millet)); as porridge. **Fish**; **Meat**; **Fruit** (bananas, coconut, oranges, pawpaw, watermelon); **Vegetables**; **Herbs** (*alefi* soup).

Asante Women
Nkontomire stew; with plantain, yam; **palm-nut soup** with *kwawu nsua & fufu*; **Fish** & shellfish (esp. crab); snails.

Akwapim women
Palm-nut soup with *kwawu nsua* or **herbs** (abeduru); **Nkontonmire** stew; **Beans**; **Fish** (*keta school boys, nsasawa*) **Fruit** (oranges, pineapples, watermelon, bananas); **Beverages** – milo, Ovaltine.
Prohibited: Ground-nut soup (gives heartburn); eggs (unspecified reason)

Ewe women
Akple; Bread; **beans**; eggs; **fish**; fufu (plantain/ cassava mix); ("lots of") **meat**

Ga women
Nkontomire and other greens (e.g., lettuce); **palm-nut soup** with fufu, banku; **Fish**; **Fruit** (all kinds).

Fanti/Efutu women
Nkontomire and other greens (e.g., bokoboko) (as sauce); **Palm-nut soup** with *kwawu nsua* (also *nsaman ntroba*, "*Ama Julie*"); **Beans** (all kinds); carrots. **Fruits** – mango, pear, pawpaw, banana. **Fish** – *keta school boys* (anchovies), *kako* (cured salted cod); Kenkey/Etew. **Beverages**: milo, Ovaltine
Prohibited: sugarcane (abortive properties), pineapple, coconut (too sweet); snails (make babies drool)

FIGURE 1 Recommended and prohibited pregnancy foods by ethnic group.

others). In Table 2 I present the cumulative pregnancy food list generated by the women under three categories: (a) raw foods, (b) cooked foods, and (c) dry/processed foods. Foods tied to specific ethnic groups are highlighted. In Figure 1, where I present a map of foods generated by ethnic group.

Some women made reference to prohibited foods. There was general agreement that excess fat and sugar was bad for pregnancy. Beyond this, reference was made to specific foods by Fante and Akwapim women. Some

TABLE 3 Prohibited Foods and Food Supplements for Pregnancy

Raw foods	Cooked foods	Dry/processed foods	Nonfoods
Fruits: oranges, pineapple, coconut, sugarcane	Ground-nut soup	High-fat; high-sugar foods	Clay (Akwapim)
	Eggs Chilli pepper (in cooked sauces)	Cooking oils	
Chilli pepper (in fresh pepper sauces)		Salt	

Akwapim women stressed that groundnut soup caused heartburn and was therefore prohibited in pregnancy. The status of other prohibited foods was not as clear-cut. For some women eggs were prohibited in pregnancy: for others eggs were recommended. One Fante woman placed extremely sweet fruits—sugarcane, pineapple, coconut—under the prohibited foods list. She observed that sugarcane had abortive functions and had to be restricted during pregnancy: her view was not common. A final category of prohibited "foods" included items such as clay and ice: their consumption by pregnant women in a variety of settings has been attributed to pica: "a perverted appetite for substances not fit as food or of no nutritional value" (Goldstein, 1998, p. 465). Because these items belong to the participant-specific pregnancy food list (i.e., food that is craved, consumed, or both during pregnancy but may not be generally recommended), it is more appropriate to discuss the context of consumption in Part 2. In Table 3 I present the list of prohibited foods.

Sources of Social Nutrition Logic

Women drew their knowledge of pregnancy and breastfeeding foods from five sources:

(a) family and friends, hereafter "lifeworlds";

(b) educational settings, typically school and university;

(c) health systems: the biomedical sphere (doctors, nurses) and traditional herbalists;

(d) media (newspapers, radio, and television); and

(e) unique pregnancy experiences (hereafter, "body-self knowledge").

The dimensions of knowledge from lifeworlds and pregnancy experiences are worth elaborating on, as these constitute the core of "social nutrition logic" and have been labelled "faulty" by nutrition experts. Knowledge drawn from lifeworlds can be categorized as cultural knowledge. The knowledge was handed down from generations through mothers and other female members of the extended family as well as from friends and close community members. This knowledge encompassed physiological, physical, as well as intersubjective and sociocultural dimensions of pregnancy experiences and as such instructed a broad repertoire of food and health practices. It was ethnically bound, so that foods specific to certain groups and regions of Ghana appeared on the list of women originally from these regions, however long they had lived in Accra (see Figure 1). All women cited their lifeworld as a primary source of knowledge for managing pregnancy.

Body-self knowledge has been defined as subjective knowledge of one's unique state of physical and psychological balance (Helman, 2000). Body-self knowledge has been reported to mediate health maintenance and illness management practices in a variety of contexts including in Ghana (Angel & Guarnaccia, 1989; Bates, Rankin-Hill, & Sanchez-Ayendez, 1997; de-Graft Aikins, 2003; de-Graft Aikins, Awuah, Pera, Mendez, & Ogedegbe, 2014). Body-self knowledge emerged as an important source of knowledge during pregnancy. This knowledge modality was particularly important for women with more than one child because body-self knowledge shaped food practices throughout all pregnancies and to a large extent mediated use of other knowledge modalities.

Functions of Recommended Foods

Most women attributed two dominant nutritional functions to the listed foods. Some foods, such as green leafy vegetables (consumed as stews or soups), were understood to "give blood" (37-year-old Asante woman) or prevent anemia. Others, such as palm nut (consumed as soups), were understood to "give body" (37-year-old Asante woman) or strengthen the pregnant body. Herbs and other food supplements such as *prekese (Tetrapleura tetraptera)*, *alefi*, and *kwawu nsua* were central to meals and were believed to augment the processes of giving blood and body or minimizing physiological disruptions such as nausea (see Part 2).

In Table 4 I juxtapose the functions attributed to traditional foods with functions attributed to these foods by local nutrition experts. Three nutrition experts were consulted in producing social nutrition logic–medical nutrition logic comparisons for Table 4.

Functions attributed to pregnancy foods by the women were similar to functions attributed by nutrition experts. The traditional foods and supplements listed functioned to prevent anemia, ensure physical strength, minimize physiological disruption, and ultimately maximize the health of babies. The functions of some foods—fruits, vegetables—were not explicitly described. Their inclusion within the recommended pregnancy food list by the majority of women, however, suggests that they perform taken-for-granted maternal health functions. These foods are themselves recommended by

TABLE 4 Functions of Pregnancy Foods and Food Supplements: Comparing Social Nutrition Logic and Medical Nutrition Logic

Social nutrition logic	Foods and food supplements	Medical nutrition logic
Foods that prevent anemia ("giving blood")	Leafy green vegetables (e.g., nkontomire); other vegetables (*kwawu nsua*)	Sources of Vitamin A & C (for healthy bones) and folic acid (formation of new cells, production of red blood cells, protein synthesis)
Foods that strengthen the body & increase fertility ("giving body")	Palm-nut soup; fish, shellfish (esp. crab) and meats; snails; blood tonics; clay; beverages (tea, milo, Ovaltine with milk & sugar)	Sources of protein (vital to formation and growth of fetal brain), iron (used by body to increase maternal hemoglobin) & calcium.
Foods that minimize physiological disruption (nausea, vomiting)	Kola nuts	High source of caffeine; prohibited in pregnancy.
Foods that maximise health of fetus	Honey	Source of fructose, a carbohydrate: fructose has lower energy value compared with sucrose, but no direct link to fetal health
Foods with uncategorized functions	Vegetables (carrots); fruits (oranges, watermelons, bananas)	Carrots source of beta-carotene (which transforms to Vitamin A); Oranges & other citrus fruits source of Vitamin C.
	Accompaniments to sauces: fufu, kenkey, banku (or the Efutu *Etew*) TuoZaafi	Fermented maize/millet meals (e.g., kenkey) increase bioavailability of B vitamins, which regulate nerves (B1), maintain mucous membranes (B2), facilitate formation of red blood cells (B6, B12)

nutritionists and maternal health experts as good sources of Vitamins A and C. Traditional sauce accompaniments such as *fufu, kenkey,* and *Tuo Zaafi,* whose functions were not outlined by the women, also have some nutritional functions as described in Table 4.

Part 2: Food Consumption Practices During Pregnancy: Physiological Changes, Bodily Demands, and Maternal Nutrition Compliance

Most women experienced physiological changes during pregnancy. Memories of these changes were acute, were linked to clearly demarcated periods in pregnancy (e.g., "first 3 months," "first 5 months," "final month") or gender of unborn child (it felt different carrying boys vs girls for some), and constituted the lens through which relationships with food was discussed. Pregnancy was a period when many gained intimate knowledge of their bodies and physiological processes. For those who had more than one child, the first pregnancy provided a sensory map for future pregnancies. Some sensed they were pregnant before conclusive medical tests because their bodies underwent clear predictable changes; others knew they were expecting girls or boys.

For many women these physiological changes were primary mediators of food consumption during pregnancy. That is to say, depending on the severity of physiological changes, one could adhere to a well-balanced nutritious diet or not. Physiological changes mediated food consumption in three main ways, corresponding to three common experiences described by the women.

Hypersensitivity and Hyperemesis

About half of the women had experienced hypersensitivity to smell, light, and motion during the first trimester. Hypersensitivity to smell was linked to nausea, spitting, and vomiting. Women who experienced nausea in their first trimester were therefore unable to eat a balanced diet because the smell of cooked (especially fried), spicy, or both foods exacerbated nausea. Most listed a restricted range of simple—"clean" (raw, steamed, boiled, roasted)—foods they could consume during this period (see Table 5). During this period, food supplements provided by antenatal clinics become central to maternal health.

TABLE 5 Foods Consumed During the First Trimester

Raw foods	Cooked foods	Dry/processed foods
"Fruits — oranges, pineapples, watermelon, and food supplements" (44, Akwapim)	"*Kobi**, *kpakpo shito***, okro (steamed)...kola nuts" (54, Ga) "pepper, fish (either fried or smoked), hot banku. Light soup. Tea with milk." (69, Ga) "fresh pepper, steamed crab, and kenkey; light soup" (47, Fante) "only dried fish" (75, Asante) "rice and bread" (69, Fante)	"Plain tea (without milk or sugar)" (64, Ga) "cereals... cocoa" (65, Krobo)
		Ice cubes and food supplements (37, Asante; 47, Akwapim) Soya milk, digestive biscuits, and food supplements" (36, Ga)

*Cured and salted tilapia; **small green aromatic chilli peppers.

255

Increased Appetite and Craving Out-of-the-Ordinary Foods

Some women experienced increased appetite throughout their pregnancy or after the difficult trimester. During periods of increased appetite, most women ate all the recommended foods, often several times a day. For example, one first-time lactating mother (36-year-old Ga woman) recalled experiencing increased appetite after the first 3 months of (nausea-induced) limited eating. She ate heavy starch and protein-based foods on average seven times a day and at unstructured times and put on 3 kg of weight: her "doctor advised weight check." Weight gain was common during periods of increased appetite and posed health risks to mother and unborn child, according to the women's doctors.

Part of the experience of increased appetite was sudden and often prolonged craving for "out-of-the-ordinary" foods. A minority of women (across the age spectrum) craved and consumed pica: Akwapim clay and ice were two common substances. In Table 6 I present the list of craved foods.

The majority of foods belonged to the general list of recommended pregnancy foods. Of the remainder, one category—the "nonfood" items clay and ice—were not recommended within lifeworlds or by health care providers. As one elderly Fante women noted, "I used to eat clay—Akwapim clay. My body craved it. Nobody told us to eat it, we just wanted it."

The second category constituted foods such as ice cream and hamburgers and energy drinks such as "Malta Guinness" that, by virtue of their high-fat and high-sugar content, belonged to the prohibited food list. Craved foods served different purposes for different women: nutritional (e.g., calcium boost in Akwapim clay for one elderly Fante woman), physiological (the nausea-reducing properties of *bisi* [kola nut] for one middle-aged Ga

TABLE 6 Foods Craved by Women During Pregnancy

Raw foods	Cooked foods	Dry/processed foods	Other
Mangoes	*Akrantie* (smoked game)	Hamburgers	Clay
Kola nuts	Fish/shellfish: crab (steamed), *kobi*, *keta school boys*, *nsasawa*, shrimp (with light soup)	Ice cream	Ice cubes
		Malt drink	
		Yogurt	
	Game: akrantie (smoked)		
	Hausa *koko* (fermented maize/millet dough porridge with spices)		
	Hausa rice		
	Okra (steamed)		
	Rice, beans with vegetables		
	Snails (steamed, added to soups)		
	Yogurt		

woman) and psychological (the comfort provided by the smell, texture, and taste of *akrantie* [smoked game] for the elderly Fante woman).

Pregnancy-Induced Illness

Three women (ages 37, 45, and 46) developed hypertension during their pregnancies, three experienced persistent heartburn when they ate spicy foods, one woman (aged 44) developed preeclampsia during her second pregnancy, and an elderly Ga woman spent all of her four pregnancies in the hospital on a vitamin-enhanced drip. Most women in this subgroup were placed on strict—low salt, low fat, no spice—diet restrictions by their doctors during their pregnancies. These diet restrictions were often difficult to maintain for all the women: most struggled to lose weight. The remaining number of women reported having had "healthy pregnancies," including those who had hypersensitivity issues in their first trimester. Two women who had had pregnancy-induced hypertension had developed adult onset hypertension, which persisted at the time of interviews.

What becomes apparent from these accounts of pregnancy experiences is that bodily processes—and by extension the pregnant body—constituted an important legitimate source of maternal nutrition knowledge. As the elderly Ga woman who spent all her four pregnancies in the hospital on a drip observed, "We all know we need a balanced diet during pregnancy, but your body will dictate what you will eat."

DISCUSSION AND CONCLUSIONS

I had four aims, based on the premise that nutrition interventions in Ghana face challenges because they fail to incorporate women's perspectives on food and nutrition and their daily food and nutrition practices: (a) to document the content, sources, and functions of women's beliefs about pregnancy foods; (b) to identify food practices during pregnancy and their mediating factors; (c) to examine the extent to which these representations and practices corresponded to or deviated from expert knowledge; and (d) to identify effective dietary interventions for pregnant Ghanaian women.

According to medical nutrition logic, noncompliance is attributed to "faulty" cultural knowledge and poor access to expert nutrition knowledge and interventions. The focus on social nutrition logic, however, highlights the complex factors underpinning the relationships pregnant women have with food and by extension its consumption or nonconsumption. Three key insights emerge from this study:

1. Women draw on pluralistic knowledge sources to make sense of pregnancy and pregnancy diets, including lay and expert knowledge.

2. Key elements of social nutrition logic and medical nutrition logic intersect. These include specific recommended and prohibited foods.
3. The pregnant body is a significant mediator of pregnancy food practices.

These findings have implications on developing effective antenatal nutrition interventions. In Figure 2, I present identified multilevel factors that mediate consumption of food and food supplements, including those advocated by maternal health experts. The current evidence suggests that medical nutrition logic is pitched solely at the structural/ideological level (lack of formal nutrition knowledge, lack of access to services) when it should also consider individual, interindividual, and group contexts of food practices. The study findings suggest that interventions that incorporate multilevel (structural, group, interindividual, individual) contexts of food beliefs and practices during pregnancy, but with sustained focus on the embodied experience of pregnancy, may yield better compliance outcomes. To conclude, I consider key challenges and opportunities for implementing multilevel interventions.

Pluralistic Knowledge on Pregnancy Foods and Nutrition

Most women drew on multiple sources of knowledge to make sense of pregnancy nutrition and food practices: lifeworlds, health systems, educational settings, the mass media, and, most importantly, their own pregnancy experiences. Processes of legitimation depended on whether the focus was on range and quality of knowledge and type and efficacy of nutrition intervention; these processes were rooted more broadly within changing

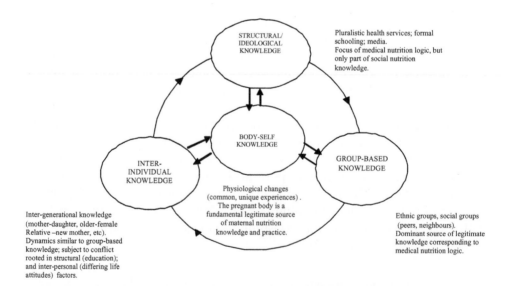

FIGURE 2 Multilevel factors mediating maternal nutrition practices.

life—and unique pregnancy—experiences. Research on medical pluralism in sub-Saharan Africa suggests that individuals and communities perceive and use pluralistic health systems as coexisting alternatives (Ben-Tovim, 1985; Nyamwaya, 1987; Prins, 1992). Ghanaian research on medical pluralistic attitudes suggests that individuals and communities evaluate pluralistic medical systems along four criteria: technical or practical knowledge of health problems, technological expertise, accessibility (geographic, economic, cultural), and ethics (de-Graft Aikins, 2005). All systems have strengths and weaknesses across these criteria, depending on the health problem (de-Graft Aikins, 2005). Since medical pluralistic attitudes and practices dominate women's experiences, the way women of childbearing age position themselves toward pluralistic nutrition knowledge—rather than towards medical nutrition logic solely—constitutes a more critical area of future research.

Social Nutrition Logic and Medical Nutrition Logic Overlap

The content of information from lifeworlds, which constituted the core of social nutrition logic (and deemed incorrect by nutritionists), corresponded in greater part to content of information from maternal health experts (deemed correct information). Five functional categories were given to recommended traditional foods and supplements. Of these, three categories corresponded to expert attributions: foods that prevented anemia (e.g., leafy green vegetables), strengthened the pregnant body (e.g., palm-nut soup and shellfish), and provided general health-enhancing functions (e.g., vegetables and fruit). Two categories were minority themes and did not have clear or positive functions according to experts: foods that minimized physiological disruption (kola nuts) and maximized the health of babies (honey). Identification of legitimation processes showed that women subjected all sources of pregnancy information to scrutiny. Thus elements of both social nutrition logic and medical nutrition logic that had proven functions were privileged.

Body-Self Knowledge: The Role of the Body in Pregnancy Food Practices

The most compelling common experience described by the women in this study was the role their bodies played in food consumption during their pregnancies. For many women the pregnant body constituted the ultimate guide to how one thought, felt, and acted about food daily during pregnancy. This guide over-rode other legitimate sources (e.g., structural, cultural) of knowledge on—the right or wrong—pregnancy foods. From the positive end, physiological changes in the pregnant body enhanced appetite for simple healthily cooked foods. From the negative end, extreme physiological changes caused either underconsumption or overconsumption of nutritious or nonnutritious food. This common experience has two broad implications. First, it implies that embodied knowledge and its everyday functions have to be prioritized and legitimized in maternal nutrition research and in antenatal care in Ghana. Second, it suggests that pregnant women whose experiences lie at opposite ends of the physiological disruption continuum (e.g., loss of appetite vs. increased appetite) are more likely to be noncompliant with maternal nutrition intervention and therefore require greater individualized medical/nutrition support. The challenge lies in developing cost-effective and practical interventions that enable over-stretched and under-resourced maternal health services to provide such vital support.

REFERENCES

Addo, A. A., Marquis, G. S., & Lartey, A. A. (2006) *Dietary intakes of Ghanaian pregnant and lactating women living in HIV affected communities.* Paper presented at the Africa Nutrition Epidemiology Conference, 15–18 August, Accra, Ghana.

Angel, R., & Guarnaccia, P. (1989). Mind, body and culture: Somatization among Hispanics. *Social Science and Medicine, 28,* 1229–1238.

Appoh, L. Y., & Krekling, S. (2004). Effects of early childhood malnutrition on cognitive performance of Ghanaian children. *Journal of Psychology in Africa, 14*(1), 1–8.

Bates, M. S., Rankin-Hill, L., & Sanchez-Ayendez, M. (1997). The effects of the cultural context of healthcare on treatment of and response to chronic pain and illness. *Social Science and Medicine, 45*(9), 1433–1447.

Ben-Tovim, D. I. (1985). Therapy managing in Botswana. *Australian & New Zealand Journal of Psychiatry, 19*(1), 88–91.

Biritwum, R. B., Gyapong, J., & Mensah, G. (2005). The epidemiology of obesity in Ghana. *Ghana Medical Journal, 39*(3), 82–85.

Clegg-Lamptey, J. N. A., & Hodasi, W. M. (2007). A study of breast cancer in Korle Bu Teaching Hospital: Assessing the impact of health education. *Ghana Medical Journal, 41*(2), 72–77.

Dake, F. A. A., Tawiah, E. O., & Badasu, D. M. (2010). Sociodemographic correlates of obesity among Ghanaian women. *Public Health Nutrition, 14*(7), 1285–1291.

de-Graft Aikins, A. (2003). Living with diabetes in rural and urban Ghana: A critical social psychological examination of illness action and scope for intervention. *Journal of Health Psychology, 8*(5), 557–572.

de-Graft Aikins, A. (2005). Healer-shopping in Africa: New evidence from a rural-urban qualitative study of Ghanaian diabetes experiences. *British Medical Journal, 331,* 737–743.

de-Graft Aikins, A. (2011) Culture, diet and the maternal body: Ghanaian women's perspectives on food, fat and childbearing. In M. Unnithan-Kumar & S. Tremayne (Eds.), *Fatness and the maternal body: Women's experiences of corporeality and the shaping of social policy* (pp. 130–154). Oxford, England: Berghahn Books.

de-Graft Aikins, A., Awuah, R. B., Pera, T., Mendez, M., & Ogedegbe, G. (2014). Explanatory models of diabetes in poor urban Ghanaian communities. *Ethnicity and Health*. Advance online publication. doi:10.1080/13557858.2014.921896

Gaskell G. (2000). Individual and group interviewing. In M. Bauer & G. Gaskell (Eds.), *Qualitative researching with text, image and sound: A practical handbook for social research* (pp. 38–56). London, England: Sage.

Ghana Statistical Service (GSS), Ghana Health Service (GHS), & ICF Macro (2009). *Ghana Demographic and Health Survey 2008*. Accra, Ghana: Authors.

Ghana Statistical Service (GSS), Noguchi Memorial Institute for Medical Research (NMIMR), & ORC Macro (2004). *Ghana Demographic and Health Survey 2003*. Calverton, MD: Authors.

Gittelson, J., & Vastine, A. E. (2003). Sociocultural and household factors impacting on the selection allocation and consumption of animal source foods: Current knowledge and application. *Journal of Nutrition, 133*, 4036S–4041S.

Goldstein, M. (1998). Adult pica: A clinical nexus of physiology and psychodynamics. *Psychosomatics, 39*(5), 465–469.

Grant, F. K. E., & Lartey, A. (2006). *Anaemia among adolescent pregnant females and its effect on infant growth*. Paper presented at the Africa Nutrition Epidemiology Conference, 15–18 August, Accra, Ghana.

Helman, C. (2000). *Culture, health and illness*. Oxford, England: Butterworth-Heineman.

Herzlich, C., & Pierret, J. (1987). *Illness and self in society*. Baltimore, MD: Johns Hopkins University Press.

Initiative for Maternal Mortality Programme Assessment (IMMPACT). (2007). *Evaluating removal of delivery fees in Ghana. Removing financial barriers helps the poorest women access needed obstetric care*. Accra, Ghana: Author/Population Reference Bureau.

Joffe, H. (1996). AIDS research and prevention: A social representational approach. *British Journal of Medical Psychology, 69*, 169–190.

Kumi-Aboagye, P. (2008). *Status of MDG 5—Evidence from the field*. Paper presented at the Maternal Mortality Consultative Meeting, July 7–8, Accra, Ghana.

Lassey, A. T., & Wilson, J. B. (1998). Trends in maternal mortality in Korle Bu Hospital, 1984–1994. *Ghana Medical Journal, 32a*, 910–916

Levine, C. E., Ruel, M. T., Morris, S. S., Maxwell, D. G., Armar-Klemesu, M., & Ahiadeke, C. (1999). Working women in an urban setting: Traders, vendors and food security in Accra. *World Development, 27*(11), 1977–1991.

Messer, E. (1989). Methods for studying determinants of food intake. In G. H. Pelto, P. J. Pelto, & E. Messer (Eds.), *Research methods in nutritional anthropology*. Tokyo, Japan: United Nations University. Retrieved from http://archive.unu.edu/unupress/unupbooks/80632e/80632E00.htm

Nettleton, S. (1995). *The sociology of health and illness*. Oxford, England: Polity.

Nyamwaya, D. (1987). A case study of the interaction between indigenous and Western medicine among the Pokot of Kenya. *Social Science and Medicine, 25*(12), 1277–1287.

Owusu, W. B., Adom, T., Opoku, Y. T., Afoakwah, N., & Ankrah, K. (2006). *Prospects for micronutrient fortification in Ghana*. Paper presented at the Africa Nutrition Epidemiology Conference, 15–18 August, Accra, Ghana.

Prins, G. (1992). A modern history of Lozi Therapeutics. In S. Feierman & J. M. Janzen (Eds.), *The social basis of health and healing in Africa* (pp. 339–365). Berkeley, CA: University of California Press.

Quarshie, K., Amoaful, E., & Armah, J. G. A. (2006). *Communications strategy for the control of malnutrition in Ghana*. Paper presented at the Africa Nutrition Epidemiology Conference, 15–18 August, Accra, Ghana.

Occupational Types and Antenatal Care Attendance Among Women in Ghana

EMMANUEL BANCHANI and ERIC Y. TENKORANG

Department of Sociology, Memorial University, St. John's, Newfoundland, Canada

Improving antenatal care is considered a priority and has been relevant toward achieving the Millennium Development Goals (MDGs), yet antenatal care attendance remains relatively low in Ghana. Guided by the Andersen and Newman framework and employing logit models, we examine associations between occupational types and antenatal care among Ghanaian women aged 15–49. Type of occupation, conceptualized as a predisposing factor, has a significant impact on the frequency and timing of antenatal care attendance at the bivariate level. The effect of occupational type was considerably mediated, however, when other socioeconomic variables such as wealth status were controlled in the multivariate models.

Improving maternal health in sub-Saharan Africa is considered important, especially because it constitutes the fifth of the United Nations' (UN's) Millennium Development Goals (MDGs). Ensuring good maternal health outcomes has become extremely relevant in Africa, given that women are increasingly participating in the labor force and are assuming the breadwinner's role for their families and households. Promoting good maternal health in most developing countries, particularly Ghana, however, has been a major challenge. Although reports of maternal mortality are high in most countries in sub-Saharan Africa, including Ghana, progress seems to be very slow in reducing this health menace (Lozano et al., 2011). Consistent with achieving the MDG 5, several studies have evaluated the benefits of antenatal care in the reduction of maternal mortality and promotion of positive pregnancy outcomes (Kabir, Iliasu, Abubakar, & Asani, 2005; Whitehouse, 2010). For instance, antenatal attendance has been associated with the detection of complications and other risk factors among pregnant women (Zanconato,

Msolombo, Guarenti, & Franchi, 2006). It is expected also that antenatal care will provide pregnant women with sufficient information to recognize and deal with complications when they occur (Gerein, Mayhew, & Lubben, 2003). Besides, in previous studies researchers have demonstrated an association between antenatal care attendance and skilled birth delivery (Adjiwanou & LeGrand, 2013; McClure, Goldenberg, & Bann, 2007). When pregnant women attend antenatal care they are not only informed about the benefits of delivering at a health facility but also are being competently managed by a health care provider. In this regard, Nikiema, Beninguisse, and Haggerty (2009) found that the number of antenatal visits increased the likelihood of institutional delivery in sub-Saharan Africa.

Some researchers have underscored the relevance of accessing antenatal care in a timely manner given that it improves birth outcomes and reduces neonatal deaths and preterm births (Brown, Sohani, Khan, Lilford, & Mukhwana, 2008; Chen, Wen, Yang, & Walker, 2007; Hollowel, Oakley, Kurinczuk, Brocklehurst, & Gray, 2011). Recently, Gross and colleagues suggested that women who attend antenatal care early receive preventive health services such as immunizations against tetanus, prophylactic treatment of malaria, and iron supplementation that are crucial toward pregnancy outcomes (Gross, Glass, Schellenberg, & Obrist, 2012). Ibrahim and colleagues (2012) found that pregnant women who had more antenatal visits and particularly in the first trimester in Indonesia experienced lower risk of neonatal mortality compared with those who had fewer visits and report later. This is corroborated by Beeckman and colleagues (2013), who argued that the timing of antenatal care is important, especially as they found lower risk of preterm births among women visiting in the first trimester of pregnancy. It is important to acknowledge, however, that the relevance of antenatal care to promoting better maternal health outcomes continues to be debated as evidenced in the works of Campbell and Graham (2006), Evans and Lien (2005), McDonagh (1996), and Villar and colleagues (2001; these four references are cited in Adjiwanou & LeGrand, 2013). Against this backdrop, we examine both the frequency and timing of antenatal care among Ghanaian women using data from the most recent version of the Ghana Demographic and Health Survey (Ghana Statistical Service [GSS], Ghana Health Service [GHS] & ICF Macro, 2009).

Research that links women's occupation to their maternal health outcomes has been limited and inconclusive. In most cases, occupation is operationalized as a binary construct (whether women are employed or not) by previous researchers (Chakraborty, Islam, Chowdhury, Bari, & Akhter, 2003; Kaaya et al., 2010). This is particularly problematic because it fails to capture heterogeneity in occupational types and how this might influence maternal health outcomes, in this case, antenatal attendance. Also, while employed women could benefit from improved resources and increased autonomy resulting in increased and timely access of antenatal services (Beaujot & Ravanera, 2009; Desai & Jain, 1994), they may also suffer negative consequences as a result of the trade-offs between working and taking care of their reproductive health needs including accessing antenatal care and doing so in a timely manner (Crawley & Liu, 2012; Morrill, 2011). Our research fills an important research gap by examining the frequency and timing of antenatal care among women belonging to different occupational types. Thus, it is an important departure from previous work that homogenized women belonging to various occupational groups whose health-seeking behaviors may be different.

THEORETICAL FRAMEWORK

Our study draws on the Andersen and Newman framework of health care utilization (Andersen, 1995; Andersen & Newman, 1973) that conceptualizes occupation as a *predisposing* factor among other variables. Although first developed to explain health service use among populations, the model has in more recent times been extended to outcomes related to mental health, dental services, home care services, cardiac rehabilitation programs, outpatient services, and hospitalization, among others (Finlayson & DalMonte, 2002). The framework includes the following three broad factors as important determinants of health care utilization.

Predisposing Factors

This refers to the sociocultural characteristics of individuals existing prior to the illness. Andersen and Newman (1995) further divided predisposing factors into three main groups including *demographic factors* (age, gender, marital status, etc.), *social structure* (education, occupation, social networks, ethnicity, culture, etc.), and *health beliefs* (attitudes and beliefs that individuals have toward the health system).

Enabling Factors

This refers to availability of services and financial resources that influence the utilization of health services. These include *personal or family resources* (such as income, health insurance, travel, etc.) and *community resources* (availability of health personnel and facilities, waiting time, etc.).

Need Factors

Need factors often appear as proximal or immediate determinants of health care utilization. These include perceived vulnerability or severity of ailment mostly informed by the total number of sick days for a reported illness; symptoms of illness; worries about health, whether or not individuals judge health problems to be sufficient enough to seek professional help; and parity at birth (Vingilis, Wade, & Seeley, 2007; Wolinsky, 1988).

Based on the Andersen and Newman model, some empirical links have been established among *predisposing, enabling,* and *need* factors and health service utilization among women in sub-Saharan Africa and elsewhere. For instance, in several studies scholars have shown a strong link between women's levels of education and health care utilization (Ochako, Fotso, Ikamari, & Khasakhala, 2011; Pell et al., 2013). It has been argued that educated mothers are more likely to take advantage of modern health care services and comply with instructions about recommended treatments than uneducated women (Abbas & Walker, 1986; Barrera, 1990; Cadwell, 1979, 1990, as cited in Elo, 1992; Munsur, Atia, & Kawahara, 2010). Maternal occupation has also been associated with antenatal care utilization in sub-Saharan Africa (Awusi, Anyanwu, & Okeleke, 2009). In Kenya, Magadi, Madise, and Rodrigues (2000) found that employed women were significantly more likely to use antenatal care services compared with unemployed women. In Ghana and elsewhere, it is documented that women who are employed have high rates of antenatal care use compared with unemployed women or housewives (Addai, 2000; Kabir et al., 2005). Sato (2012) found that income has a positive effect on the choice of modern health care in Ghana. In addition, some authors find that the ability to pay for antenatal care services is associated with the level of income among women in sub-Saharan Africa (Awusi et al., 2009; Bonfrer, Poel, Grimm, & van Doorslaer, 2012; Kevany, Murima, & Singh, 2012; Pell et al., 2013). Like income, Monheit (2000, p. 11) notes that "health insurance plays a critical role in insuring timely access to medical care, in protecting families from financial hardship due to expensive and unanticipated medical events, and in enhancing social welfare through risk pooling."

Some researchers also find that religion is associated with preventive health care including maternal health (Aaron, Levine, & Burstin, 2003; Benjamins & Buck, 2008). Benjamins and Buck (2008) argue that religious groups tend to regulate the health behaviors of their members through information sessions, thus encouraging positive attitudes toward health-seeking behaviors. Similar to religion, some researchers have identified demographic variables such as marital status, age, and parity at birth as important determinants of antenatal care. Married women are more likely to utilize antenatal care services compared with unmarried or single women (Glei, Goldman, & Rodriguez, 2003). Younger women between the ages of 20 to 35 years are more likely to utilize antenatal care services than women below 20 and those older than 35 years (Arthur, 2012; Dairo & Owoyokun, 2010). Parity, the number of previous live births, is associated with the use of antenatal care services. Results from other studies show that women are more likely to use antenatal services for their first pregnancy than subsequent pregnancies in sub-Saharan Africa (Rai, Singh, Kumar, & Singh, 2013). Guided by

Andersen and Newman's model, we examine the independent effects of occupational types on the frequency and timing of antenatal care among Ghanaian women.

METHODS

Data and Sampling

Data for this study are drawn from the 2008 Ghana Demographic and Health Survey (GDHS), which is the fifth in such surveys of the GDHS program (see www.dhsprogram.com for more information). The 2008 GDHS is a household-based survey implemented in a representative probability sample of more than 12,323 households, selected nationwide. It is the fifth national-level population and health survey undertaken in Ghana since 1988. The 2008 GDHS utilized a two-stage sample design. The first stage involved selecting sampling points or clusters from an updated master sampling frame constructed from the 2000 Ghana Population and Housing Census. The second stage involved the systematic sampling of 30 of the households listed in each cluster. A total of 4,916 women ages 15 to 49 were identified and interviewed nationwide, with an individual women's response rate of 97%. The sample for this study was restricted to 2,117 women ages 15 to 49 who attended antenatal care within the 5 years preceding the survey.

Ethics

Data and survey instruments were reviewed by the ethics review boards of the host country, Macro (a U.S.-based organization that collaborates and provides technical assistance to the DHS), and other implementing partners. An informed consent statement was read out to respondents who participated in the study. Participation in the study was completely voluntary, and respondents had the right to refuse to answer any questions or stop the interview at any point.

Measures

Two dependent variables were used to measure women's antenatal attendance: the *frequency of antenatal visits* and *timing of first antenatal visits*. These variables were transformed into dichotomous variables. The first dependent variable is from the question, "How many times did you receive antenatal care during this pregnancy? This was coded as "0" for fewer than four antenatal care visits and "1" for at least four antenatal care visits. Antenatal care attendance is defined as the number of visits with a health care professional (obstetrician, midwife, or generalist), whether in the hospital, community, or home (Beeckman, Louckx, & Putman, 2010). The World

Health Organization (WHO, 1994) recommends four antenatal visits in order to enjoy the full benefits of care.

The second dependent variable, timing of antenatal care, comes from the question, "How many months pregnant were you when you first received antenatal care for this pregnancy? This was then coded "0" for visits beyond the first trimester and "1" for visits within the first trimester. This is justified because the new standard guidelines from the WHO recommend that women initiate antenatal care attendance during the first trimester of pregnancy (WHO, 2006).

The independent variables in the analysis were selected based on Andersen and Newman's framework that identifies *predisposing, enabling,* and *need* factors as influential to antenatal care attendance. Occupation, which is considered the focal independent variable for this study, is conceptualized as a *predisposing* factor among other variables such as educational level, region, religion, ethnicity, age, marital status, and place of residence. Wealth and health insurance are conceptualized as *enabling* factors and parity at birth as a *need* factor. The focal independent variable, occupational status of respondents, is operationalized as "not working = 0," "professional/managerial/clerical = 1," "sales = 2," "self-employed = 3," and "services and skilled labor = 4." Other predisposing factors are coded as follows: education ("no education = 0," "primary education = 1," and "secondary/higher education = 2"), region of residence ("Greater Accra = 0," "Central = 1," "Western = 2," "Volta = 3," "Eastern = 4," "Ashanti = 5," "Brong Ahafo = 6," "Northern = 7," "Upper East = 8," and "Upper West = 9"), ethnicity ("Akan = 0," "Ga/Dangbe = 1," "Ewe = 2," and "other northern ethnic groups = 3"), religion ("Christian = 0," "Muslim = 1," "Traditionalist = 2," and "no religion = 3"), marital status ("never married = 0," "currently married = 1," and "formerly married = 2"), place of residence ("urban = 0," and "rural = 1"), and age of respondents introduced as a continuous variable Wealth as an enabling factor was operationalized as ("poorest = 0," "poorer = 1," "middle = 2," "richer = 3," and "richest = 4"). Health insurance was categorized according to whether the person was a registered member with the NHIS. This was coded as "yes = 1," and "no = 0." The only *need* factor parity at birth is coded as follows: "no births = 0," "one birth = 2," "two births = 2," and "three births = 3."

Data Analysis

A binary logistic regression is used to examine the impact of occupational status and other selected covariates on both the timing and frequency of antenatal care attendance among Ghanaian women. A binary logit model was used due to the dichotomous nature of the dependent variables (Worster, Fan, & Ismaila, 2007). Generally, a logistic model estimates the probability or likelihood of an event occurring through the maximum likelihood function. The coefficients from logit models may be transformed into exponentiated betas also known as the odds ratios indicating the likelihood of an event occurring as opposed to the event not occurring (Hosmer, Lemeshow, & Sturdivant, 2013). A major assumption underlying most standard regression techniques, including logit models, which require particular attention, however, is the assumption of independence (see Raudenbush & Bryk, 2002). The hierarchical/multistage nature of the DHS data where women are nested within households and clusters presents a good case for violating this assumption and potentially biasing the standard errors and parameter estimates. STATA 12.SE, which provides an outlet for handling this problem, is used by imposing on our models a "cluster" variable, usually the identification numbers of respondents at the cluster level. This in turn adjusts the standard errors producing statistically robust parameter estimates (Cleves, Gould, & Gutierrez, 2004; Tenkorang & Owusu, 2010). An odds ratio greater than one indicates a higher likelihood of accessing antenatal care within the first trimester or at least four times compared with not doing so, while an odds ratio less than one indicates a lower likelihood of attending antenatal care within the first trimester or at least four times. Model fits were determined using the Hosmer and Lameshow chi-square statistic.

RESULTS

In Table 1 we present descriptive statistics for the predictor and outcome variables used in this study. The majority of Ghanaian women (76.78%) make the recommended antenatal visits (at least four), and the majority also visited in the first trimester of pregnancy (57.65%). Regarding occupation, it is clear that 10.49% indicated they are not working (unemployed), 2.78% are in the professional/managerial category, 32.49% are in the sales category, and 8.85% are in the skilled labor category. Quite a substantial proportion of women reported they had secondary/higher education (40.25%), compared with those with no education (35.99%). Respondents are almost evenly distributed across the various wealth quintiles, with 29.40% of women identified as "poorest," 22.10% as "poorer," 18.26% as "richer," and 12.69% as "richest." Approximately, 9.69% of women are located in the Greater Accra Region, where the capital is also located. This sharply contrasts with the 14.89% and 14.28% of women hailing from the Ashanti and Northern regions, respectively. As we introduced demographic variables into the analysis, we see that on average women in the sample are about 30 years of age. The majority of the women are currently married (88.86%), identify as Christians (67.93%), belong to the Akan ethnic group (39.03%), and live in the rural areas (64.47%). It is quite interesting to find that majority of Ghanaian women are not enrolled on the NHIS (58.99%) and that the average number

TABLE 1 Univariate Analysis of Antenatal Care Attendance Among Women in Ghana

Dependent variables	%
Number of antenatal visits	
Fewer than four visits	23.22
At least four visits	76.78
Timing of antenatal visits	
First trimester	42.39
Beyond first trimester	57.61
Independent Variables	
Occupational types	
Not working	10.49
Professional/managerial/clerical	2.78
Sales	32.49
Self-employed	38.04
Services	7.63
Skilled labor	8.85
Educational level	
No education	35.99
Primary education	23.76
Secondary/higher education	40.25
Ethnicity	
Akan	39.03
Ga/Dangbe	4.73
Ewe	12.70
Northern languages	40.02
Other languages	3.51
Age (years in mean)	30.18
Religion	
Christians	67.93
Muslims	19.46
Traditionalists	7.83
No religion	4.78
Region of residence	
Greater Accra	9.69
Central	7.35
Western	8.85
Volta	8.43
Eastern	8.75
Ashanti	14.89
Brong-Ahafo	9.64
Northern	14.28
Upper East	8.33
Upper West	9.78
Marital status	
Never married	5.43
Currently married	88.86
Formerly married	5.71
Place of residence	
Urban	35.53
Rural	64.47
Wealth status	
Poorest	29.40
Poorer	22.10
Middle	17.56

(Continued on next page)

TABLE 1 Univariate Analysis of Antenatal Care Attendance Among Women in Ghana (*Continued*)

Dependent variables	%
Richer	18.26
Richest	12.69
Health insurance	
No	58.99
Yes	41.01
Parity (mean of children ever born)	3.5

of children ever born by a Ghanaian woman was estimated as 3.5 births, which is almost equivalent to current estimates of the total fertility rate for the country.

Results for the bivariate analysis are shown in Table 2. The bivariate findings indicate that several *predisposing* factors are related to the frequency and timing of antenatal care among pregnant women in Ghana. As postulated in the theoretical model, occupation is statistically associated with both the number of antenatal visits and the timing of first antenatal care among Ghanaian women. Specifically, women in the professional/managerial/clerical group are three times more likely to go for antenatal care and two times more likely to visit within the first trimester of pregnancy compared with the nonworking women. Also, compared with the unemployed, women in the services and skilled labor categories are 69% more likely to make their antenatal visits within the first trimester of pregnancy. Consistent with previous research, this study finds that education is strongly associated with both the likelihood and timing of accessing antenatal care. Compared with those with no education, women with secondary/higher education are three times more likely to make the recommended number of visits (at least four visits) and 67% more likely to visit within the first trimester of pregnancy. Turning to ethnicity, the results show clearly that women who identify with the northern ethnic groups are 46% significantly less likely to make the recommended number of visits (at least four four antenatal visits) and 27% less likely to visit within the first trimester of pregnancy compared with the Akans. Age of respondents is not significantly related to the number and timing of antenatal care at the bivariate level, but religion is. Compared with Christians, who are in the majority, Traditionalists and women with no religious affiliation are less likely to make the recommended number of visits (at least four antenatal visits). Also, Muslims and Traditionalists are less likely to go for their first antenatal visit within the first trimester of pregnancy compared with Christians. There are regional differences in the number and timing of antennal care. Women who reside in the regions other than the Greater Accra regions are significantly less likely to make the recommended number of visits (at least four antenatal visits). Regarding the timing of antenatal

TABLE 2 Bivariate Analysis of Antenatal Care Attendance Among Women in Ghana

Independent variables	Number of visits	Timing of visits
Occupational types		
Professional/managerial/clerical	3.398*	2.781**
	(1.852)	(0.957)
Sales	1.236	1.181
	(0.245)	(0.188)
Self-employed	0.474***	0.829
	(0.0880)	(0.130)
Services	1.977*	1.686*
	(0.598)	(0.370)
Skilled labor	1.080	1.689*
	(0.274)	(0.355)
Educational level		
Primary education	1.260	1.383**
	(0.158)	(0.165)
Secondary/higher education	3.524***	1.673***
	(0.458)	(0.173)
Ethnicity		
Ga/Dangbe	0.745	0.805
	(0.189)	(0.174)
Ewe	0.825	0.899
	(0.144)	(0.131)
Northern languages	0.543***	0.724**
	(0.0639)	(0.0731)
Other languages	0.647	0.911
	(0.181)	(0.230)
Age	1.013	0.996
	(0.00721)	(0.00615)
Religion		
Muslim	0.898	0.643***
	(0.123)	(0.0730)
Traditionalist	0.222***	0.425***
	(0.0374)	(0.0750)
No religion	0.425***	0.728
	(0.0919)	(0.158)
Region of residence		
Central	0.340***	0.947
	(0.104)	(0.215)
Western	0.289***	0.890
	(0.0844)	(0.192)
Volta	0.270***	0.706
	(0.0792)	(0.153)
Eastern	0.277***	0.641*
	(0.0809)	(0.135)
Ashanti	0.555*	0.830
	(0.159)	(0.157)
Brong-Ahafo	0.372***	0.661*
	(0.110)	(0.137)
Northern	0.198***	0.245***
	(0.0534)	(0.0476)
Upper East	0.184***	0.765
	(0.0530)	(0.166)

(Continued on next page)

TABLE 2 Bivariate Analysis of Antenatal Care Attendance Among Women in Ghana (Continued)

Independent variables	Number of visits	Timing of visits
Upper West	0.520*	1.038
	(0.159)	(0.220)
Marital status		
Currently married	1.114	1.102
	(0.247)	(0.218)
Formerly married	1.022	1.028
	(0.307)	(0.277)
Place of residence		
Rural	0.322***	0.735**
	(0.0408)	(0.0691)
Wealth status		
Poorer	1.547***	1.318*
	(0.205)	(0.167)
Middle	2.079***	1.362*
	(0.312)	(0.183)
Richer	5.091***	1.749***
	(0.948)	(0.234)
Richest	10.68***	3.283***
	(3.062)	(0.542)
Health insurance		
Yes	2.475***	1.326**
	(0.283)	(0.121)
Parity	0.906***	0.900***
	(0.0198)	(0.0182)

Exponentiated coefficients; robust standard errors in parentheses.
$*p < .05, **p < .01, ***p < .001.$

care, it is clear that women in the Eastern, Brong-Ahafo, and Northern regions are significantly less likely to make their first antenatal visit within the first trimester of pregnancy compared with those in the Greater Accra region. Similar to region of residence, place of residence is significantly associated with antenatal care utilization. Compared with those residing in the urban areas, women in the rural areas are significantly less likely to make the recommended number of visits (at least four antenatal visits) and are less likely to make the first visit within the first trimester of pregnancy.

Enabling and *need factors* as conceptualized by Andersen and Newman are strong and significant predictors of both the number and timing of antenatal visits among women in Ghana. As shown in Table 2, women in the richer and richest wealth quintiles are significantly more likely to make the recommended number of visits (at least four visits) and make this visit within the first trimester of pregnancy compared with those in the poorest wealth quintile. Results also show that women enrolled on the NHIS are 2.5 times more likely to make the recommended number of antenatal visits (at least four antenatal visits) and are 33% more likely to make this visit within the first trimester of pregnancy compared with those not enrolled. It is also clear from the table that women who had more children are about 10% less likely to make the recommended number of visits and to make their first visit within the first trimester of pregnancy compared with those with fewer children.

While bivariate results presented above are useful, they may be limited especially as they do not take into consideration confounding and mediating effects. Multivariate models presented in Tables 3 and 4 consider these effects. In all, six multivariate models are constructed (three each for *number of visits* and *timing*). Model 1 examines the effects of occupation on the number of visits and timing of antenatal care with other *predisposing factors* such as (education, marital status, residence, age, etc.) controlled. Models 2 and 3 add *enabling* (wealth and health insurance) and *need factors* (parity at birth), respectively.

Results from Model 1 in Tables 3 and 4 indicate that although somewhat attenuated, occupation is significantly associated with the number of visits for antenatal care and the timing of the first visit. In particular, women who work in the service sector are significantly more likely to make the recommended number of visits compared with the unemployed. Further, it is observed that women in skilled labor, those who work as professionals/managers/clerks, and those in the service sector are all significantly more likely to make their first visit earlier (within the first trimester of pregnancy) rather than later. The effect of occupation, however, is significantly attenuated after controlling for enabling factors (wealth and health insurance) in Model 2. Further analysis (not shown) indicates that wealth mediated the effects of occupation. It is observed, for instance, that it is only the odds ratio for women belonging to the skilled labor category that remained significant even after enabling factors had been controlled.

Several other factors remained statistically significant in the final model. We find, for instance, that compared with the poorest and respondents with no education, wealthier women and those with secondary/higher education not only made the recommended number of visits but also the first antenatal visit within the first trimester of pregnancy. It is worth noting that while women enrolled on the National Health Insurance Scheme (NHIS) were significantly more likely to make the recommended number of antenatal visits, being on the NHIS did not make any difference regarding the timing of antenatal care. Parity at birth is strongly related to both number of visit and timing, as women with a higher number of children were significantly less likely to make the recommended number of visits and make the first visit within the first trimester of pregnancy. As expected, older women were more likely to make the recommended number of visits, and Traditionalists were less likely to do so compared with Christians. It was intriguing, however, to have found that women from the Upper West region were significantly more likely to have made the recommended number of visits compared with those

TABLE 3 Multivariate Analysis of Number of Antenatal Care Visits Among Women in Ghana

Independent variables	Model 1	Model 2	Model 3
Occupational types			
Professional/managerial/clerical	1.835	1.262	1.175
	(1.020)	(0.738)	(0.688)
Sales	1.232	1.123	1.140
	(0.251)	(0.235)	(0.237)
Self-employed	0.799	0.883	0.913
	(0.174)	(0.195)	(0.204)
Services	1.927*	1.696	1.640
	(0.603)	(0.543)	(0.527)
Skilled labor	1.177	1.091	1.037
	(0.311)	(0.297)	(0.282)
Educational level			
Primary education	0.997	0.964	0.944
	(0.160)	(0.157)	(0.153)
Secondary/higher education	2.238***	1.817**	1.665**
	(0.423)	(0.353)	(0.320)
Ethnicity			
Ga/Dangbe	0.911	0.966	0.949
	(0.279)	(0.309)	(0.305)
Ewe	1.299	1.414	1.390
	(0.291)	(0.312)	(0.307)
Northern languages	0.740	0.761	0.722
	(0.181)	(0.186)	(0.174)
Other languages	0.760	0.719	0.693
	(0.273)	(0.260)	(0.248)
Age	1.028**	1.025**	1.059***
	(0.00878)	(0.00861)	(0.0148)
Religion			
Muslim	1.018	1.038	1.020
	(0.197)	(0.205)	(0.203)
Traditionalist	0.396***	0.428***	0.452***
	(0.0748)	(0.0795)	(0.0851)
No religion	0.560*	0.615*	0.620
	(0.138)	(0.152)	(0.152)
Region of residence			
Central	0.671	0.881	0.911
	(0.280)	(0.373)	(0.382)
Western	0.518	0.635	0.659
	(0.213)	(0.266)	(0.276)
Volta	0.469	0.608	0.587
	(0.183)	(0.245)	(0.237)
Eastern	0.452*	0.515	0.518
	(0.163)	(0.193)	(0.194)
Ashanti	0.901	1.063	1.098
	(0.351)	(0.423)	(0.437)
Brong-Ahafo	0.827	0.965	0.963
	(0.357)	(0.431)	(0.430)
Northern	0.834	1.073	1.126
	(0.338)	(0.460)	(0.485)
Upper East	0.793	0.858	0.829
	(0.339)	(0.389)	(0.377)

(Continued on next page)

TABLE 3 Multivariate Analysis of Number of Antenatal Care Visits Among Women in Ghana (*Continued*)

Independent variables	Model 1	Model 2	Model 3
Upper West	2.095	2.509*	2.629*
	(0.941)	(1.172)	(1.236)
Marital status			
Currently married	1.394	1.160	1.205
	(0.363)	(0.316)	(0.328)
Formerly married	0.945	0.863	0.862
	(0.321)	(0.298)	(0.295)
Place of residence			
Rural	0.536***	0.773	0.795
	(0.0882)	(0.138)	(0.143)
Wealth status			
Poorer		1.085	1.057
		(0.180)	(0.177)
Middle		1.159	1.129
		(0.240)	(0.234)
Richer		2.374**	2.221**
		(0.650)	(0.611)
Richest		3.251**	2.918**
		(1.205)	(1.098)
Health insurance			
Yes		1.776***	1.771***
		(0.233)	(0.230)
Parity			0.868**
			(0.0377)
N	2117	2117	2117
ll	−1008.5	−985.5	−979.6

Exponentiated coefficients; robust standard errors in parentheses.
*$p < .05$, **$p < .01$, ***$p < .001$.

in the Greater Accra region. A discussion of the results described above is provided in the next section of the article.

DISCUSSION

The need to improve maternal health in the developing world and sub-Saharan Africa remains top priority for both national and international actors. This need, as boldly enshrined in the UNs' MDGs, asked that countries in sub-Saharan Africa including Ghana reduce maternal mortality and infant and child deaths by the year 2015 (UN, 2008, 2013; WHO, 2008, 2010). Besides, it was recommended that universal access to reproductive health be achieved in the same year. These recommendations were reechoed in a recent high-level plenary meeting held by the General Assembly of the UN in New York (Development Alternatives with Women for a New Era, 2012). The recommendations were made against the backdrop that maternal

TABLE 4 Multivariate Analysis of the Timing of Antenatal Care Visits Among Women in Ghana

Independent variables	Model 1	Model 2	Model 3
Types of occupation			
Professional/managerial/clerical	2.142*	1.780	1.672
	(0.712)	(0.625)	(0.591)
Sales	1.131	1.116	1.135
	(0.186)	(0.187)	(0.189)
Self-employed	0.956	1.054	1.111
	(0.177)	(0.196)	(0.208)
Services	1.581*	1.463	1.420
	(0.322)	(0.304)	(0.294)
Skilled labor	1.566*	1.575*	1.509
	(0.349)	(0.350)	(0.334)
Educational level			
Primary education	1.030	1.000	0.975
	(0.145)	(0.141)	(0.138)
Secondary/higher education	1.130	0.981	0.881
	(0.168)	(0.151)	(0.138)
Ethnicity			
Akan	0.872	0.917	0.902
	(0.236)	(0.258)	(0.254)
Ga/Dangbe	0.972	1.012	0.978
	(0.180)	(0.192)	(0.188)
Ewe	1.264	1.270	1.203
	(0.226)	(0.229)	(0.219)
Northern languages	1.336	1.266	1.218
	(0.376)	(0.366)	(0.350)
Age	1.000	0.998	1.031**
	(0.00674)	(0.00677)	(0.0105)
Religion			
Muslim	0.853	0.865	0.865
	(0.137)	(0.140)	(0.141)
Traditionalist	0.681*	0.701	0.742
	(0.128)	(0.134)	(0.142)
No religion	0.805	0.850	0.839
	(0.183)	(0.196)	(0.195)
Region of residence			
Central	1.110	1.405	1.455
	(0.265)	(0.351)	(0.367)
Western	1.012	1.262	1.315
	(0.246)	(0.316)	(0.333)
Volta	0.831	1.102	1.087
	(0.188)	(0.275)	(0.274)
Eastern	0.738	0.937	0.956
	(0.176)	(0.237)	(0.242)
Ashanti	0.881	1.101	1.128
	(0.182)	(0.242)	(0.249)
Brong-Ahafo	0.753	0.985	0.981
	(0.186)	(0.264)	(0.266)
Northern	0.298***	0.400***	0.412**
	(0.0753)	(0.107)	(0.112)

(Continued on next page)

TABLE 4 Multivariate Analysis of the Timing of Antenatal Care Visits Among Women in Ghana *(Continued)*

Independent variables	Model 1	Model 2	Model 3
Upper East	0.773	1.011	0.983
	(0.237)	(0.349)	(0.341)
Upper West	1.136	1.500	1.583
	(0.327)	(0.458)	(0.490)
Marital status			
Currently married	1.368	1.209	1.249
	(0.303)	(0.271)	(0.282)
Formerly married	1.117	1.059	1.043
	(0.317)	(0.303)	(0.297)
Place of residence			
Rural	0.904	1.159	1.189
	(0.112)	(0.156)	(0.161)
Wealth status			
Poor		1.115	1.089
		(0.171)	(0.168)
Middle		1.212	1.189
		(0.216)	(0.215)
Richer		1.531*	1.442
		(0.303)	(0.288)
Richest		2.816***	2.547***
		(0.736)	(0.666)
Health insurance			
Yes		1.092	1.084
		(0.113)	(0.112)
Parity			0.863***
			(0.0303)
N	2024	2024	2024
ll	−1313.9	−1302.4	−1293.7

Exponentiated coefficients; robust standard errors in parentheses.
$^*p < .05$, $^{**}p < .01$, $^{***}p < .001$.

mortality remained unacceptably high in developing countries including those in sub-Saharan Africa, that large disparities still exist in providing pregnant women with skilled medical personnel and assistance during labor, and that the majority of deaths resulting from pregnancy complications are in fact avoidable (Adegoke, Utz, Msuya, & van de Broek, 2012; Gerein, Green, & Pearson, 2006).

After almost a decade of launching the MDGs, it has become clear that the majority of countries in sub-Saharan Africa including Ghana are unable to meet these targets. Currently, Ghana ranks forty-first on the world maternal mortality rate index with a maternal mortality ratio of 350 deaths per 100,000 live births (WHO, 2012). Although the ratios are a significant reduction from previous years, the WHO and other international bodies adjudged the current rates as relatively high, especially when countries in the developed world such as Canada and the United States have recorded maternal mortality ratios of 12 and 21 deaths per 100,000 live births, respectively. The Ghana government over the years has responded to calls by these international bodies to reduce maternal, infant, and child deaths by initiating numerous policies, some of which I have discussed in the literature review. Worth mentioning, however, is the recently introduced NHIS, which not only reduced personal costs and increased greater access to health care but also made access to maternal health services free, including easy access to antenatal care for pregnant women in Ghana.

Similar to policymakers, researchers interested in maternal and reproductive health outcomes in sub-Saharan Africa and Ghana have attempted to understand the high rates of maternal, child, and infant mortality including access to antenatal care (Alvarez, Gil, Hernandez, & Gil, 2009; Bour & Bream, 2004; Khan, Wojdyla, Say, Gulmezoglu, & Van, 2006). The bulk of the research in the past focused on how socioeconomic, demographic, and cultural differences influence access to antenatal care (Kevany et al., 2012; Pell et al., 2013; Tsegay et al., 2013). In these studies, education, income, and occupation were used as proxies for socioeconomic status. It is argued here that the operationalization of occupation as a binary construct (whether women are employed or not) by previous researchers is problematic as it fails to capture heterogeneity in occupational types and how this might influence maternal health outcomes, in this case, antenatal attendance among Ghanaian women. Further, while women engaged in professional/skilled labor may benefit from improved financial resources that might affect access to antenatal care positively, the tensions that exist between time allocated for professional duties and household activities may negatively affect such women meeting their reproductive and health needs including accessing antenatal care. Thus, using the Andersen and Newman framework, which conceptualized occupation as a *predisposing* factor, among other *enabling* and *need* factors controlled, this study examined the effects of occupational types on both the frequency and timing of first antenatal care among Ghanaian women. Findings generally support the Andersen and Newman framework as efficacious in determining antenatal care access among women in Ghana. Occupation as a *predisposing* factor was statistically associated with both the frequency and timing of antenatal care. At the bivariate level, for instance, women categorized as professional/managerial/clerical and those identifying as belonging to the service sector were more likely to make the recommended number of antenatal visits and did so within the first trimester of pregnancy compared with unemployed women. While self-employed women were less likely to make the recommended number of visits, women categorized as "skilled" were more likely to visit in the first trimester of pregnancy. The multivariate models, on the other hand, suggested that when other variables were controlled occupation lost its significance. Further analysis indicated that both education and wealth mediated the effects of occupation on the frequency and timing of antenatal care, respectively. Together, these findings demonstrate that in Ghana occupational differences regarding both the frequency and timing of antenatal care are artefacts of educational and income/wealth differences. It is mostly the case that women engaged in the so-called professional/managerial/clerical, skilled, and service jobs are those in the higher educational and wealth brackets (see Gyimah, Takyi, & Tenkorang, 2008; Gyimah, Tenkorang, Takyi, Adjei, & Fosu, 2010). Thus, the findings provide some qualified support for the thesis that career-oriented women may be benefiting from the advantages that education and wealth may confer, compared with their unemployed counterparts. Several studies have underscored the positive effects of education and wealth on maternal health outcomes in sub-Saharan Africa (Arthur, 2012; Assefa, Berhane, & Worku, 2012; Kevany et al., 2012; Nketiah-Amponsah, Senadza, & Arthur, 2013). Education creates awareness and informs women about the merits of seeking antenatal care and doing it quite early during pregnancy, but access to care is made possible when women are financially resourced and can afford it. Thus, the finding that educated and wealthier women are more likely to make the recommended number of antenatal visits than uneducated and poorer women is consistent with previous research (see Adewoye, Musah, Atoyebi, & Babatunde, 2013; Awusi, 2009; Kevany et al., 2012; Magadi, Madise, & Rodrigues, 2000; Myer & Harrison 2003; Sato, 2012).

Similar to income that enables access to antenatal care, this study confirmed health insurance as also crucial to antenatal care attendance among Ghanaian women. Women enrolled in the NHIS were more likely to have made the recommended number of antenatal visits compared with those not enrolled. It was quite interesting to find, however, that enrollment on the NHIS had no significant association with the timing of antenatal care. We propose two different explanations as to why the NHIS increases the likelihood of the number of antenatal visits and yet does not influence the timing of the first antenatal visit. First, the NHIS can only impact the timing of antenatal visits if women are aware they are pregnant, and many women in sub-Saharan Africa do not even realize they are pregnant until the second trimester, making early antenatal care through NHIS unlikely (Gross et al., 2012; Myer & Harrison, 2003). Second, the majority of women enroll for NHIS when they are faced with a health need. In this case, there are numerous administrative bottlenecks that delay enrollment, so that by the time a woman realizes she is pregnant, travels to a clinic, completes a pregnancy test, waits for the positive result, travels to the NHIS office, waits in line, completes the paperwork with the agent, and receives her temporary enrolment card, she may very well be beyond her first trimester (Dixon, Tenkorang, Luginaah, Kuuire, & Boateng, 2013).

There are also variations in antenatal care utilization among the regions as shown in the study. For instance, women in the Upper West region are more likely to make the recommended number of visits than women in the Greater region. A possible reason could be attributed to the free maternal health care policy that was implemented in the region earlier. Thus, women in this region might have taken advantage of the policy and are able to make the recommended number of visits. Moreover, the Upper West is one of the poorest regions in Ghana, and the introduction of the free maternal health policy in the region meant that it took away the financial barriers that previously hindered women from accessing antenatal care.

Previous research that examined the relationship between parity and antenatal care has been inconclusive. While some found that women with higher parity attended antenatal care more often (McCray, 2004), others found high parity associated with decreased attendance for antenatal services (Rai et al., 2013). Moreover, women with large family sizes may face resource constraints that will limit their ability to utilize maternal health services including antenatal care (Chakraborty et al., 2003). This study confirms the latter findings of higher parity leading not only to decreased antenatal care attendance but also to visits that go beyond the first trimester of pregnancy. Here we argue that it is very likely that as women give birth to more children they gain some experience and familiarity with common ailments that keep them from visiting the doctor during the pregnancy period. In contrast, first timers may lack such familiarity, and their frequent visits may just reflect concerns and inexperience in dealing with some of what may appear as "minor" complications during pregnancy.

Regarding pregnancy complications, previous research indicates that older women are very vulnerable (Karabulut, Ozkan, Bozkurt, & Kayan, 2013). It is thus not surprising to have found that older women were not only more likely to have experienced increased antenatal care attendance but visited within the first trimester of pregnancy. Alternatively, older women may be knowledgeable and aware of the benefits of attending antenatal care and doing so in a timely manner. Although the findings are insightful, there are some limitations worth considering.

Limitations

The DHS data are cross sectional, meaning that data were collected contemporaneously. It is therefore difficult to make causal connections between predictor and outcome variables. Thus, our findings are limited to mere associations, and extreme caution should be taken in making causal inferences between dependent and independent variables. Also, the results should be interpreted with caution due to the possibility of underreporting among women who may have difficulty in recollecting information about their pregnancy histories. In this regard, memory could be faulty and women could have difficulty in recalling accurately all past events associated with their antenatal care attendance. Due to data limitations, this study could not consider some proximal reasons why women attend antenatal care in Africa such as reasons related to pregnancy complications. There is also no information about formal service availability and quality of services rendered and how that may impact utilization of antenatal services. Furthermore, this study only examined individual-level factors as determinants of antenatal care utilization among women in Ghana. There are other studies that employ multilevel models to show the relevance of structural factors (Zere, Kirigia, Duale, & Akazili, 2012). We could not control for such structural variables due to data limitations. Despite these limitations, this study offers several conclusions and policy recommendations.

CONCLUSIONS AND POLICY RECOMMENDATIONS

An important conclusion from this work is that occupational differences in both the likelihood and timing of accessing antenatal care are largely a re-flection of educational and wealth differences. It was also discovered that educated and wealthier women were more likely to make the recommended number of antenatal visits and do so within the first trimester of pregnancy. This provides support for enacting policies that encourage women's empow-erment in sub-Saharan Africa, including Ghana. Such policies will include creating educational and employment opportunities for women in Ghana. It is expected that creating such opportunities will improve the economic circumstances of Ghanaian women and improve maternal health outcomes. For instance, providing women with formal education may not only unleash their economic potential but also keep them informed about the benefits of accessing antenatal care and doing so in a timely manner. This can be achieved through health promotion programs targeting women with little or no education in the communities about the importance of antenatal care attendance among women.

We also provide some support for the recently introduced NHIS as an effective tool for increasing antenatal care attendance among Ghanaian women. Over the past few years, the NHIS has seen large increases in enrollment, with some studies suggesting that the scheme has benefited its members by protecting against the financial burden of health care for both in-patient and out-patient treatment (Health Systems 20/20 Project, 2009; Nguyen Rajkotia & Wang, 2011). Some studies show that the NHIS is failing in meeting its propoor mandate because the wealthy are more likely to enroll than the poor (see Dixon, Tenkorang, & Luginaah, 2011). It is important for government and other stakeholders to consider and examine the barriers that prevent poorer women from enrolling, especially when our study shows that enrollment has implications for maternal health outcomes including antenatal care attendance.

More importantly, through this study we reveal that higher parity at birth is negatively associated with antenatal care use. It is important to ensure that programs and policies are enacted to focus on women with more births since they are at risk during pregnancy. It is important to consider how antenatal services could reach these categories of women to ensure that their pregnancies can be managed to safe delivery.

REFERENCES

Aaron, K. F., Levine, D., & Burstin, H. R. (2003). African American church participation and health care practices. *Journal of General Internal Medicine, 18,* 908–913.

Addai, I. (2000). Determinants of use of maternal–child health services in rural Ghana. *Journal of Biosocial Science, 32,* 1–15.

Adegoke, A., Utz, B., Msuya, S. E., & van de Broek, N. (2012). Skilled birth attendants: Who is who? A descriptive study of definitions and roles from nine sub-Saharan African countries. *PLoS ONE, 7,* 7. doi:10.1371/journal.pone.0040220

Adewoye, K. R., Musah, I. O., Atoyebi, O. A., & Babatunde, O. A. (2013). Knowledge and utilization of antenatal care services by women of child bearing age in Ilorin-East local government area, North Central Nigeria. *International Journal of Science and Technology, 3,* 188–193.

Adjiwanou, V., & LeGrand, T. (2013). Does antenatal care matter in the use of skilled birth attendance in rural Africa: A multi-country analysis. *Social Science & Medicine, 86,* 26–34.

Alvarez, J. L., Gil, R., Hernandez, V., & Gil, A. (2009). Factors associated with maternal mortality in sub-Saharan Africa: An ecological study. *BioMed Central Public Health, 9,* 462. doi:10.1186/1471-2458-9-462

Andersen, R. (1995). Revisiting the behavioral model and access to medical care: Does it matter? *Journal of Health and Social Behavior, 36,* 1–10.

Andersen, R. M., & Newman, J. F. (1973). Social and individual determinants of medical care utilization in the United States. *Milbank Memorial Quarterly, 51,* 95–124.

Arthur, E. (2012). Wealth and antenatal care use: Implications for maternal health care utilisation in Ghana. *Health Economics Review, 2,* 14.

Assefa, N., Berhane, Y., & Worku, A. (2012). Wealth status, mid upper arm circumference (MUAC) and antenatal care (ANC) are determinants for low birth weight in Kersa, Ethiopia. *PLoS ONE, 7,* 6. doi:10.1371/journal.pone.0039957

Awusi, V. O., Anyanwu, E. B., & Okeleke, V. (2009). Determinants of antenatal care services utilization in Emevor village, Nigeria. *Benin Journal of Postgraduate Medicine, 11,* 21–26.

Beaujot, R., & Ravanera, Z. R. (2009). Family models for earning and caring: Implications for child care and for family policy. *Canadian Studies in Population, 36,* 145–166.

Beeckman, K., Louckx, F., Downe, S., & Putman, K. (2013). The relationship between antenatal care and preterm birth: The importance of content of care. *European Journal of Public Health, 23,* 366–371.

Beeckman, K., Louckx, F., & Putman, K. (2010). Determinants of the number of antenatal visits in a metropolitan region. *BioMed Central Public Health, 10,* 527. doi:10.1186/1471-2458-10-527

Benjamins, M. R., & Buck, A. C. (2008). Religion: A sociocultural predictor of health behaviors in Mexico. *Journal of Aging and Health, 20,* 290–305.

Bonfrer, I., Poel, E. V., Grimm, M., & van Doorslaer, E. (2012). *Does health care utilization match needs in Africa? Challenging conventional needs measurement* (iBMC working paper W2012.02). Rotterdam, Netherlands: Erasmus University Rotterdam Institute of Health Policy & Management.

Bour, D., & Bream, K. (2004). An analysis of the determinants of maternal mortality in sub-Saharan Africa. *Journal of Women's Health, 13*(8), 926–938.

Brown, C. A., Sohani, S. B., Khan, K., Lilford, R., & Mukhwana, W. (2008). Antenatal care and perinatal outcomes in Kwale district, Kenya. *BioMed Central Pregnancy and Childbirth, 8,* 2. doi:10.1186/1471-2393-8-2

Chakraborty, N., Islam, M. A., Chowdhury, R. I., Bari, W., & Akhter, H. H. (2003). Determinants of the use of maternal health services in rural Bangladesh. *Health Promotion International, 18,* 327–337.

Chen, X., Wen, S. W., Yang, Q., & Walker, M. C. (2007). Adequacy of prenatal care and neonatal mortality in infants born to mothers with and without antenatal high-risk conditions. *Australian and New Zealand Journal of Obstetrics and Gynaecology, 47,* 122–127.

Cleves, M. A., Gould, W. W., & Gutierrez, R. G. (2004). *An introduction to survival analysis using STATA* (Rev. ed.). College Station, TX: Stata Press.

Crawley, J., & Liu, F. (2012). Maternal employment and childhood obesity: A search for mechanisms in time use data. *Economics and Human Biology, 10,* 352–364.

Dairo, M. D., & Owoyokun, K. E. (2010). Factors affecting the utilization of antenatal care services in Ibadan, Nigeria. *Benin Journal of Postgraduate Medicine, 12,* 3–13.

Desai, S., & Jain, D. (1994). Maternal employment and changes in family dynamics: The social context of women's work in rural South India. *Population and Development Review, 20,* 115–136.

Development Alternatives with Women for a New Era. (2012). DAWN welcomes historic CPD resolution on sexual and reproductive health and rights for adolescents and youth. [Press release]. Retrieved from http://www.dawnnet.org / uploads / documents / DAWN % 20Press % 20Release % 20on % 20 CPD45.pdf

Dixon, J., Tenkorang, E. Y., & Luginaah, I. (2011). Ghana's National Health Insurance Scheme: Helping the poor or leaving them behind? *Environment and Planning C: Government and Policy, 29,* 1102–1115.

Dixon, J., Tenkorang, E. Y., Luginaah, I. N., Kuuire, V. Z., & Boateng, G. O. (2013). National health insurance scheme enrollment and antenatal care among women among women in Ghana: Is there any relationship? *Tropical Medicine and International Health, 19*(1), 98–106.

Elo, I. T. (1992). Utilization of maternal health care services in Peru: The role of women's education. *Health Transition Review, 2,* 49–69.

Finlayson, M., & DalMonte, J. (2002). Predicting the use of occupational therapy services among people with multiple sclerosis in Atlantic Canada. *Canadian Journal of Occupational Therapy, 69,* 239–248.

Gerein, N., Green, A., & Pearson, S. (2006). The implications of shortages of health professionals for maternal health in sub-Saharan Africa. *Reproductive Health Matters, 14,* 40–50.

Gerein, N., Mayhew, S., & Lubben, M. (2003). A framework for a new approach to antenatal care. *International Journal of Gynecology and Obstetrics, 80,* 175–182.

Ghana Statistical Service (GSS), Ghana Health Service (GHS), & ICF Macro. (2009). *Ghana Demographic and Health Survey 2008.* Accra, Ghana: Authors.

Glei, D. A., Goldman, N., & Rodriguez, G. (2003). Utilization of care during pregnancy in rural Guatemala: Does obstetrical need matter? *Social Science & Medicine, 57,* 2447–2463.

Gross, K., Alba, S., Glass, T. R., Schellenberg, J. A., & Obrist, B. (2012). Timing of antenatal care for adolescent and adult pregnant women in south-eastern Tanzania. *BioMed Central Pregnancy and Childbirth, 12,* 16.

Gyimah, S. O., Takyi, B., & Tenkorang, E. Y. (2008). Denominational affiliation and fertility behaviour in an African context: An examination of couple data from Ghana. *Journal of Biosocial Science, 40,* 445–458.

Gyimah, S. O., Tenkorang, E. Y., Takyi, B. K., Adjei, J., & Fosu, G. (2010). Religion, HIV/AIDS and sexual risk-taking among men in Ghana. *Journal of Biosocial Science, 42,* 531–547.

Health Systems 20/20 Project and Research and Development Division of the Ghana Health Service. (2009). *An evaluation of the effects of the National Health Insurance Scheme in Ghana.* Bethesda, MD: Author, Abt Associates Inc.

Hollowel, J., Oakley, L., Kurinczuk, J. J., Brocklehurst, P., & Gray, R. (2011). The effectiveness of antenatal care programmes to reduce infant mortality and preterm birth in socially disadvantaged and vulnerable women in high–income countries: A systematic review. *BioMed Central Pregnancy and Childbirth, 11,* 13. doi:10.1186/1471-2393-11-13

Hosmer, D. W., Lemeshow, S., & Sturdivant, R. X. (2013). *Applied logistic regression.* Hoboken, NJ: Wiley.

Ibrahim, J., Yorifuji, T., Tsuda, T., Kashima, S., & Doi, H. (2012). Frequency of antenatal care visits and neonatal mortality in Indonesia. *Journal of Tropical Pediatrics, 58,* 184–188.

Kaaya, S. F., Mbwambo, J. K., Kilonzo, G. P., van den Borne, H., Leshabari, M. T., Fawzi, M.C.S., & Schaamal, H. (2010). Socio-economic and partner relationship factors associated with antenatal depressive morbidity among pregnant women in Dar es Salaam, Tanzania. *Tanzania Journal of Health Research, 12,* 1–12.

Kabir, M., Iliasu, Z., Abubakar, I. S., & Asani, A. (2005). Determinants of utilization of antenatal care services in Kumbotso village, Northern Nigeria. *Tropical Doctor, 35,* 110–111.

Karabulut, A., Ozkan, S., Bozkurt, A. I., & Kayan, S. (2013). Perinatal outcomes and risk factors in adolescent and advanced age pregnancies: Comparison with normal reproductive age women. *Journal of Obstetrics and Gynaecology, 33,* 346–350.

Kevany, S., Murima, O., & Singh, B. (2012). Socio-economic status and health care utilization in rural Zimbabwe: Findings from Project Accept (HPTN 043). *Journal of Public Health in Africa, 3*(13), 46–51.

Khan, K., Wojdyla, D., Say, L., Gulmezoglu, A. M., & Van, L. P. F. (2006). WHO analysis of causes of maternal death: A systematic review. *Lancet, 367,* 1066–1074.

Lozano, R., Wang, H., Foreman, K., Rajaratnam, J. K., Naghavi, M., Marcus, J. R., . . . Murray, C. J. L. (2011). Progress towards Millennium Development Goals 4 and

5 on maternal and child mortality: An updated systematic analysis. *Lancet, 378,* 1139–1165.

Magadi, M. A., Madise, N. J., & Rodrigues, N. (2000). Frequency and timing of antenatal care in Kenya: Explaining the variations between women of different communities. *Social Science & Medicine, 51,* 551–561.

McClure, E. M., Goldenberg, R. L., & Bann, C. M. (2007). Maternal mortality, stillbirth and measures of obstetric care in developing and developed countries. *International Journal of Gynecology and Obstetrics, 96,* 139–146.

McCray, T. M. (2004). An issue of culture: The effects of daily activities on prenatal care utilization patterns in rural South Africa. *Social Science and Medicine, 59,* 1843–1855.

Monheit, A. C. (2000). Race/ethnicity and health insurance status: 1987 and 1996. *Medical Care Research and Review, 57,* 11–35.

Morrill, M. S. (2011). The effects of maternal employment on the health of school-age children. *Journal of Health Economics, 30,* 240–257.

Munsur, A. M., Atia, A., & Kawahara, A. (2010). Relationship between educational attainment and maternal health care utilization in Bangladesh: Evidence from the 2005 Bangladesh household income and expenditure survey. *Research Journal of Medical Sciences, 4,* 33–37.

Myer, L., & Harrison, A. (2003). Why do women seek antenatal care late? Perspectives from rural South Africa. *Journal of Midwifery and Women's Health, 48,* 268–272.

Nguyen, H. T. H., Rajkotia, Y., & Wang, H. (2011). The financial protection effect of Ghana National Health Insurance Scheme: Evidence from a study in two rural districts. *International Journal for Equity in Health, 10,* 4.

Nikiema, B., Beninguisse, G., & Haggerty, J. L. (2009). Providing information on pregnancy complications during antenatal visits: Unmet educational needs in sub-Saharan Africa. *Health Policy and Planning, 24,* 367–376.

Nketiah-Amponsah, E., Senadza, B., & Arthur, E. (2013). Determinants of utilization of antenatal care services in developing countries: Recent evidence from Ghana. *African Journal of Economic and Management Studies, 4*(1), 58–73.

Ochako, R., Fotso, J., Ikamari, L., & Khasakhala, A. (2011). Utilization of maternal health services among young women in Kenya: Insights from the Kenya Demographic and Health Survey, 2003. *BioMed Central Pregnancy and Childbirth, 11,* 1. doi:10.1186/1471-2393-11-1

Pell, C., Menaca, A., Were, F., Afrah, N. A., Chatio, S., Manda-Taylor, L., Pool, R. (2013). Factors affecting antenatal care attendance: Results from qualitative studies in Ghana, Kenya and Malawi. *PLoS ONE, 8,* 1, doi:10.1371/journal.pone.0053747

Rai, R. K., Singh, P. K., Kumar, C., & Singh, L. (2013). Factors associated with the utilization of maternal health care services among adolescent women in Malawi. *Home Health Care Services Quarterly, 32,* 106–125.

Raudenbush, S. W., & Bryk, A. S. (2002). *Hierarchical linear models: Applications and data analysis methods* (2nd ed.). Thousand Oaks, CA: Sage.

Sato, A. (2012). Does socio-economic status explain use of modern and traditional health care services? *Social Science & Medicine, 75,* 1450–1459.

Tenkorang, E. Y., & Owusu, G. A. (2010). Correlates of HIV testing among women in Ghana: Some evidence from the Demographic and Health Surveys. *AIDS Care: Psychological and Socio-medical Aspects of AIDS/HIV, 22,* 296–307.

Tsegay, Y., Gebrehiwot, T., Goicolea, I., Edin. K., Hailemariam, L., & Sebastain, M. S. (2013). Determinants of antenatal and delivery care utilization in Tigray region, Ethiopia: A cross-sectional study. *International Journal for Equity in Health, 12,* 30. doi:10.1186/1475-9276-12-30

United Nations (UN). (2008). *Achieving the Millennium Development Goals in Africa. Recommendations of the MDG Africa Steering Group.* Retrieved from http://www.mdgafrica.org/pdf/MDG%20Africa%20Steering%20Group%20Recommendations%20-%20English%20-%20HighRes.pdf

United Nations (UN). (2013). *The Millennium Development Goals report 2013.* New York, NY: Author. Retrieved from http://www.un.org/millenniumgoals/pdf/report-2013/mdg-report-2013-english.pdf

Vingilis, E., Wade, T., & Seeley, J. (2007). Predictors of adolescent health care utilization. *Journal of Adolescence, 30,* 773–800. doi:10.1016/j.adolescence.2006.10.001

Whitehouse, K. (2010). Organization of antenatal care. *InnovAiT: The Royal College of General Practioners Journal for Associates in Training, 3*(9), 528–538.

Wolinsky, F. (1988). *Seeking and using health services. The sociology of health* (2nd ed.). Belmont, CA: Wadsworth.

World Health Organization (WHO). (1994). *Antenatal care: Report of a technical working group. WHO/FRH/MSM/968 1994.* Geneva, Switzerland: Author.

World Health Organization (WHO). (2006). *Provision of effective antenatal care: Integrated management of pregnancy and childbirth (IMPAC). Standards for maternal and neonatal care.* Geneva, Switzerland: Author. Retrieved from http://www.who.int/reproductivehealth/publications/maternal_perinatal_health/effective_antenat al_care.pdf

World Health Organization (WHO). (2008). *Ouagadougou declaration on primary health care and health system in Africa: Achieving better health for Africa in the New Millennium.* Brazzaville, Republic of the Congo: Regional Office for Africa, Author.

World Health Organization (WHO). (2010). *Towards reaching the health–related millennium development goals: Progress report and the way forward: Report of the Regional Director.* Brazzaville, Africa: Regional Office for Africa, Author.

World Health Organization (WHO). (2012). *World health statistics.* Geneva, Switzerland: Author.

Worster, A., Fan J., & Ismaila. (2007). Understanding linear and logistic regression analyses. *Canadian Journal of Emergency Medicine, 9,* 111–113.

Zanconato, G., Msolomba, R., Guarenti, L., & Franchi, M. (2006). Antenatal care in developing countries: The need for a tailored model. *Seminars in Fetal and Neonatal Medicine, 11,* 15–20.

Zere, E., Kirigia, J. M., Duale, S., & Akazili, J. (2012). Inequities in maternal and child health outcomes and interventions in Ghana. *BioMed Central Public Health, 12,* 252. doi:10.1186/1471-2458-12-252

Modernization and Development: Impact on Health Care Decision-Making in Uganda

DEBRA ANNE KAUR SINGH

Kimanya-Ngeyo Foundation for Science and Education, Jinja, Uganda

JAYA EARNEST

International Health Program, School of Nursing and Midwifery, Curtin University, Bentley, Western Australia, Australia

MAY LAMPLE

Kimanya-Ngeyo Foundation for Science and Education, Jinja, Uganda

Uganda has faced numerous challenges over the past 50 years from overcoming political conflict and civil unrest, to rapid population growth, to combating the HIV epidemic and ever-growing health needs. Women in Uganda have had a major role to play in the health of families and communities. The researchers' purpose in this study, undertaken in rural Uganda, was to a) identify a people-centered definition of development, b) compare it to the process of modernization, and c) investigate how these processes have changed the role women play in decision-making, in areas directly and indirectly related to their health and that of their families. Twenty-two men and women participated in focus group discussion and completed questionnaires. Based on our analysis of discussions it appears that both modernization and development have impacted health positively and negatively. Key themes distilled from interviews included that modernization has led to the breakdown of families; increased maternal responsibility for children; diminished land and economic resources; and an erosion of cultural values and practices that had previously provided stability

We acknowledge Robinah, Julius, and Emmanuel for their assistance in the field during data collection. We also thank the community members for giving so generously of their time. We are thankful to the International Health Program, School of Nursing and Midwifery, Curtin University for funding for this study.

for the society. In terms of development, women play an increas-
ing role in decision-making processes in the household and are
gaining increasing respect for their expertise in a number of areas,
notably health care. We propose a movement of grassroots discourse
on modernization. Development, and its effect on health, is neces-
sary if the positive aspects of Ugandan culture and those of similar
emerging societies are not to be lost (International Covenant on
Economic, Social and Cultural Rights, 1966).

The World Health Organization (WHO) defines health as follows:

> A state of complete physical, mental and social well-being and not merely
> the absence of disease or infirmity; it is a fundamental right. ... This
> definition implies that the health of a person may be broader than solely
> physical needs. (WHO & United Nations Children's Fund [UNICEF], 1978,
> p. 1)

The Declaration of Alma Ata defines primary health care as follows:

> Essential health care based on practical, scientifically sound and socially
> acceptable methods and technology made universally accessible to in-
> dividuals and families in the community through their full participation
> and at a cost that the community and country can afford to maintain at
> every stage of their development in the spirit of self-reliance and self-
> determination. (WHO & UNICEF, 1978, p. 3)

The WHO and UDHR definitions of health incorporate an understanding
that not just physical well-being but also mental and social well-being are
important.

For the purpose of this article, drawing on the above definitions, we
have defined health care as basic, affordable, preventative, and curative
services that are of a quality that will, in the majority of cases, lead to an
accurate diagnosis and cure for commonly encountered illnesses.

Thus defined, health care in Uganda varies considerably depending on
where one is living in the country. For most rural people in Uganda, access
to quality affordable health care does not exist (Konde-Lule, Gitta, Okuonzi,
Onama, & Forsberg, 2010). In their study of three rural districts of Uganda,
Konde-Lule and colleagues (2010) found that 95.7% of all 445 facilities surveyed were private, while 4.3% were public. Traditional practitioners (TPs)
and general merchandise shops that sold medicines comprised 77.1% of
all providers. Although they had limited infrastructure and skills, TPs and
shops were often located in the villages and therefore were easily accessible
(Konde-Lule et al., 2010). The authors note that while "private health care is
versatile... the quality of private care, especially among informal providers,
is often unsatisfactory" (Konde-Lule et al., 2010, pp. 6–7). The majority of

health care available in Uganda is fee-for-service. Although government facilities are theoretically free of charge, costs are often incurred for transport to the clinic or hospital, and to ensure that the patient is attended to in a timely fashion, and for medication and for basic necessities, including food, water, and supplies.

The suggestion provided by the Earth Institute (2011) recognizing, "the need to systematically and professionally train lay community members to be part of the health workforce has emerged not simply as a stop-gap measure, but as a core component of primary health care systems in low-resource settings" (p. 2). This suggestion would be effective in resource-poor countries such as Uganda. In addition to the need for improved health care delivery, there are a number of other determinants of health that need to be addressed in Uganda. These determinants include poverty, agriculture and farming, food choices, family planning and reproductive health, and female engagement in health decision-making. Thus there is a need to examine the association among gender roles, female education, autonomy, and health.

WOMEN AND HEALTH

The education of a girl has long-term and more sustainable implications for the health of her future family and subsequently community. Education of a future mother leads to improvement of child health through the provision of more effective care in the home and more appropriate use of treatment and prevention services from the health care system (Hadden & London, 1996). Education also contributes to delayed onset of motherhood, reduced maternal mortality, the decision to have fewer children with increased spacing, as well as improved economic and income generating opportunities to increase income through work options outside the home. Female education is associated with longer life expectancies, lower death rates, and improved child health and nutrition (Caldwell, 1990; Hadden & London, 1996; Karlsen et al., 2011). The link between female education and fertility in Uganda is consistent with the findings in other countries in the developing world, with contraceptive use increasing with the number of years of education (Bbaale & Mpuga, 2011b).

Bayisenge (2010) notes that 54% of 20–24 year olds in Uganda are married or in de facto relationships before they are 18. This impacts the possibilities of young adolescent girls completing their education and increases childbirth related risks. The World Bank (2005) also found that school girls enter sexual relationships as a way of getting necessities that parents cannot afford due to poverty, and that sexual defilement, and sexual coercion of young girls, followed by financial compensation to the parents is widespread in Uganda and across Africa.

There are numerous ways that women contribute to family health. Women play a major role in the nutrition of the family. Where land is available, women do most of the digging, weeding, and harvesting and cook the food for the family. They also choose to plant subsistence crops, where men more often choose to grow cash crops. Unfortunately, studies from the developing world have documented that once any excess crop has been sold, the woman is unlikely to have access to the funds generated from the sale of the cash crops (World Bank, 2005). This has implications for health care when, for the most part, additional funds will be required for either transport to a facility, fees for a private clinic, or to purchase medications. This may be contrasted with developed societies where women either have access to their own funds or where high quality health care services are provided free by the government and are more easily accessible to where they are residing.

Although women contribute to the health of their families, we found in the literature that they are frequently excluded from critical decisions about health care. For example, the choice of what to do when a child is sick is also often not in her hands. The World Bank (2005) found that Ugandan women had greater decision-making power at the household level compared with women in many other countries of sub-Saharan Africa, except in the area of deciding whether to seek health care for children.

When developing and commencing this research, the plan was to focus exclusively on issues that contribute to health and to investigate the role women play in decision-making around these issues. In this regard, we focused on health care from the perspective of prevention and treatment. We focused on how decisions are made in the family during periods of illness in an attempt to understand decision-making dynamics within the family.

During focus group discussions, however, we realized that there was considerable turmoil occurring at an individual, family, and community level in rural Uganda. Social changes were perceived to be happening at a rapid rate, and respondents remarked repeatedly about the loss of cultural practices that previously had provided stability. Participants noted that cultural practices were being replaced by the promise of a "modern" life that was not realistic given the currently available resources and opportunities for young people. Of particular note was the economic strain experienced by families. The following statement from an article entitled "Planning for Instability in Kampala" discusses riots in Kampala and provides some insight into the complex situation that has affected the entire country:

> In November, 2009 . . . the Uganda Bureau of Statistics noted that the annual rate of inflation for food crops was 49.5%. Export of food produced in Uganda to Sudan and Kenya has fueled the inflation, which has made life more difficult for people who buy food with wages, but has caused hunger and malnutrition among those without regular wages (and the)

youth unemployment rate in Kampala is over 32.2%. The combination of extreme rises in the cost of food, a dearth of opportunities for earning a livelihood, and the contraction of the informal economy with an economic downturn, create a dire situation for urban youth. (Hanson, 2009, p. 3)

Thus, drawing on participant voices in the FGDs, in trying to understand what was happening in the villages in which our participants were living, we decided to examine the two main processes affecting village life: modernization and development.

MODERNIZATION AND DEVELOPMENT

Modernization is a widely contested topic. The definition encompasses governance, social systems, human resource development through education, economic structures, and rates of growth (Charlton & Andras, 2003). Economic definitions are common, and for the most part modernization is seen as a transition from traditional, agricultural based societies to societies that are based on trade and industry (Irwin, 1975). In "The Modernization Imperative," Charlton and Andras (2003) argue that modernization at the societal level operates under the following assumptions: the future will take care of itself, economics should be the dominant force, the individual takes precedence over family and community, and communities can live with a loss of moral impetus and culture that is often contained in what is perceived as backward traditional society (Encyclopedia Britannica, 2012).

Modernization is considered inevitable, and proof of its deemed superiority is provided through the trend of rural urban drift by able-bodied rural populations, despite often appalling conditions in cities (Charlton & Andras, 2003; Mulumba & Olema, 2009). Proponents of modernization value educational advancement and social and geographic mobility and perceive a flexible attitude toward life and work as beneficial. There are, however, opponents to modernization. Hezel (1987) provides a description of the breakdown of culture and traditional roles in Micronesia and how this has impacted society, particularly young men. He mentions that while the role of young women has stayed much the same, young men no longer engage in deep-sea fishing, farming, building houses and canoes, and conducting warfare. As a result, young men suffer from dislocation resulting in high rates of delinquency, alcohol abuse, and juvenile arrest and also have four times the rates of mental illness than young women (Hezel, 1987).

There is also opposition amongst some groups including ecological modernization theorists who are pessimistic about the "future will take care of itself" scenario. Huber (2000) suggests that the answer is to slow down or change the course of modernization to such a point that society or individuals can plan for the future. This slowing is achieved by making the world a simpler place that can be more safely controlled (Charlton & Andras, 2003). This opposition to modernization is also held by over 200 million peasant farmers in 70 countries in Africa, Asia, Europe, and the Americas, who are finding a voice in the sustainable development discourse through organizations such as La Via Campesina and Navdanya (Navdanya, 2009). They believe that food sovereignty is the right of people and that small scale sustainable production rather than large scale monocultural farms benefit both communities and the environment (La Via Campesina, 2012).

While development is also commonly defined from an economic perspective (Marshall, 1985), we believe a definition that attempts to encompass the multifaceted nature of the human being—a people-centered definition—is more useful. According to the International Development Research Council, when development is looked at as "change that improves the conditions of human well-being so that people can exercise meaningful choices for their own benefit and that of society" (Ryan, 1995, as quoted in Beemans, 1995, p. v), it places people at the centre of the development process. According to the Institute for the Study of Global Prosperity (2008), "When viewed as capacity building, development is concerned principally with the generation, application, and diffusion of knowledge. . . . Specifically, . . . the world's inhabitants . . . must be engaged in applying knowledge to create well-being, thereby generating new knowledge and contributing in a substantial and meaningful way to human progress" (p. 7).

MODERNIZATION, DEVELOPMENT, AND HEALTH

The processes of modernization and development have health implications, both positive and negative. Negative health impacts of modernization include increased poverty as extended family support and traditional knowledge are lost, poor nutrition due to deterioration in the quantity and quality of land deteriorates, health consequences of increased high density living in city slums, increased sexually transmitted infections (STIs) and risk taking behavior, disintegration of families, and increased alcohol use as young men lose their traditional roles (Ramin, 2009). Positive impacts include greater access to private and public health facilities, improved access to tests and drugs, and improved knowledge of and access to preventative care such as immunizations.

In terms of development, changes that lead to improved health of families include increased female education, increased paid employment, greater autonomy for women in decision-making including family planning, and more equality and respect in marriages and in the community (Bbaale & Mpuga, 2011a; Hadden & London, 1996). Making the distinction between development and modernization, while overly simplistic, acknowledges that not all change is positive. This cross-section study undertaken in rural Uganda has attempted to identify changes at community and family level in areas that are related to female decision-making that may impact health.

METHODOLOGY

Study Design and Methods

This cross-sectional, qualitative exploratory study was undertaken to gain insights into the rural community in which the first author and lead researcher was living. The main objective of the study was to investigate how the processes of modernization and development have changed the role women play in decision-making in areas directly and indirectly related to their health and that of their families.

The study was conducted in two districts of central Uganda—Jinja and Buikwe. Some of the participants, however, were also from Northern, Western, and Eastern Uganda. Thus information derived in the focus groups describes experiences from a number of regions in Uganda. The inclusion criteria were that participants both male and female were over 18 years and currently living in a rural area. Snowball sampling was used to recruit participants from five villages using contacts from key informants. In appreciation for their participation they were reimbursed for transport costs (not more than $5) and a snack and drink or a meal, depending on the time of the day when the focus group took place. This study protocol was approved by the Human Research Ethics Committee at Curtin University in Western Australia.

The focus group questions and questionnaire were initially trialed with a cultural reference group made up of three older women (two from Central Uganda and one from Eastern Uganda). The members of the group were well respected and experienced community members with an awareness of Ugandan women's issues because of their professions: a judge, a community development consultant, and an administrator in a development organization. Feedback from the cultural reference group and the key informants helped to modify the FGD and interview questions and enhance the validity of the study. A graduate student conducted the focus groups with the assistance of the key informants, who also acted as translators. The principal investigator (D.S.), and first author, transcribed the conversations during the focus group discussions. The focus groups took approximately 90 minutes to complete. Table 1 provides the main themes and types of questions that were asked in the focus groups.

Analysis

The data were transcribed during the focus groups with pseudonyms attached to each respondent. A multidisciplinary team then used thematic

TABLE 1 Themes Discussed in the Focus Group

Theme	Specific topic
Roles of men and women at home	Work, raising children, agriculture, use of funds
Agriculture and food choices	Decisions on what is grown, sold, utilized at home
Education	Intergenerational change in education choice
	Barriers to education for girls and boys
Marriage	Decision-making of partner choice and marriage
	Procedures, spacing of children, family planning
	Intergenerational differences in marriage
Health choices	Decision-making for treating family members
	Acceptability of female unilateral decision-making
	Intergenerational change in health choices

analysis. Instances of discussion about "modernization" and "development" were checked for, and codes were created to reflect the interviewees' statements. Emerging codes were systematically developed from the data. The researchers discussed emerging categories and themes. Recoding was done on the basis of group consensus. Standard descriptive statistics (frequencies and percentages) were used to summarize the responses to the demographic data and questionnaire questions that were of a closed-ended nature. Cross-tabulations of question responses against gender were performed to identify any differences between male and female respondents:

> Boys especially (are affected by) peer groups, some enjoy alcohol, and they won't go to school.... They take jobs like brick making (which) needs no qualifications, on landing sites, fishing, selling sand and they forget education. (*Woman, focus group of women over 45 years*)

RESULTS

Table 2 provides a summary of the characteristics of the participants.

Family Planning

When asked about who decides when, and if, to use family planning, there were quite different responses from older and younger participants and men and women.

Modernization and culture: Children as a means of relationship security, no child a possible ground for divorce. Responses include the following:

> They decide together, (they) may consult on what is needed and decide later is better. Both decide otherwise if no child he will divorce her. (*Woman, focus group of women over 45 years*)

TABLE 2 Summary of Participant Characteristics

Characteristic	Male N	Female %	Total N	Total %	N	%
Religion						
Christian	8	36	9	41	17	77
Muslim	2	9	1	5	3	14
Baha'i	1	5	1	5	2	9
Location						
Village	11	50	11	50	22	100
Marital status						
Single	3	14	4	18	7	32
Married	7	32	5	23	12	55
Divorced	1	5	0	0	1	5
Widowed	0	0	2	9	2	9
Age						
18–23	2	9	4	18	6	27
24–28	4	18	2	9	6	27
45–55	2	9	5	23	7	32
Over 55	3	14	0	0	3	14
Children						
Yes	8	36	9	40	17	77
No	3	14	2	9	5	23
Education						
Primary	3	14	1	5	4	18
Secondary	6	27	7	32	13	59
Postsecondary	2	9	3	14	5	23
Education status						
Studying	1	5	1	5	2	9
Left school	10	45	10	45	20	91
Reason						
School fees	10	45	7	32	17	77
Other	1	5	4	18	5	23
Who decided						
Parents	7	32	8	36	15	68
Self and family	2	9	1	5	3	14
Self	1	5	0	0	1	5
Still studying	1	5	1	4	2	10
School (pregnancy)	0	0	1	5	1	5

The mother feels she should produce for you, especially a baby boy, she uses it as security. It is the man who decides on the children. If the lady refuses (to have children), then the marriage is in trouble. If she doesn't produce, then he can get another wife. Family planning should be the man's decision. Spacing makes the marriage not secure. (*Man, focus group of men 18 to 28 years*)

Development: Family planning as a means of addressing the lack of resources. Responses include the following:

At present, you have to decide. In the past you might have a wife that is used to the long ago—she may just continue to conceive. Now many people are using family planning. The problem is the cost of living. You will not manage to feed, educate and provide health and clothes (for many children). Men are feeling the pressure of having too many children, even more than women. In the past years, the people had a big land, now it is very small land and it is difficult to feed, educate, provide clothes, etc. There is no good employment. (*Man, focus group of men over 45 years*)

Health Choices

Health decisions, other than family planning, seem to be an area where women are considered to have expertise. When asked who makes the decisions on where and when to take a child for health care, the focus group members replied the following.

Modernization: Women as the main decision-makers and caregivers for family health. Respondents replied:

> When in good terms, it is the husband and wife (who decide where to seek health care). When on not good terms, it is the woman. She can take the child to the hospital. (*Man, focus group of men 18 to 28 years*)

> The mother will treat with tablets and will decide on what to do if the husband is not there. If he is there, they will decide together; if he is drunk, she will take the responsibility. (*Woman, focus group of women over 45 years*)

When asked, "If a woman decided to go to the clinic or take her child to a clinic without discussing this with her husband, would this cause a problem in the family?" the following are amongst the responses given:

> There is no problem. You need to communicate. If you don't have money and you need a lot of money for the treatment—why go to an expensive clinic? He will quarrel if she chooses the expensive one. Men do not always communicate well if they have the money or they don't. They need to communicate and they will tell them to take to government or a private clinic (according to the available funds). (*Man, focus group of men over 45 years*)

Development: Women as decision-makers and changes in increased health care choices. In the discussions it appeared that women have a well-recognized role in decision-making when a child in the family becomes unwell:

> Children falling sick worries the parent. It is better to discuss with people who have once been parents. The woman is the main one who gives the

care. The women take the responsibility. (*Woman, focus group of women 18 to 28 years*)

Even if the man is not around, they will give the money when she has taken the child. The man backs off—he doesn't know how to cope. (*Woman, focus group of women 18 to 28 years*)

When asked about how health care choices have changed since the time of their parents, the participants mentioned increased access to prevention and treatment with clinics and hospitals and greater government involvement:

They used local herbs because they were far from hospitals. The government has helped with vaccinations, Village Health Teams, clinics, and hospitals and are working well with the communities. (*Woman, focus group of women over 45 years*)

Transport, communication, clinics are close by and there are now many hospitals. They used local herbs—they squeezed them and put in water and washed the baby. Very few people have the knowledge now—the knowledge is lost. (*Man, focus group of men over 45 years*)

Government hospitals are there. Clinics are there. Before they would not test (for HIV), but now they test. In the past they would hide their children and not immunize their children; now this is not the case. (*Woman, focus group of women 18 to 28 years*)

Agriculture and Food Choices

Agriculture and the way that food is distributed can potentially impact significantly on the nutritional status and health of the family. The focus group participants were asked about who makes the decisions about what gets grown, sold, and used at home. The following are some of the responses.

Modernization: Changing roles, loss of land fertility, poor harvest, hunger. Responses include:

Growing potatoes is turning into a woman, so a man who used to grow potatoes is laughed at by friends. Now it is changing; they grow what they want to and now the land is less and it [is] used for sugar cane. Now people leave their home to go and find money. (*Man, focus group of men 15 to 28 years*)

(Men) have to cater for your children, shelter, nutrition, education, and health. With us we formerly never had to buy food, but in the past we had 5 acres of land, but now it is shared with many families. Cost of living has become very high and the health care in the time I was born it was free. These days there are private—before there were only government (facilities). Now most of us are starving. (*Man, focus group of men over 45 years*)

They went on to explain that part of the problem is the lack of fertile land:

Formerly with father and mother—(they) just plant(ed) groundnuts without spraying it, plant, and weed it, and nowadays without spraying there is not enough yield. The soil has lost its fertility and there are so many pests. There was more land, but now maize, beans, potatoes (sweet) and matoke. (We now) don't grow ground nuts, cassava, soya beans, millet. (*Woman, focus group of men over 45 years*)

Development: Mutual decision-making. Regarding mutual decision-making, one man said:

In the past it was the man who decides—cassava, cash crop. But now family members sit together and decide what will be grown. (*Man, focus group men 18 to 28*)

Vision of development expressed by the participants. In the course of the focus groups a number of people provided statements related to the way they would like their society to move forward. A number of these statements were related to equality of women and men:

(We) prefer to have fewer children and having one wife. When you have 3 or 4 wives and 20 children, then there is little land and then the grandsons are coming. (*Man, focus group of men 18 to 28 years*)

Wife and husband make decisions together; it was the man in the past. He was the owner of the family, These days, the owner is the woman. They say that man and woman are equal and it has affected the way they feel. (*Man, focus group of men over 45 years*)

Girls can do anything. Most of the women and girls are coming out, to prove they are equal. Putting aside culture—equal education, medication, and making decisions. Girls should not be left aside, not be considered the inferior sex. (*Woman, focus group of women 18 to 28 years*)

DISCUSSION

Through this study we explored women's and men's views of how decisions are made in the family for issues related to health. Gender roles played in the family: agriculture and food choices, family planning, education, and health choices were discussed from the perspective of modernization and development, where relevant. In addition, statements that were related to a vision for the future were also included. Many of the themes that were discussed were inter-related and had an impact on family life.

Throughout the conversations, participant voices revealed that changes in families were evident. It was sometimes difficult to label these changes as either modernization or development. Many seemed to be the result of increasing population pressures, reducing land per capita and changes in the global and local economy resulting in a higher and somewhat unsustainable cost of living. There was increasing access to family planning, but social pressures, cultural factors, and lack of communication between the sexes and generations prevented its effective use. While life was becoming more challenging for most rural people, there were definite indicators of development with women having a more significant role to play in decision-making processes in the home and increasing respect for their expertise in a number of areas including health care. The participants also shared that there was greater access to preventative and curative medical services through private and government facilities that were closer to home than in the time of their parents.

Gender Roles, Family Planning, and Agriculture

Thus we noted that there is a blurring of some of the previously distinct gender roles, although women continue to be the primary caregivers to children. During the conversations we found that increasingly women were taking responsibilities in the families and that men were feeling pressure to provide support, but they were finding this more and more difficult due to economic realities and lack of land. Perhaps, as a result of this sense of failure, men were more often absent from the families and made poor choices with the little money that was available that did not benefit the family. Amongst these choices included increased alcohol consumption, gambling, and relationships with other women. This impacted on family health due to reduced access to income and the increased chances of STIs. Another area with important health implications was the issue food security, which was mentioned on several occasions. Some of the identified problems included a lack of and infertility of the land, limits to the range of crops being grown, increasing cost of living, limited job opportunities, and the use of cash crops and subsequent inability to purchase food for the family after a short period of time.

The outcome of these pressures increased family conflict experienced by the majority of households. Women felt that men were not fulfilling their responsibilities; trust had eroded with both women and men hiding funds from each other. Women increasingly have a voice and demand their rights and will take husbands to local authorities so that they can be held accountable for violence and irresponsible behavior. While both older and younger men acknowledged the critical importance of family planning, it was apparent that women felt compelled to keep having children so that their husbands did not take another wife. Polygamy is still common, however, but is less desirable as men feel the strain of supporting many children.

In light of economic pressures that exist in Uganda, we ask if there needs to be more cooperation and mutual support in partnerships since it may be unrealistic to expect men to find the money that is needed for school fees and health care in a changing economic environment. This does not, however, justify the misuse of funds.

Development and Status of Women

Some signs of development in the rural areas where focus groups participants came from were the increasing access to education and health care, although the cost and quality of the available health and education facilities were questionable.

Women were also more respected for their knowledge in certain areas, particularly in health, and there was more decision-making power given to women generally. The general status of women and the way they saw their role seemed also to be changing rapidly. Women were making more decisions either unilaterally or with their husbands when it came to what to plant, what to sell, what to cook, how to distribute food, and how to use the funds. Interestingly, older women had a confidence about their roles in these areas that younger women did not seem to. Women were also the most reliable in the care of children and making health decisions.

Men often deferred to their wives decisions on health issues, except when they felt that funds were not available to support their choices in health care. Interestingly, the results of our small exploratory study differed from the findings of a World Bank report that stated that Ugandan women had little role in health care decision-making for their children (World Bank, 2005). On the contrary, there seemed to be a deference to women when it came to caring for and deciding upon the best course of action for sick children. All participants visualized a future around an increasing respect and role for women outside the house and the acknowledgment of their diverse capabilities.

LIMITATIONS

This was a small study with only 22 participants. The themes and challenges that emerged were consistent, for the most part, throughout all of the focus groups. Methodological limitations include a possible interviewer bias with the first author, who, although working and living in the area for nearly a decade, was not Ugandan, and thus was an outsider. To minimize this effect, similar questions were asked in various formats and sections of the focus groups and questionnaires and cross checked for consistency. Finally, two individuals went through the content of each focus group transcription to check for the validity of the themes as a form of member checking, and a cultural reference group was consulted on a number of issues. Language barriers were also an issue. Some participants preferred to speak in English, while others were more comfortable speaking in the local language. We encouraged the participants to speak in the local language; however, because of the cultural mix, not everyone was as well versed in Lusoga or Luganda as the others. There was translation between the predominant local language and English, however, and it was probable that some minor subtleties were missed.

RECOMMENDATIONS BASED ON PARTICIPANT PERCEPTIONS

Based on the analysis of participant responses, a number of avenues for further investigation and consultation are proposed:

1. *Enabling a grassroots community discourse:* Making a distinction between modernization and development enables the community to appreciate that choices can be made and that not all change that appears "modern" is useful to Uganda. A grassroots discourse will enable the community to create a common vision for development in Uganda and may counteract some of the more subtle, destructive changes of modernization.
2. *Relationship building:* Men and women need to examine the multitude of factors that are causing increasing family hardships and disunity. When they are able to work together, they can find solutions that benefit the family without creating an environment of discontent that can encourage irresponsible decisions around existing funds. Trust between partners is a fundamental requirement for this new relationship.
3. *Health care provision as a means of female empowerment:* Because women are valued in provision of health care, it would make sense that they take a lead role in health care provision. Engaging more women as village health team members and community health workers at the village level would provide them with a forum through which their existing knowledge, which is already valued at family level, could benefit the community.
4. *Wider role of women:* With women increasingly sharing their opinions and being heard, the stage is set for furthering their roles in the wider community as women take up more responsibility in the workplace and have greater access to means that can improve the situation of their families.

CONCLUSION

Based on the findings of the study, it is clear that change is inevitable, but we question if the process of change could become more conscious. Attempting to emulate cultures heavily influenced by materialism, individualism, and self-interest may not be the best choice for Uganda where the role of community and the extended family is greatly valued. Can we imagine the process of modernization taking a different path? If modernization is a force with a life of its own, then it requires individuals (both men and women) and communities to make conscious decisions about the direction they would like modernization to take. From the definitions used in this article, we suggest that development takes place when men and women themselves begin to create and apply knowledge consciously to improve their lives and when they are empowered to make meaningful choices about the way they would like their society to develop. Issues of family relationships, consultation, and decision-making, and the equality of men and women all need to be further addressed as part of these community and family conversations. A starting point for community development is through generation and application of knowledge using female community health education workers. It potentially would provide young women with a voice and confidence as they are seen as knowledge bearers. We acknowledge that there are gaps in our understanding, but by respecting and listening to the voices of men and women in rural communities, we can set realistic goals and formulate plans that respect culture and can lead inclusive strategies that not only improve health and well-being but also sustainable development.

REFERENCES

Bayisenge, J. (2010). Early marriage as a barrier to girls education: A development challenge in Africa. In C. Ikekeonwu (Ed.), *Girl-child education in Africa* (pp. 43–66). Nigeria: Catholic Institute for Development, Justice & Peace (CIDJAP) Press. Retrieved from http://www.ifuw.org/fuwa/docs/Early-marriage.pdf

Bbaale, E., & Mpuga, P. (2011a). Female education, contraceptive use, and fertility: Evidence from Uganda. *Consilience: The Journal of Sustainable Development*, 6(1), 20–47.

Bbaale, E., & Mpuga, P. (2011b). Female education, labor force participation and choice of employment type: Evidence from Uganda. *International Journal of Economics and Business Modeling*, 2(1), 29–41. Retrieved from http://www.bioinfo.in/contents.php?id=37

Caldwell, J. (1990). Cultural and social factors influencing mortality in developing countries. *The Annals of the American of Political and Social Science, 510*, 44–59.

Charlton, B., & Andras, P. (2003). *The modernization imperative*. Exeter, UK: Imprint Academic. Retrieved from http://www.hedweb.com/bgcharlton/modernization-imperative.html

Earth Institute, Columbia University. (2011). *One million community health workers: Task force report*. Retrieved from http://millenniumvillages.org/files/2011/06/1mCHW_TechnicalTaskForceReport.pdf

Encyclopedia Britannica. (2012). *Modernization*. Retrieved from http://www.britannica.com/EBchecked/topic/387301/modernization

Hadden, K., & London, B. (1996). Educating girls in the third world: The demographic, basic needs, and economic benefits. *International Journal of Comparative Sociology, 37*(1–2), 31.

Hanson, H. (2009, November). *Planning for instability in Kampala*. Paper presented at the Association for African Studies annual meeting, New Orleans, LA.

Hezel, F. (1987). The dilemmas of development: The effects of modernization on three areas of island life. In S. Stratigos & P. Hughes (Eds.), *The ethics of development: The Pacific in the 21st Century* (pp. 60–74). Port Morseby, Papua New Guinea: University of Papau New Guinea Press. Retrieved from http://www.micsem.org/pubs/articles/socprobs/frames/dildevfr.htm

Huber, J. (2000). Towards industrial ecology: Sustainable development as a concept of ecological modernization. *Journal of Environmental Policy and Planning, 2*, 269–285.

Institute for the Study of Global Prosperity. (2008). *Science, religion and development: Some initial considerations*. Retrieved from http://ww.globalprosperity.org/library

International Covenant on Economic, Social and Cultural Rights. (1966, December 16). Retrieved from http://www2.ohchr.org/english/law/cescr.htm

Irwin, P. (1975). An operational definition of societal modernization. *Economic Development and Cultural Change, 23*, 595–613.

Karlsen, S., Say, L., Souza, J., Houge, C., Calles, D., Gülmezoglu, A., & Raine, R. (2011). The relationship between maternal education and mortality among women giving birth in health care institutions: Analysis of the cross-sectional WHO global survey on maternal and perinatal health. *BMC Public Health, 11*, 606. Retrieved from http://www.biomedcentral.com/1471-2458/11/606/

Konde-Lule, J., Gitta, S., Okuonzi, S., Onama, V., & Forsberg, B. (2010). Private and public health care in rural areas of Uganda. *BMC International Health and Human Rights, 10*, 29. Retrieved from http://www.biomedcentral.com/1472-698X/10/29/

La Via Campesina. (2012). *La via campesina, international peasant's movement*. Retrieved from http://viacampesina.org/en/

Marshall, S. (1985). Development, dependence, and gender inequality in the third world. *International Studies Quarterly, 29*, 217–240.

Mulumba, D., & Olema, W. (2009). *IMMIS—African migration and gender in a global context: Implementing migration studies. Policy analysis report: Mapping migration in Uganda*. Retrieved from http://www.immis.org/wp-content/uploads/2010/05/Policy-Analysis-Report-Uganda.pdf

Navdanya. (2009). *Navdanya*. Retrieved from http://www.navdanya.org/

Ramin, B. (2009). *Slums, climate change and human health in sub-Saharan Africa*. Retrieved from www.who.int/bulletin/volumes/87/12/09-073445/en/index.html

Ryan, W. (1995). Culture, spirituality and economic development: Opening a dialogue. *IDRC*. Retrieved from http://www.idrc.ca/EN/Resources/Publications/Pages/IDRCBookDetails.aspx?PublicationID=274

World Bank. (2005). *Uganda from periphery to center: A strategic country gender assessment. Office of the sector director poverty reduction and economic management Africa region* (Report no. 30136-UG). Retrieved from http://www. wds.worldbank.org/external/default/WDSContentServer/WDSP/IB/2005/03/25/ 000090341_20050325085641/Rendered/PDF/301360UG.pdf

World Health Organization (WHO), & United Nations Children's Fund (UNICEF). (1978, September). *Report of the international conference on primary health care, Alma Ata*. Retrieved from http://whqlibdoc.who.int/publications/ 9241800011.pdf.

Policy Strategies to Improve Maternal Health Services Delivery and Outcomes in Anambra State, Nigeria

MABEL EZEONWU

School of Nursing and Health Studies, University of Washington Bothell, Bothell, Washington, USA

Pregnancy and childbirth present major health risks for Nigerian women. Key maternal mortality measures indicate that the risks are high. Despite improvement efforts, the country has made insufficient progress in reaching the United Nations' millennium development goal of decreasing maternal mortality by 75% by 2015. The author in this qualitative descriptive study explores the perspectives of experienced nurse leaders on policy strategies to improve maternal health in Nigeria. In this study, the author suggests that removal of financial barriers to access and utilization of health services, spousal and family inclusiveness in plan of care, and health systems-related physical and human infrastructural improvements constitute critical policy approaches.

In this qualitative study, the author discusses nurses' perspectives on pragmatic approaches to improve maternal health outcomes in Anambra State, Nigeria. Although the United Nations' millennium development goal #5 is to decrease maternal mortality by 75% between 1990 and 2015, Nigeria is moving very slowly toward achieving this goal. The country's maternal mortality ratio has only decreased by 24% since 1990 (United Nations Population Fund [UNFPA], 2011). With a low contraceptive prevalence (modern type) of 15% (UNFPA, 2011), a total fertility rate of 5.5, and only 39% of live births attended by skilled personnel (World Health Organization [WHO], 2012), the risk of maternal mortality and morbidity remains high. Evidence shows that nurses and midwives are core to maternal health services delivery, and they play pivotal roles in preventing maternal mortality in poor countries (Bhutta, Lassi, & Mansoor, 2010; UNFPA, 2006; WHO, 2005; Wirth, 2008). Furthermore, nurses and midwives constitute 45% to 60% of the entire health workforce in sub-Saharan Africa (Dovlo, 2007) and are the professional workforce that is consistently present with women at the critical period preceding birth, during birth, and 24 hours after birth. The views of experienced nurse leaders at the frontlines of maternal health care delivery are therefore critical to any maternal health policy discussions. This study is pertinent to a global interdisciplinary audience since maternal health issues present significant public health and economic burdens to all societies. In addition, it is imperative that policymakers from diverse professional backgrounds in different countries are informed by the experiences of people on the field as they deliberate on policies directed at improving maternal health.

BACKGROUND

Nigeria is the most populous country in Africa, with a population of 169 million people (WHO, 2013a). Anambra State is located in the southeast region and is home to 4.2 million people (Anambra State Government, 2013a). It is the second most densely populated state in Nigeria after Lagos State. The state has clusters of numerous rural villages with an estimated 1,500 to 2,000 persons living within every square kilometer (National Bureau of Statistics, 2012). Although state-specific maternal health data are not available, the country-level data are believed to adequately reflect the maternal health status of the state.

Nigeria's maternal mortality ratio (MMR) is one of the highest in the world at 630 deaths per 100,000 live births. The lifetime risk of maternal death is one in 29 considering the high cumulative exposure to pregnancies (WHO, 2012). These are too high, particularly in comparison with developed countries. For the United States and United Kingdom, for example, the MMRs are 21 and 12, respectively with corresponding lifetime risks of maternal death of one in 2,400 and one in 4,600 (WHO, 2013b). Previous reports show that obstetric complications are common in Nigeria and often lead to maternal or fetal death (Ezeonwu, 2011). In most cases, life threatening conditions are not identified, treated, referred, or followed up appropriately by trained providers during the course of the pregnancy, delivery, and postpartum sometimes resulting in disability or death. For example, in most developing countries including Nigeria, hemorrhage accounts for most deaths (WHO, 2012) even though it is mostly preventable.

Merson, Black, and Mills (2012) posit that in order to reduce maternal deaths to a significant level in low- and middle-income countries, emphasis on reducing overall fertility levels and the frequency of high-risk pregnancies are unlikely to be sufficient. This is because (a) there are economic and social incentives for having more children and (b) there are limitations to trying to reduce high-risk pregnancies. The global consensus on effective intervention aims to ensure, first, that every pregnancy is wanted through universal access to voluntary contraception; and, second, that every child-birth is safe and attended by skilled personnel with midwifery competencies (Gilmore & Gebreyesus, 2012). In other words, reducing the mortality risk for each and every pregnancy must be emphasized (Merson et al., 2012).

A critical question for policymakers follows: How could the mortality risk for each and every pregnancy be reduced? According to the United Nations Children's Fund [UNICEF] (n.d.), the most important interventions for safe motherhood are to make sure that (a) a trained provider with midwifery skills is present at every birth; (b) transport is available to referral services; and (c) quality emergency obstetric care is available. These interventions present significant challenges for Nigeria due to poor physical infrastructures and absence of skilled providers at the majority of deliveries. The most recent Demographic and Health Survey reveals that a significant number of Nigerian women aged 15–49 reported that they received antenatal care from "no one." These include 71.0% of women who belong to the lowest wealth quintile, 63.7% of women with "no education," and 46.9% of rural dwellers (National Population Commission [NPC] [Nigeria] and ICF Macro, 2009). The data demonstrate the complexity of maternal health issues and the need for interdisciplinary and multisectorial policy approaches.

On a positive note, among the small segments of women who sought some form of obstetric care, Akpabio, Edet, Etifit, and Robinson-Bassey (2014) report that those who preferred and patronized modern health care practitioners (skilled providers) far out-numbered those who preferred and patronized the traditional birth attendants (TBAs) in Cross River State, Nigeria. Evidence also shows that among all skilled providers in Nigeria, nurses and midwives are most preferred (Ezeonwu, 2011; NPC [Nigeria] and ICF Macro, 2009). These data make the case for realistic and effective policies to use the most effective trained providers to target and reach the most vulnerable women irrespective of their abilities to pay, education levels, and where they reside.

METHODS

Research Design

In this descriptive study, a qualitative approach was used to explore the perspectives of nurse leaders in Nigeria on effective strategies to improve maternal health outcomes. Interview data collected included specific policy recommendations to improve maternal health services delivery and outcome. Content analysis was used to analyze data collected through semistructured face-to-face interviews. The study was approved by the Institutional Review Board of the University of Washington.

Recruitment

In order to obtain broad policy recommendations from participants, I recruited and interviewed a convenience sample of nurse experts from diverse backgrounds, including five nurse educators who were directors or principals of their respective nursing and midwifery schools; five health administrators who managed and directed nursing and health services at their respective hospitals; and two top management staff of the Nursing and Midwifery Council of Nigeria (NMCN). Physical access factors in Nigeria, such as road conditions, transportation, and weather influenced participant recruitment because some local roads that lead to potential participant locations were eroded and unsafe to walk or drive on due to heavy rains.

In order to be included in the study, participants had to be over 18 years of age and speak and understand English. In addition, they should either be nurse educators who direct their nursing and midwifery schools, hospital administrators who direct the relevant health facility, or members of the management staff of the NMCN who were active representatives of the governing body of the council. All 12 participants were females, with 32 average years of service. They have extensive leadership, educational, and practice experiences acquired through their career locales: government and mission schools; private, mission, and government hospitals and clinics; specialist hospitals; voluntary agencies; government agencies; the Nursing and Midwifery Council; and private practices.

Prior arrangements for interviews were not made due to communication difficulties. The interviews were conducted on the spot without prior contact. I walked into the facilities where potential participants worked. After identifying each potential participant, I introduced myself and my study and provided detailed information about the study procedures. Questions regarding the study were answered, and written informed consent was obtained from each participant. The interviews were conducted in participants' respective offices primarily in Anambra State. Members of the council, however, were interviewed in their offices located outside the state.

Data Collection

In addition to completing a basic demographic questionnaire, participants responded to interview questions that centered on practical and effective strategies to improve maternal health in the country. Examples of open-ended interview questions included the following: (a) What are your views on ways to improve maternal health outcomes in the country? (b) If you had all the resources to change and improve things around maternal health, what would be your priorities? The interviews lasted between 45 and 80 minutes. Detailed notes were taken, and all interviews were audiorecorded except for those of two participants who declined voice recordings.

Data Analysis

All identifiers were removed, and data were coded appropriately. All recorded face-to-face interview data and field notes were transcribed verbatim and analyzed using qualitative content analysis procedures and processes outlined by Elo and Kyngas (2007) and Graneheim and Lundman (2004). Interview texts were read multiple times. Units of analysis were extracted from the whole interview texts and condensed into one text. Important sentences, keywords, or phrases that characterize policy strategies were identified and highlighted. Categories and subcategories of data were created by sorting common ideas in the text and carefully coding them based on their differences and similarities. The words and phrases within the categories and subcategories were reduced by crossing out repetitions or similar words or phrases. Policy themes and subthemes emerged, which accounted for all the data in the interview transcript. Three senior researchers from my institution reviewed and agreed with the coding and analysis processes.

FINDINGS

Based on the participants' extensive experiences and years of professional immersion in the Nigerian health care system, several strategies to improve maternal health outcomes in Anambra State Nigeria were suggested and highlighted in Table 1.

TABLE 1 Themes and Subthemes Related to Policy Suggestions to Improve Maternal Health Outcomes

Main themes	Subthemes
Free health care	No charges for provider visits, hospitalizations/birthing, drugs, and other supplies
Broad outreach and education	Spousal, family, and community inclusiveness (in reproductive health and maternal plan of care)
Stronger health system to improve access to quality maternal care	Physical infrastructural improvement
	• Physical access to care
	• Equipment, supplies, and blood products availability
	Workforce improvement
	Nursing quality improvement

Free Health Care: Provider Visits, Hospitalizations/Birthing, Drugs, and Other Supplies

All participants in this study concurred that cost is a critical determinant of maternal health services utilization in the country. They reported that poverty affects rural women disproportionately because most of them have minimal or no education and therefore slim opportunities for financial security. In order to improve antenatal clinic turn-out, they asserted that women must have assurance and a good sense of security that they will not be turned away because of their inability to pay for services and that they will not go home with outrageous charges that they will not be able to clear. One participant said that free treatments should be offered to poor rural women. Another said, "Free cost of delivery, free drugs, and free everything, improve attendance." The most common threaded word related to health care cost among all participants was *free*. This included free antenatal visits, delivery, and postnatal care; free treatment for all pregnancy-related problems; free tests, immunizations, and drugs particularly antimalarial and antiretroviral therapies; and free contraceptives.

In response to how the country could afford free reproductive and maternal health services, respondents stated that the government's priorities should simply change. Suggestions ranged from stopping all corruption and embezzlement of government money particularly by government officials to increasing the budgetary allocations to the health sector. They pointed out that although Nigeria is one of the world's largest producers and exporters of crude oil, the oil revenue does not go into meeting public needs. One participant stated, "This is the richest country with the greatest number of poor people." Another participant summed it up this way: "The government should invest in health care."

Broad Outreach and Education: Spousal, Family, and Community Inclusiveness

Responses from nurse leaders clearly showed that reproductive and pregnancy-related matters are not just a woman's problem but the collective problem of everyone in the community, particularly spouses and other family members. They noted that in addition to reaching out to women through a one-on-one approach, the extended family members and the larger community (mothers-in-law; sisters-in-law; and young, old, male, and female audiences) should be targeted by delivering health talks at social and religious gatherings. All participants believed that spouses should be included in obstetric plan of care and that they should always accompany their women to antenatal visits particularly for HIV/AIDS education and testing and family planning. A participant described this approach as "public enlightenment" and an important cultural breakthrough because men are not involved in childbirth and discussions related to sexuality including contraception in Nigeria. They emphasized the importance of grassroots education and creating awareness of the importance of family planning, sexually transmitted diseases such as HIV/AIDS, and dietary needs during pregnancy. Risks and consequences of not getting antenatal care from trained providers and early recognition of complications were some of the health messages that the communities should receive, according to participants.

Another aspect of general community outreach emphasized by participants included supporting and empowering women and wives to go to school and acquire degrees. They noted that women are still living under the shadow of men, and the belief that men should be the main financial provider for their family is hurting women and society. As a paternalistic society, participants emphasized that focusing on and diffusing the pervasive culture of male dominance and superiority will help support the maternal health agenda. It will support each woman's efforts to pursue education and get good jobs to support themselves and their families. A participant noted that the "re-orientation of the culture so that men will allow their wives to reach their maximum potential" is very important for women, the profession, and the entire population.

Stronger Health System to Improve Access to Quality Maternal Care

PHYSICAL INFRASTRUCTURAL IMPROVEMENT

Physical access to care. According to participants, in order to utilize available services, mothers should be able to easily access the locations where the services are provided. The nurse experts explained that the distance between rural women and health facilities, often located in the urban areas, negatively affects maternal health outcomes in different ways. For example, some women in the rural areas are often overwhelmed by the challenges of distance and cost of care, and they simply settle with an unlicensed provider or a TBA in their villages. They also stated that most remote villages could only be accessed with *okada*—a popular commercial motorcycle transportation system in Nigeria. One participant pointed out that "in case of emergency, you cannot carry a pregnant, dying woman on *okada*," thus stressing the severity of the problem. They recommended that the government should as a matter of urgency do the following: (a) build and maintain health facilities in every locality, closer to the people to discourage the use of TBAs; (b) provide basic amenities particularly pipe-borne water and electricity to attract trained providers to stay and practice in those rural areas; and (c) improve and maintain the deplorable roads in the rural areas (often washed away during each rainy season) and support appropriate transportation options for easier and quicker access to higher-level facilities in emergency situations.

Availability of equipment, supplies, and blood products.   The majority of health centers and maternity homes in Nigeria lack basic care supplies and drugs, and most hospitals are ill-equipped to deliver high-level care to patients, according to the nurse leaders. They noted the dearth of sophisticated care equipment: scanning and diagnostic imaging machines; basic supplies including gloves, needles, tapes, intravenous fluids, and tubes; and emergency obstetric drugs. A participant said, "Yes, the equipment, the hospital should be well equipped so that when a person comes, we see that we have the things to resuscitate or get the person recovered from the illness. Not when a person comes, we say, 'Ahh, we are looking for this, we don't have that.'" They strongly recommended that health facilities be provided with adequate funding to procure and stock needed items in order to save lives. Participants also pointed out that postpartum hemorrhage remains one of the major causes of maternal death and yet, in most emergency cases, the needed drugs and blood are not available. Family members are sent out to look for blood or blood products for a dying woman even in emergency situations. Participants suggested that blood banks be located and fully stocked in every health facility that delivers high-level obstetric services.

WORKFORCE IMPROVEMENT

Participants noted that improving maternal health outcomes starts with building a strong health workforce. They believed that nurses and midwives are the most popular and effective workforce in maternal health services delivery in the country, and efforts should be channeled toward improving nursing and midwifery education and workforce development. Although they recognized the efforts of the Nursing and Midwifery Council in reintroducing the basic midwifery program and ensuring regular reviews and reaccreditations of all the schools in the country, they reiterated that a lot more needs to be done to train and retain this critical workforce in order to deliver appropriate and adequate maternal health care to the growing population. A participated stated, "We need enough strength of staff in the hospitals. When people go to the hospitals, they would like to see the doctor and the nurse as quickly as possible. And the nurses should know what they're doing. We need well-trained nurses and midwives." All the experts were regretful and emphatic in their views about the total neglect that the nursing and midwifery profession receives. They recommended adequate funding of nursing and midwifery education as a fundamental step, with funds directed to improving physical infrastructures in schools, recruitment, training, and retention. Participants pointed out that professional training of nurses and midwives would be effective with good investment in the following:

- Adequate accommodation (classroom, laboratory, and office spaces) to promote teaching and learning;

- Properly equipped buildings with appropriate lighting, chairs, and tables to support student comfort;
- Adequate and appropriate teaching aids such as projectors, computers, and laptops;
- Books and periodicals (hard copies and electronic copies);
- Properly equipped demonstration laboratories for skills training;
- Adequately equipped training facilities (hospitals, health centers, and maternity homes) to enhance practical experiences for students; and
- Functional communication mechanisms (stable Internet and phone networks).

In addition to the physical infrastructures within and around academic institutions, the experts also stated that efforts directed at recruitment, training, and retention of nurse and midwife educators are crucial in order to strengthen the profession and keep experienced nurses from migrating overseas. Participants' recommendations follow:

- Training and employing more professorial staff to offset teaching staff shortages;
- Increasing the salaries, wages, and working conditions of nurse educators to (a) retain academic staff in order to maintain a steady supply of the nursing workforce and (b) entice and convince young nurses to pursue a nursing and midwifery education pathway as a financially and professionally rewarding career option;
- Providing professional development and continuing education opportunities for academic staff, clinical staff, and nursing students in the form of workshops, seminars, and conferences both within and outside the country;
- Creating opportunities for international collaborations.

In addition to improving the schools and the working conditions of academic staff, nurse and midwife clinicians who provide direct care should be supported and compensated well, according to the nurse leaders. They pointed out that rural dwellers are disproportionately affected by health problems and yet there are not enough providers to address those issues due to the unattractiveness of the wages and the working conditions in rural areas. A participant stated that those problems will be minimized if the government saturates the communities and villages with highly skilled nurses and midwives. Another participant said, "Improving the remuneration for nurses and midwives will make them work in the rural areas where the majority of the masses are." All of the experts' comments show that paying nurses and midwives higher salaries and providing them with professional development opportunities will improve their morale since they outnumber the physicians and do more in terms of maternal care. They are confident that the goal of improved maternal health outcomes would be achieved if a critical mass of trained and well-compensated nurse providers stay in the country and make their ways to the hinterlands.

Nursing Quality Improvement

Participants noted that due to the weak health system, the professional regulatory mechanism designed to oversee the qualification standards and licenses of health practitioners and health facilities is also weak. For nursing, poor quality assurance tarnishes the image of the profession and also affects the health of patients. They expressed with certainty that nursing would reclaim its respectful position as soon as unqualified personnel are barred from practicing. One expert stated, "Reducing the number of frustrated quacks who are in practice is critical in order to reduce the risks of maternal deaths and to maintain practice standards for the profession." The quacks in this context refer to individuals who work as nurses in the health care system despite the fact that they were unable to pass the qualifying examinations in order to meet the licensing standards of the NMCN. The participant believes that the "three strikes, you are out" assessment system of the Nursing and Midwifery Council, in which those who fail the qualifying examination three times must start all over, is not only bad for individuals but is bad policy for the profession and the country in general, pointing out that the complex system forces the individuals to drop out. She explained that such individuals still end up practicing on their own in the villages, delivering babies without license, and possibly get recruited by private hospitals and clinics. A major suggested change to the council's examination practice is to retain all academically at-risk students within the system and professionally support them to practice at a lower level, while they work their way up through the examination retake processes to fully qualify.

DISCUSSION

The persistent unimpressive maternal health indicators in Nigeria and the country's lethargic progress toward achieving Millennium Development Goal #5 show that policymakers must pay attention to fundamental issues that hinder maternal health improvement efforts. As this study suggests, strategic policies should focus on providing free maternal and reproductive health services particularly in the rural areas—the hub of poverty. Previous studies show relationships among poverty, rural residence, and maternal health. For example, Bhutta, Cabral, Chan, and Keenan (2012) reported that much of the global burden of maternal mortality is among women who are poor, uneducated, of indigenous origin, and from marginalized or rural populations. Ezeonwu (2011) also found that poverty has a significant negative effect on maternal health because poor women are deterred from accessing and utilizing professional skilled services. Among adolescents who constitute a key segment of Nigerian population, Rai, Singh, and Singh (2012) reported that even when appropriate services are in place, poverty was a key determinant in the way they utilized maternity services. Gilmore and Gebreyesus (2012) recommended that financial restrictions to contraceptive access, especially for the poorest women and those who are pregnant during adolescence, should be addressed by offering free or nearly free services at the point of care.

The recommendation for free maternal health care is justified because Nigeria is one of the world's largest producers of crude oil. Despite the huge revenue from petroleum export, expenditure on health remains low. For example, in 2010 the general government expenditure on health as a percentage of the total government expenditure was only 4% and the per capita total expenditure on health was $59.00 (WHO, 2012). This leaves the citizens with high out-of-pocket costs for health care. Since families and individuals make tough choices between investing their very meager income on basic human needs (food, shelter, and clothing) and health care, a health care option that employs the services of skilled attendants, though desirable, however, will rank lower for mothers particularly when there are cheaper alternatives such as the TBAs.

A simple but logical policy approach to increase demand for skilled services among poor women is for the government to subsidize the cost of skilled services and, in this context, make such services free or offered at lower prices than the TBAs. For the poor, increasing access to care depends on reducing financial barriers to receiving care, particularly out-of-pocket costs (WHO, 2012). Evidence shows that the delivery exemption policy in Ghana resulted in increased use of antenatal care in the country (Aboagye & Agyemang, 2013). In South Africa, eliminating user fees for maternal and child health care also led to increased use of antenatal and child health services (WHO, 2005). Broader exemption policies that include reproductive and maternal health services should be fully considered for Nigerian women.

Efforts to increase the demand for and utilization of skilled services by eliminating cost must be augmented by targeted education and outreach to women and their support system to ensure that they understand the importance of antenatal care, skilled attendance at delivery, and postnatal care. The findings of this study show that spousal, family, and community inclusiveness in the plan of care are fundamental to improving reproductive and maternal health outcomes. In support of this finding, a recent study conducted in Malawi suggests that involving men, as well as the extension of antenatal care services to men, can help overcome obstacles to improving maternal health at the community level (Aarnio, Chipeta, & Kulmala, 2013).

In their report on maternal and newborn health roadmaps, Ekechi, Wolman, and De Bernis (2012) pointed out that working with individuals, families, and communities, and ramping up human resources are the top two strategies for reducing maternal mortality. Furthermore, the WHO (2010) *Making Pregnancy Safer Initiative* emphasized the importance of the collective roles of women, their partners, families, and the larger community in improving health. It recommended that both improvement of maternal and newborn health services and actions at the community level are required to ensure that women and their newborns have access to skilled care when they need it. Intense outreach, education, and engagement of the whole community will help improve outcomes for mothers.

Nigeria experiences several health systems-related physical and human infrastructural deficits that directly and indirectly diminish maternal health improvement efforts. The findings of this study consistently suggest that the Nigerian government should prioritize and invest in health care. According to a WHO (2012) report, supportive legislation is a key first step in improving access to quality care, and it must be followed by sustained political commitment and strong support from stakeholders so that policies are translated into actions on the ground. A clear maternal policy agenda that includes support for nursing and midwifery must be articulated in all the 36 states in Nigeria including Anambra State in order to meet the overwhelming health needs. Such a policy agenda must address the country's weak health system particularly in (a) maintaining a robust financing mechanism and (b) ensuring access to quality maternal care provided by well-trained and adequately paid workforce at well-maintained health facilities.

Although Nigeria has made some efforts in fixing the health system, they are not enough to make a significant impact on maternal health. For example, the Federal Executive Council developed and approved the National Strategic Health Development Plan that outlines a broad framework to strengthen the national health system and improve the health status of Nigerians (Nigerian Federal Ministry of Health, 2010). Concrete actions, however, are needed to implement appropriate policies and programs that are associated with the plan including those that relate to maternal health access and associated point of care and workforce supply chain infrastructure. Also, in December 2009, the government launched the Midwives Service Scheme in which new, unemployed, and retired midwives were recruited and deployed to primary health care facilities in rural areas (Abimbola, Okoli, Olubajo, Abdullahi, & Pate, 2012). This program encountered challenges including funding, unavailability of qualified midwives, and retention. There was attrition related to inadequate social amenities, language barriers between the midwives and the local community, and working in hard-to-reach rural areas. Improving maternal health requires a comprehensive package that includes physical infrastructure and workforce development.

Adequate health workforce is a critical part of health systems since all other programs depend on it. In resource-poor settings such as in Nigeria, nurses and midwives, who are the most patronized and versatile health workforce, can provide skilled and effective maternal health services. Ezeonwu (2013) outlined challenges to nursing and midwifery training and retention including health systems issues that negatively impact the students' ability to learn and the educators' ability to teach such as poorly equipped schools, poor remunerations, high unemployment, and transnational migration. With nurse density-to-population ratios of 1.6 per 1,000 for Nigeria (WHO, 2013c) and one per 1,843 for Anambra State (Anambra State Government, 2013b), it is difficult to adequately cover the health needs of the population, particularly those in rural areas. This study found that for the country's tide to turn in the direction of positive maternal outcomes, nursing and midwifery schools must be supported in order to produce enough highly skilled and qualified personnel.

Historical evidence aligns with this study's findings that nursing training and retention policies should be emphasized in maternal health improvement strategies. For example, increased midwife registrations and retention, followed by strengthening and equipping district hospitals in Thailand since the 1960s, reduced maternal mortality (WHO, 2005). Harrison (2003) reported that in the early 1940s, the state of maternal health was unsatisfactory in the Niger Diocese (within the Niger Delta in Nigeria), and the British colonial government through the Church Missionary Society decided to address the problem. The plan was to "raise the standard of midwifery work and to try to bring it nearer to that of similar work in England and other countries" (Harrison, 2003, p. 582). Policy changes included overhauling the maternity homes by providing adequate infrastructure, upgrading the midwifery training, and approving decent salaries and wages for midwives "to reflect their importance and to allow them to concentrate on their jobs rather than worry about money" (p. 582). According to the report, in 1950, more midwives were trained, antenatal attendance was high, and the maternal mortality rate was low. These important pieces of history clearly show that building a strong nursing and midwifery workforce is central to any maternal health policy in developing countries.

It is evident that nursing has not received the adequate political and financial support it needs in order to make a greater impact on maternal health outcomes. For example, instead of directing resources to nursing and midwifery training and retention, the Nigerian government had focused on training community health extension workers and deploying them to the rural areas even though they will not replace the irreplaceable skilled services of nurses and midwives during the perinatal period (Ezeonwu, 2011). Also, Nigeria is among the top three recipients of official development assistance (ODA) and private foundations' funds in sub-Saharan Africa between 2005 and 2007 (Esser & Bench, 2011). Kaiser Family Foundation's breakdown of the ODA's *access to care* funding category (as cited in Esser & Bench, 2011) shows that the funding went to medical education/training, medical research, basic health care (nonimmunizations), and health education. It is unclear how much of the funding, if any, went to nursing and midwifery education since the profession was never mentioned in the report. This underscores the findings of this study that nursing is neglected despite the central role it plays in maternal health services delivery. Nursing education often falls through the cracks because it has historically been overshadowed by medical education.

Evidence also shows that HIV/AIDS, malaria, tuberculosis, and hunger and malnutrition are funding priorities for major donor agencies and foundations (Esser & Bench, 2011; Kaiser Family Foundation, 2007; Shiffman, 2007). Such prioritization of disease-based medical interventions and medical education, though critical, has not turned the page for the overall health of women in developing countries including those in rural Anambra State, Nigeria. Without enough well-trained nurses to care for and administer new and improved drugs or vaccines to patients with HIV/AIDS, malaria, and tuberculosis, for example, those priority projects and programs will be stalled. Maternal health problems also contribute to global health burdens. A broader health policy approach that also prioritizes women's health is therefore essential. Such a policy must include the expansion and strengthening of the health workforce, particularly nursing, in order to provide adequate skilled maternal care to all women, even in the most remote areas of the world.

CONCLUSION

For Nigeria to make faster progress in improving maternal health outcomes, strategic policies should focus on reducing and removing all financial restrictions to maternal health services access and utilization. The emphasis on cost is essential due to the persistent poverty among women particularly in the rural villages. Policymakers must embrace the principle that a woman's financial and educational status and where she lives should have no bearing on maternal and reproductive health services that are available to her. Furthermore, nurses and midwives are at the center of maternal health care delivery. They however operate under the shadow of physicians as reflected in the overall differential benefits and professional support and recognition through various major funding mechanisms. Adequate funding of nursing education would be a big step forward. Integrating nurses' expert knowledge and views—as core maternal health providers in health policies—will help improve health outcome for mothers not only in Nigeria but also in other developing countries.

ACKNOWLEDGMENTS

The author is most grateful to Drs. Debbie Ward, Bobbie Berkowitz, and Catherine Carr for their support during this research.

FUNDING

This study was supported by the Women's Health Nursing Research Training Grant, NINR T32NR07039, and the Hester Mclaws Scholarship, University of Washington School of Nursing.

REFERENCES

Aarnio, P., Chipeta, E., & Kulmala, T. (2013). Men's perceptions of delivery care in rural Malawi: Exploring community level barriers to improving maternal health. *Health Care for Women International*, *34*(6), 419–439. doi:10.1080/07399332.2012.755982

Abimbola, S., Okoli, U., Olubajo, O., Abdullahi, M. J., & Pate, M. A. (2012). The midwives service scheme in Nigeria. *PLOS Medicine*, *9*(5), e1001211, 1–5. doi:10.1371/journal.pmed.1001211

Aboagye, E., & Agyemang, O. S. (2013). Maternal health-seeking behavior: The role of financing and organization of health services in Ghana. *Global Journal of Health Sciences*, *5*(5), 67–79. doi:10.5539/gjhs.v5n5p67

Akpabio, I. I., Edet, O. B., Etifit, R. E., & Robinson–Bassey, G. C. (2014). Women's preference for traditional birth attendants and modern health care practitioners in Akpabuyo community of Cross River State, Nigeria. *Health Care for Women International*, *35*(1), 100–109. doi:10.1080/07399332.2013.815751

Anambra State Government. (2013a). *Welcome to Anambra State*. Retrieved from http://anambrastate.gov.ng/oldsite/

Anambra State Government. (2013b). *Ministry of Health*. Retrieved from http://anambrastate.gov.ng/ministries.html

Bhutta, Z. A., Cabral, S., Chan, C., & Keenan, W. J. (2012). Reducing maternal, newborn, and infant mortality globally: An integrated action agenda. *International Journal of Gynecology and Obstetrics*, *119*(2012), S13–S17. doi:10.1016/j.ijgo.2012.04.001

Bhutta, Z. A., Lassi, Z. S., & Mansoor, N. (2010). *The systematic review on human resources for health interventions to improve maternal health outcomes: Evidence from developing countries*. Retrieved from http://www.who.int/pmnch/activities/human_resources/hrh_maternal_health_2010.pdf

Dovlo, D. (2007). Migration of nurses from sub-Saharan Africa: A review of issues and challenges. *Health Services Research*, *42*(3), Part II, 1373–1388. doi:10.1111/j.1475-6773.2007.00712.x

Ekechi, C., Wolman, Y., & De Bernis, L. (2012). Maternal and newborn health road maps: A review of progress in 33 sub-Saharan African countries, 2008–2009. *Reproductive Health Matters*, *20*(39), 164–168. doi:10.1016/S0968-8080(12)39630-4

Elo, S., & Kyngas, H. (2007). The qualitative content analysis process. *Journal of Advanced Nursing, 62*(1), 107–115. doi:10.1111/j.1365-2648.2007.04569.x

Esser, D. E., & Bench, K. K. (2011). Does global health funding respond to recipients' needs? Comparing public and private donors' allocations in 2005–2007. *World Development, 39*(8), 1271–1280.

Ezeonwu, M. C. (2011). Maternal birth outcomes: Processes and challenges in Anambra State, Nigeria. *Health Care for Women International, 32*(6), 492–514. doi:10.1080/07399332.2011.555827

Ezeonwu, M. C. (2013). Nursing education and workforce development: Implications for maternal health in Anambra State, Nigeria. *International Journal of Nursing and Midwifery, 5*(3), 35–45. doi:10.5897/IJNM12.014

Gilmore, K., & Gebreyesus, T. A. (2012). What will it take to eliminate preventable maternal deaths? *Lancet, 380*, 87–88. Retrieved from http://dx.doi.org/10.1016/S0140-6736(12)60982-9

Graneheim, U. H., & Lundman, B. (2004). Qualitative content analysis in nursing research: Concepts, procedures and measures to achieve trustworthiness. *Nurse Education Today, 24*, 105–112.

Harrison, K. A. (2003). Reproductive health struggles in Nigeria. *Lancet, 362*(9383), 582.

Kaiser Family Foundation. (2007). *A global look at public perceptions of health problems, priorities, and donors: The Kaiser/Pew Global Health Survey.* Retrieved from http://www.pewglobal.org/files/pdf/259.pdf

Merson, M. H., Black, R. E., & Mills, A. J. (2012). *Global health: Diseases, programs, systems and policies* (3rd ed.). Burlington, MA: Jones & Bartlett Learning.

National Bureau of Statistics. (2012). *Anambra State information.* Retrieved from http://www.nigerianstat.gov.ng/information/details/Anambra

National Population Commission (NPC) [Nigeria] & ICF Macro. (2009). *Nigeria Demographic and Health Survey 2008.* Abuja, Nigeria: Author. Retrieved from http://nigeria.unfpa.org/pdf/nigeriadhs2008.pdf

Nigerian Federal Ministry of Health. (2010). *National strategic health development plan 2010–2015.* Retrieved from http://www.health.gov.ng/images/PolicyDoc/NSHDP.pdf

Rai, R. K., Singh, P. K., & Singh, L. (2012). Utilization of maternal health care services among married adolescent women: Insights from the Nigeria Demographic and Health Survey, 2008. *Women's Health Issues, 22*(4), e407–414. doi:10.1016/j.whi.2012.05.001

Shiffman, J. (2007). Generating political priority for maternal mortality reduction in five developing countries. *American Journal of Public Health, 97*(5), 796–803.

United Nations Children's Fund (UNICEF). (n.d.). *Millennium development goal #5: Improve maternal health.* Retrieved from http://www.unicef.org/mdg/maternal.html

United Nations Populations Fund (UNFPA). (2006). *Investing in midwives and others with midwifery skills to save the lives of mothers and newborns and improve their health.* Retrieved from http://www.unfpa.org/webdav/site/global/shared/documents/publications/2008/midwives_eng.pdf

United Nations Populations Fund (UNFPA). (2011). *The state of the world's midwifery.* Retrieved from http://www.unfpa.org/sowmy/resources/docs/main_report/en_SOWMR_Full.pdf

Wirth, M. (2008). Professionals with delivery skills: Backbone of the health system and key to reaching the maternal health millennium development goal. *Croatian Medical Journal, 49*(3), 318–333. doi:10.3325/cmj.2008.3.318

World Health Organization (WHO). (2005). *The world health report 2005: Make every mother and child count*. Retrieved from http://www.who.int/whr/2005/whr2005_en.pdf

World Health Organization (WHO). (2010). *Working with individuals, families and communities to improve maternal and newborn health*. Retrieved from http://whqlibdoc.who.int/hq/2010/WHO_MPS_09.04_eng.pdf

World Health Organization (WHO). (2012). *Building a future for women and children: The 2012 report on the countdown to 2015*. Retrieved from http://www.countdown2015mnch.org/documents/2012Report/2012-Complete.pdf

World Health Organization (WHO). (2013a). *WHO African region: Nigeria*. Retrieved from http://www.who.int/countries/nga/en/

World Health Organization (WHO). (2013b). *Maternal mortality country profiles*. Retrieved from http://www.who.int/gho/maternal_health/countries/en/index.html

World Health Organization (WHO). (2013c). *Health workforce: Aggregated data*. Retrieved from http://apps.who.int/gho/data/node.main.A1442?lang=en

Gender Equality as a Means to Improve Maternal and Child Health in Africa

KAVITA SINGH and SHELAH BLOOM

Department of Maternal and Child Health, Gillings School of Global Public Health; and MEASURE Evaluation, Carolina Population Center, University of North Carolina at Chapel Hill, Chapel Hill, North Carolina, USA

PAUL BRODISH

MEASURE Evaluation, Carolina Population Center, University of North Carolina at Chapel Hill, Chapel Hill, North Carolina, USA

In this article we examine whether measures of gender equality, household decision making, and attitudes toward gender-based violence are associated with maternal and child health outcomes in Africa. We pooled Demographic and Health Surveys data from eight African countries and used multilevel logistic regression on two maternal health outcomes (low body mass index and facility delivery) and two child health outcomes (immunization status and treatment for an acute respiratory infection). We found protective associations between the gender equality measures and the outcomes studied, indicating that gender equality is a potential strategy to improve maternal and child health in Africa.

In this article we explore the question of whether gender equality is associated with key health outcomes predictive of maternal and child mortality in Africa. In much of sub-Saharan Africa, health services are not easily available to all women because of distance or cost. If women with higher decision making and more positive gender norms have greater ability to access existing maternal and child health services than their counterparts,

This study was funded by the United States Agency for International Development (US-AID) through a cooperative agreement (GHA-A-00-08-00003-00) with MEASURE Evaluation. The views expressed in this article do not necessarily reflect those of USAID. The authors are grateful to the Carolina Population Center (R24 HD050924) for general support.

then the promotion of gender equality could be seen as a means to give women access to potentially life-saving care and treatment for themselves and their children.

Despite some progress, maternal and under-5 mortality remain high in developing countries. Millennium Development Goal (MDG) 5 aims to reduce by three-fourths the maternal mortality ratio from 1990 to 2015. The decrease from 400 maternal deaths per 100,000 live births in 1990 to World Health Organization's (WHO's) estimate of 260 maternal deaths per 100,000 live births in 2008 represents only a 35% decline (WHO, 2010). MDG 4 aims to reduce by two-thirds the under-5 mortality rate from 1990 to 2015. The decline from 87 under-5 deaths per 1,000 live births in 1990 to (United Nations Children's Fund [UNICEF], 2012) estimate of 51 under-5 deaths per 1,000 live births in 2011 represents only a 41% decline. Africa in particular carries a high burden of maternal and under-5 mortality, accounting for an estimated 15% of the world's population but 50% of under-5 deaths and 58% of maternal deaths. Few countries in Africa are on track to meet either MDG4 or MDG5.

While MDG4 and 5 have a maternal and child health focus, MDG3 pertains to gender equality and women's empowerment. While the promotion of gender equality is important in and of itself, global health organizations are also considering gender equality as a key strategy to improve health not just for women but also for their children. An example of such a strategy is seen with the United States' Global Health Initiative, which has seven pillars, the first of which is "Focus on women, girls and gender quality." UNAIDS and UNICEF also have a gender focus as a means to protect the health and well-being of women and children.

In this study we seek to understand the role of specific constructs of gender equality, namely, women's autonomy and gender norms, on maternal and child health outcomes in Africa. *Autonomy* is defined as the ability to make decisions through control over information and resources, and it includes the ability to act upon those decisions (Basu & Basu, 1991; Dyson & Moore, 1983). Autonomy within the household or household decision making has been shown to be particularly important for the study of individual health outcomes and behaviors (Basu & Basu, 1991; Bloom, Wypij, & Das Gupta, 2001; Jejeebhoy, 2000). Household decision making is often dependent on the social context (i.e., cultural norms and social institutions) in which a woman lives (Mason, 2003), thus the importance of attitudes toward gender norms.

Studies in Asia have demonstrated a clear positive relationship between gender equality and a woman's ability to seek and advocate for services for herself and her children (Beegle, Frankenberg, & Thomas, 2001; Bloom et al., 2001; Mistry, Galal, & Lu, 2009; Visaria, 1993). Few researchers have explored the significance of gender equality for African women and children, and only a handful have explored associations between gender equality and the particular maternal health (facility delivery and low body mass index [BMI]) and child health outcomes (treatment for an acute respiratory infection, or ARI, and full vaccination for children) that we explore here. Researchers studying women in the slums of Nairobi, Kenya, found that among poor and middle-income households, gender measures were weakly associated with facility delivery (Fotso, Essendi, & Ezeh, 2009). Woldemicael (2010) found for women in Ethiopia and Eritrea that gender measures were not significantly associated with facility delivery after controlling for socioeconomic factors. They were, however, associated with a child being fully vaccinated. Researchers studying women in Northern Nigeria also found a gender measure, decision making, to be associated with a child being fully vaccination (Babalola, 2009). Hindin (2000) found that women in Zimbabwe who did not have a say in household decisions were more likely to have low BMI than women who did have some say. Researchers studying women in Nigeria have recently found that gender equality is significantly associated with whether a woman has a facility delivery (Singh, Bloom, Haney, Olorunsaiye, & Brodish, 2012) and whether her child is fully immunized (Singh, Haney, & Olorunsaiye, 2013).

The rationale for studying the specific health outcomes chosen for this study is their close theoretical association with maternal and child mortality, which are the focus of MDG4 and MDG5. The promotion of *skilled delivery* is widely regarded as a key strategy to reduce maternal mortality (Campbell, Graham, & Series, 2006; WHO, 2004). Low BMI is often a sign of chronic energy deficiency (CED), which can lead to increased risk for both mortality and morbidity. In addition, CED during pregnancy can lead to low birth weight babies, who have greater risk of mortality than normal weight babies. Low birth weight is actually one of the strongest predictors of neonatal, infant, and under-5 deaths. Thus low BMI has consequences for a woman herself, her birth outcomes, and her ability to take care of her family. Although two million under-5 deaths are prevented through immunizations, tragically, 2.5 million children still die every year from vaccine-preventable diseases (WHO, UNICEF, & World Bank, 2009). Finally, pneumonia, the most common and severe form of an ARI is the leading cause of mortality for children under 5, resulting in 1.8 million deaths per year or 18% of under-5 deaths (WHO, 2011). Thus we seek to understand whether gender equality enables women to access immunization services for their children and treatment for the leading cause of under-5 mortality.

METHODS

Data

We looked at diverse African countries for which recent Demographic and Health Surveys (DHS) data were available—Democratic Republic of the

Congo (2008), Egypt (2008), Ghana (2008), Liberia (2007), Mali (2006), Nigeria (2009), Uganda (2006), and Zambia (2007; ICF International, 2012). The DHS surveys include questions on household characteristics, socioeconomic variables, and maternal and child health, among other topics. Questions are largely standardized across countries, and standardized training, data collection, and data processing procedures are used. We restricted the full sample to currently married women with a birth in the last 5 years.

GENDER EQUALITY VARIABLES

The DHS datasets include several gender equality measures including questions on decision making and attitudes regarding inequalities in gender roles. We used four specific questions to create a household decision-making variable: decisions regarding health care, the purchase of major household goods, the purchase of daily goods, and visits to family/friends. (These questions were asked in all eight countries with the exception of decisions regarding health care, which was not asked in Liberia.) We categorized women who made all decisions either alone or jointly as having high decision-making authority, while those not involved in all four (or three in the case of Liberia) decisions we categorized as having low decision-making authority.

We also included in the analysis an indicator regarding attitudes toward gender norms. The DHS includes questions about the acceptability of a form of gender-based violence, wife beating, under specific circumstances (a wife going out without telling her husband, neglecting the children, arguing with her husband, refusing to have sex with her husband, and burning food). We categorized respondents who indicated that a husband is not justified in beating his wife for any of these reasons as believing wife beating is not acceptable. We classified those who indicated that wife beating is justified for at least one of the items on the list as indicating that it is acceptable.

OUTCOME MEASURES

Facility delivery. We classified delivery of the last child in the past 5 years as either a facility or nonfacility delivery. Facility deliveries comprised the response categories hospital, clinic, and health center. Nonfacility deliveries included other sites, such as the home. We used the delivery site for the youngest child if a woman had more than one birth in the past 5 years.

BMI. We categorized women (who were not currently pregnant and who had not been pregnant in the past 3 months) as having either low or normal BMI. We excluded women having high BMI because high BMI is also a negative outcome and associations between gender equality measures and high BMI would not have strong programmatic or policy recommendations. BMI was calculated by the formula:

$$BMI = weight\,(in\,kg)/height\,(in\,meters)^2.$$

Following international standards, we classified women with a BMI below 18.5 as having low BMI, and those with a BMI between 18.5 and 24.9 as having normal BMI.

Fully immunized child. We defined a fully immunized child as a child between 12 and 23 months who received three doses of oral polio vaccine, three doses of diphtheria, pertussis, and tetanus, one dose each of Bacille Calmette-Guerin, and measles vaccine before 12 months of age.

Treatment for an ARI. We calculated a treatment fraction for children with an ARI. We calculated this fraction as the number of children under age 2 who were sick with cough and had difficulty breathing in the past 2 weeks and who were taken for treatment to a health facility, divided by the number of children under age 2 who were sick with cough and had difficulty breathing in the past 2 weeks.

SOCIODEMOGRAPHIC FACTORS

We studied several covariates likely to be associated with the outcomes: age, parity, residence (urban/rural), education level, wealth, and working status (whether worked outside the home in the past 12 months). Unfortunately, the dataset did not include potentially important community-level factors such as distance to the nearest health facility.

Analysis

We pooled data across the eight countries and used multilevel logistic regression analysis to analyze the data. Using multilevel analysis we could determine whether, after accounting for differences and similarities among the countries, the gender measures were associated with the outcomes. We used a random intercepts model approach with country at the second level and all other variables at the first level. (We could not use a random slopes and intercepts model because we did not have enough observations at the second level.) We applied sampling weights and accounted for the cluster sampling approach of the DHS. We used Stata's generalized linear latent and mixed models (GLLAMM) command for the analysis. This program fits GLLAMMs, which are a class of multilevel latent variable models that includes multilevel generalized linear models or generalized linear mixed models (Rabe-Hesketh & Skrondal, 2012). We included (in model 1) only the key gender equality measures in the regression, and then we added the socioeconomic variables into Model 2 to determine if the associations remained after adding in these control variables.

RESULTS

In Table 1 we present the descriptive statistics of the socioeconomic and gender variables for the full sample of 50,246 currently married women with a birth in the past 5 years. About 43% percent of women had no education, compared with 57% who had at least a primary education. Sixty-nine percent of the sample were rural residents, compared with 31% who were urban residents. Sixty-three percent of women were currently working, while about 43% were in the two lowest wealth quintiles. In terms of the

TABLE 1 Maternal, Socioeconomic and Gender Measures, Pooled Data for Eight Countries

Explanatory variable	%
Maternal background characteristics	
Age	
15–19	6.14
20–24	22.02
25–34	47.25
35+	24.59
Parity	
1	17.07
2–3	34.58
4+	48.35
Education	
None	43.47
Primary	27.04
Secondary+	29.49
Residence	
Urban	30.66
Rural	69.34
Working	
No	36.86
Yes	63.14
Wealth index	
Poorest	21.71
Poor	21.62
Middle	20.09
Rich	19.25
Richest	17.33
Gender equality measures	
Household decision-making authority	
High	46.85
Low	53.15
Attitudes toward wife beating	
Never acceptable	43.30
Acceptable	56.70
Number of observations	50,246

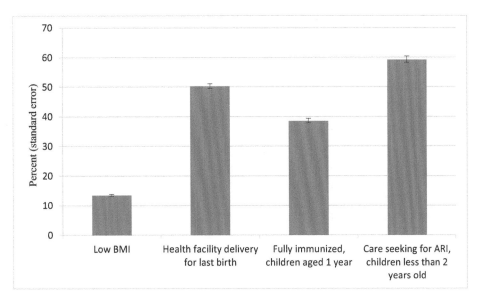

FIGURE 1 Summary statistics for four maternal and child health outcomes, pooled data for eight countries ($n = 50{,}246$) (color figure available online).

gender measures, 47% of women in the sample had high household decision-making authority, and 43% believed that wife beating is never acceptable.

In Figure 1 we plot descriptive statistics for the outcome variables. For the maternal health outcomes, about 14% of women had low BMI and 50% delivered their last child in a health facility. For the child health outcomes, 38% of children under 1 year were fully immunized, and 60% of children under 2 years who had been sick with an ARI were taken for treatment.

In Table 2 we show the multilevel logistic regression results. As expected, we find associations between education and wealth such that wealthier and more educated women tend to have better health outcomes for themselves and their children. Wealth was strongly associated with facility delivery, with an odds ratio (OR) of 6.93 ($p < .001$) in Model 2 for women in the highest wealth quintile compared with the lowest wealth quintile. Women who were currently working were significantly less likely to be of low BMI and more likely to have a facility delivery than women who were not currently working. In terms of the gender measures, high household decision making was significantly associated with a lower odds of having low BMI (OR = 0.78, $p < .05$) and a higher odds of taking a child sick with an ARI to a health facility (OR = 1.31, $p < .01$). Women who believed that wife beating is not acceptable were significantly less likely to have low BMI (OR = 0.88, $p < .001$), more likely to have a facility delivery (OR = 1.10, $p < .001$), and more likely to have a 1-year-old child who is fully immunized (OR = 1.27, $p < .001$).

TABLE 2 Parameter Estimates[a] (Odds Ratio) for the Multilevel Models for Four Maternal and Child Health Outcomes

Explanatory variable	Low BMI (n = 23,535) OR (95%CI)	Facility delivery (n = 49,468) OR (95% CI)	Fully immunized (n = 14,150) OR (95% CI)	ARI care (n = 3,468) OR (95% CI)
Fixed effects				
Household decision-making authority				
Low (RC)	1.00	1.00	1.00	1.00
High	0.78 (0.63,0.97)*	1.25 (0.92,1.72)	1.31 (0.92,1.87)	1.31 (1.12,1.54)***
Attitudes toward wife beating				
Acceptable (RC)	1.00	1.00	1.00	1.00
Never acceptable	0.88 (0.84, 0.92)***	1.10 (1.05,1.16)***	1.27 (1.16,1.40)***	1.11 (0.99,1.25)
Age				
15–19	1.35 (1.20,1.53)***	0.74 (0.61,0.90)**	0.62 (0.40,0.95)*	0.68 (0.46,1.00)*
20–24	1.10 (1.02,1.18)*	0.79 (0.67,0.93)**	0.89 (0.72,1.09)	0.75 (0.63,0.90)**
25–34 (RC)	1.00	1.00	1.00	1.00
35+	0.95 (0.76,1.19)	1.13 (0.99,1.30)	1.06 (0.98,1.16)	0.96 (0.76,1.22)
Parity				
1 (RC)	1.00	1.00	1.00	1.00
2–3	0.92 (0.78,1.09)	0.61 (0.53,0.69)***	0.94 (0.79,1.12)	1.02 (0.81,1.27)
4+	1.01 (0.84,1.22)	0.46 (0.36,0.57)***	0.86 (0.65,1.15)	0.79 (0.62,1.02)

	Model 1	Model 2	Model 3	Model 4
Education				
None (RC)	1.00	1.00	1.00	1.00
Primary	0.76 (0.65,0.90) ***	1.96 (1.27,3.01) **	1.49 (0.91,2.44)	1.29 (1.01,1.65) *
Secondary+	0.63 (0.51,0.78) ***	3.51 (1.83,6.73) ***	2.50 (1.36,4.61) **	1.29 (0.86,1.94)
Residence				
Urban (RC)	1.00	1.00	1.00	1.00
Rural	0.98 (0.86,1.11)	0.49 (0.33,0.73) ***	0.96 (0.86,1.06)	1.24 (0.83,1.86)
Working				
No (RC)	1.00	1.00	1.00	1.00
Yes	0.88 (0.78,0.99) *	1.33 (1.09,1.61) **	1.20 (0.98,1.46)	1.06 (0.88,1.27)
Wealth index				
Poorest (RC)	1.00	1.00	1.00	1.00
Poor	0.87 (0.72,1.05)	1.29 (1.11,1.50) **	1.13 (0.85,1.51)	1.07 (0.82,1.40)
Middle	0.77 (0.57,1.03)	1.71 (1.18,2.48) **	1.45 (1.02,2.05) *	1.17 (0.81,1.69)
Rich	0.65 (0.49,0.85) **	3.04 (1.84,5.00) ***	1.58 (0.82,3.02)	1.56 (0.97,2.49)
Richest	0.64 (0.41,0.98) *	6.93 (3.98,12.06) ***	2.36 (1.18,4.71) *	2.08 (1.16,3.70) *
Random effects				
Country-level variance[b]	1.86 *	1.74 ***	4.64 ***	1.63 ***
Log likelihood	−8803.99	−25251.61	−6657.08	−2080.47
AIC	17624	50517	13330	4175
Log likelihood ratio test (χ^2)[c]	226.09 ***	12154.63 ***	711.38 ***	65.23 ***

RC = reference category.

[a] Parameters for predictors (fixed effects) are reported as odds ratio; for random effects, the parameter is the variance.

[b] Significance of random effects evaluated by comparing model with a similar one in which random effects have been constrained to be zero.

[c] Compared to null model with no covariates.

*p < .05 **p < .01 ***p < .001.

CONCLUSIONS

There is a global focus on the promotion of gender equality and women's empowerment as seen in MDG3; however, few previous studies have explored associations of gender equality and maternal and child health outcomes in African countries (Babalola, 2009; Fotso et al., 2009; Hindin, 2000; Singh et al., 2012, 2013; Woldemicael, 2010). Notably this study is unique in that it looks not just at one country but at Africa as a region.

After controlling for socioeconomic variables including wealth and education, we find that household decision making was significantly associated with two of the four outcomes. Women with high decision making were less likely to have low BMI and more likely to take a child sick with an ARI for treatment. The measure capturing attitudes toward wife beating was significantly associated with three of the four outcomes. Women who felt that wife beating is not acceptable were less likely to be of low BMI, more likely to have a facility delivery, and more likely to have a fully immunized child. Thus there is potential for the promotion of gender equality to improve maternal and child health by increasing the ability of a woman to access services for herself and her children. While developing countries are aiming to improve accessibility of services, which is essential, the concurrent promotion of gender equality can enable women to access existing services. The promotion of gender equality may also enable women not only to access services but also to achieve better overall health, as evidence by the protective effect of both gender measures against low BMI.

Also important are the significant associations among the outcomes and education, working status, and wealth. These socioeconomic variables are key inputs into the causal pathway linking equality to improved health outcomes. For example, it may be difficult for a woman in the lowest wealth quintile to have autonomy because the concept of autonomy implies that an individual has choice. A woman in dire poverty may not have much choice—the ability to obtain a treatment for a sick child may not be feasible because of a complete lack of resources. Thus the significance of the gender measures after controlling for these key inputs implies that a focus on gender equality, in addition to a focus on education and poverty reduction, can do more to improve maternal and child health than a focus on education and poverty reduction alone.

A key limitation of this analysis is the lack of a variable measuring accessibility or distance to the nearest health facility. In some cases a woman may have high decision making and positive gender attitudes, but the nearest health facility is too far away. We believe this limitation is somewhat mitigated by the inclusion of the residence (urban/rural) variable, which may account for some of the differences in accessibility. Another limitation is endogeneity, particularly for the low BMI analysis, such that a woman may have low decision making and thus little say in her health, or the converse could be true: a woman may have low decision-making because she is not in good health.

Despite the limitations of this analysis, we find the global focus on gender equality as a means to improve maternal and child health outcomes is warranted. A programmatic and policy focus on gender has particularly important implications for improving maternal and child health outcomes in Africa, where the burden of maternal and under-5 mortality is so high. By enabling women to have the autonomy to have a say in their own health and an ability to obtain and advocate for potentially life-saving services for both themselves and their children, we can enable countries to see vast improvements in the health status of their citizens. Studies have shown that women who are more highly educated and those with independent sources of income or cash demonstrate higher levels of empowerment than other women (Bloom et al., 2001). Micro-credit schemes that extend small business loans to women have been successful in giving women a consistent source of independent income and in raising empowerment levels in Asia and Africa (Norwood, 2011; Rao, 2011). Programs such as Stepping Stones in South Africa have changed gender norms that contribute to gender-based violence, and this change was correlated with a reduced incidence of intimate partner violence (Jewkes, Dunkle, Nduna, & Shai, 2010). In the countries studied, a combination of programs aimed at providing women with an independent means or support along with those seeking to influence a change toward more equitable gender norms should raise levels of women's empowerment and eventually impact maternal and child health outcomes positively.

REFERENCES

Babalola, S. (2009). Determinants of the uptake of the full dose of Diphtheria-Pertussis-Tetanus vaccines (DPT3) in Northern Nigeria: A multilevel analysis. *Maternal and Child Health Journal, 13*, 550–558. doi:10.1007/s10995-008-0386-5

Basu, A. M., & Basu, K. (1991). Women's economic roles and child survival: The case of India. *Health Transition Review, 1*, 83–103.

Beegle, K., Frankenberg, E., & Thomas, D. (2001). Bargaining power within couples and use of prenatal and delivery care in Indonesia. *Studies in Family Planning, 32*, 130–146. doi:10.1111/j.1728-4465.2001.00130.x

Bloom, S. S., Wypij, D., & Das Gupta, M. (2001). Dimensions of women's autonomy and the influence on maternal health care utilization in a North Indian city. *Demography, 38*(1), 67–78. doi:10.2307/3088289

Campbell, O.M.R., Graham, W. J., & Series, L.M.S. (2006). Maternal survival 2—Strategies for reducing maternal mortality: Getting on with what works. *Lancet, 368*(9543), 1284–1299. doi:10.1016/S0140-6736(06)69381-1

Dyson, T., & Moore, M. (1983). On kinship structure, female autonomy, and demographic behavior in India. *Population and Development Review, 9*(1), 35–60. doi:10.2307/1972894

Fotso, J. C., Essendi, H., & Ezeh, A. C. (2009). Maternal health in resource-poor urban settings: How does women's autonomy influence the utilization of obstetric care services. *Reproductive Health, 6*, 1742–1755.

Hindin, M. J. (2000). Women's power and anthropometric status in Zimbabwe. *Social Science & Medicine, 51*, 1517–1528. doi:10.1016/s0277-9536(00)00051-4

ICF International. (2012). *Demographic and health surveys (various, 2006–2009)*. Calverton, MD: Author.

Jejeebhoy, S. J. (2000). From women's autonomy in rural India: Its dimensions, determinants, and the influence of context. In H. Presser & G. Sen (Eds.), *Women's empowerment and demographic processes: Moving beyond Cairo*. New York, NY: Oxford University Press.

Jewkes, R. K., Dunkle, K., Nduna, M., & Shai, N. (2010). Intimate partner violence, relationship power inequity and incidence of HIV infection in young women in South Africa: A cohort study. *Lancet, 376*(9734), 41–48.

Mason, K. (2003). *Measuring empowerment: A social demographers view*. Washington, DC: The World Bank.

Mistry, R., Galal, O., & Lu, M. (2009). Women's autonomy and pregnancy care in rural India: A contextual analysis. *Social Science & Medicine, 69*, 926–933. doi:10.1016/j.socscimed.2009.07.008

Norwood, C. (2011). Women, microcredit, and family planning practices: A case study from rural Ghana. *Journal of Asian and African Studies, 46*, 169–183.

Rabe-Hesketh, S., & Skrondal, A. (2012). *Multilevel and longitudinal modeling using stata* (3rd ed., vol. I & II). College Station, TX: Stata Press.

Rao, S. (2011). Work and empowerment: Women and agriculture in South Asia. *Journal of Development Studies, 47*, 294–315.

Singh, K., Bloom, S., Haney, E., Olorunsaiye, C., & Brodish, P. (2012). Gender factors and facility delivery: Nigeria and MDG5. *African Journal of Reproductive Health, 16*, 122–128.

Singh, K., Haney, E., & Olorunsaiye, C. (2013). Maternal autonomy and attitudes towards gender norms: Associations with childhood immunizations in Nigeria. *Maternal and Child Health Journal, 17*, 837–841. doi:10.1007/s10995-012-1060-5

United Nations Children's Fund (UNICEF). (2012). *Committing to child survival: A promised renewed*. New York, NY: Author.

Visaria, L. (1993). Female autonomy and fertility behaviour: An exploration of Gujarat data. In *Proceedings of International Population Conference of International Union for the Scientific Study of Population, Montreal* (vol. 4, pp. 263–275). Liege, Belgium: IUSSP.

Woldemicael, G. (2010). Do women with higher autonomy seek more maternal health care? Evidence from Eritrea and Ethiopia. *Health Care for Women International, 31*, 599–620. doi:10.1080/07399331003599555

World Health Organization (WHO). (2004). *Making pregnancy safer: The critical role of the skilled birth attendant. A joint statement by WHO, ICM and FIGO*. Geneva, Switzerland: Author.

World Health Organization (WHO). (2010). *Trends in maternal mortality: 1990 to 2008: Estimates developed by WHO, UNICEF, UNFPA, and the World Bank.* Geneva, Switzerland: Author.

World Health Organization (WHO). (2011). *Pneumonia fact sheet.* Retrieved from http://www.who.int/mediacentre/factsheets/fs331/en/index.html

World Health Organization (WHO), United Nations Children's Fund (UNICEF), & World Bank. (2009). *State of the world's vaccines and immunization* (3rd ed.). Geneva, Switzerland: World Health Organization.

Rethinking How to Promote Maternity Care-Seeking: Factors Associated With Institutional Delivery in Guinea

ELLEN BRAZIER and RENÉE FIORENTINO

EngenderHealth, New York, New York, USA

SAIDOU BARRY, YAYA KASSE, and SITA MILLIMONO

EngenderHealth, Conakry, Guinea

This article presents findings from a study on women's delivery care-seeking in two regions of Guinea. We explored exposure to interventions promoting birth preparedness and complication readiness among women with recent live births and stillbirths. Using multivariate regression models, we identified factors associated with women's knowledge and practices related to birth preparedness, as well as their use of health facilities during childbirth. We found that women's knowledge about preparations for any birth (normal or complicated) was positively associated with increased preparation for birth, which itself was associated with institutional delivery. Knowledge about complication readiness, obstetric risks, and danger signs was not associated with birth preparation or with institutional delivery. The study findings highlight the importance of focusing on preparation for all births—and not simply obstetric emergencies—in interventions aimed at increasing women's use of skilled maternity care.

While there is consensus on skilled attendance during childbirth as an important intervention for improving maternal survival, rates of skilled attendance remain low, particularly in sub-Saharan Africa, and evidence is lacking on effective interventions for increasing women's access to and use of these services. Birth preparedness/complications (BP/CR) interventions offer an intuitively appealing strategy for increasing women's use of institutional delivery care. Evidence on the effectiveness of these interventions, however, is mixed. In this article, we explore women's knowledge related to both birth preparedness and complications readiness, as well as the association of each with care-seeking preparations and behaviors. We will suggest that increased attention should be given during antenatal consultations and through community interventions to promoting and supporting preparation for birth—not simply raising awareness about danger signs and complication readiness.

While global and regional estimates of maternal mortality have been the focus of considerable debate in recent years (Byass & Graham, 2011; Hogan et al., 2011; Lozano et al., 2011; World Health Organization [WHO], 2010), there is agreement on the essential strategies for improving maternal health outcomes. Increasing access to skilled care during childbirth and during obstetric emergencies—along with access to family planning and safe abortion care—were recently reaffirmed as critical for sustaining progress made since the launch of the Millennium Development Goals (MDGs) in 2000 and for addressing the "unfinished business" of the fifth MDG to improve maternal health (Langer, Horton, & Chalamilla, 2013).

Despite consensus about priority maternal health interventions, evidence is lacking on how best to increase use of skilled maternity care for the approximately 144 million women who give birth each year. In sub-Saharan Africa, rates of skilled attendance have changed little since the launch of the MDGs in 2000 (United Nations [UN], 2012). Researchers analyzing data from 54 Countdown to 2015 countries have shown that wealth inequalities remain far greater for skilled attendance at birth than any of the other proven interventions for maternal, newborn, and child health for which national data are available (Barros et al., 2012).

Initiatives promoting birth preparedness and complication readiness (BP/CR) have been described as "one of the conceptually compelling and logical means" of ensuring timely receipt of skilled and emergency obstetric care (Stanton, 2004). In the extant literature, however, operational definitions of BP/CR have varied widely, contributing to a diversity of approaches and little consistent evidence of intervention effectiveness or on essential elements of these interventions; some researchers have focused primarily on preparations for obstetric emergencies (e.g., heightening awareness of danger signs, identifying a facility where emergency obstetric care is available, setting aside money for an emergency, identifying a potential blood donor, and arranging for emergency transport; McPherson, Khadka, Moore, & Sharma, 2006; Moran et al., 2006; Mutiso, Qureshi, & Kinuthia, 2008). Other researchers have explored both complication readiness and planning for normal delivery without making a clear distinction between the two (Agarwal, Sethi, Srivastava, Jha, & Baqui, 2010; Ekabua et al., 2011; Hailu, Gebremariam, Alemseged, & Deribe, 2011; Kabakyenga, Ostergren, Turyakira, & Pettersson, 2012; Kakaire, Kaye, & Osinde, 2011; Magoma et al., 2013; Mullany, Becker, & Hindin, 2007; Turan, Tesfagiorghis, & Polan, 2011), and several have included women's use of antenatal care (ANC), the content of those consultations, or both, among measures of birth preparedness (Kakaire et al., 2011; Karkee, Lee, & Binns, 2013; McPherson et al., 2006).

In a recent cluster randomized trial in rural Tanzania, use of institutional delivery care was found to be higher in intervention clusters where ANC providers offered individualized support to pregnant women in developing a birth plan to prepare for delivery and possible complications (Magoma et al., 2013). Similarly, in a prospective cohort study in one district of Nepal, Karkee and colleagues (2013) found that the number of birth preparations made during pregnancy was positively associated with use of institutional delivery care. Evidence on the association between BP/CR and women's care-seeking during childbirth from other research, however, is inconclusive. The results of other intervention studies, which used measures of BP/CR such as women's knowledge about danger signs/risks, their use of antenatal care during pregnancy, and their preparation for newborn care and items for the newborn, showed that there was weak or no association between BP/CR interventions and women's use of skilled maternity care (Kumar et al., 2008; McPherson et al., 2006; Mullany et al., 2007).

In the face of existing evidence, it remains unclear which elements of birth preparedness and complications readiness interventions are important in supporting and motivating women to seek institutional delivery care during birth. In this article, we investigate this question further by differentiating between women's knowledge about birth preparations and their knowledge about complications readiness and obstetric risks, while exploring factors associated with their levels of preparation for a recent birth and their use of institutional delivery care. Using a subset of data from an evaluation study conducted in Guinea, we explore the influence of exposure to BP/CR messages from two sources (antenatal care consultations and community-level sources) on women's knowledge related to birth preparedness and complications readiness, their levels of preparation for childbirth, and, ultimately, their care-seeking during delivery (see Figure 1).

METHODS

Study Area

Located in West Africa, the Republic of Guinea is one of the world's poorest countries, ranked 178th out of 187 countries on the 2011 Human

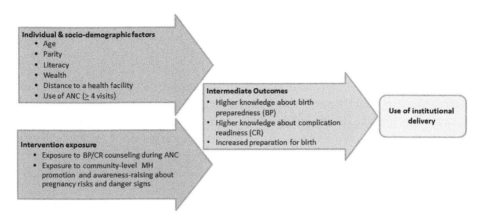

FIGURE 1 Conceptual model of causal pathway between intervention exposure, intermediate outcomes, and behavioral outcomes.

Development Index (United Nations Development Program [UNDP], 2011). Estimates of maternal mortality are high, ranging from 610 to 860 maternal deaths per 100,000 live births (Hogan et al., 2011; Lozano et al., 2011; WHO, 2010). Women's use of institutional delivery is low (46% nationally).

The study was conducted mid-2011 in two prefectures of Guinea: Kissidougou prefecture in Faranah Region in southeastern Guinea, and Labé prefecture in Labé region in the north of the country. Both regions of the country have poor maternal health indicators, with only 29.0% and 26.9% of births, respectively, taking place in health facilities (Institute National de la Statistique [INS], 2012).

Selected villages in Kissidougou and Labé prefectures had been the focus of a 5-year project to prevent and address obstetric fistula. Funded by USAID and led by EngenderHealth, the Fistula Care project focused on increasing local surgical capacity to repair fistula and on the prevention of obstetric fistula through improved labor monitoring at selected health facilities and through supporting village safe motherhood committees (VSMCs) to promote the use of skilled care throughout pregnancy and childbirth. Established in selected periurban communities in each prefecture, the VSMCs were trained to raise awareness about obstetric risks, danger signs, and causes of obstetric fistula and to promote the use of ANC during pregnancy and institutional delivery care during childbirth. The volunteers serving on the VSMCs received training on these topics, as well as a flipchart for use in leading health education sessions at the community level and in conducting household-level pregnancy monitoring visits. The community-level intervention was launched in Kissidougou in late 2007 and expanded to Labé in 2009. After the initial establishment and training of the VSMCs, quarterly review meetings were conducted for all members of the VSMCs in each region to reinforce volunteers' skills and knowledge about maternal health and to provide a forum for each committee to report on their awareness-raising and pregnancy-monitoring activities.

Study Design and Sample

Data were collected through a population-based household survey of women of reproductive age in 30 villages across the two regions as part of a retrospective evaluation of the community-level intervention. In each village, households were randomly selected for interview using household lists developed by the National Institute of Statistics for the 2011 national census. In each household, an interview was conducted with the household head to gather information on all household residents and household assets. In addition, up to two women of reproductive age (15–49 years) were interviewed.

Interviews with women focused on their knowledge about maternal health and BP/CR and their perceptions of community norms related to these topics. Basic demographic information on respondents' schooling, literacy, employment, ethnicity, and religion were also collected. Among women who had had a live birth or stillbirth within the 5 years prior to the study, questions explored their exposure to community- and facility-level interventions promoting maternal health and BP/CR, as well as their birth preparedness practices and their care-seeking during pregnancy, delivery, and the postpartum period.

Ethical Considerations

The Comité National d'Ethique pour la Recherche en Santé of Guinea (National Ethics Committee for Health Research) reviewed the study protocol and survey tools and provided ethical clearance for the study. Informed consent was obtained from all survey respondents.

Data Collection and Management

Data collection and entry were conducted by a consultant research firm, StatView International, based in Conakry. Data collection took place over a 6-week period between July and August 2011. At least two attempts were made to interview selected households, and a total of 1,846 households were successfully interviewed. A total of 2,335 women of reproductive age were interviewed, of whom 1,333 had given birth within the previous 5 years, and 763 had given birth within the past 24 months.

In view of the potential for recall errors regarding preparation for births to increase with time (Solnes Miltenburg, et al., 2013; Stanton, 2004), our analysis of factors associated with birth preparedness and use of maternal health services focused on women who had given birth with the past 24 months.

Variables in the Study

Given that women attending health facilities do not have the ability to influence the type or qualification of the service provider on duty, we defined institutional delivery (as opposed to skilled attendant) as the key outcome variable for measuring maternal health care-seeking behaviors. Institutional delivery was defined as giving birth in a hospital, health center, or health post (public or private/mission).

Other intermediate outcome variables were created to measure women's knowledge related to maternal health and their level of preparation for their most recent birth. We created two knowledge indexes to measure women's knowledge related to birth preparedness and complication readiness. The Birth Preparedness (BP) Knowledge Index measured women's knowledge about important birth preparations for any delivery (as opposed to preparations specifically for an emergency). The BP Knowledge Index was based on whether respondents cited the following as important preparations for birth: deciding on the place of delivery; discussing delivery plans with their husband/family members; saving money for delivery; making arrangements for transport to the place of delivery; and obtaining "approval" for delivery plans from household decisionmakers. Women received a score of 1 for each birth preparation that they were able to mention spontaneously. A cut-off value of 2 (i.e., ≥ 2) was used to create a dichotomous variable for "high" vs. "low" individual knowledge about birth preparedness.

The Complications Readiness (CR) Knowledge Index measured women's knowledge about risks and danger signs related to pregnancy and childbirth, and their knowledge about preparedness for obstetric emergencies. It was based on whether respondents agreed that every pregnancy was risky; knew at least three danger signs during pregnancy and childbirth; knew at least three danger signs during the postpartum period; and mentioned identifying a possible blood donor among important preparations for birth. A score between 0 and 4 was assigned to each woman, and a cut-off value of ≥ 3 was used to create a dichotomous variable for "high" vs. "low" individual knowledge related to CR.

The Birth Preparedness Behavioral Index measured the number of preparations that women reported (unprompted) that they had made for their most recent birth, including whether they had discussed institutional delivery with their partner; discussed transport; discussed how to pay for the delivery; identified a possible blood donor; or set aside money for the delivery. A score between 0 and 4 was assigned to each woman, based on her responses, and a cut-off value of ≥ 3 was used to create a dichotomous variable for "high" vs. "low" BP.

Two composite variables were created to allow for exploration of the association between intervention factors and the dependent variables described above. Because the clinical and counseling content of ANC has been shown to influence care-seeking during childbirth (Barber 2006; Bloom, Lippeveld, & Wypij, 1999; Mpembeni et al., 2007), a composite variable was developed to summarize the counseling provided to women during their ANC visits. The BP/CR Counseling Index was based on whether women reported that, during any of their ANC visits, they were advised to deliver at a health facility; advised about danger signs during pregnancy and delivery; and advised on any of the following delivery preparations: saving money, arranging for transport, discussing delivery plans with family members, or identifying a blood donor. Based on their responses to these questions, scores between 0 and 3 were assigned to each woman, and a cut-off value of ≥ 2 was used to create a dichotomous variable for "high" vs. "low" exposure to counseling on birth preparedness.

A second intervention exposure index was the Community Exposure Index, which measured each woman's exposure to community-level maternal health promotion activities carried out by the VSMCs, local health and hygiene committees, or other community-level health agents. The Community Exposure Index was derived based on whether a woman agreed that there was a local committee involved in promoting maternal health through community discussions and pregnancy monitoring visits; mentioned (unprompted) a community health committee or agent as a main source of maternal health information and help; and had personally attended a community discussion on maternal health during the past year. Based on their responses to these questions, scores between 0 and 3 were assigned to each woman, and a cut-off value of ≥ 2 was used to create a dichotomous variable for "high" vs. "low" exposure to community-level maternal health promotion activities.

Principal components analysis (Filmer & Pritchett, 2001) was used to compute wealth quintiles based on data related to household assets, which included consumer items (e.g., radio, television, bicycle, etc.) and dwelling characteristics (flooring materials, type of drinking water source, toilet facilities, etc.). Each household was assigned a standardized score for each asset, with the score determined by household ownership of that asset. Scores were summed for each household, and individuals were ranked according to the total score of the household in which they resided. The full sample (2,335 women) was divided into population quintiles, which represent the poorest 20% of the population, second poorest 20%, middle 20%, fourth poorest 20%, and least poor 20% of the population, respectively.

Statistical Analysis

Data were analyzed in SPSS (version 20.0). Descriptive analyses and frequencies were run for all variables of interest. Bivariate analyses were performed to explore the association of intervention exposure and sociodemographic factors with (a) intermediate knowledge outcomes related to birth

TABLE 1 Participant Characteristics ($N = 763$)

Characteristic	Mean	Standard deviation
Age (in years)	28.2	7.4
Age at time of most recent birth (in years)	27.3	7.4
Wealth quintile	3.0	1.4
Parity	3.9	2.3

Characteristic	Number	Percent (%)
Region		
Kissidougou	401	52.6
Labé	362	47.4
Religion		
Muslim	620	81.3
Christian	143	18.7
Any education	243	31.8
Literacy (can read with difficulty or easily)	157	20.6
Currently married	719	94.2
Wealth quintile		
Poorest	161	21.1
Second poorest	153	20.1
Middle	147	19.3
Fourth poorest	161	21.1
Least poor	139	18.2
Employed in remunerated activity	468	61.4
Member of community group	418	54.8
Ever travelled outside village	187	24.5
Live within 2 km of maternity care facility	366	48.0
Live more than 5 km of maternity care facility	169	22.1
Live within 30 minutes of maternity care facility	315	41.3
BP/CR Counseling Index (High)	309	44.8
Community Exposure Index (High)	304	39.8
Complication Readiness (CR) Knowledge Index (High)	108	14.2
Birth Preparedness (BP) Knowledge Index (High)	237	31.1
Birth Preparedness Behavioral Index (High)	262	34.3
At least one ANC visit	616	80.7
At least four ANC visits	434	57.0
Delivered in a health facility	396	51.9

preparedness and obstetric risks and (b) behavioral outcomes related to birth preparedness and delivery in a health facility.

Multivariate logistic regression models were used to explore the association between intervention exposure and intermediate knowledge outcomes on behavioral outcomes of interest while controlling for known predictors (wealth, literacy, distance to a health facility, age, and parity). A cut-off value of $p < 0.1$ was used as the criterion for including predictor variables in the multivariate regression models.

RESULTS

Characteristics of the women in our sample are shown in Table 1. Just over half of study participants (52%) were residents of Kissidougou region, while

47% were from Labé. The mean age of women in the sample was 28 years (+/−7 years), and mean parity was 3.9. Almost all study participants were married, and the majority had never attended school. Literacy was low, with 79% reporting that they could not read at all; only 14% reported that they could read easily. Distances to health facilities that provided delivery care were relatively small, with almost half of the women reporting that they lived within 2 kilometers of such a facility.

Almost half (45%) of the women in the sample had a high score on the BP/CR Counseling Index, meaning that, during their most recent pregnancy, they recalled receiving more comprehensive counseling on place of delivery, important birth preparations, and obstetric risks and danger signs. Similarly, 40% had a high score on the Community Exposure Index, indicating that they had personally been exposed to community-level awareness-raising sessions about maternal health risks, pregnancy monitoring visits, or both conducted by community health cadres or volunteers.

Only 31% of respondents had a high score on the BP Knowledge Index, and only 14% had a high score on the CR Knowledge Index. Thirty-four percent of women in our sample had made three or more preparations for their most recent birth, and had a high score on the BP Behavioral Index. The majority of respondents (81%) had attended ANC at least once during their most recent pregnancy, and 57% had attended at least four ANC visits. Just over half (52%) had delivered in a health facility.

Results of bivariate analyses exploring the association of selected sociodemographic and intervention factors with high scores on the BP and CR Knowledge Indexes are shown in Table 2. Both intervention exposure indexes (i.e., the BP/CR Counseling Index and the Community Exposure Index) were positively and significantly associated with high scores on the two knowledge indexes. Few of the sociodemographic variables were associated with high scores on either knowledge index, with the exception of wealth, which was inversely related to knowledge. Literacy was significantly associated with knowledge about birth preparedness, but not associated with CR knowledge. Both intervention exposure indexes were positively associated with high scores on the BP Behavioral Index (see Table 3). The BP/CR Counseling Index was positively associated with institutional delivery, whereas the association between exposure to community-level maternal health promotion activities and institutional delivery was borderline in significance ($p = 0.07$). A high score on the BP Knowledge Index was significantly associated with institutional delivery; however, no such association was observed for the CR Knowledge Index.

We used multivariate logistic regression to assess the association between intervention exposure and intermediate knowledge outcomes on (a) birth preparedness and (b) institutional delivery, while controlling for individual and sociodemographic factors (e.g., literacy, wealth, and distance to a health facility) that were significantly associated with the respective

TABLE 2 Bivariate Associations of Sociodemographic, Individual, and Intervention Factors With BP and CR Knowledge

Characteristic	BP knowledge (high) N = 763		CR knowledge (high) N = 763	
	N (%)	OR (95% CI)	N (%)	OR (95% CI)
Age (≥ 25 years)	160 (0.9)	1. 1 (0.8, 1.5)	76 (10.0)	1.3 (0.8, 1.9)
Literacy	45 (5.9)	1.7 (1.1, 2.5)*	14 (1.8)	0.9 (0.5, 1.6)
Parity (≥ 2)	207 (27.1)	1.4 (0.9, 2.3)	91(11.9)	1.0 (0.6, 1.8)
Wealth (wealthiest two quintiles)	77 (10.1)	0.7 (0.5, 0.9)**	27 (3.5)	0.5 (0.3, 0.7)**
Distance to health facility ≤ 2 km	115 (15.1)	1.0 (0.7, 1.3)	47 (6.2)	0.7 (0.5, 1.1)
At least 1 ANC visit	186 (24.4)	1.0 (1.0, 1.0)	95 (12.4)	0.4 (0.0, 4.1)
At least 4 ANC visits	145 (19.0)	1.3 (1.0, 1.8) p = .09	62 (8.1)	1.0 (0.7, 1.5)
BP/CR Counseling Index (High)	120 (15.7)	2.0 (1.4, 2.7)***	62 (8.1)	2.4 (1.5, 3.7)***
Community Exposure Index (High)	130 (17.0)	2.5 (1.8, 3.4)***	56 (7.3)	1.8 (1.2, 2.7)**

*$p \leq .05$; **$p \leq .01$; ***$p \leq .001$.

TABLE 3 Bivariate Associations of Sociodemographic, Individual, Intervention, and Intermediate Outcome Variables With Birth Preparedness and Institutional Delivery

Characteristic	Birth preparedness (high) N = 763		Institutional delivery N = 763	
	N (%)	OR (95% CI)	N (%)	OR (95% CI)
Age (≥ 25 years)	176 (23.1)	1.1 (0.8, 1.5)	257 (33.7)	0.9 (0.7, 1.2)
Literacy	44 (5.7)	1.4 (0.9, 2.2)	111 (14.5)	2.7 (1.9, 4.0)***
Parity (≥ 2)	223 (29.2)	1.1 (0.7, 1.7)	326 (42.7)	0.8 (0.5, 1.1)
Wealth (wealthiest two quintiles)	107 (14.0)	1.1 (0.5, 1.6)	185 (24.2)	1.9 (1.4, 2.6)***
Distance to health facility ≤ 2 km	131 (17.2)	1.1 (0.8, 1.6)	234 (30.7)	2.8 (2.1, 3.8)***
At least 1 ANC visit	211 (27.7)	1.0 (0.9, 1.0)	309 (40.4)	1.0 (0.9, 1.0)
At least 4 ANC visits	166 (21.8)	1.7 (1.2, 2.3)**	243 (31.8)	1.5 (1.1, 1.9) **
BP/CR Counseling Index (High)	159 (20.8)	4.7 (3.3, 6.6)***	196 (25.7)	2.4 (1.7, 3.2)***
Community Exposure Index (High)	134 (17.6)	2.0 (1.5, 2.8)***	170 (22.3)	1.3 (1.0, 1.8) p = .07
CR Knowledge Index (High)	45 (5.9)	1.4 (0.9, 2.1)	61 (8.0)	1.2 (0.8, 1.9)
BP Knowledge Index (High)	126 (16.5)	3.0 (2.2, 4.2)***	145 (19.0)	1.7 (1.3, 2.4)**
BP Behavioral Index (High)	—	—	184 (24.1)	3.6 (2.6, 5.0)***

*$p \leq .05$; **$p \leq .01$; ***$p \leq .001$.

TABLE 4 Multivariate Regression Results—Factors Associated With Increased Birth Preparedness

Variables (reference category)	Model 1 adjusted OR (95% CI)	Model 2 adjusted OR (95% CI)
Intervention exposure variables		
BP/CR Counseling Index (high vs. low score)	4.3 (3.0, 6.1)***	4.0 (2.8, 5.8)***
Community Exposure Index (high vs. low score)	1.6 (1.1, 2.3)*	1.4 (1.0, 2.0)
ANC use (≥ 4 ANC visits during pregnancy vs. < 4 ANC visits)	1.6 (1.1, 2.3)*	1.6 (1.1, 2.3)*
Intermediate outcome variables		
BP Knowledge Index (high vs. low score)	—	2.2 (1.5, 3.2)***

*$p \leq .05$; **$p \leq .01$; ***$p \leq .001$.

outcomes of interest in our bivariate analyses. We controlled for high ANC attendance (≥ 4 visits) in view of the fact that women who attend ANC more frequently may be more inclined to seek professional care during delivery.

We present multivariate regression results for birth preparedness in Table 4. Because none of the sociodemographic or individual variables (e.g., wealth, literacy, parity, or age) met specified criteria ($p < 0.1$) for inclusion in the model, they were excluded, along with the CR Knowledge Index. In the first model, in which we controlled for increased use of ANC (≥ 4 visits), receipt of counseling on BP and exposure to community-level maternal health promotion activities were both significantly associated with higher preparation for childbirth. In a second model, the BP Knowledge Index was added. The effect of the Community Exposure Index was attenuated in the expanded model; however, the BP/CR Counseling Index remained positively and significantly associated with increased preparation for childbirth, as did a high score on the BP Knowledge Index and receipt of at least four ANC visits (see Table 4).

Similar analyses were performed using institutional delivery as the outcome variable (Table 5). In the first model, the two intervention exposure variables were included, along with sociodemographic and individual variables that met criteria for inclusion. The BP Knowledge Index and the BP Behavioral Index were included in an expanded model to explore their association with institutional delivery (Model 2). In this expanded model, exposure to BP/CR Counseling during ANC remained significantly associated with institutional delivery, along with wealth, literacy, and distance to a health facility. Women's level of birth preparation was also significantly

TABLE 5 Multivariate Regression Results: Factors Associated With Institutional Delivery

Variables (reference category)	Model 1 adjusted OR (95% CI)	Model 2 adjusted OR (95% CI)
Intervention exposure variables		
BP Counseling Index (high vs. low score)	2.3 (1.6, 3.2)***	1.8 (1.2, 2.6)**
Community Exposure Index (high vs. low score)	1.3 (0.9, 1.9)	1.1 (0.8, 1.7)
Sociodemographic & individual variables		
Wealth (two wealthiest quintiles vs. three poorest quintiles)	1.9 (1.3, 2.7)**	2.0 (1.4, 3.0)**
Literacy (able to read easily or with difficulty vs. cannot read at all)	2.4 (1.5, 4.1)**	2.4 (1.4, 4.3)**
Distance ($\leq$ 2 km of maternity care vs. > 2 km)	2.6 (1.8, 3.6)***	2.7 (1.9, 3.9)***
ANC use ($\geq$ 4 ANC visits during pregnancy vs. < 4 ANC visits)	1.4 (1.0, 1.9)	1.3 (0.9, 1.8)
Intermediate outcome variables		
BP Knowledge Index (high vs. low score)	—	1.3 (0.9, 2.0)
BP Behavioral Index (high vs. low score)	—	2.5 (1.7, 3.8)***

$^*p \leq .05;\ ^{**}p \leq .01;\ ^{***}p \leq .001.$

associated with institutional delivery in the full model; women making at least three preparations for childbirth were twice as likely to deliver at a facility as those who made fewer birth preparations. The effect of women's knowledge about birth preparedness was attenuated and not significant, however, a finding that is to be expected given the strong positive association between birth preparedness knowledge and levels of birth preparedness (see Table 4).

Study Limitations

This study has several limitations. It has been noted by Stanton (2004) that women's retrospective self-reported preparations for childbirth may be influenced by the care they receive during childbirth, and that such self-reports may be subject to increased recall errors as time elapses. We had no means of independently verifying that reported preparations had been made for the births under question. In addition, it is important to acknowledge that women's knowledge related to birth preparedness and obstetric complications may be informed by experiences during their most recent pregnancy or birth. Because this study used a retrospective design, we cannot be sure that respondents' BP/CR knowledge at the time of the survey was consistent with their knowledge at the time of the birth in question.

Third, the study did not include assessments of the capacity of local health facilities and maternity staff to provide care for normal and complicated deliveries. Clients' perceptions of service quality are known to influence their care-seeking behaviors; however, we were not able to control for service quality across the study areas. Finally, as noted earlier, the study was conducted in two periurban areas of Guinea, and the sample is not nationally representative.

DISCUSSION

Interventions promoting BP/CR are intuitively appealing; however, the influence of such interventions on women's preparation for birth and their use of institutional delivery care is unclear. To date, in program design and intervention research, operational definitions of birth preparedness have varied widely, with some such interventions focused primarily on preparations for any delivery (normal or complicated) and other interventions focusing primarily on readiness for both maternal and newborn complications. Research and evaluations related to BP/CR interventions have yielded mixed evidence on the efficacy of such interventions; while some studies have indicated that BP/CR interventions are effective in increasing use of skilled delivery care (Magoma et al., 2013), others—and particularly studies of interventions that focused primarily on complications readiness—have not shown any positive association with institutional delivery (Kumar et al., 2008; McPherson et al., 2006). Nonetheless, many researchers call for increased attention to educating pregnant women about obstetric risks and danger signs in order to increase their use of skilled maternity care and to prevent delays in care-seeking for complications (Ekabua et al., 2011, Hailu et al., 2011, Kabakyenga et al., 2012; Kakaire et al., 2011; Mutiso et al., 2008).

The findings of this study help to further elucidate the pathway between BP/CR interventions, household preparation for birth, and women's use of institutional delivery care. We found that facility- and community-level interventions promoting BP/CR were both positively associated with increased knowledge about both birth preparedness and complication readiness. Complication readiness knowledge (i.e., knowledge about obstetric risks and danger signs), however, was not associated with increased preparation for childbirth or with women's use of health facilities for delivery.

In contrast, women's knowledge about routine birth preparations (e.g., deciding place of delivery, saving money for delivery, making arrangements for transport, etc.) was positively associated with their practice of birth preparedness, which was itself strongly associated with institutional delivery.

Importantly, neither literacy nor wealth status were significantly associated with higher preparation for birth. In view of the strong association between birth preparation and use of institutional delivery, these findings are noteworthy as they suggest that promoting birth preparedness among poor and low-literate women can be an important strategy for addressing wealth disparities in use of professional maternity care.

Other researchers (Barber, 2006; Bloom, et al., 1999; Kabakyenga et al., 2012; Mpembeni et al., 2007) have highlighted the positive relationship between the quantity of ANC (measured in terms of number of visits) and women's use of institutional delivery care. Our findings underscore the importance of the counseling that women receive during these visits. In our multivariate models, receiving BP/CR counseling had a stronger association with women's preparation for birth and their use of institutional delivery than did receipt of four or more ANC visits.

The above findings have important implications for the design of both community- and facility-level interventions to improve maternal survival. During the past two decades, considerable efforts have been made in community-level interventions to raise awareness of pregnancy-related risks and danger signs in order to address the "three delays" (Thaddeus & Maine, 1994) that contribute to maternal mortality and morbidity. A key assumption behind such interventions is that knowledge about obstetric risks and danger signs will motivate the use of professional maternity care and will reduce delays in recognizing life-threatening obstetric complications when they arise and in reaching and receiving appropriate care. In our study, exposure to community-level maternal health promotion efforts was associated with increased knowledge about obstetric risks and danger signs. This knowledge, however, was not associated with preparation for birth or with women's use of institutional delivery.

These findings raise questions about the utility of focusing on danger signs and risk awareness in community-level interventions to promote women's use of professional maternity care. Instead, such interventions might be better focused on promoting household preparations for accessing skilled maternity care during all births and on catalyzing changes in social and gender norms related to birth preparedness, including increasing the involvement of male partners, which other research has highlighted as important (Iliyasu, Abubakar, Galadanci, & Aliyu, 2010; Kakaire et al., 2011; Mullany et al., 2007).

Similarly, based on the study findings, we suggest that ANC providers' limited time for counseling might be best devoted to advising on place of delivery and specific preparations that should be made for any birth—normal or complicated. Almost two decades have passed since the antenatal risk screening approach has been discredited, and it is widely agreed that every birth should be attended by a skilled health professional (Campbell & Graham, 2006). Nevertheless, many women who attend antenatal care are not advised to deliver at a health facility. In our sample of women with recent births, fully 50% reported that they were not advised on any preparation for childbirth (i.e., setting aside money, arranging for transport, discussing and agreeing on plans with family members, etc.) during any of their ANC visits, and 44% reported that they were not advised to deliver in a health facility. The findings from our study suggest that focusing on risks and danger signs during ANC counseling may have little or no effect on routine care-seeking. The findings also raise questions about whether focusing on risks and danger signs may have the unintended effect of reinforcing outdated perceptions that home births are safe for "normal" pregnancies and deliveries.

Finally, we suggest that women's planning for and use of maternal health services may not be motivated by fear or concerns about risks—a finding that is consistent with conclusions from a meta-analysis of more than 350 HIV prevention interventions, which concluded that interventions designed to induce fear were not effective, compared with interventions that were designed in accordance with theories of reasoned action and planned behavior (Albarracín, Durantini, & Earl, 2006). Focusing on birth preparedness can offer women and their families specific, concrete actions they can take to ensure access to professional care during childbirth, whereas focusing on risks and danger signs does not appear to achieve the same results.

Consistent with these findings, it is worth noting that simply knowing pregnancy risks and danger signs will not be sufficient to overcome the formidable barriers posed by large geographic distances and limited means of transport—particularly in contexts where the limited availability and quality of basic obstetric care at primary health care facilities result in the practice of "bypassing" local health facilities because of the poor quality of care available (Kruk et al., 2009). Indeed, in such settings, advance decision-making, planning, and preparation for institutional delivery offer the only means of accessing such care when labor begins.

ACKNOWLEDGMENTS

The authors thank Abigail Greenleaf for her review of the literature on birth preparedness, as well as Evelyn Landry, EngenderHealth, and Mary Ellen Stanton and Erin Mielke for reviewing and commenting on drafts of this article.

FUNDING

This study was funded through the U.S. Agency for International Development (USAID), under associate cooperative agreement GHS-A-00-07-00021-00. Views expressed here do not necessarily reflect those of USAID.

REFERENCES

Agarwal, S., Sethi, V., Srivastava, K., Jha, P., & Baqui, A. (2010). Birth preparedness and complication readiness among slum women in indoor city, India. *Journal of Health and Population Nutrition, 4*, 383–391.

Albarracín, D., Durantini, N., & Earl, A. (2006). Empirical and theoretical conclusions of an analysis of outcomes of HIV-prevention interventions. *Current Directions in Psychological Research, 15*(2), 73–78.

Barber, S. (2006). Does the quality of prenatal care matter in promoting skilled institutional delivery? A study in rural Mexico. *Maternal and Child Health Journal, 10*(5), 419–425.

Barros, A., Ronsmans, C., Axelson, H., Loaiza, E., Bertoldi, A. D., França, G., ... Victora, C. G. (2012). Equity in maternal, newborn, and child health interventions in Countdown to 2015: A retrospective review of survey data from 54 countries. *The Lancet, 379*, 1225–1233.

Bloom, S., Lippeveld, T., & Wypij, D. (1999). Does antenatal care make a difference to safe delivery? A study in urban Uttar Pradesh, India. *Health Policy and Planning, 14*(1), 38–48.

Byass, P., & Graham, W. J. (2011). Grappling with uncertainties along the MDG trail. *The Lancet, 378*, 1119–1120.

Campbell, O., & Graham, W. (2006). Strategies for reducing maternal mortality: Getting on with what works. *The Lancet, 368*, 1284–1299.

Ekabua, J., Ekabua, K., Odusolu, P., Agan, T., Iklaki, C., & Etokidem, A. (2011). Awareness of birth preparedness and complication readiness in southeastern Nigeria. *ISRN Obstetrics and Gynecology, 2011*, 1–6. doi:10.5402/2011/560641.

Filmer, D., & Pritchett, L. (2001). Estimating wealth effects without expenditure data—or tears: An application to educational enrollments in states of India. *Demography, 38*(1), 115–132.

Hailu, M., Gebremariam, A., Alemseged, F., & Deribe, K. (2011). Birth preparedness and complication readiness among pregnant women in Southern Ethiopia. *PLoS ONE, 6*, 1–7.

Hogan, M. C., Foreman, K. J., Naghavi, M., Ahn, S. Y., Wang, M., Makela, S. M., ... Murray, C. R. L. (2011). Maternal mortality for 181 countries, 1980–2008: A systematic analysis of progress towards Millennium Development Goal 5. *The Lancet, 375*, 1609–1623.

Iliyasu, Z., Abubakar, I., Galadanci, H., & Aliyu, M. (2010). Birth preparedness, complication readiness and fathers' participation in maternity care in a northern Nigerian community. *African Journal of Reproductive Health, 14*, 21–32.

Institute National de la Statistique (INS). (2012). *Enquête démographique et de santé et à indicateurs multiples (EDS-MICS IV)*. Conakry, Guinea: Author, Ministère du Plan, Ministère de la Santé et de l'Hygiène Publique, MEASURE DHS, ICF International.

Kabakyenga, J., Ostergren, P., Turyakira, E., & Pettersson, K. (2012). Influence of birth preparedness, decision-making on location of birth and assistance by skilled birth attendants among women in south-western Uganda. *PLoS ONE, 7*(4), e35747. doi:10.1371/jo

Kakaire, O., Kaye, D., & Osinde, M. (2011). Male involvement in birth preparedness and complication readiness for emergency obstetric referrals in rural Uganda. *Reproductive Health, 8*, 12–19.

Karkee, R., Lee, A. H., & Binns, C. W. (2013). Birth preparedness and skilled attendance at birth in Nepal: Implications for achieving millennium development goal 5. *Midwifery, 29*, 1206–1210.

Kruk, M., Mbaruku, G., McCord, C., Moran, M., Rockers, P., & Galea, S. (2009). Bypassing primary care facilities for childbirth: A population-based study in Tanzania. *Health Policy and Planning, 24*, 279–288.

Kumar, V., Mohanty, S., Kumar, A., Misa, R., Santosham, M., Awasthi, S., . . . Singh, P. (2008). Effect of community-based behavior change management on neonatal mortality in Shivgarh, Uttar Pradesh, India: A cluster-randomised controlled trial. *The Lancet, 372*, 1151–1162.

Langer, A., Horton, R., & Chalamilla, G. (2013). A manifesto for maternal health post-2015. *The Lancet, 381*, 601–602.

Lozano, R., Wang, H., Foreman, K. J., Rajaratnam, K. J., Naghavi, M., Marcus, J. R., . . . Murray, C. J. L. (2011). Progress towards Millennium Development Goals 4 and 5 on maternal and child mortality: An updated systematic analysis. *The Lancet, 378*, 1139–1165.

Magoma, M., Requejo, J., Campbell, O., Cousens, S., Merialdi, M., & Filippi, V. (2013). The effectiveness of birth plans in increasing use of skilled care at delivery and postnatal care in rural Tanzania: A cluster randomized trial. *Tropical Medicine & International Health, 18*(4), 435–443.

McPherson, R., Khadka, N., Moore, J., & Sharma, M. (2006). Are birth-preparedness programmes effective? Results from a field trial in Siraha district, Nepal. *Journal of Health, Population and Nutrition, 4*, 479–488.

Moran, A., Sangli, G., Dineen, R., Rawlins, B., Yaméogo, M., & Baya, B. (2006). Birth-preparedness for maternal health: Findings from Koupéla District, Burkina Faso. *Journal of Health, Population and Nutrition, 24*(4), 489–497.

Mpembeni, R. N. M., Killewo, J. Z., Leshabari, M. T., Massawe, S. N., Jahn, A., Mushi, D., & Mwakipa, H. (2007). Use pattern of maternal health services and determinants of skilled care during delivery in Southern Tanzania. *BioMed Central Pregnancy and Childbirth, 7*, 29. doi:10.1186/1471-2393-7-29

Mullany, B., Becker, S., & Hindin, M. (2007). The impact of including husbands in antenatal health education services on maternal health practices in urban Nepal: Results from a randomized controlled trial. *Health Education Research, 22*, 166–167.

Mutiso, S., Qureshi, Z., & Kinuthia, J. (2008). Birth preparedness among antenatal clients. *East African Medical Journal, 85*, 275–283.

Solnes Miltenburg, A., Roggeveen, Y., van Elteren, M., Shields, L., Bunders, J., van Roosmalen, J., & Stekelenburg, J. (2013). A protocol for a systematic review of birth preparedness and complication readiness programs. *Systematic Reviews, 2*(11), 1–8. Retrieved from http://www.systematicreviewsjournal.com/content/pdf/2046-4053-2-11.pdf

Stanton, C. (2004). Methodological issues in the measurement of birth preparedness in support of safe motherhood. *Evaluation Review, 28*, 179–200.

Thaddeus, S., & Maine, D. (1994). Too far to walk: Maternal mortality in context. *Social Science and Medicine, 38*(8), 1091–1110.

Turan, J. M., Tesfagiorghis, M., & Polan, M. (2011). Evaluation of a community intervention for promotion of safe motherhood in Eritrea. *Journal of Midwifery and Women's Health*, *56*, 8–17.

United Nations (UN). (2012). *The Millennium Development Goals Report*. New York, NY: Author.

United Nations Development Program (UNDP). (2011). *Human Development Report. Sustainability and equity: A better future for all*. New York, NY: Author.

World Health Organization (WHO). (2010). *Trends in maternal mortality: 1990 to 2008*. Geneva, Switzerland: Author, World Bank, United Nations International Children's Emergency Fund (UNICEF), United Nations Population Fund (UNFPA). Retrieved from http://whqlibdoc.who.int/publications/2010/9789241500265_eng.pdf

Teenage Sexuality, HIV Risk, and the Politics of Being "Duted": Perceptions and Dynamics in a South African Township

NOKUTHULA HLABANGANE

*Department of Anthropology and Archaeology, University of South Africa,
Pretoria, South Africa*

*HIV risk among teenagers is argued to be entangled with a plethora
of other risks so that HIV-related risk may not be a paramount
consideration. Teenage sexuality is a subject fraught with such
consideration. This article is an ethnographic rendition of teenage
sexuality in action in a South African township.*

Young people know how to prevent HIV; what continues to drive the
epidemic is not their response to the message but how they view their
educational, social and economic circumstance. Through collective effort
we can give young people a chance to think of their futures in a different
way so that they can become drivers of change in our society.

—*LoveLife, 2010*

South Africa has the highest HIV/AIDS rate in the world. In many cases
HIV risk is measured through unidimensional surveys in the tradition of the
knowledge, attitude, practices, and behavior (KAPB) health belief model and
thus fails to highlight the qualitative nuances of everyday sexual considerations (see Pelto and Pelto, 1997, and Pool and Geissler, 2007, for a similar
analysis). Bolton (1999) argues that the urgency to resolve HIV-related questions has engendered practices that are detrimental to the social sciences
in general and to anthropology in particular. These include the tendency to
artificially extricate sexual behavior, for instance, from the relations of power
and meaning that animate it. Here, the focus of analysis becomes individual
sexual behavior rather than the systems of relations that underlie and shape

it. Studies on teenage sexuality have also tended to emphasize individual behavior.

Sexuality embodies the tension between agency and structure. So while I posit apartheid legacies as exemplified in family structure, access to material resources and the general environment that makes Soweto, the research setting, I endeavor to juxtapose the deterministic potential of this structure against individual and intersubjective agency. Further, the topic of sexuality is ubiquitous and, therefore, demands that we make and recognize the links that may not be as apparent but are central to its credible analysis. The choice of the age group under study is informed by the assumption that this age group offers a window of a changing sexuality from sexual experimentation and the attendant contradictions to a consolidation, so to speak, of "teenage sexuality." Participants have in common their age grouping; identify as heterosexual; and are also exposed, to varying extents, to the contextual factors that make the place Soweto with its particular history. The rationale for including both boys and girls in conversation is that they imply one another. To understand teenage sexuality necessarily means that the gender influence be made explicit. Therefore, to understand the sexual character and expression of girls, one has to bring into relief the sexual character and expression of boys and vice versa.

Qualitative data gathering strategies including focus group discussions (FGDs) in the first instance and individual in-depth interviews later were employed. Efforts were made to retain FGDs participants for the longitudinal individual in-depth interviews. The broad, entry-point questions that were asked during the FGDs were revisited in the individual interviews to explore them further. Other emerging concerns were allowed expression in the individual interviews. In all, 12 FGDs were carried out in three different locations that were chosen for their alleged socioeconomic complexion. The FGDs were both gender biased (females only and males only) and gender mixed (males and females together). Of those who participated in FGDs, 23 participated in the longitudinal, in-depth individual interviews. Data were interpreted through the paradigms espoused by grounded theory (Glaser, 1992), including relying on my social competence in the research setting. Data for this research were collected intermittently between June 2008 and December 2009 as part of doctoral research.

This article is an attempt to solicit the voices of young people and explore their everyday encounters with the reality of HIV/AIDS. In particular, I recognize and highlight the myriad "risks" embedded in the lives of the young people in Soweto, South Africa. The informants of this study are 14–19-year-old boys and girls who reside in Soweto, Johannesburg, South Africa. They, more than their White counterparts, inspire labels such as "Black youth at risk," "the lost generation," and "youth crying out for help." They reflect the brutal history of South Africa. They embody the political economy of South Africa in the same way that Fassin (2007) argues that a microreading of his subjects' narratives is not just because beyond the utterances by individual subjects lies a history of systematic exploitation, brutalization, and deprivation. Stillwaggon (2006, p. 157) characterizes the stories of so-called AIDS sufferers as "individual effects of multilevel causes." She goes further to argue that "by accepting the wrong paradigm, the AIDS discourse has failed to ask the right questions, and failed to understand the complexity of AIDS" (p. 157). Frayser (1985) also suggests that when important life questions are taken care of and, thus, taken for granted, the individual is better able to pursue individual interests. In other words, there is a need to elevate HIV/AIDS (risk) analysis by framing it in its complexity; the idea of HIV risk as embedded in individual sexual behavior wherein lasting solutions could be found is no longer viable. A new paradigm for understanding HIV/AIDS risk that goes beyond individual complicity is needed.

The lack of a broad-based systematic effort to understand the content and dynamics of teenage sexuality is despite the fact that each day 7,000 people between the ages of 15 and 24 are infected with HIV worldwide, resulting in 2.6 million new infections per year, 1.7 million of which occur in Africa (UNAIDS, 2002). Similarly, most new infections in South Africa occur among young people (McClure, Gray, & Rybczyk, 2004). The Nelson Mandela Human Science Research Council's (NMHSRC) household survey conducted in 2002 in South Africa highlighted the vulnerability of this age group to HIV infection, with 10% of the study population (which is representative of the wider South African population) already living with HIVAIDS (Shisana & Simbayi, 2002). The authors of this study recommended a systematic investigation of teenage sexuality if appropriate interventions are to be instituted for this age group, identifying a number of contributory factors such as statutory rape, sexual coercion, child sexual abuse and intergenerational sex. The findings of the NMHSRC study were corroborated by the Reproductive Health Research Unit a few years later. In this study, the HIV prevalence rate was 4.8% among boys and 15.5% among girls aged between 15 and 24 (Pettifor, Rees, Steffenson, Hlongwa-Madikizela, & McPhail, 2005).

TOWARD UNDERSTANDING SEXUAL RISK: A GENDERED PERSPECTIVE

Risk has always been synonymous with sex. Vance (1992) and feminist thinkers, generally, take the view that women are not safe in sexual relations. Feminists argue that women lack the social, economic, political, and cultural clout to influence sexual relationships to their advantage. This age-old argument is carried in De Beauvoir's (1952) characterization of women as "the second sex." Similarly, ideas about women being Other (De Beauvoir) speak to the assertion that "Access to power is based on a hierarchy where male is preferred over female (Ayieri, 2010, p. 13). From this point of view, 'normal' is defined from the perspective of the heterosexual [white] male and other perspectives are peripheral" (Ayieri).

Teenage sexuality is also conceptualized as reckless and risk prone (see, for instance, Campbell and McPhail, 2002, about young people's views on condom use for such an analysis). The reality of HIV/AIDS has further high-lighted the risky nature of sex. Therefore, any consideration of sexuality is not complete without considering questions of disproportional vulnerability to HIV risk, risk perception, and risk aversion. HIV vulnerability is exacer-bated by the lack of power of individuals and communities to minimize or modulate their risk. The HIV risk status of individuals and communities is thus compounded by neglect and marginalization. The politics of HIV risk perception and aversion have gone full circle in many respects. In particular, in South Africa the advent of HIV/AIDS has met with a number of stumbling blocks. Notably are the so-called AIDS denialism and the concomitant lack of political will to tackle the epidemic head-on.

Life in Soweto, and townships like it, is characterized by want and deprivation, resulting in a general feeling of vulnerability that engenders high levels of risk tolerance. Young people have daily encounters with risk to the extent that their decisions may be influenced by a hierarchy of risks. Sexual risk is but one of such risks; and it may not be foremost in their assessment of danger. This may especially be the case for boys who are more likely to be party to the other risky/dangerous elements of life in Soweto. Girls, on the other hand, were more in touch with and aware of sexual risk because they are the main victims of sexual violence. They related a sense of widespread sexual risk. Three female participants related rape experiences, two by people whom they knew and trusted. These are common stories (see Jewkes and Abrahams, 2002, and Vetten et al., 2008 for a detailed exposition of rape and sexual coercion in South Africa). Also common is the sense of being at risk from sexual assault not only from strangers but also from males in general.

The female participants were aware of their rights to safety and bodily integrity and the recourse that is open to them in the form of the justice system. They also had a keen sense that practical access to judicial recourse was difficult, however, and they did not trust this system. Following the jus-tice system route may also be hampered by a sense of shame and self-blame characteristic of such an experience. The girls who participated in this re-search expressed an awareness that how they dressed or carried themselves has nothing to do with possible sexual assault. They also had not inter-nalized the negative images that males seem to have of them. In Soweto, Leclerc-Madlala's (2002) characterization of the female body perceived as essentially dirty and contaminating did not apply. For example, the notion that menstrual blood is "dirty" and can harm a sexual partner did not apply. Consideration was rather given to comfort and hygiene in its simplest form in this regard. This rejection of negative social connotations informed the fighting spirit that the female participants displayed. They were not unduly burdened by the said "inferior" status that supposedly emanates from their sex as females. In particular, the female participants rejected responsibility for the conduct of their male counterparts, understanding sexual assault as a violation that deserved punishment.

Interestingly and perhaps very telling of their ownership of the HIV epidemic is that the notion that men can force themselves on women because "she drank my money" (Wojcicki, 2002) is outdated in view of the possibility that the woman may be infected with HIV, as a participant related:

> Like he said, many boys do not know that if they buy alcohol and expect payment in return, what does the person from whom he expects payment has on her. Let us say AIDS—he does not know. So if he expects me to pay him, I would not mind doing that because I know I have AIDS and I do not want to die alone. So I think: "This person wants me to pay him, I will pay him and if he suggests that we use a condom, I will say I do not eat a sweet with its wrapping on." I will insist on "skin-to-skin" and I won't stop with him. So the "mentality" that boys have that they will expect payment for things that they buy us is outdated. (*Thato, 17-year-old female, mixed gender FGD, Mofolo*)

In other words, men have to consider possible HIV infection if they want to force themselves on women. So while the young women felt vulnerable to sexual assault by men, they recognized and highlighted the danger that such acts may pose to the men. These arguments underscore Bujra's (2000) assertion that although women have always had a fair dose of mistrust for men, HIV/AIDS has also engendered a sense that male authority over women cannot go unchallenged.

Girls are said to be "eaten" and are not endowed with the ability to also "eat" in return. As they are eaten, however, they are "loose" because they were supposed to resist being "eaten." They thus pose a sexual risk to their partners. A recurring argument is that although women are seen as essentially *femme fatale*, they are also gullible because they can be sweet-talked into anything (hence they need the guidance and protection of some man). Girls dismissed this view of them as limited, however, and to the detriment of men. In other words, girls were quick to assert their agency in relationships with their male counterparts. Research has, generally, overlooked this agency, on the whole painting girls as victims except when they actively seek the proverbial 3Cs—clothes, cellphones and cash—,from "sugar daddies" (Leclerc-Madlala, 2003). Implicit in such research is the notion that young women, who purportedly lack negotiation skills to secure favorable bases for a sexual relationship, are necessarily always taken advantage of by such relationships. Such a view fails to appreciate that while girls in their individual capacity may be taken advantage of against their will, they are part of families that may play a protective role. Boys, in particular, pointed out that their treatment of girls is sometimes mediated by consideration of

the potential reaction of, say, a "gun-touting uncle," as one male participant declared. The idea that girls are necessarily always taken advantage of
by sexual relations resonates with the implicit notion ingrained in research
on teenage sexuality that girls should always and inevitably resist sexual
involvement with their male counterparts. This notion highlights a commod-
ification of women that renders them objects to be pawned between men.
Competition in sexual relationships, however, was not confined to males
competing for female attention. Females were not hapless in this process;
they may also do their own cheating;

> Yes, you may think that you are the only one, but you may never know
> (for sure). You do not stay at her house and you may not spend all the
> time with her during the day. You would never know all her comings
> and goings. (*Noma, 17-year-old female, mixed FGD, Pimville*)

Here, again, we see an assertion of wills on the nature of the relationship,
pointing to both the lack of trust between the parties concerned and the all-
too-often downplayed agency of girls in setting the tone of the relationship.

There was also a mutual lack of trust between boys and girls (even when
they were in relationship). This lack of trust extended to the consideration
that a sexual partner is a potential conduit for disease and thus a threat. One
way to get around this was to stay with the tried and familiar with the hope
of exerting control on an otherwise unpredictable terrain:

> For the record, I do not go out with girls I meet at parties. I cannot
> sleep with a person I have no idea who else she slept with and then I
> also sleep with her. I proposition girls from my neighbourhood and from
> school. That is where I look. I know that I meet her at school every day.
> Even if she gives me a challenge, tomorrow we have an understanding.
> Imagine being given a challenge by a girl at a party! That is ridiculous. I
> know that I will meet this other one at school. I would buy her lunch.
> Being given a challenge at a party, I would be drunk obviously. (*Keke,
> 18-year-old male, all male FGD, Mofolo*)

Keke's input above, while on the surface, shows a particular street wisdom,
falls into the proverbial shortcoming that HIV risk is visible and can thus be
avoided by employing "safe" measures that eliminate risk. I would like to
argue that while Sowetans, as perhaps most South Africans, do adopt a "you
never know, so it is better to be safe than sorry" attitude (cf. Sobo, 1993),
the idea that one can make calculated assessment of another's HIV status
persists. This remains one of the primary drivers of the spread of HIV among
young people, especially. I argue that while HIV does constitute a primary
concern, this concern is tempered by some distance to the immediacy of the
threat on this age cohort. This point is also made by Varga and Makubalo
(1996) when they contend that young people have not internalized HIV risk.

To this end, I go on to argue that the incubation period from HIV to AIDS further informs the lack of ownership of young people's vulnerability to HIV. The incubation period means that young people do not have real-life examples of peers afflicted by the epidemic.

The distrust expressed by boys talks to the fear of being trapped into (undeserved) fatherhood. This was compounded by a sense that their traditional hold on girls was being compromised by girls who were taking matters into their own hands. The girls were not waiting to be cheated on but were doing their own cheating. The distrust between girls and boys is perhaps pronounced in this time of HIV and is fueled by fears of potential HIV infection as shown below:

> Even if she is old [as opposed to being young and gullible], when you suggest this [whatever this is], she says yes. Something must make you wary, why is this girl saying yes to everything? You may say, "Let us go and sleep, we won't use a condom." She agrees to everything. You have to ask yourself, "Why is she so quick to agree to everything?" (*Bonolo, 19-year-old male, all male FGD, Mofolo*)

Further,

> Even if she does want to do these things, she will want to argue first. (*Bongane, 19-year-old male, all male FGD, Mofolo*)

Similarly,

> *Bonolo (19-year-old male, all male FGD, Mofolo)*: But the one who does not want to argue—be wary, something must be wrong. She has lit a cable.
> *Moderator*: What does that mean?
> *Thabiso (19-year-old male, all male FGD, Mofolo)*: She is tracking. She wants to infect you.

The discussion continues:

> Those who agree to sleep with you without a condom are dangerous. If I say to a girl, "Let us not use a condom" and she agrees without hesitation, I become suspicious. What is this? Why is she agreeing to all this? Is she afraid of me, or what? (*Baholo, 18-year-old male, all male FGD, Mofolo*)

The theme above reiterates a recurring concept in sexual relations that accords disproportional responsibility for the well-being of the relationship to girls. This is in the same vein that girls and women are not only expected to manage their own sexuality but also that of boys and men, which is said to be urgent and uncontrollable (Varga, 2004). Such expectations are despite the fact that women may not necessarily always have the ability to control their own but men's sexuality as well. So, when a girl is being invited to a sexual encounter, she is given the responsibility to mediate this with reason and caution lest she is regarded with suspicion. The rationale is that a girl who is seen to be unnecessarily eager to engage in a sexual encounter may have a sinister agenda to "off-load" an infection onto an unsuspecting male. The advent of HIV/AIDS has resurrected notions of women as contaminating and dangerous to men's sexual health (Bujra, 2000; Esplen, 2007; Leclerc-Madlala, 2002). These sentiments were expressed by the fearful male participants, and the female participants did not necessarily assimilate and own them. This is generally not how the girls thought of themselves: by virtue of being women they possess polluting properties. This, however, did not stop them from acknowledging that they can also potentially infect a man with HIV and other sexually transmitted diseases should they be infected, as shown above. The fears that the possibility of condomless sex invoke also refer to the age-old fear that a man can be trapped into (undeserved) fatherhood. This, in fact, may be a bigger consideration than HIV infection. This is in the same vein that girls may put more consideration on preventing a pregnancy by using contraceptives than on HIV infection (Varga, 2004).

So while I argue for girls' agency in sexual relationships, it is relative; it is not absolute. Holland and colleagues (1994) attribute the ambiguous position that girls find themselves in to the romanticized notion that love entails trust and the concomitant need to please one's sexual partner sometimes at one's expense. The ability of girls to "pick and choose" sexual partners is curtailed by the societal attitude that discourages a sexually knowing girl who can negotiate on her own behalf. They also point to the gap between knowledge and practice—what Holland and colleagues (1994) call a "disembodied sexuality"—where girls do not practice what they know to be good and safe for their sexual well-being.

The following series of extracts is presented together to underscore several interlinked points (they represent a conversation where one comment elicited another). Two points in particular are being made in the conversation; local ideas of what kind of girl poses HIV risk and the politics of opportunity that go beyond the former considerations:

> You look at the girl's status—you can see if a girl is running around (promiscuous) and the other one is more home-bound—the woman of the house. (*Wanda, 18-year-old male, mixed gender FGD, Pimville*)

> Let me tell you, the innocent ones are the most promiscuous. (*Mbali, 16-year-old female, mixed gender FGD, Pimville*)

> I am quiet and listening, but my view is that sometimes when an opportunity for sex presents itself and you do not have a condom and you

decide to go ahead (and have sex anyway). The consideration of how a girl is (what type of a girl she is) has little to do with it. (*Sthe, 19-year-old male, mixed gender FGD, Pimville*)

If we have condoms, we will use them and if not ... (*Unaccounted for voice*)

Let me add—you know, the innocent-looking ones are the ones who bring troubles. Miss Innocent stays at home every day and gets pregnant, and the one who is fly does not. (*Lebo, 17-year-old female, mixed gender FGD, Pimville*)

The above extracts also introduce the idea that while a girl's "risk profile," so to speak, may be read from her perceived sexual comportment, this is not cut and dried. Those who may be perceived to be "innocent" may actually prove to be more "dangerous." Again, the notion of taking advantage of an opportunity to have sex with little regard to the safety of such an encounter is brought to the fore. According to Sthe above, such a consideration does not also extend to the "kind" of girl she is. The paramount consideration is to take advantage of the opportunity for a sexual encounter.

WILLFUL TRANSGRESSION—BEYOND A REDUCTIONIST VIEW OF SEXUAL RISK

The politics of condom use and concomitant risk behaviors are complicated, defying the all-too-easy utilitarian analyses to which they have been subjected:

Moderator: So, whose responsibility is it to ensure that condoms are used?

Keke (18-year-old male, all male FGD Mofolo): But the truth is that we boys are obstinate. I could say I do not have a condom on me and the girl then says, "Well, bad luck." I would push it, trying to get my way by saying, "Look, we are both ready." Obviously, she will end up doing it without really wanting to just to satisfy me and after she has satisfied me, I no longer care about her.

Moderator: After she has satisfied you, you no longer care for her?

Keke: Yes, that is the life of boys. She should play hard to get. We like a challenge.

Keke's input above points to the gender-based assertion of wills in sexual relationships. Risk is here carried in the sense of being in the thick of things where rational thought is deliberately suspended. So, while the boy would want to test and push sexual boundaries, the girl, on the other hand, is expected to fight very hard to maintain these boundaries:

> There are things that you do and you do not want your parents to know about. . . . It is like when you have stolen, would you agree that you have stolen? (*Mthokozisi, 18-year-old male, all male FGD, Pimville*)

> Guys even when we were still very young we were told that when you sleep with a girl without a condom you will make a child, so there is no mistake about it! (*Bobo, 16-year-old male, all male FGD, Pimville*)

> We do these things knowing well enough—let us say we are from a party and we are drunk from whatever—you cannot think when you are that drunk, worry about condom. . . . We might resort to the "morning-after" pill. (*Sthe, 19-year-old male, all male FGD, Pimville*)

Embedded in the extracts above is a connotation of risk beyond reason—willful transgression. This is one of the discussions that I felt the participants were no longer talking to me but to each other, showing the centrality of the issues under discussion to their everyday concerns. The question of willful transgression in relation to risk-taking behavior has not received much attention. Instead, commentators have concentrated on the purported lack of knowledge that informs risk-taking behavior. Willful transgression relates to a number of considerations: in particular, that it is ingrained human nature to want to transgress social boundaries and that this tendency may be accentuated in young people whose "larger-than-life" streak has not been punished and thus checked by life experience. Perhaps the difference in susceptibility between young people who take measured, life-affirming decisions and those who are "careless" with their lives is a world view that is tolerant of high levels of risk, itself a reflection of life experiences. From this point of view, it may be instructive to expand opportunities for young people that allow them to express themselves in ways that are not detrimental to their well-being.

RISKY RELATIONSHIPS

Both Bolton (1999) and Watney (1999) argue for a holistic interpretation of HIV sexual risk. Bolton argues for research that is sensitive to the nuances embedded in sexual decision-making and sexual performance, while Watney argues for safe sex as community practice. The sexual choices that individuals make may be indicative of their needs in particular relationships. For instance, Holland and colleagues (1998) write about the "bastard" male syndrome, where young males move from one relationship to another with little thought; rejection from any of the girls is met with indifference because this does not impact on their sense of self. Much like Mthokozisi's tongue-in-cheek comment below that signals what in the township is euphemistically called "living in the fast lane":

> At this time, there is no longer time to fix things [*laughter*]. You just "hit and run." Really there is no time to fix anything—you go forward. (*Mthokozisi, 18-year-old male, all male FGD, Pimville*)

Holland and colleagues (1998) juxtapose this with another type of male who invests himself in a few relationships with girls and may thus feel a personal rejection when the relationships do not work out. From this point of view, one may argue that depending on the particular needs of the individuals involved and the nature of the relationship, concerns of risk would vary.

For instance there is a somewhat rigid characterization of a sexual relationship as a one-night stand, "jolling," or being in relationship in popular discourse in Soweto (cf. Mkhwanazi, 2010). One-night stands are purely about sex and are likely to emanate in settings like parties and street bashes where alcohol use is rife. "Jolling" is a common arrangement that is trickier to characterize as it embodies a somewhat nebulous relationship as is shown by Collette's contribution below:

> No, it was just simple jolling. We were just playing. That thing to say I also have a boyfriend. ... You see, that boy I was jolling with would not have insisted that we do this or that (because we were just "jolling"). (*Collette, 18-year-old female, individual interview, Mofolo*)

Thabiso related a similar opinion:

> It is not my priority that when we are jolling, we should have sex. But it is something that could happen after some time. You do not know the person, you need to know the person first. (*Thabiso, 19-year-old male, individual interview, Mofolo*)

While the term is nebulous, in my view, it connotes a somewhat stable liaison that may call for exclusivity, but at the same time, by its nebulousness leaves room for engaging in other sexual relationships. In other words, extra-affair liaisons can be justified in a "jolling" relationship. This is, however, not the case with "being in relationship," which connotes more seriousness and permanence and thus exclusivity. A "jolling" relationship is at once in line with the idea of "passing time" as on the whole posited by the male participants in an attempt to dismiss the importance of a relationship (that may have gone sour due to some alleged misdeed by the girl).

Both the questions of emotional involvement and condom use cannot be imposed on any of these arrangements in any straightforward way. It

would thus be shortsighted to claim that a particular "type" of relationship would necessarily and automatically result in a particular type of sexual behavior. For instance, the participants argue that they are likely to use condoms in casual relationships. There are extenuating factors to this, however, such as disinhibition when drunk. The same argument against a utilitarian individual who always makes health-affirming decisions applies to the other "types" of relationships. While an individual may not always and necessarily make life-affirming sexual decisions, there is also ingrained caution against making reckless decisions that are akin to "living in the fast lane." The significance of this lies in the notion that one's clever antics would render one "an example"—a "clever" who is ultimately a victim of these supposedly clever antics. In the same vein, one is cautioned against indulging in pleasurable pursuits—*ubumnandi*—that may result in dire long-term consequences. Here we see sexual risk behavior being cautioned, drawing from everyday wisdom.

Thus different relations engender different expectations that influence sexual decisions and inform HIV risk perception. This is reflected in notions that have come to connote condom use. In particular, notions of trust are said to confound consistent condom use. For instance, Varga (1997) argues that, in many cases, sex workers contract HIV in nonprofessional sexual relations from which they derive a sense of belonging and intimacy. In the same vein, longer-standing relationships may, in fact, pose more risk to the individuals involved as condom use becomes more lax as trust becomes part of the relationship. If sexual relations are a quest for intimacy, safer sex tampers with this (Taylor, 1990). In the same vein, Bujra (2000) argues that "to trust is to court risk." Watney (1999) suggests that safer sex not only be made a community practice, thus eliminating its context specificity, but also that it should be made erotic. Eroticizing safer sex is a step toward affirming the affective nature of sexual relations. Grafting condom use into an erotic script may begin to tamper with the connotations of trust and suspicion that beset safer sex. This may also help sustain condom use over time. Condoms have become part of the sexual discourse of young people; whether they use them or not is a loaded consideration. On the whole, as illustrated in this article, condoms are associated with HIV risk elimination.

PEER PRESSURE AND THE POLITICS OF BEING "DUTED"

The influential role of peer pressure in teenage sexual decision making has been highlighted (Eaton, Flisher, & Aaro, 2003). This discussion is being taken further, however, to explore factors that facilitate resilient behavior in a hostile environment. In this section, I explore some of the ways in which the destructive influence of peer pressure is mitigated. Using extracts from interviews, I show the importance of home influence in this regard as well as draw from ingrained notions of "personhood" whose influence plays a cautionary role. Both Thabo and Lehlohonolo (below) highlight the importance of the steadying influence of home life. This, they argue, mitigates the effects of peer pressure. For instance, Thabo lauds the values that one learns from home that are protective from peer pressure. This is generally the same argument that Lehlohonolo makes:

> I think there is no peer pressure. Your attitude and the environment in which you grew up—your home—where you were raised are important. Those two allow you to take responsibility for your own life. If at home they give you lessons to live by, that should protect you from pressure from other people. (*Thabo, 18-year-old male, mixed gender FGD, Mofolo*)

> We are not the same as people. There are those who do things and get called to order at their homes and there are those who are a law unto themselves. There is no way that such people would be the same. This one they will call a fool and other derogatory names because he does not want to live the life that they want him to live. He has chosen what he thinks is good for his life. (*Lehlohonolo, 18-year-old male, mixed gender FGD, Mofolo*)

Noteworthy is the point that Lehlohonolo makes: "We are not the same." Fundamentally, the distinguishing factor is home influence, together with personal characteristics. I argue that home influence stands a better competing chance against peer influence if home has demonstrated a caring and containing role in the upheavals of life. Therefore, the importance of a functional family structure in lending resilience to growing children who are faced with many competing influences cannot be overemphasized.

This can help the notion of a "diseased penis" that Themba below raises and in a similar token a diseased vagina:

> To be frank, there is this notion that there is a diseased penis that you avoid by all means. Same with girls. You just think, here is a pool of dirt and disease I would not go near. As a person you see this is death (and you seek to avoid it). (*Themba, 19-year-old male, all male FGD, Motsoaledi*)

The notion of not behaving "like a person" is invoked in other transgressions such as rape, murder, *and* the lack of wisdom to avoid "a diseased penis" where one is suspected. Heald (1995, p. 495) puts it thus: "The kind of propriety in social life that these rules speak to is the *mark of an adult*; indiscrimination is seen as characteristic of children and animals, while deliberate transgression is the sign of witchcraft." Therefore, systems that denigrate and disempower take away one's "personhood," encouraging animal-like behaviors that undermine the need to self-preserve and be of value to society.

Wilson (2006) similarly argues that people who feel that society has let them down feel they owe society nothing. Such systems do not give individuals a chance to aspire to excellence, thus achieving the epitome of *ubuntu*. They are implicated in micropractices becoming macropractices (cf. Comaroff & Comaroff, 1992). I argue that researchers have a moral and intellectual responsibility to highlight these sometimes-not-so-apparent links.

The argument about the ontology of a person is taken further by Thabiso below, who makes a distinction between things that one can allow oneself to be pressured into doing by peers and what one chooses to do. A line is drawn when one is being "duted with out-of-order things" because this speaks about one's character (and the upbringing one had) and is more likely to lose one favor with peers than the other way around:

> In terms of "dutying" each other, *sometimes it is guys just testing you*—do not use a condom etc., *just to see if you have a "backbone"* and if we duty you on something "out-of-order" and you do it, *then we know there is not much to you.* But if we duty you and you stick to your guns, then we can see that you are a dog and no, this one is a dog he does not play ball and *that way you gain the respect of the guys.* Yes, it is like that, we are like that we do not duty each other with "out-of-order" things. *If we happen to, and you do it, we just see that this one is empty and we laugh at you, calling you names that you are a fool and it would be clear that you were being played.* (Thabiso, 19-year-old male, individual interview, Mofolo)

The idiom of being "duted" is a common one in Soweto. It is derived from the English word "duty"—to work. It can be infused into all the languages found in Soweto as it does not belong to any one of them. I would even venture to say it is uniquely used by teenagers. I cannot imagine adults invoking this word in conversation with each other, although they may use it with their teenage children. The idea of being "duted" carries connotations of being made to slog mindlessly against one's wishes. It connotes a prize to be paid to remain popular with the group. My sense is that only those who allow themselves to be "duted," in the first place, will attract being "duted" further. In other words, if one lacks the "backbone" to put one's foot down once and for all, then one will always be seen as a potential candidate for being made to slog to prove group loyalty. This is at once seen as a game—"Go get that girl and let's make a spectacle out of that transaction," but also proof of one's ability to take up a challenge—a dare (to prove a particular masculinity). Being "duted" can take many forms; it can be a spur of the moment "let us derive some fun out of this, there is not much at stake here other than having fun" and perhaps protracted when one is being influenced to partake in an activity that may have far-reaching consequences such as crime or unsafe sex. On one level peer pressure applies to issues that can be characterized as mere games and on another it applies to serious issues. Research that indiscriminately cites peer influence as central to teenage sexuality fails to see these levels.

While being "applauded" by peers can be a virtue, there is a greater call to not "overdo" it. A peer who has a habit of "overdoing it" soon gains a reputation of being mindless, a bad influence and a liability, and thus "futureless," resulting in peers writing him off. This communicates a sense that it is all very well to be part of a group and go with group mentality, but ultimately one is on one's own. Both the boys and the girls who participated in this research had a keen sense of this because this may be the ultimate "weapon" that parents may use to dissuade their children against group mentality. Internalizing this is also a measure of one's maturity.

A point needs to be made about risky behavior and ideas about one's future prospects. The participants have a keen sense that teenage years can make or break one's future prospects. This sense is engendered by an awareness of the many distractions in the daily fabric of Soweto life and the many examples of "failed" people in the community. The participants also communicated a sense of "growing toward," implying that one's behavior has to be more responsible as one matures as shown below:

> You know, I would do things that I would regret later. I would go "clubbing" with my friends while I have not reported this to my mother. I am beginning to change, I am experiencing and seeing things differently. I no longer have the same views on things. I used to take things for granted that if others are doing this, so can I and not really think of the consequences for me. (*Yanga, 17-year-old female, individual interview, Motsoaledi*)

Therefore, a holistic understanding of teenage HIV risk can be arrived at only by looking at the structural barriers that lead to despondence and thus making "careless" decisions about one's life. The nature of family dynamics that may decide whether the teenager will heed the advice of his/her elders is as important. Group dynamics that seek to put a prize to belonging and the factors that may ultimately sway individual behavior one way or the other are as important. Psychologists may chalk these to up to issues of self-esteem and locus of control.

Peer pressure is just as important for/in female relationships, although the dynamics may be different as girls seem to have a (socially) built-in mistrust of one another. Girls may be in competition with one another for the available and not-so-available boys because it remains an ideal to have a boyfriend, which proves one's attractiveness to the opposite sex. According to Chumisa below, the ingrained competitive spirit that characterizes relationships between girls has potential to mediate the effects of peer pressure among girls:

Boys really look after each other—unlike us girls. We really do not plot together. There is always the suspicion that perhaps your friend wants your boyfriend if she gives you certain advice. We just say there is nothing to the allegations made by the friend, whereas boys listen to each other. They say, "Friend, this girl is cheating on you." Sometimes it may happen that my boyfriend propositions my friend or my boyfriend's friend propositions me. What will happen is that us girls will fight over it and end up not talking to each other, whereas the guys even when they know about what happened between his friend and his girlfriend remain good friends without any real tension. (*Chumisa, 17-year-old female, all female FGD, Pimville*)

Peer pressure is thus tampered for girls, not least by the competition for boys as well as the more private performance of sexual relationships. Girls usually go it alone, whereas the group dynamics that may influence risky behavior among boys talk to the public display of masculinity that is central to their image of themselves and their ability to keep up with the "in crowd."

CONCLUSION

In this article I highlighted the complexity of teenage HIV sexual risk in Soweto, emphasizing the social factors that bear on HIV risk definition, perception, management, and susceptibility. From this point of view, I consider the agency of the participants, itself rooted and shaped by a particular sociocultural context. In particular, I highlight the gender-based assessment and management of HIV risk. For instance, the male perception of women as potential carriers of HIV infection and the resultant lack of trust were highlighted. This male dynamic was also attributed to the weakening of the traditional male hold on women; women who did not conform to particular expectations of acceptable female comportment were viewed with suspicion. The female participants, however, were not hapless victims of this assessment. They actively wrestled for an active and equal position with their male counterparts. For instance, they pointed to the irony that rape, while posing HIV danger to them, may equally pose danger to the male perpetrators. Their overall attitude to the male/female relationship was summed up as "who is fooling who?" The disproportional vulnerable social position of women in general was not, however, in the process, discounted. The intricacies of how power dynamics influence whether a particular risky behavior is actualized or not were also highlighted. The argument around "being duted with out-of-order things" explains not only the agency of young people in deciding which risks to take or not to take, it also explains the hierarchical assessment of risk in the research setting of Soweto.

My review of data clearly points to the centrality of risk in the fabric of life in the township. To this end, I argue that HIV infection may be a culmination of vulnerability to all sorts of other risks and may not be the sole and paramount concern of growing people in South Africa. It is imperative for research and interventions to work with a dynamic and complex frame of risk to HIV infection. This is so as we acknowledge that sexual experimentation is an integral part of growing up. Furthermore, I identify "types" of sexual relationships in Soweto. Sexual risk cannot be inferred from these types as they are flexible and are all subject to the fallible nature of sexual risk assessment and management by fallible individuals, made even more fallible by the place that they occupy in the political economy of a transforming South Africa.

ACKNOWLEDGMENTS

This is my own unaided work that is drawn from my doctoral thesis awarded by the Department of Social Anthropology, University of the Witwatersrand, 2013 under the supervision of Shahid Vawda.

REFERENCES

Ayieri, E. (2010). Sexual violence in conflict: A problematic international discourse. *Feminist Africa, 14*, 7–20.

Bolton, R. (1999). Mapping Terra Incognita: Sex research for HIV prevention—An urgent agenda for the 1990s. In R. Parker & P. Aggleton (Eds.), *Culture, society and sexuality: A reader* (pp. 434–456). London, England: UCL.

Bujra, J. (2000). Risk and trust: Unsafe sex, gender and AIDS in Tanzania. In P. Caplan (Ed.), *Risk revisited* (pp. 59–84). London, England: Pluto.

Campbell, C. & MacPhail, C. (2002). Peer education, gender and the development of critical consciousness: Participatory HIV prevention by South African youth. *Social Science & Medicine, 55*, 331–345.

Comaroff, J., & Comaroff, J. (1992). *Ethnography and the historical imagination*. Boulder, CO: Westview.

De Beauvoir, S. (1952). *The second sex: Woman as other*. New York, NY: Vintage Books. (Original work published 1949)

Eaton, L., Flisher, A. J., & Aaro, L. E. (2003). Unsafe sexual behaviour in South African youth. *Social Science and Medicine, 56*, 149–165.

Esplen, E. (2007). *Women and girls living with HIV/AIDS: Overview and annotated bibliography*. London, England: University of Sussex.

Fassin, D. (2007). *When bodies remember: Experiences and politics of AIDS in South Africa*. Berkeley, CA: University of California Press.

Frayser, S. (1985). *Variations of sexual experiences: An anthropological perspective on human sexuality*. New Haven, CT: Human Relations Area Files.

Glaser, B. G. (1992). *Basics of grounded theory analysis: Emergence vs. forcing*. Mill Valley, CA: Sociology Press.

Heald, S. (1995). The power of sex: Some reflections on the Cladwell's "African sexuality" thesis. *Africa, 65*, 489–505.

Holland, J., Ramazanoglu, C., Scott, S., Sharpe, S., & Thomson, R. (1991). Pressure, resistance, empowerment: Young women and the negotiation of safer sex. *Youth Research*, *9*(2), 15–26.

Holland, J., Ramazanoglu, C., Scott, S., Sharpe, S., & Thomson, R. (1992). Risk, power and the possibility of pleasure: Young women and safer sex. *AIDS Care*, *4*(3), 273–283.

Holland, J., Ramazanoglu, C., Scott, S., Sharpe, S., & Thomson, R. (1994). Power and desire: The embodiment of female sexuality. *Feminist Review*, *46*, 21–38.

Holland, J., Ramazanoglu, C., Scott, S., Sharpe, S., & Thomson, R. (1998). *The male in the head: Young people, heterosexuality and power*. London, England: Tufnell.

Jewkes, R., & Abrahams, N. (2002). The epidemiology of rape and sexual coercion in South Africa: An overview. *Social Science and Medicine*, *55*, 1231–1244.

Leclerc-Madlala, S. (2002). On the virgin cleansing myth: Gendered bodies, AIDS and ethnomedicine. *African Journal of AIDS Research*, *1*(2), 87–95.

Leclerc-Madlala, S. (2003). We do sex to have money: Modernity and meaning in contemporary relationships. Unpublished article. Department of Anthropology, University of Natal, South Africa.

LoveLife. (2010). *HIV prevention for young people: Moving from what-to-change to want-to-change* (Fact sheet). Retrieved from http://www.lovelife.org.za. research/reports.php

McClure, C. A., Gray, G., & Rybczyk, G. K. (2004). Challenges to conducting HIV preventative vaccine trials with adolescents. *Journal of Acquired Immune Deficiency Syndromes*, *36*(2) 726–733.

Mkhwanazi, N. (2010). Understanding teenage pregnancy in a post-apartheid South African township. *Culture, Health and Sex*, *12*, 347–358.

Pelto, J. P., & Pelto, G. H. (1997). Studying knowledge, culture and behaviour in Applied Medical Anthropology. *Medical Anthropology Quarterly*, *11*, 147–163.

Pettifor, A., Rees, H. V., Steffenson, A. E., Hlongwa-Madikizela, L., & McPhail, C. (2004). *HIV and sexual behaviour among young South Africans: A national survey of 15–24 year old Johannesburg, South Africa*. Johannesburg, South Africa: University of the Witwatersrand, RHRU.

Pool, R., & Geissler, W. (2007). *Medical anthropology: Understanding public health*. Berkshire, England: Open University Press.

Shisana, O., & Simbayi, L. (2002). *Behavioural responses of South African youth to the HIV/AIDS epidemic: A nationwide survey*. Pretoria, South Africa: HSRC.

Sobo, E. (1993). Inner-city women and AIDS: The psychosocial benefits of unsafe sex. *Culture, Medicine and Psychiatry*, *17*, 455–485.

Stillwaggon, E. (2006). *AIDS and the ecology of poverty*. Oxford, England: Oxford University Press.

Taylor, C. C. (1990). Condoms and cosmology: The fractal person and sexual risk in Rwanda. *Social Science and Medicine*, *31*, 1023–1028.

UNAIDS. (2002). *Report on the global HIV/AIDS epidemic*. Geneva, Switzerland: Author.

Vance, C. S. (Ed.). (1992). *Pleasure and danger: Exploring female sexuality*. Boston, MA: Routledge & Kegan Paul.

Varga, C. (1997). The conundrum: Barriers to condom use among commercial sex workers in Durban, South Africa. *African Journal of Reproductive Health*, *1*(1), 74–88.

Varga, C. (2004). Sexual decision-making and negotiation in the midst of AIDS: Young adults' sexual interaction—Results from a diary study. *Lancet, 363,* 1415–1421.

Varga, C. A., & Makubalo, L. (1996). Sexual (non)negotiation among Black African teenagers in Durban. *Agenda, 28,* 31–38.

Vetten, L., Jewkes, R., Fuller, R., Christofides, N., Loots, L., & Dunseith, O. (2008). *Tracking justice: The attrition of rape cases through the criminal justice system in Gauteng.* Johannesburg, South Africa: Tshwaranang Legal Advocacy Centre, South African Medical Research Council and the Centre for the Study of Violence and Reconciliation.

Watney, S. (1999). Safer sex as community practice. In L. Parker & P. Aggleton (Eds.), *Culture, society and sexuality: A reader* (pp. 405–416). London, England: Routledge.

Wilson, F. (2006). On being a father and poor in South Africa today. In L. Richter & R. Morrell (Eds.), *Baba: Men and fatherhood in South Africa* (pp. 26–37). Cape Town, South Africa: HSRC.

Wojcicki, J. M. (2002). She drank his money: Survival sex and the problem of violence in taverns in Gauteng province, South Africa. *Medical Anthropology Quarterly, 16,* 267–293.

Emotional and Psychosocial Aspects of Menstrual Poverty in Resource-Poor Settings: A Qualitative Study of the Experiences of Adolescent Girls in an Informal Settlement in Nairobi

JOANNA CRICHTON

School of Social and Community Medicine, University of Bristol, Bristol, UK

JERRY OKAL

Population Council, Nairobi, Kenya

CAROLINE W. KABIRU

African Population and Health Research Center, Nairobi, Kenya

ELIYA MSIYAPHAZI ZULU

African Institute for Development Policy (AFIDEP), Nairobi, Kenya

We introduce the concept of "menstrual poverty" to categorize the multiple deprivations relating to menstruation in resource-poor settings across the Global South, and we examine how this affects the psychological well-being of adolescent girls in an urban informal settlement in Kenya. We use qualitative data collected through 34 in-depth interviews and 18 focus group discussions with girls, women, and key informants. Menstrual poverty involved practical

This project was carried out in partnership with the Division of Reproductive Health at the Kenyan Ministry of Public Health and Sanitation. The authors acknowledge the financial support (grant HD4) by the UK Department for International Development (DfID) for the Realising Rights Research Programme Consortium. The views expressed are not necessarily those of DfID. We are also grateful to the Kenyan Ministry of Education and the City Council of Nairobi for their support. We give special thanks to the community members, pupils, teachers, and nurses who participated in the study. We thank Judi Kidger, Beki Langford, and Rachel Hodgins for commenting on a previous draft of this article. We appreciate the contributions of APHRC staff.

and psychosocial challenges affecting girls at home and at school. Its emotional impacts included anxiety, embarrassment, fear of stigma, and low mood. Further research is needed on how menstrual poverty affects girls' psychological and educational outcomes.

Across the Global South, poverty causes multiple material and psychosocial deprivations for girls and women during menstruation (Adinma & Adimna, 2008; Ali & Rizvi, 2009; El-Gilany, Badawi, & El-Fedawy, 2005; Garg, Sharma, & Sahay, 2001; Mahon & Fernandes, 2010; Rashid & Michaud, 2000; Sommer, 2009a, 2009b), leading to experiences of embarrassment, shame, anxiety, and stigma (McMahon et al., 2011; Sommer, 2009a, 2009b). There are good reasons to prioritize research on the emotional and psychological impacts of menstrual poverty on adolescent girls. Puberty is a time of rapid, simultaneous, and substantial change across biological, psychological, cognitive, and social domains (Mendle, Turkheimer, & Emery, 2007). The biological processes initiated in puberty interact with the social context to affect an individual's emotional and social development, with implications for their mental and physical health in adolescence and adulthood (Patton & Viner, 2007).

In this article, we seek to address two limitations with existing research. First, researchers studying resource-poor contexts have focused on documenting challenges with managing menstruation in particular contexts, without making comparisons between contexts. Such comparisons are needed to develop understanding of the international phenomenon of menstrual poverty and to design interventions to adequately address its health, psychological, and educational impacts. Second, researchers have previously focused on practical and hygiene-related aspects of menstrual poverty, and the psychological and educational impacts are poorly understood (McMahon et al., 2011; Sommer, 2009a, 2009b). Researchers in North America have begun to investigate the psychosocial and psychological aspects of menarche (onset of menstruation) and subsequent menstruation among adolescent girls in that context (Chang, Hayter, & Wu, 2010; Greif & Ulman, 1982; Koff & Rierdan, 1995; McPherson & Korfine, 2004; Ruble & Brooks-Gunn, 1982; Swenson & Havens, 1987), but these aspects have rarely been considered in developing countries, where practical and social challenges with menstruation are likely to be much greater. Marván and Trujillo (2009) have moved this agenda to a new context by examining psychosocial aspects of menstruation in Mexico, but they did not examine the impact of menstrual poverty.

We aim to address these literature gaps in two ways. First, we argue that the categories of deprivation relating to menstruation and poverty are similar across sub-Saharan Africa, North Africa, South Asia, and other resource-poor settings, and propose the concept of "menstrual poverty" to encourage comparative and theoretical approaches and to galvanize and focus future research efforts to address them. Second, we aim to take a first step toward bridging Northern and Southern research agendas by using qualitative data to examine the impact of menstrual poverty on the emotional well-being of adolescent girls in an informal settlement in Nairobi, Kenya.

LITERATURE REVIEW

Across sub-Saharan Africa, North Africa, and South Asia, adolescent girls and women experience multiple challenges with managing menstruation. In our review of the literature, we found that, although the challenges vary qualitatively and in severity in different contexts (for example, between rural and urban areas [El-Gilany et al., 2005; Khanna, Goyal, & Bhawsar, 2005; Sommer, 2009b]), the same categories of deprivation exist in all contexts. Our literature searches, however, did not identify a single comparative study examining the characteristics and impacts of poverty on menstruation in resource-poor contexts. We therefore propose the concept of "menstrual poverty," which we define as the combination of multiple practical and psychosocial deprivations experienced by menstruating girls and women in resource-poor settings. We present the various aspects of this concept in Figure 1. In the first section of Figure 1, we show how material deprivations, including inability to afford the cost of acceptable and reliable methods for managing menstrual flow (Adinma & Adinma, 2008; El-Gilany et al., 2005; Garg et al., 2001; Khanna et al., 2005; Sommer, 2009a), lack of access to adequate water and sanitation facilities, and lack of privacy required for dealing with menstruation lead to discomfort and hygiene risks (Ali & Rizvi, 2009; El-Gilany et al., 2005; Khanna et al., 2005; Rashid & Michaud, 2000; Sommer, 2009a). Moving to the second section of Figure 1, girls in diverse settings such as Egypt, India, Nigeria, Pakistan, and Tanzania experience psychosocial deprivations including lack of information, support, and guidance before menarche and with subsequent menses (Adinma & Adinma, 2008; Ali & Rizvi, 2009; Crichton, Ibisomi, & Gyimah, 2012; Deo & Ghattargi, 2005; El-Gilany et al., 2005; Garg et al., 2001; Khanna et al., 2005; Sommer, 2009a, 2009b). In the third section of Figure 1, we list the contextual factors in which these deprivations occur, which include taboos around menstrual blood and discussing menstruation, cultural restrictions, social norms and expectations, and gender-discriminatory environments (Adinma & Adinma, 2008; Ali & Rizvi, 2009; Crichton et al., 2012; El-Gilany et al., 2005; Garg et al., 2001; Khanna et al., 2005; Sommer, 2009a, 2009b).

Some researchers have gone beyond documenting problems to examining the impacts on girls' physical and emotional health and well-being. Menstrual poverty undermines women's and girls' participation in physical, social, and economic activities. For instance, some researchers have investigated the potential effects of menstrual poverty on menstrual hygiene (Ali &

Material deprivations

Lack of access to acceptable and reliable methods for managing

menstrual flow

Poor quality or inaccessible toilets

Inadequate water and bathing facilities

Lack of privacy

Lack of disposal facilities

Psychosocial deprivations

Lack of information and emotional and practical support before

menarche and during subsequent menstruation from parents,

guardians, and family members

Limited access to accurate and comprehensive information and

guidance about menstruation in schools and communities

FIGURE 1 Menstrual poverty in the Global South.

Rizvi, 2009; Khanna et al., 2005) and on skin and reproductive tract infections (Khanna et al., 2005; Morison et al., 2005; Wasserheit, Harris, Chakraborty, Kay, & Mason, 1989). Problems managing menstruation have been found to cause periodic absence or school dropout among menstruating girls, although the evidence is inconclusive and more research is needed (Ali & Rizvi, 2009; Lloyd, Mensch, & Clark, 1998; McMahon et al., 2011; Oster & Thornton, 2009; Scott, Dopson, Montgomery, Dolan, & Ryus, unpublished; Sommer, 2009b).

To our knowledge, only three peer-reviewed papers have examined the emotional and psychological impacts of menstrual poverty in any detail. First, Rashid and Michaud (2000) described how lack of privacy and washing facilities in the context of cultural concepts of menstrual blood being polluting led to feelings of distress and shame among adolescent girls during the 1998 floods in Bangladesh. Second, Sommer (2009b) observed that limited access to sanitary facilities, menstrual supplies, and credible sources of information on puberty and lack of gender sensitivity in schools lead to experiences of embarrassment, shame, and stigma among girls in Tanzania (Sommer, 2009a, 2009b). Third, McMahon and colleagues (2011) found that menstruation leads to feelings of shame, guilt, fear, and powerlessness among young women in rural Kenya. Munthali and Zulu (2007) also briefly report that Malawian girls who received adequate briefing on menstruation before menarche were better prepared and reacted more positively to the experience. Researchers in Pakistan and India have noted high levels of negative feelings about menarche and subsequent menses in surveys (Ali & Rizvi, 2009; Deo & Ghattargi, 2005; Khanna et al., 2005). For example, 44% of girls in urban areas in India reported being scared by first menstruation and 13% by subsequent menstruation (Deo & Ghattargi, 2005). These studies used crude measures of emotional aspects of menstruation, however, and did not examine the reasons for these feelings, beyond hypothesizing that they are due to lack of information and guidance prior to menarche.

Menarche and subsequent menstruation are important aspects of puberty for girls, with implications for their social adjustment, psychological well-being, and personal development. Research from industrialized countries, particularly in North America, has demonstrated the significance of psychosocial dynamics of menarche and subsequent menstruation for the emotional well-being of adolescent girls. Adequate practical and emotional guidance and support before menarche and during menstruation are important for girls to adjust positively to menstruation (Chang et al., 2010; Greif & Ulman, 1982; Koff & Rierdan, 1995; Marván & Trujillo, 2009; McPherson & Korfine, 2004; Orringer & Gahagan, 2010; Ruble & Brooks-Gunn, 1982; Swenson & Havens, 1987).

In cultures all over the world, menstruation is a stigmatizing condition, where menstruating women have a "discreditable" status, which is not immediately observable, but individuals tend to behave in ways to keep the stigma concealed (Kowalski & Chapple, 2000; Roberts, Goldenberg, Power, & Pyszczynski, 2002). This stigma affects women's perception about their interpersonal relationships (Kowalski & Chapple, 2000; Roberts et al., 2002) and can lead to prejudice and peer antagonism (McMahon et al., 2011; Sommer, 2009a). The impacts of psychosocial problems with menstruation during adolescence have developmental implications that may continue into adulthood. For example, there is evidence that negative experiences of menarche are associated with menstrual shame and negative body image in adulthood, which in turn can undermine sexual negotiation and lead to sexual risk taking (Schooler, Ward, Merriwether, & Caruthers, 2005; Stubbs, 2008). As Sommer (2009a) points out, girls in resource-poor settings experience the challenges of adjustment to puberty in a social and economic context that makes it hard for them to manage the potentially stigmatizing aspects of menstruation in private. The psychological impacts of this, however, have not been studied in detail.

In this study, we seek to address these knowledge gaps by using qualitative investigation of the emotional and psychosocial aspects of menstrual poverty among adolescent girls in Korogocho, an urban informal settlement in Nairobi, Kenya. We begin by examining girls' experiences of menstrual poverty including lack of access to sanitary pads, problems with hygiene and privacy, and lack of support and guidance. We then examine how menstrual poverty relates to social stigma. Next, we examine girls' descriptions of the effects of these challenges on their emotional well-being during menstruation. Finally, we examine coping strategies used by girls for dealing with menstrual poverty. In our discussion section, we relate these findings to the international literature on menstruation in resource-poor settings and on the psychosocial aspects of menstruation in industrialized countries, and identify implications for interventions and further research in this area.

Research Setting

This study was carried out in Korogocho, one of many informal "slum" settlements in Nairobi city. Korogocho has a high population density, estimated at 63,318 inhabitants per square kilometer (African Population and Health Research Center [APHRC], 2006). As with other informal settlements, it has high levels of poverty and unemployment, limited and inadequate sanitation and waste disposal facilities, overcrowding, and poor health outcomes (APHRC, 2002; Emina et al., 2011; Kyobutungi, Ziraba, Ezeh, & Yé, 2008). Few homes have direct water supply or sanitation facilities, and many residents have to pay for containers of water and use of communal toilets and washing facilities (Mudege & Zulu, 2010). Water shortages are common and persistent. Residents sometimes go without water for bathing and laundry, or have to use water contaminated with sewage and industrial effluent (Undie, John-Langba, & Kimani, 2006). A typical family in the slums of Nairobi lives in a one-room house, and the room serves as a bedroom, sitting room, and often a cooking room as well. Sanitary pads and cotton wool are readily available for purchase from retail outlets in the community. Sanitary pads cost approximately U.S. $1 for a pack, however, which is difficult to afford for many in Nairobi slums, where 83% of residents rely on unstable informal incomes, 27% are economically inactive, and between 55% and 33% live below the household poverty line (estimated at 2,913 Kenyan shillings or approximately U.S. $40 per month) between 2006 and 2009 (Emina et al., 2011).

As of 2005, the majority of girls (80%) aged 6–13 years in Korogocho were enrolled in primary school (Epari, Ezeh, Mugisha, & Ogollah, 2008).

Most schools in Korogocho are privately run and nonformal, many of which are not registered with the Ministry of Education. The quality of water and sanitation facilities in these schools often falls below government standards (Keidar, Berry, Ezeh, & Donchin, 2008).

METHODS

Procedure

In our study, we combined inductive and deductive approaches to data collection and analysis (Fereday & Muir-Cochrane, 2006). This involved assessment of concurrency between our data and existing literature on menstruation, while allowing themes to emerge from open-ended interview questions and careful reading of participants' voiced experiences and views. After analysis, we carried out a more systematic literature review to search for publications on the main themes arising from our study. We carried out searches of English-language publications in the bibliographic databases Medline and PubMed using combinations of the search terms adolescents, menarche, menstruation, menstrual hygiene products, poverty, stigma, health, well-being, psychological development, puberty, psychosocial, and anxiety.

We carried out 15 in-depth interviews (IDIs) and 10 focus group discussions (FGDs) with adolescent girls aged 12 to 17 years, 14 IDIs and eight FGDs with adult women, and five key informant interviews with five teachers and a community nurse. Data collection was carried out as part of a wider project examining menstrual attitudes, practices, and problems among both girls and women. Although we were primarily concerned with girls' experiences of menstruation, we found the interviews with adult women to be important sources of data for two reasons. First, nine of the adult IDIs and four of the focus groups featured testimony from mothers of adolescent girls, providing insights into their perspectives on their daughters' behavior and well-being and information on their concerns and practices as parents. Second, women of all ages provided valuable insights into the social context in which menstruation occurs (for example, on taboos and social norms around menstruation and menarche and attitudes toward adolescence and puberty). The key informant interviews provided important overviews about challenges to menstrual well-being in the community and school approaches to dealing with menstruation.

Data collection for this qualitative phase of the study was carried out in May and June 2008. We worked with teachers to identify adolescent girls in schools and with community members to identify women and out-of-school girls through door-to-door recruitment. We used purposive quota sampling (Ulin, Robinson, & Tolley, 2005) to ensure our sample reflected variations in age (12–14, 15–17 age groups), schooling status (in school, out of school), and ethnicity in Korogocho. Focus groups were separated according to age group and in- or out-of-school status to help participants feel at ease and to encourage discussion.

A total of 87 girls and 69 women participated in FGDs. Participants included the most populous ethnic groups in Korogocho: the Luo, Luhya, Kamba, Kikuyu, and Somali. Semistructured topic guides were used for the IDIs and FGDs. These guides were translated into Kiswahili and back-translated into English. The guides were pretested during a pilot study and revised accordingly. Questions were asked on attitudes and social norms, menstrual practices and problems, and the impacts on physical and mental well-being. The mothers of postmenarcheal girls were also asked questions about their experiences and opinions as mothers. Questions were open-ended, seeking information on both positive and negative menstrual experiences. Fieldworkers were experienced in working with young people on sensitive topics and were provided with further training about menstruation and puberty.

In-depth interviews (IDIs) and FGDs were conducted in Kiswahili or English according to informants' preference. These interviews were used for collecting participants' personal experiences and hygiene practices, including potentially stigmatizing issues such as hygiene problems. Focus groups generated wider ranging and more nuanced discussions about the social context. All interviews were audio-digitally recorded and transcribed verbatim and simultaneously translated from Kiswahili to English. Participants were prepared to talk about menstruation and were willing to be audio-recorded once they understood the confidential nature of the study. In addition, a number of participants mentioned that they appreciated the chance to talk about menstruation, because social norms often proscribe such discussions.

Data Analysis

Transcripts were stored in and analyzed using Nudist 6.0 QSR software. Two of us (J.C. and J.O.) conducted thematic analysis of the transcripts (Boyatzis, 1998; Patton, 1990; Silverman, 1993). We began by separately reading four interview and four focus group transcripts and developing lists of themes and subthemes. We then worked together to critically review and synthesize these lists and create a codebook, reading through four transcripts together and discussing their interpretation. Next, we each read and coded half the transcripts, editing the codebook where necessary. We made notes of emerging issues and questions as we carried out the coding process, discussing these observations periodically. Finally, all of us read through a sample of J.C.'s and J.O.'s coding. Where differences occurred, this allowed the researchers to discuss and clarify the themes and hierarchy. Seven themes and 57 subthemes were identified, covering the social, psychological, and socioeconomic aspects of menstruation, and girls' perceptions and experiences.

Ethical Approval and Confidentiality

Ethical approval for the study was provided by Kenya Medical Research Institute's (KEMRI) Ethical Review Committee. All participants gave informed consent before being interviewed. To ensure confidentiality, informed consent forms were stored in a locked filing cabinet and digital recordings and transcripts were password protected.

FINDINGS

Menstrual Poverty in Korogocho

We summarize the material and psychosocial deprivations involved in menstrual poverty in Korogocho in the second column of Table 1. We provide examples of other places where these categories of menstrual poverty have been documented in the third column of the table.

Material Deprivation

The material deprivations were a combination of problems with access to sanitary products, lack of access to good quality water and sanitation facilities, and problems with privacy. Almost all participants described sanitary pads as their preferred method for managing menstrual flow, describing them as convenient, hygienic, and reliable. Almost all girls had used sanitary pads before and most reported using sanitary pads in their last 3 periods. Nearly half, however, used cloths or a combination of sanitary pads and cloths to save money. Cloths, socks, and cotton wool were commonly used but were seen as involving greater risk of dampness, discomfort, and leakage than sanitary pads. Some participants used pads but changed them infrequently, for example, making use of just two or three pads during a whole period lasting 3 or more days. Some women and girls complained that using cloths or infrequent changes of pads irritates their skin and causes rashes.

Because of overcrowding and limited access to toilets and sanitation facilities, many girls lacked the privacy needed for changing pads and cloths. Privacy appeared to be a greater concern for younger girls than adult women, because they often shared the house with parents and siblings and had less control over the physical space within their homes. One female teacher noted:

> It is a problem because these houses are single rooms and the whole family is there including the father. It becomes hard for them to go and change [sanitary products] and then they also don't have toilet facilities. ... Maybe they will wait until night [when their family are asleep]. (KII4, Female head teacher, informal primary school)

TABLE 1 Menstrual Poverty in Korogocho and Other Resource-Poor Contexts

Aspects of menstrual poverty	Findings from Korogocho, Kenya (this study)	Country examples from literature review
Practical deprivations		
Lack of access to acceptable and reliable methods for managing menstrual flow	Sanitary pads preferred by all participants but difficult for many to afford. Many girls and women use cloths or a combination of pads and cloths, or change their pads infrequently. Some use cotton wool, socks, or tissue paper. Participants complain of experiencing dampness, discomfort, and itching/rashes due to lack of access to sanitary pads.	Nepal (Oster & Thornton, 2009) Urban SE Nigeria (Adinma & Adinma, 2009) Rajistan, India (Khanna, Goyal, & Bhawsar, 2005) Delhi, India (Garg et al., 2001) Pakistan (Ali & Rizvi, 2009) Egypt (El-Gilany et al., 2005) Rural Kenya (McMahon et al., 2011) Rural and urban Tanzania (Sommer 2009a, 2009b) Rural and urban Bangladesh (Rashid & Michaud, 2000)
Poor quality or inaccessible toilets and water and bathing facilities	Communal toilets and bathing facilities inadequate for size of population and some are subject to user charges. Lack of facilities for hand washing in schools and communities. Most homes without water, toilet, or bathing facilities. Water often purchased in small quantities at a high price. Water subject to supply shortages and contamination.	Rural Kenya (McMahon et al., 2011) Rural and urban Tanzania (Sommer 2009a, 2009b) Rural and urban Bangladesh during 1998 floods (Rashid & Michaud, 2000)
lack of privacy	Many families live in one-room houses, leaving girls little opportunity to bathe, change pads or cloths, or wash and dry cloths at home. Toilets in schools and communities do not always have adequate or lockable doors.	Egypt (El-Gilany et al., 2005) Rural and urban Tanzania (Sommer 2009a, 2009b) Rural and urban Bangladesh during 1998 floods (Rashid & Michaud, 2000)
Lack of facilities for disposing of cloths and pads	Lack of refuse collection facilities. Used sanitary pads and cloths lying around in the streets.	Rural Ghana (Scott et al., unpublished)
Psychosocial deprivations		
Limited access to information and guidance before menarche	Most girls knew about menstruation before menarche, but the information they had was often vague or inaccurate. Many mothers avoid discussing menstruation with their daughters. In some cases, girls failed to inform their mothers or guardians that they had started menstruating because of embarrassment or lack of close relationships.	Pakistan (Ali & Rizvi, 2009) Delhi, India (Garg et al., 2001) Rajistan, India (Khanna, Goyal, & Bhawsar, 2005)

Lack of information and emotional and practical support during subsequent menstruation from parents, guardians, and family members.	Many mothers and guardians avoided discussing menstruation with their daughters after menarche or gave them limited and inaccurate information. Many focused on practical aspects of menstruation and responsibilities of girls, rather than providing emotional support. Some girls do not receive from mothers any practical support with managing menstruation.	Urban and rural Tanzania (Sommer 2009a, 2009b) Kenya (Crichton, Ibisomi & Gyimah, 2012; Wamoyi, Fenwick, Urassa, Zaba, & Stones, 2010)
Lack of knowledge; Limited access to accurate and comprehensive information and guidance about menstruation in schools and communities	Teachers and mothers interviewed in the study had limited and sometimes inaccurate knowledge about menstruation, for example, not knowing where menstrual blood comes from or believing that normal aspects of menstruation are a sign of health problems. Inadequate coverage of menstruation and puberty in school curricula. Some teachers provide informal, practical guidance to female pupils on their own initiative.	Urban and rural Tanzania (Sommer, 2009a, 2009b) Urban SE Nigeria (Adinma & Adinma, 2008) Egypt (El-Gilany et al., 2005) Pakistan (Ali & Rizvi, 2009) Urban and rural India (Deo & Ghattargi, 2005)

Emotional and psychosocial impacts of menstrual poverty

Social stigma	Girls and teachers mentioned incidents of menstruation-related bullying by pupils. Girls expressed fear of stigma due to discovery of their menstruating status, leakage, and odor.	Urban and rural Tanzania (Sommer, 2009a, 2009b) Rural Kenya (McMahon et al., 2011)
Embarrassment, anxiety, fear of being stigmatized, low mood	Girls in our study linked menstrual poverty with fear of stigma and feelings of embarrassment, anxiety, and low mood. A few girls reported acute distress.	Urban and rural Tanzania (Sommer, 2009a, 2009b) Rural Kenya (McMahon et al., 2011) Rural Ghana (Scott et al., unpublished) Rural and urban Bangladesh (Rashid & Michaud, 2000) Urban and rural India (Deo & Ghattargi, 2005)
Feeling isolated from others/reduced socializing	Some girls and teachers described how difficulties managing menstruation lead some girls to isolate themselves from social activities.	Pakistan (Ali & Rizvi, 2009) Rural Ghana (Scott et al., unpublished)
Negative impacts on education	Girls were often anxious and distracted in class and their concentration and participation was affected. Most girls tried not to miss school, but girls reported occasional absenteeism due to both difficulties managing menstruation and menstrual cramps.	Urban and rural Tanzania (Sommer, 2009a, 2009b) Rural Kenya (McMahon et al., 2011) Rural Ghana (Scott et al., unpublished)

Difficulties with disposing of pads in toilets and the risk that the next person using the toilet would see a pad or menstrual blood in blocked toilets was repeatedly cited as a source of concern. This would elevate the risk of discovery and break taboos about seeing other people's menstrual blood, as expressed in the following excerpts:

> When you throw it in the toilet, the next person will know it was you and tell others. (FGD 13, girls aged 12–14)

> If you go to the toilet and see it on the floor or the toilet basin, it is not good. It messes your day when you see it. It is a private thing and not for all to see. (FGD 18, women aged 30–38)

Psychosocial Deprivation

The psychosocial deprivations described by girls, women, and teachers in our study involved a lack of access to accurate information, and limited emotional and practical guidance and support (see the second section of Table 1). Most girls had heard about menstruation from family members, teachers, or friends before menarche, but the information they received was often vague or inaccurate. Although most knew that menstruation is related to the reproduction system, many did not know what menstrual blood is:

> I hear people say it is impurities which are coming out of the body, but I don't understand how it becomes impure and why in the form of blood only? (IDI 15, out of school girl aged 17)

The female primary teachers we interviewed lamented that there were limited opportunities within the curricula to provide formal education on menstruation and that they did not have sufficient knowledge to do so. One teacher had inaccurate health knowledge including the beliefs that dark-colored menstrual blood is a sign of health problems and that girls with heavy flow should not bend at the waist during menstruation because this causes blood clots.

Many girls we interviewed described mothers or other family members as their preferred sources of support regarding menstruation. The support girls wanted from their relatives included practical help with menstrual flow management and guidance and emotional support to ease adaptation to menarche, such as reassurance that their experiences were normal. Some mothers we interviewed tried to mitigate the impacts of poverty on their daughters by using cloths themselves and saving up the money needed to buy pads for their daughters. Some girls received little advice or guidance before or after menarche, however, and some delayed or avoided discussing the onset of menstruation with family members. Many mothers said they found it uncomfortable, embarrassing, or shameful to discuss menstruation with their daughters and some avoided it altogether. The pressures of urban poverty limited mothers' time and motivation for supporting their daughters with menstruation, and some girls described their mothers as unavailable, harsh, or unhelpful. In some cases lack of money for sanitary pads led to conflict between girls and their parents. In the following example, the participant described lack of support from her mother as one of her greatest concerns relating to menstruation:

> *Interviewer:* Is it easy to talk to your parents about menstruation, for example, your mother?

> *Participant:* No. . . . When she is under pressure it is not easy for her to listen to you. She can easily start abusing you instead. . . . I worry who to tell because there are some mothers who when told about periods don't care and you are forced to go and tell someone else about it to assist you [with sanitary pads]. (IDI 25, girl aged 12)

Menstrual Poverty and Stigma

We summarize our findings on the emotional and psychosocial impacts of menstrual poverty in Table 1 (second column, third section). Problems with leakage, hygiene, and lack of privacy all contribute to challenges keeping one's menstruating status secret, leading to embarrassment and exposure to stigma. All participants stated that it is very important to prevent other people from seeing one's menstrual blood. Some teachers described accidents where female pupils stained their clothes during menstruation as "misbehaving," emphasizing the transgression of social taboos. Participants described living with constant anxiety during their periods because of fear of leakage and body odor because infrequent change of menstrual products was widely regarded as a major source of stigma and embarrassment. Concerns about body odor and the importance of bathing were repeatedly mentioned by parents, teachers, and girls. Many participants described social expectations to use sanitary pads and bathe three times a day during menstruation:

> If you don't have pads, and maybe that day there is water shortage, you will definitely start smelling and if your parent or the people living with you smell that bad odor, they will complain and you will feel embarrassed to say you are the cause. (FGD 8, girls aged 12–14, formal primary school)

In some cases, girls who are not able to hide their menstruating status are gossiped about or bullied by other pupils:

Last week there was an embarrassment here. . . . One girl had her periods, so it is like the boys knew about it. They were jeering at her, so she decided to stay at home for 2 days until the period was over. (KII 3, female head teacher, formal primary school)

Effects of Menstrual Poverty on Emotional Well-Being

Girls described lack of reliable access to menstrual products as a major cause of physical discomfort, embarrassment, anxiety, fear of being stigmatized, and low mood (See Table 1). Participants used language like "feeling bad," feeling "stressed", or "fearful" and "wanting to cry" to describe the emotional distress they experienced. For many students, negative feelings associated with menstrual poverty caused particular anxiety during school days:

> When you are at school, it is better to use pads because it is protective and you don't keep asking for permission from the teacher every now and then to go and change in the toilet. You can wait until break time; that is when you can go to change. Also if your menstrual flow is heavy, the pad helps you to stay a bit longer before you go to change, whereas if it were the cloth, it kind of soaks very fast and can embarrass you. . . . [Later in the interview, talking about when participant cannot access pads:] I feel uncomfortable and worse when it is [a] school day. That is the time I wish I could be at home so that I don't have to worry about my clothes being stained and other people laughing at me. (IDI 16, girl aged 14)

> *Interviewer:* What about a girl who has nothing to use but has gone to school, what happens to her?

> *Participant 3:* She can get assistance from a fellow girlfriend.

> *Interviewer:* How do girls feel when they are in such situation?

> *Participant 7:* You feel embarrassed and stressed; you just want to cry. (FGD 3, girls aged 12–14)

In some cases, participants described feeling tired or sick in the context of the anxiety, hinting at particularly high levels of emotional distress involved:

> I feel tired [when menstruating], I don't want to meet people, and you don't know how to leave the place because you are not sure if you have stained your dress. . . . You feel so bad because you were not expecting your periods and they have come and it makes you feel very sick. . . .

> You are afraid; you don't want to play with others and are scared the
> pad or cloth will fall to the floor in front of people. (IDI 29, girl aged 13)

Although teachers reported that some girls miss school because of lack
of sanitary pads, most girls we interviewed said they rarely or never miss
school because of their periods. Many said, however, that they felt inhib-
ited because of anxiety about staining their clothes or odor, for example.
keeping very still while sitting in class, worrying about moving or standing
up, and avoiding physical games and sports. Participants explained how this
affected some girls' ability to socialize with their peers and undermined their
concentration in class. A male teacher in one of the informal schools noted
that female pupils "don't concentrate because they are cautious about the
menstruation and are worried they could have soiled their clothes. She has
to be in and out of class to check" (KII2, Male teacher, informal school):

> They feel as if they have been isolated from the rest of the people and
> they become lonely. Some can easily be depressed and their school
> performance affected badly. (FGD 10, girls aged 12–14 out of school)

Limitations in gender sensitivity in the school environment, including
lack of privacy in some school toilets, added to discomfort and fear of
discovery:

> The toilets have no good doors, and anyone can see you when you are
> changing. (IDI 25, girl aged 12)

The effect of menstruation on education was not only due to anxiety or
fear of exposing menstrual blood. Menstrual cramps were described as another problem affecting school attendance and concentration in class. Some
girls said that they take analgesics when they have menstrual cramps and, in
one school, teachers said they provide painkillers to menstruating girls when
required. In some cases, however, girls said that they never took medication
when affected by pain because of lack of knowledge or lack of money to
buy them:

> [The menstrual cramps] are so severe that I am not able to eat my meals.
> . . . I am not able to concentrate in class. . . . I have never known if there
> is any medicine to take. (IDI 3, girl aged 14)

In a few cases, girls described having positive experiences of menstruation. In the following example, feeling positive about menstruation required
having access to sanitary pads and feeling confident about how to keep
menstruation secret:

When I am at home, I don't like sitting in the house. I prefer going outside when I have my pad on and I am not afraid to play with my friends. (IDI 26, girl aged 14)

Strategies for Coping With Menstrual Poverty

A few girls and a larger number of the women described taking a pragmatic approach to menstrual poverty, trying to avoid upsetting thoughts about it, or taking a positive view of what they learned from the experience:

Interviewer: What do you usually feel when you cannot afford the pads and have to resort to using a cloth to manage your periods?

Participant: I cannot put a lot of my thoughts on that because I don't like being stressed. I simply take the piece of cloth and use it to manage the periods. (IDI 13, adult woman)

Interviewer: Right now [those who do not have access to pads] feel bad, but in the future what effects will it have on their lives?

Participant: It is ok because she has been through a lot and she is familiar with problems so that when she gets money she knows how to use it. (FGD 10, out of school girls aged 12–14)

Some girls who lacked support at home reported taking proactive measures to get practical help with menstruation, for example, befriending and seeking help from neighbors or other family members. Schools emerged as important sources of support for girls who did not receive sufficient support with menstruation at home. Not all girls felt confident enough to confide in teachers, however, and this form of support was not accessible to out-of-school girls. School teachers described taking informal approaches to guiding girls with managing menstruation, explaining about the practicalities of menstrual flow management, and advising girls to use socks if they did not have access to sanitary pads. Girls also mentioned the helpfulness of informal advice and assistance from some teachers. One teacher believed she and her colleagues had an important role in increasing girls' confidence, demonstrating the benefits of repeated guidance and support with managing menstruation:

Previously it has been that way, such that you find a girl on her own [during menstruation] but now, after [teachers are] talking to them frequently, they are not isolating themselves. In fact girls who were isolating themselves by not playing with the others were doing so because they were not able to manage their periods. (KII 3, Principal, female, formal primary school)

One girl mentioned that being encouraged to talk about menstruation in school helped her to overcome her initial shyness about discussing the issue:

> I remember there was a time that happened [discussion about menstruation] where all class seven and eight girls were put together. Girls talked until I realized I didn't have such a big problem and so I stopped being shy. I also talk about it these days. (IDI 16, girl aged 14)

DISCUSSION

In this article, we sought to take a first step toward international comparative research on the impacts of poverty on the well-being of menstruating girls and women. We introduced the concept of "menstrual poverty" to refer to the multiple material and psychosocial deprivations experienced by menstruating girls and women in resource-poor settings. We also highlighted the emotional and psychosocial impacts of menstrual poverty on adolescent girls through a qualitative study involving adolescent girls and women in an urban poor context in Nairobi City, Kenya.

Menstrual Poverty in Korogocho and Other Contexts

Our study found that girls and women in Korogocho experience similar material and psychosocial deprivations to those documented in other studies in low-income contexts in South Asia and sub-Saharan and North Africa.

As in other contexts, menstrual poverty in Korogocho involved multiple material deprivations, including limited access to sanitary pads and lack of privacy and water and sanitation facilities in communities and schools. These material deprivations led to physical discomfort, inconvenience, hygiene problems, and risk of embarrassment and stigma. Poor quality water and sanitation facilities affect menstrual well-being in Tanzania and Bangladesh (Rashid & Michaud, 2000; Sommer, 2009a, 2009b). Many girls and women reported using a mixture of methods, depending on what they could afford at the time, including cloths or socks when they did not have money to purchase pads. Although this was not a quantitative study, we produced tallies of interview transcripts, which revealed that most girls reported using sanitary pads at some point during their past three periods, a much higher proportion than in contexts such as an urban informal settlement in Delhi, where only 3% of women report using sanitary pads or clean cotton cloth (Garg et al., 2001).

Second, many girls in our study experienced psychosocial deprivations including limited access to information and lack of emotional and practical support with menstruation from parents and other family members. Limited and inaccurate knowledge about menstruation, including inability to explain the reproductive processes involved in menstruation, has been observed in Tanzania, Nigeria, Egypt, Pakistan, and India (Adinma & Adinma, 2008; Ali & Rizvi, 2009; Deo & Ghattargi, 2005; El-Gilany et al., 2005; Sommer, 2009a, 2009b). Most girls in our study reported receiving at least some information about menstruation before menarche, suggesting that levels of menstrual preparedness in Korogocho are much higher than in South Asian contexts where between 50% and 97% of girls receive no information about menstruation prior to menarche (Ali & Rizvi, 2009; Garg et al., 2001; Khanna et al., 2005). Many of our participants, however, reported that they lacked access to accurate information about menstruation. Some of the reasons for lack of parent support were communication taboos and lack of awareness and knowledge on the part of mothers. These barriers to parental support have also been identified in Bangladesh, Tanzania, India, Malawi; and Egypt (El-Gilany et al., 2005; Garg et al., 2001; Munthali & Zulu, 2007; Rashid & Michaud, 2000; Sommer, 2009a, 2009b). In addition, our study found that poverty and deprivation in the cash-based urban economy limit women's time and motivation to engage with their daughters. Mother–daughter communication about menstruation in Korogocho is investigated in more detail in Crichton and colleagues (2012).

One advantage of grouping together conceptually the multiple deprivations involved in menstrual poverty is that it enabled us to examine how these deprivations interrelate in the ways they affect girl's health and well-being. For example, lack of privacy and problems with hygiene become all the more problematic in contexts where there are particularly strong taboos against discussing menstruation, preventing parental support and guidance. We also believe that the concept is useful for facilitating comparison of the differences in the quality and severity of each category of menstrual poverty between different contexts, such as the variations in levels of menstrual preparedness and access to sanitary pads between Korogocho and other contexts, particularly in South Asian, noted above. One area where there is particular variation between contexts is regarding social norms around personal hygiene during menses. Girls and mothers in Korogocho emphasized the importance of good personal hygiene during menstruation. This included social expectations to use sanitary pads instead of cloths and to bathe up to three times a day, practices that are often made difficult or impossible by urban poverty. Attitudes toward washing during menses vary widely in different resource-poor contacts. Social norms against bathing during menses have been observed in contexts including Pakistan (Ali & Rizvi, 2009), Muslim communities in India (Garg et al., 2001), Egypt (El-Gilany et al., 2005), Korea, and the Philippines (World Health Organization [WHO], 1981). To our knowledge, widespread social norms around frequent washing during menses have not previously been noted by researchers, although a 10-country study observed that some women in each of their study contexts held such beliefs (WHO, 1981). Social norms around frequent washing are important because people who cannot conform to them due to poverty may experience embarrassment and exposure to stigma.

Our study revealed that the social context had important influences on how menstrual poverty related to emotional well-being. Participants described the existence of stigma against those who failed to keep menstruation secret, for example, through stains on their clothes or odor. Menstruation-related stigma appears to be present in all societies around the world (Kowalski & Chapple, 2000; Roberts et al., 2002; Sommer, 2009a). In this study and numerous contexts including West Africa, Southern Africa, and South Asia (Adinma & Adinma, 2008; Ali & Rizvi, 2009; Garg et al., 2001; Munthali & Zulu, 2007; Rashid & Michaud, 2000), menstrual blood was commonly perceived as dirty or polluting, which may add to the feelings of embarrassment and shame experienced by girls affected by menstrual poverty. The strong social norms around sanitary pads being "correct" and "hygienic", and the widespread view that using cloths is unhygienic, may have led those who had difficulties accessing sanitary pads to internalize negative perceptions.

Emotional and Psychosocial Aspects of Menstrual Poverty: A Neglected Research Topic

The second main contribution of our study is the exploration of the emotional and psychosocial impacts of menstrual poverty, which are only beginning to be addressed by researchers. Our study provides testimony that negative emotional and psychosocial impacts of menstrual poverty are an important concern for girls and involve fear of stigma and feelings of embarrassment, anxiety, and low mood. Anxiety during menstruation has barely been addressed in existing research from resource-poor settings, and its relationship with menstrual poverty has not been examined in detail (Deo & Ghattargi, 2005; McMahon et al., 2011; Sommer, 2009a). In some cases, a high severity of emotional distress was suggested by comments that participants felt tired or "sick" or wanted to cry because of the anxiety. Hormone-related symptoms of fatigue and mood symptoms including tension and depressed mood are highly prevalent among menstruating girls and women regardless of social context or menstrual poverty (Wong & Khoo, 2010; Yonkers, Shaughn O'Brien, & Eriksson, 2008). Participants in this study, however, directly linked anxiety about menstrual poverty with emotional distress in their descriptions of menstrual experiences. Girls affected by menstrual poverty in Korogocho and other settings are making the turbulent transitions involved in puberty in an economic and social context that makes it difficult for them to keep their menstruating status secret (Sommer, 2009a, 2009b). For young girls affected by menstrual poverty, menstruation involves a large and avoidable additional psychological burden that others of the same age do not have to bear.

Both teachers and pupils explained that discomfort and anxiety during menstruation undermines girls' schooling experience. Similar to accounts of girls in Tanzania (Sommer, 2009a), girls in Korogocho described experiencing fear of discovery of their menstruating status because of lack of access to pads on schooldays and in some cases due to lack of privacy for changing and disposal of menstrual products. Anxiety about discovery and stigma was exacerbated by isolated events of male and female pupils teasing and bullying girls who are discovered to be menstruating. Unlike the Tanzania study (Sommer, 2009b), many girls in Korogocho found teachers to be approachable and supportive during menstruation. The teachers we interviewed were concerned about girls' problems during menstruation and had initiated informal discussions about menstruation with female pupils and provided practical support and advice. Most girls said that they tried not to miss school during menstruation, but menstrual poverty did cause occasional absenteeism and more frequently undermined girls' concentration in class.

Strengths and Limitations

This article provides an important contribution to knowledge because it is one of the first studies to focus on the psychological implications of menstrual deprivations caused by poverty in resource-poor settings. The qualitative nature of this study means that it provides powerful evidence of the emotional distress experienced by adolescent girls as described in their own words. Another advantage of qualitative research is that it enables new, unexpected themes to emerge (Glaser & Strauss, 1967; Patton, 1990). The article was based on a wider study of menstrual practices and problems among girls and women in Korogocho, but the emotional impacts of menstrual poverty emerged as an important source of concern for girls. This study allowed us to identify that anxiety is an important outcome of menstrual poverty for some adolescent girls in resource-poor settings. A limitation of using open-ended questioning and nonrepresentative sample, however, was that it provided an indication of the kinds of emotional impacts of menstrual poverty but not their prevalence or severity. Also, the open-ended nature of the questions, our reliance on adolescents' own reports, and the cross-sectional nature of the study means that we were not able to measure the psychological impacts of menstrual poverty. Finally, our literature search examined only English-language publications, so we may have missed publications on this topic in other languages.

Future Research

The categories of menstrual poverty described by participants in Korogocho are similar to those found in a range of resource-poor urban and rural contexts in sub-Saharan Africa, North Africa, and South Asia, suggesting that the types of emotional distress found among menstruating girls in Korogocho might also be present in those contexts. Future cross-country comparative research could examine whether sociocultural and economic variations around the world cause variation in the type and extent of the psychological impacts of menstrual deprivation within and between regions.

Further research is also needed to measure the types and severity of emotional impacts of menstrual poverty during adolescence, and the longer-term educational, psychological, and developmental implications. For example, use of standardized psychological measures would enable researchers to measure the severity and prevalence of emotional distress caused by menstrual poverty.

Research from industrialized countries, especially the United States, offers insights into potential directions and approaches for examining longer-term mental health impacts and for designing and evaluating interventions to address them. Researchers have examined preparation and support before and during menarche, girls' experience of menstruation, and positive adjustment to puberty (Chang et al., 2010; Greif & Ulman, 1982; Koff & Rierdan, 1995; McPherson & Korfine, 2004; Ruble & Brooks-Gunn, 1982; Swenson & Havens, 1987). They have also found that emotional support and access to information about puberty can help young people to acquire the knowledge and skills needed for avoiding sexual risk taking (Short & Rosenthal, 2008; Stubbs, 2008). Similar research is very important in contexts where there are taboos against parent–child communication and limited access to information as in many resource-poor settings. Researchers in the United States have found evidence that negative experience of menarche are associated with menstrual shame and negative body image in adulthood, which in turn can undermine sexual negotiation and lead to sexual risk taking (Schooler et al., 2005; Stubbs, 2008). Researchers could consider whether the relationships between menstrual poverty and body shame contribute toward sexual risk taking among adolescent girls and women in resource-poor settings. Researchers have also noted the impact of psychosocial factors in adolescence such as interpersonal difficulties and parenting style in contributing to longer-term developmental problems such as depression and anxiety disorders (Short & Rosenthal, 2008). There is a need for researchers to consider whether the psychosocial and emotional aspects of menstrual poverty lead to developmental problems, and how this can be mitigated by interventions. Such research is necessary because risk and protective factors in these contexts are likely to be different from the industrialized countries such as the United States where associations between menstrual well-being and developmental impacts have been studied (Ndugwa et al., 2010).

Finally, this study contributes to the limited evidence available on the impact of menstrual poverty on girls' education (Ali & Rizvi, 2009; Lloyd et al., 1998; McMahon et al., 2011; Oster & Thornton, 2009; Scott et al., unpublished; Sommer, 2009b). Our study provides evidence that menstrual poverty and its psychological impacts lead to negative schooling experiences among menstruating pupils. Further research is needed to examine whether this impacts on their academic performance.

Policy Implications

Interventions for enhancing well-being during menstruation need to be multifaceted, in order to address the multiple and interrelated deprivations involved in menstrual poverty. This requires a combination of addressing menstruation in water hygiene and sanitation programs, improving gender sensitivity, information provision, and social and emotional care relating to menstruation in schools and communities, and efforts to improve access to effective, culturally acceptable, and sustainable methods for managing menstrual flow (McMahon et al., 2011). Given the resource constraints involved, there is a need to look beyond conventional commercial sanitary products to those that are low-cost, locally produced, or reusable. In Kenya, such projects include efforts to train girls to make their own reusable sanitary pads (Access Collective, 2011) and to assess the acceptability of reusable menstrual cups in informal settlements (APHRC, 2009).

The coping strategies used by girls and others in the community to mitigate the effects of menstrual poverty offer some insights into potential school- and community-based initiatives for addressing the emotional burden of menstrual poverty. The informal conversations and support teachers offered to students could be strengthened and replicated in other settings, and include promoting more positive attitudes toward menstruation, sharing practical tips, and creating opportunities to discuss menstruation. Such discussions need to be carefully facilitated to ensure that stigmatizing views are not reinforced, and this is especially important in settings with inequality in degrees of menstrual poverty. Our study found that the information and support provided by teachers was limited to informal advice on practical management of menstruation, and some teachers lacked accurate knowledge about menstruation. It is pertinent that teachers receive improved training about puberty, and that schools provide accurate information about menstruation and address the complex emotional and physical changes that girls deal with during puberty by providing comprehensive sexuality education from an early age. Teachers and community members must promote more positive perceptions about girls' capacity to participate and perform well in school and other activities during menstruation, and for initiatives to reduce bullying and stigma. Community-based initiatives are needed to meet the needs of out-of-school girls. Given the multiple and interrelated problems surrounding menstruation in urban informal settlements, such interventions have the potential to promote psychological well-being and positive adjustment during puberty, improve performance in school, increase self-efficacy, and reduce sexual risk taking.

REFERENCES

Access Collective. (2011). *Access Health Project Mwezi*. Retrieved from http://access-collective.com/health

Adinma, E. D., & Adinma, J. I. (2008). Perceptions and practices on menstruation amongst Nigerian secondary school girls. *African Journal of Reproductive Health, 12*(1), 74–83.

African Population and Health Research Center (APHRC). (2002). *Population and health dynamics in Nairobi's informal settlements. Report of the Nairobi Cross-sectional Slums Survey (NCSS) 2000*. Nairobi, Kenya: Author.

African Population and Health Research Center (APHRC). (2006). *Averting preventable maternal mortality: Delays and barriers to the utilization of emergency obstetric care in Nairobi's informal settlements*. Nairobi, Kenya: Author.

African Population and Health Research Center (APHRC). (2009). *Attitudes towards, and acceptability of, menstrual cups as a method for managing menstruation: Experiences of women and schoolgirls in Nairobi, Kenya* (APHRC Policy Brief No. 21). Nairobi, Kenya: Author.

Ali, T. S., & Rizvi, S. N. (2009). Menstrual knowledge and practices of female adolescents in urban Karachi, Pakistan. *Journal of Adolescence, 33*, 531–541.

Boyatzis, R. (1998). *Transforming qualitative information: Thematic analysis and code development*. Thousand Oaks, CA: Sage.

Chang, Y.-T., Hayter, M., & Wu, S.-C. (2010). A systematic review and meta-ethnography of the qualitative literature: Experiences of the menarche. *Journal of Clinical Nursing, 19*, 447–460.

Crichton, J., Ibisomi, L., & Gyimah, S. O. (2012). Mother-daughter communication about sexual maturation, abstinence and unintended pregnancy: Experiences from an informal settlement in Nairobi, Kenya. *Journal of Adolescence, 35*, 21–30. doi:10.1016/j.adolescence.2011.06.008

Deo, D. S., & Ghattargi, C. H. (2005). Perceptions and practices regarding menstruation: A comparative study in urban and rural adolescent girls. *Indian Journal of Community Medicine, 30*(1), 21–30. Retrieved from http://www.indmedica.com/journals.php?journalid=7&issueid=28&articleid=306&action=article

El-Gilany, A.-H., Badawi, K., & El-Fedawy, S. (2005). Menstrual hygiene among adolescent schoolgirls in Mansoura, Egypt. *Reproductive Health Matters, 13*(26), 147–152.

Emina, J., Beguy, D., Zulu, E. M., Ezeh, A. C., Muindi, K., Elung'ata, P., Otsola, J. K., & Yé, Y. (2011). Monitoring of health and demographic outcomes in poor urban settlements: Evidence from the Nairobi Urban Health and Demographic Surveillance System. *Journal of Urban Health, 88*(Suppl. 2), 200–218.

Epari, C., Ezeh, A. C., Mugisha F., & Ogollah, R. (2008). *Oh! So 'we' have been under-reporting Nairobi's primary school enrolment rates?* (APHRC Working Paper, No. 35). Nairobi, Kenya: APHRC.

Fereday, J., & Muir-Cochrane, E. (2006). Demonstrating rigor using thematic analysis: A hybrid approach of inductive and deductive coding and theme development. *International Journal of Qualitative Methods*, *5*(1), 80–92.

Garg, S., Sharma, N., & Sahay, R. (2001). Socio-cultural aspects of menstruation in an urban slum in Delhi, India. *Reproductive Health Matters*, *19*(17), 16–25.

Glaser, G. & Strauss, L., (1967). *The discovery of grounded theory: Strategies of qualitative research*. London, UK: Weidenfeld and Nicolson.

Greif, E. B., & Ulman, K. J. (1982). The psychological impact of menarche on early adolescent females: A review of the literature. *Child Development*, *53*, 1413–1430.

Keidar, O., Berry, E. M., Ezeh, A. C., & Donchin, M. (2008). *Determining appropriate entry point for health promoting schools intervention in Nairobi informal settlements* (APHRC Working Paper, No. 42). Nairobi, Kenya: APHRC.

Khanna, A., Goyal, R. S., & Bhawsar, R. (2005). Menstrual practices and reproductive problems: A study of adolescent girls in Rajasthan. *Journal of Health Management*, *7*(1), 91–107.

Koff, E., & Rierdan, J. (1995). Early adolescent girls' understanding of menstruation. *Women Health*, *22*, 1–21.

Kowalski, R. M., & Chapple, T. (2000). The social stigma of menstruation: Fact or fiction? *Psychology of Women Quarterly*, *24*, 74–80.

Kyobutungi, C., Ziraba, A. K., Ezeh, A., & Yé, Y. (2008). The burden of disease profile of residents of Nairobi's slums: Results from a Demographic Surveillance System. *Population Health Metrics*, *6*(1).

Lloyd, C. B., Mensch, B. S., & Clark, W. H. (1998). *The effects of primary school quality on the educational participation and attainment of Kenyan girls and boys*. Nairobi, Kenya: Population Council.

Mahon, T., & Fernandes, M. (2010). Menstrual hygiene in South Asia: A neglected issue for WASH (water, sanitation and hygiene) programmes. *Gender and Development*, *18*(1), 99–113.

Marván, M. L., & Trujillo, P. (2009) Menstrual socialization, beliefs, and attitudes concerning menstruation in rural and urban Mexican women. *Health Care for Women International*, *31*(1), 53–67.

McMahon, S. A., Winch, P. J., Caruso, B. A., Obure, A. F., Ogutu, E. A., Ochari, I. A., & Rheingans, R. D. (2011). 'The girl with her period is the one to hang her head: Reflections on menstrual management among schoolgirls in rural Kenya. *BMC International Health and Human Rights*, *11*(7).

McPherson, M. E., & Korfine, L. (2004). Menstruation across time: Menarche, menstrual attitudes, experiences and behaviors. *Women's Health Issues*, *14*, 193–200.

Mendle, J., Turkheimer, E., & Emery, R. E. (2007). Detrimental psychological outcomes associated with early pubertal timing in adolescent girls. *Developmental Review*, *27*, 151–171.

Morison, L., Ekpo, G., West, B., Demba, E., Mayaud, P., Coleman, R., Bailey, R., & Walraven, G. (2005). Bacterial vaginosis in relation to menstrual cycle, menstrual protection method, and sexual intercourse in rural Gambian women. *Sexually Transmitted Infections*, *81*, 242–247.

Mudege, N., & Zulu, E. M. (2010). Discourses of illegality and exclusion: When water access matters. *Global Public Health*, *13*, 1–13.

Munthali, A. C., & Zulu, E. M. (2007). The timing and role of initiation rites in preparing young people for adolescence and responsible sexual and reproductive behavior in Malawi. *African Journal of Reproductive Health, 11*, 150–167.

Ndugwa, R. P., Kabiru, C. W., Cleland, J., Beguy, D., Egondi, T., Zulu, E. M., & Jessor, R. (2010). Adolescent problem behavior in Nairobi's informal settlements: Applying problem behavior theory in Sub-Saharan Africa. *Journal of Urban Health, 88*(Suppl. 2), 298–317.

Orringer, K., & Gahagan, S. (2010). Adolescent girls define menstruation: A multiethnic exploratory study. *Health Care for Women International, 31*, 831–847.

Oster, E., & Thornton, R. (2009). *Menstruation and education in Nepal* (NBER Working Paper Series, No. W14853). Cambridge, MA: National Bureau of Economic Research.

Patton, M. (1990). *Qualitative evaluation and research methods.* Newbury Park, CA: Sage.

Patton, G. C., & Viner, R. (2007). Pubertal transitions in health. *Lancet, 369*, 1130–1139.

Rashid, S. F., & Michaud, S. (2000). Female adolescents and their sexuality: Notions of honour, shame, purity and pollution during the floods. *Disasters, 24*(1), 54–70.

Roberts, T.-A., Goldenberg, J. L.,, Power, C., & Pyszczynski, T. (2002). "Feminine protection": The effects of menstruation on attitudes towards women. *Psychology of Women Quarterly, 26*, 131–139.

Ruble, D. N., & Brooks-Gunn, J. (1982). The experience of menarche. *Child Development, 53*, 1557–1566.

Schooler, D., Ward, L. M., Merriwether, A., & Caruthers, A. S. (2005). Cycles of shame: Menstrual shame, body shame, and sexual decision-making. *Journal of Sex Research, 42*, 324–334.

Scott, L., Dopson, S., Montgomery, P., Dolan, C., & Ryus, C. (Unpublished). Impact of providing sanitary pads to poor girls in Africa. University of Oxford Study. Retrieved from http://doublex.eyedivision.info/wp-content/uploads/2010/09/University-of-Oxford-Sanitary-Pad-Study1.pdf.

Short, M. B., & Rosenthal, S. L. (2008). Psychosocial development and puberty. *Annals of the New York Academy of Science, 1135*, 36–42.

Silverman, D. (1993). *Interpreting qualitative data.* London, UK: Sage.

Sommer, M. (2009a). Where the education system and women's bodies collide: The social and health impact of girls' experiences of menstruation and schooling in Tanzania. *Journal of Adolescence, 33*, 521–529.

Sommer, M. (2009b). Ideologies on sexuality, menstruation and risk: Girls' experiences of puberty and schooling in northern Tanzania. *Culture, Health and Sexuality, 11*, 383–398.

Stubbs, M. L. (2008). Cultural perceptions and practices around menarche and adolescent menstruation in the United States. *Annals of the New York Academy of Sciences, 1135*, 58–88.

Swenson, I., & Havens, B. (1987). Menarche and menstruation: A review of the literature. *Journal of Community Health Nursing, 4*, 199–210.

Ulin, P. R., Robinson, E. T., & Tolley, E. E. (2005). *Qualitative methods in public health: A field guide for applied research.* San Fransisco, CA: Jossey-Bass.

Undie, C., John-Langba, J., & Kimani, E. (2006). The place of cool waters: Women and water in the slums of Nairobi, Kenya. *Wagadu: A Journal of Transnational Women's and Gender Studies, 3*, 40–60.

Wamoyi, J., Fenwick, A., Urassa, M., Zaba, B., & Stones, W. (2010). Parent-child communication about sexual and reproductive health in rural Tanzania: Implications for young people's sexual health interventions. *Reproductive Health, 12*(7), 6.

Wasserheit, J. N., Harris, J. R., Chakraborty, J., Kay, B. A., & Mason, K. J. (1989). Reproductive tract infections in family planning population in rural Bangladesh: A neglected opportunity to promote MCH-FFI programs. *Studies in Family Planning, 20*, 69–80.

Wong, L. P., & Khoo, E. M. (2010). Dysmenorrhea in a multiethnic population of adolescent Asian girls. *International Journal of Gynaecology & Obstetrics, 108*, 139–42.

World Health Organization (WHO). (1981). A cross-cultural study of menstruation: Implications for contraceptive development and use. *Studies in Family Planning, 12*(1), 3–16.

Yonkers, K. A., Shaughn O'Brien, P. M., & Eriksson, E. (2008). Premenstrual syndrome. *Lancet, 371*(9619), 1200–1210.

Effects of a Teenage Pregnancy Prevention Program in KwaZulu-Natal, South Africa

MYRA TAYLOR

Department of Public Health Medicine, University of KwaZulu-Natal, Durban, South Africa

CHAMPAK JINABHAI

Faculty of Health Sciences, Durban University of Technology, Durban, South Africa

SIYABONGA DLAMINI

Department of Public Health Medicine, University of KwaZulu-Natal, Durban, South Africa

RESHMA SATHIPARSAD

School of Social Work and Community Development, University of KwaZulu-Natal, Durban, South Africa

MATTHIJS S. EGGERS and HEIN DE VRIES

Department of Health Communication, Maastricht University, Maastricht, The Netherlands

Researchers aimed to determine the effects of a teenage pregnancy (TP) prevention program for 816 high school students attending 16 KwaZulu-Natal, South African schools through a randomized control trial. Data were collected at baseline and at the 8-month follow-up in 2009. Results were calculated using multivariate analyses of program effects employing Mplus 6, and indicated significantly healthier attitudes, including intentions to abstain from sex whilst at school, plans to communicate with partners about teenage pregnancy, and increased reports of condom use. Researchers thus provide some support for the effectiveness of a TP prevention program that should be further strengthened in a comprehensive approach that includes schools and families.

Teenage pregnancy (TP) is an international concern, and both developed and developing countries are seeking solutions so that we can provide our young women with a better future and their children with adequate care. In this article we describe the effects of an intervention program targeting high school students in KwaZulu-Natal, South Africa, that resulted in healthier attitudes about TP, increased intentions to delay sexual initiation and to communicate with partners, and increased use of condoms. The limitations and challenges are also described.

BACKGROUND

TP has several detrimental effects such as increased chances of dropping out of school and increased risk of sexually transmitted infections (STIs), preterm birth, mental health problems, and economic family burden (Kanku & Mash, 2010). A South African review reported a pregnancy rate of 71 per 1000 women (15–19 years; Panday, Makiwane, Ranchod, & Lestoala, 2009). The need for barrier methods to prevent transmission of HIV and other STIs emphasizes the need for male involvement (Harrison, Newell, Imrie, & Hoddinott, 2010), and the importance of targeting both sexes to promote abstinence or consistent condom use. Many scholars have also reported lack of gender equity and the urgent need to address gender norms in a society of male privilege, despite South Africa's Bill of Rights (Jewkes, Vundule, Maforah, & Jordaan, 2001; Sathiparsad & Taylor, 2011; Wood, Maforah, & Jewkes, 1998). School settings are ideal places to effectively reach teens to motivate them to engage in TP prevention behaviors (Bennett & Assefi, 2005; DiCenso, Guyatt, Willan, & Griffith, 2002; Kirby, 2011).

Researchers employed a Cochrane systematic review of educational interventions to prevent unintended pregnancies amongst youth, 27 of which were undertaken at schools, and found that multicomponent interventions combining educational and contraceptive interventions were successful (Oringanje, Meremikwu, Eko, Esu, & Meremikwu, 2009). The literature also includes a report of the benefits of improving knowledge, changing beliefs and attitudes, and increasing the intentions of teens to protect themselves, either through sexual abstinence or by using contraception (Kirby, 2011). South Africa has progressive social and health policies that permit young women from the age of 12 to independently decide on contraception and abortion, and these services should be free and available at local health facilities (Department of Health, 2012a). There are problems however, both with the awareness amongst teens of the availability and the accessibility of services such as contraception, the morning after pill, and abortion (Willan, 2013). School settings offer an opportunity to provide students attending high school with the information and skills that can assist them to improve their sexual and reproductive health. Over the past two decades there have been wide-ranging efforts to promote the health of teens attending school. These include the "Lifeskills" module in South African schools, which, as part of the Life Orientation syllabus, is an examinable subject that includes sexual health (James et al., 2004). This has not, however, proved effective in reducing the number of teen pregnancies (Panday et al., 2009). An additional issue is that discussion of sex and sexuality in the home is taboo (Jewkes, Morrell, & Christofides, 2009; Swartz & Bhana, 2009). Focused sexual and reproductive health educational programs are therefore required to change adolescent attitudes about early sexual debut and sexual risk behavior in order to reduce TP. In this study researchers thus investigated whether a prevention intervention program could change attitudes and influence the intentions to practice safe sexual behavior amongst high school students in the province of KwaZulu-Natal, in order to reduce TP.

CONCEPTUAL FRAMEWORK

The researchers adapted the I-Change model (de Vries et al., 2003), and used this as the conceptual framework because this had proved helpful in our previous studies that investigated high school students' sexual behavior (sexual abstinence and condom use; Dlamini et al., 2008; Taylor et al., 2007). The premise of the adapted model is that constructs such as students' positive and negative attitudes about TP are contributory demotivating and motivating factors, respectively, that can influence their intentions to prevent TP. We were interested in investigating the high number of teen pregnancies (between a quarter and a third of female teens become pregnant; Panday et al., 2009), and if poverty (using a measure of socioeconomic status [SES]) was a factor amongst these teens that influenced their attitudes to teen pregnancy. Arising from the focus discussions, which explored gender norms, the role of students' attitudes in motivating their intentions to prevent teen pregnancy was investigated. The researchers also used the I-Change model since this takes cognisance of the current behavior of the student, so that in this study the researchers designed an intervention that targeted both abstinent and sexually experienced teens (Figure 1).

METHODS

We undertook a randomized controlled trial of 16 high schools selected from the KwaZulu-Natal Department of Education's list of 1,580 high schools. We selected schools in 2009 from two (urban and rural) of 11 districts in the province of KwaZulu-Natal. We used geographical stratification to randomly allocate schools to experimental or control groups. We then invited students in one randomly selected grade 8 class (their first year at high school) at each school to participate in the study. Of the selected schools, eight schools

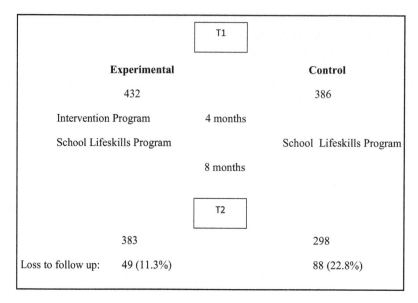

FIGURE 1 Grade 8 students in intervention and control groups at 16 KwaZulu-Natal, South African schools. T1, $n = 818$, T2, $n = 681$.

(four experimental and four control) were in the predominantly rural district of Ugu (population 790,000), and eight were in the metropolitan area of eThekwini (population 3.2 million).

The student respondents were requested to complete a self-completed structured questionnaire, based on prior elicitation research from focus groups with teens attending six urban and rural high schools. These focus groups had explored reasons for TP and possible ways to address this issue. The researchers used these data to develop the questionnaire, translated it into isiZulu, and back-translated this for clarity. In the year prior to the study the researchers piloted the questionnaire in a school not included in this study. We coded the questionnaires to ensure confidentiality, and each student completed a questionnaire at baseline (T1) and 8 months later (T2). Research assistants explained the study purpose, the importance of valid responses, and the strict confidentiality. They were also present to clarify if learners were uncertain about answering any question. The students each placed completed questionnaires in an envelope that each student then sealed. The researchers obtained ethical clearance from the University of KwaZulu-Natal and permission from the KwaZulu-Natal Department of Education, in addition to the principals from each school. Parents and students provided written informed consent. There were no refusals from the selected schools or students.

Outcome Variables

Outcome variables are presented in Table 1. We used a Likert scale ranging from 1 (*strongly disagree*) to 5 (*strongly agree*).

TABLE 1 Outcome Variables

Item	Statement
Positive attitudes to TP (pros) 6 statements: Cronbach $\alpha = 0.72$.	If I fall pregnant/cause a pregnancy it proves I am fertile and can have a child. There is a chance that I'll keep my boyfriend/girlfriend. I will get the child support grant. I don't need to attend school. I will be regarded as an adult. I can have sex more often.
Negative attitudes to TP (cons) 8 statements: Cronbach $\alpha = 0.72$.	My parents will be angry with me. My teachers will be angry with me. My family will be ashamed of me. People will make rude/unkind comments. I won't be able to go back to school. I will lose my family's trust. I will lose my friends. There's a chance that I'll lose my boy/girlfriend.
TP intentions 4 statements: Cronbach $\alpha = 0.73$ (these statements were analyzed separately to better discriminate the students' responses).	I intend to abstain from sex whilst at school. I intend to communicate with my partner about TP. I intend to prevent myself from becoming pregnant/causing a pregnancy. I intend to use condoms consistently.

The researchers assessed sexual behavior by three questions ($0 = no$, $1 = yes$): "Have you ever had sex? Do you use condoms? Have you ever been pregnant/caused a pregnancy?" In addition, condom use consistency was assessed by asking students, "How often do you use condoms with your regular partner?" The students provided answers on a 4-point scale, ranging from 1 (*never*) to 4 (*always*). Students were also asked, "At what age did you first have sex? What was the age of your partner? Have you ever been forced to have sex?"

Covariates

We assessed students using the sociodemographic variables of age, gender, and SES, and for the latter we used a family affluence scale based on whether the household had a television or cell phone (1), a television and a cell phone (2) or no television or cell phone (0). We also requested information about home language, religion, with whom they lived and the number of nights that students went to bed hungry the previous week.

Program

The researchers developed the program, which consisted of 12 weekly lessons using an interactive variety of activities including role plays, small and large group discussions, debates, and viewing of videos made especially for the discussions with students, which were implemented by two pairs of young male and female trained facilitators (Taylor et al., 2012). The program objectives were to provide information, address students' attitudes, and encourage intentions to prevent TP. The researchers, who comprised an interdisciplinary team, developed the material for the program based on the formative research undertaken in the previous 2 years. The researchers then piloted this at two schools not included in the randomized controlled trial (RCT). The topics discussed were Knowing Yourself, The Choice is Yours, Relationships, Making Choices, Body Development, Contraception, Peer Pressure, Culture, Parenthood, Responsibility, and Human Rights, following principles outlined by Kirby (2011). Gender norms were a core component of all the modules.

Analysis

The researchers used descriptive statistics to describe the study sample and used t-tests and chi-square analysis to detect differences between groups. We calculated the intervention effects with multivariate linear and logistic regression analysis in Mplus 6, and we included as covariates age, gender, SES, sexual experience, and baseline scores. We corrected all intervention effects for the cluster effect of students within schools using Mplus 6. Effects were considered significant when $p < .05$. See Figure 2.

RESULTS

Baseline (T1)

The 816 students comprised similar proportions of males (mean age: 14.6 years; $SD = 1.4$) and females (mean age: 13.9 years; $SD = 1.1$) with similar demographic characteristics. Sixty percent of students were Christian. A third of students lived with both parents, but slightly more (36%) lived in single-parent households with their mothers (36.0%), and fewer lived with their fathers. Many children lived with grandparents and other relatives and friends. The researchers noted that at baseline there were differences between the experimental and control group for hunger (see Table 2). The schools in the study were situated in areas of low SES—a quarter of the students had gone to bed hungry the previous week, and 21.2% of households lacked a television (not in table).

Most students were not sexually experienced (12.7% had ever had sex). Of these 104 sexually experienced students, 91 were males (87.5%) who had initiated sex at a mean age of 12.6 years ($SD = 2.9$), whereas females had been slightly older (mean age 13.0 years, $SD = 3.6$). The students had initiated sex with partners who were usually about 15 years of age, which

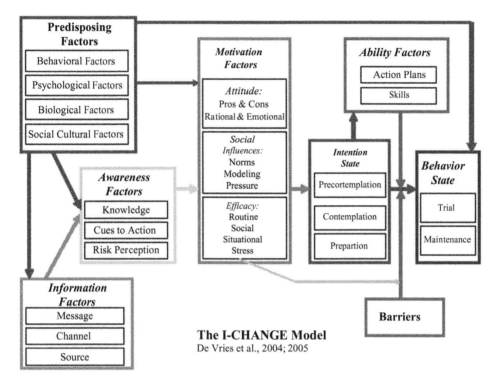

The I-CHANGE Model
De Vries et al., 2004; 2005

FIGURE 2 The I-Change model.

suggests that their sexual partners were fellow schoolgoers. Thirty percent of these sexually experienced students had ever been forced to have sex, but no statistically significant gender or urban/rural differences were found.

The students' mean scores for attitudes toward the perceived advantages of TP (the pros) were the lowest of all the scores (2.32 and 2.40 for the experimental and control groups, respectively). Students in both groups thus considered pregnancy among teens a disadvantage, but students in the control group had the more negative attitude (3.69 vs. 3.51, $p < .01$), and were also more intent on preventing TP (3.59 vs. 3.17, $p < .01$) and on using condoms consistently (3.90 vs. 3.71, $p < .05$). We adjusted for these baseline differences in the follow-up analysis. Over 60% of sexually experienced students used male condoms, but both groups failed to use condoms consistently (see Table 2).

We found that drop-out (16.6%) by students participating in the RCT was associated with being in the control group, female, and of an older age (Figure 1). Although school attendance in South Africa is compulsory, there is no monitoring of nonattenders or follow-up of missing children at many schools, but another driver, is that due to the high rate of unemployment many parents move in search of work (Statistics South Africa, 2013).

TABLE 2 Sample Characteristics and Program Effects

| | Baseline (T1) | | Follow-up (T2) | | |
| | Control | Experimental | Control | Experimental | Intervention effect |
Characteristic	($N = 385$)	($N = 431$)	($N = 296$)	($N = 383$)	B
Gender (% male, N)	50.1% (193)	50.6% (218)	51.4% (152)	51.4% (197)	—
Mean age (*SD*)	14.22 (1.41)	14.25 (1.26)	14.36 (1.29)	14.43 (1.19)	—
Mean SES (*SD*)	1.71 (0.55)	1.72 (0.52)	2.21 (0.42)	2.25 (0.49)	—
Home language (% IsiZulu, N)	99.2% (382)	98.8% (427)	97.3% (290)	99.2% (380)	—
Religion:					
Christian	61.2% (233)	57.1% (242)	73.1% (215)	59.1% (221)*	—
African traditional	20.2% (77)	19.8% (84)	10.5% (31)	19.3% (72)*	—
Other	19.6% (75)	23.1% (98)	16.4% (48)	21.6% (81)	—
With whom do you live:					
Both parents	34.9% (130)	33.4% (141)	34.1% (101)	33.8% (129)	—
Either parent	41.7% (155)	42.6% (180)	37.5% (111)	40.8% (156)	—
How many times did you go to bed hungry in the last week (Mean [*M*], *SD*)	0.57 (1.14)	0.40 (0.99)*	0.32 (0.93)	0.41 (1.12)	—
Attitudes to TP (*M, SD*) [a]:					
Pros ($\alpha = .72$)	2.40 (0.88)	2.32 (0.85)	2.45 (0.85)	2.26 (0.82)**	−0.13 (0.13)
Cons ($\alpha = .94$)	3.69 (0.96)	3.51 (1.00)**	3.83 (0.93)	3.81 (0.87)	0.01 (0.09)
Intent to abstain whilst at school (*M, SD*)[a]	3.92 (1.27)	3.99 (1.29)	3.97 (1.20)	4.18 (1.12)*	0.17 (0.07)*
Intent to communicate partner TP (*M, SD*)[a]	3.92 (1.17)	3.88 (1.16)	3.95 (1.01)	4.11 (0.96)*	0.17 (0.07)*
Intent to prevent pregnancy (*M, SD*)[a]	3.59 (1.35)	3.17 (1.42)***	4.00 (1.10)	3.89 (1.13)	−0.06 (0.10)
Intent to use condoms consistently (*M, SD*)[a]	3.90 (1.16)	3.71 (1.24)*	3.96 (1.04)	3.80 (1.15)	−0.11 (0.09)
Ever had sex (%, N)	11.3% (43)	14.4% (61)	15.9% (47)	21.4% (82)	0.21 (0.11)
Condom use (%, N)[c]	63.9% (23)	62% (31)	36.7% (11)	54.2% (39)	0.98 (0.37)**
Condom use consistency (*M, SD*)[bc]	2.48 (1.37)	2.69 (1.39)	2.66 (1.28)	2.34 (1.29)	−0.25 (0.21)
Been pregnant or caused a pregnancy (%, N)[c]	7.3% (3)	3.4% (2)	4.4% (2)	6.3% (5)	0.27 (2.99)

*$p < .05$; **$p < .01$; ***$p < .001$.
[a]Ranging from 1 (*strongly disagree*) to 5 (*strongly agree*).
[b]Ranging from 1 (*never*) to 4 (*always*).
[c]Subsample consisting of only those who reported to have had sex.

Effects of Intervention Program (T2)

Positive changes from intervention. At T2 significantly fewer students in the experimental group had positive attitudes toward TP (2.26 vs. 2.45, $p < .01$), and their intentions to abstain from sex whilst at school had also strengthened when compared with the control group (4.18 vs. 3.97, $p < .05$). The intervention effects resulted in more students expressing intentions to communicate with their partner about TP (4.11 vs. 3.97, $p < .05$) and to use condoms (54.2% vs. 36.7%, $p < .01$), but the sample of students in the control group reporting condom use had halved (Table 2).

Lack of significant change. We found that although the mean scores regarding intentions to prevent pregnancy and to use condoms consistently increased amongst students in the experimental group, this increase was matched in the control group. Thus, although the program appeared to significantly increase condom use, it did not impact on condom use consistency (Table 2).

DISCUSSION

The researchers found program effects for improved attitudes to prevent TP, intentions to abstain from sex, and intentions to communicate about TP with the partner and for actual condom use.

Demographic Factors

Our sample of students were in grade 8, had just started high school, and comprised both sexes because most schools in KwaZulu-Natal are coeducational, and both sexes are affected by TP. In initiating a program to reduce TP, we thus aimed to address the needs of young teens starting to become sexually active, but such programs also need to be reinforced as more teens become sexually active and require easily accessible contraception. A recent policy initiative of the Department of Health envisages sending teams of school health nurses to high schools, and provision of contraceptives could be linked with the "Lifeskills program that is part of the school curriculum (Departments of Health and Basic Education, 2012).

Improved Attitudes of Teens Concerning Prevention of TP

In a social context where TP is common, we were interested in reducing the perceptions of teens about the advantages of TP. The school intervention program through its varied activities provided the young teens with an opportunity to consider TP more realistically and reconsider their attitudes. Harrison (2010) has noted that younger teens are less likely to engage in protected sex due to limited knowledge, fear, uncertainty, or lack of negotiating ability, emphasizing the importance of delaying sexual initiation until teens are better prepared. Buthelezi and colleagues (2007) describe the physical and emotional changes that occur in adolescence and the stress and social pressures that result from moving from primary to high school. Furthermore, adolescence is a time of exploration and experimentation, with sexuality being a major area of development and change (Harrison, 2010). This phase provides an opportunity to discuss with teens issues relating to intimate relationships and sexually responsible behavior. The intervention program was thus successful in changing the attitudes of the grade 8 students in the experimental group, in reducing students' beliefs that teen pregnancy has advantages, and in explaining the consequences of TP for students.

Sexual initiation may not be voluntary, however, and sexual abuse in South Africa has been shown to be prevalent and significantly associated with HIV infection. The lack of condom use results from the inequitable gender norms where females are unable to insist on the use of condoms (Dunkle et al., 2004). In our study almost a third of teens had been forced to have sex, and there are few counsellors available to assist such students, indicating an unmet need in schools for social workers (Sathiparsad & Taylor, 2005).

Change in Students Intentions Toward Preventing TP

Amongst the abstinent students, the TP program appeared to reinforce sexual abstinence whilst at school and to promote condom use amongst the sexually active. The use of condoms consistently was not achieved by this program and requires more attention. Studies have indicated that although condoms are used initially, such use is more common with occasional than regular sexual partners. Inconsistent condom use among these teens is congruent with the findings of Makiwane and Mokomane (2010) in their study of sex between South African youth. Peer pressure is a concern, but, in addition to the risk of TP, the high rate of HIV in South African communities emphasizes the importance of consistent condom use. Amongst women attending antenatal clinics in South Africa, the HIV prevalence amongst 15–19 year olds was 18.8% (Department of Health, 2012b). There are many social pressures on students, however, including lack of parental guidance and supervision and living in poverty, that may negatively influence students' sexual behavior (Brook, Morojele, Zhang, & Brook, 2006).

The program was successful in increasing students' intentions to communicate with partners about TP. This is an important finding because due to existing gender norms females often lack agency in sexual decision making. The program effects suggest that teens participating in the program learned skills that would enable them to discuss with their partner the need to prevent pregnancy. This is a step in the right direction, because, in a previous study, James and colleagues (2005) reported that students were unable to communicate with their partners about the use of condoms.

The absence of effects on intentions to prevent pregnancy is unexpected because both groups increased significantly, and media exposure or other sexual education efforts might have had confounding effects. Further, no effects were found for reported TP, but, because of low pregnancy prevalence rates in our sample, this lack of effect can perhaps be attributed to low power.

The results of this study indicated that similar numbers of students in both groups initiated sex during the course of the study, confirming that programs providing sex education that are implemented at school do not increase sexual activity (Kirby, 2011).

Targeting Students' Sexual Behavior

The literature highlights the need for a comprehensive approach rather than a focus only on abstinence, and in this intervention program there was emphasis on responsible sexual behavior and condom use (Bennett & Assefi, 2005; Kirby, 2011). The intervention program included both primary and secondary abstinence, but it also included the benefits of dual protection and the consistent use of condoms by sexually active teens. Overall, the program was well received and used recommended strategies (Kirby, 2011).

Program Implementation

Our program was developed to address concerns expressed by teens in the prior focus group discussions and to empower them to understand the biological, psychosocial, and economic pressures related to TP. The program aimed to assist them to clarify aspects such as their attitudes toward TP and intentions to avoid becoming pregnant or causing a TP, and to offer them the implementation skills to achieve these goals. The program was implemented carefully by two teams of male/female facilitators of similar culture to the students, and they visited the schools once each week to implement the 12 sessions as planned.

Limitations

It is difficult to measure TP over the short term, and the outcome measures selected for this study were therefore change in attitude, intentions, and sexual behavior. Although in this study the administrators of the questionnaire emphasized the confidentiality of the students' responses and the important of valid answers, these are self-reports.

Implementation was not always optimal due to the many participants in one class (sometimes >60 learners), hindering active participation. Future effects may also be improved by using a slightly shorter and more targeted approach addressing salient beliefs (Dlamini et al., 2008; Taylor et al., 2007). A limitation was the high drop-out rate over the 8- month period. Although attendance is compulsory, school nonattendance is a variable with no sanctions. South Africa's child support grant—besides supporting new families—also contributes to positive attitudes toward pregnancies (Kanku & Mash, 2010). Furthermore, South African's context is characterized by high levels of sexual activity and also sexual violence (Department of Health, 2012b; Dunkle et al, 2004).

Students in schools not receiving our TP prevention program (the control group) received the compulsory classroom-based Lifeskills program and media messages regarding TP, both of which were also available to the experimental group. At the end of the RCT, the control schools were provided with the "Prevention of Teenage Pregnancy Programme."

These findings necessitate a comprehensive approach toward the prevention of TP that needs to target not only the micro but also the macro level (Kanku & Mash, 2010; Kirby, 2011; Vundule, Maforah, Jewkes & Jordaan, 2001). The HIV/AIDS epidemic in South Africa has caused the death of many parents, and their children often lack the care and support that adolescents require due to the social disintegration of families. Further, the lack of youth-friendly clinics in South Africa reduces access to contraceptive services (Dickson-Tettiah, Pettifor, & Moleko, 2001), requiring new community initiatives facilitating access (Pillay, 2012).

Implications—Summary Statement

The program results indicate effects on condom use and intentions to abstain and communicate about TPs. TPs also result in financial benefits, however, from the child support grant for poor families. Consequently, South African TP prevention requires an ecological approach also improving economic conditions.

ACKNOWLEDGMENTS

We thank the KwaZulu-Natal Department of Education Community (principals, parents, and students) and the research team.

FUNDING

We thank our funders, SANPAD, for their support.

REFERENCES

Bennett, S. E., & Assefi, N. P. (2005). School-based teenage pregnancy prevention programs: A systematic review of randomized controlled trials. *Journal of Adolescent Health, 36*, 72–81.

Brook, D. W., Morojele, N. K., Zhang, C., & Brook, J. S. (2006). South African adolescents: Pathways to risky sexual behaviour. *AIDS Education and Prevention, 18*, 259–272.

Buthelezi, T., Mitchell, C., Moletsane, R., De Lange, N., Taylor, M., & Stuart, J. (2007). Youth voices about sex and AIDS: Implications for life skills education through the "Learning Together" project in KwaZulu-Natal, South Africa. *International Journal for Inclusive Education, 11,* 445–459.

Department of Health. (2012a). *National Contraception and Fertility Planning Policy and Service Delivery Guidelines.* Pretoria, South Africa: Author.

Department of Health. (2012b). *National antenatal HIV and syphilis prevalence survey 2011.* Pretoria, South Africa: Author.

Departments of Health and Basic Education. (2012). *Integrated school health policy.* Pretoria, South Africa: Author.

de Vries, H., Mudde, A., Leijs, I., Charlton, A., Vartiainen, E., Buijs, G., … Kremers, S. (2003). The European Smoking Prevention Framework Approach (EFSA): An example of integral prevention. *Health Education Research, 18,* 611–626

DiCenso, A., Guyatt, G., Willan, A., & Griffith, L. (2002). Interventions to reduce unintended pregnancies among adolescents: Systematic review of randomised controlled trials. *British Medical Journal, 324,* 1426–1435.

Dickson-Tettiah, K., Pettifor, A., & Moleko, W. (2001). Working with public sector clinics to provide adolescent-friendly services in South Africa. *Reproductive Health Matters, 17,* 160–169.

Dlamini, S. B., Taylor, M., Nyawo, N. N., Huver, R., de Vries, H., & Sathiparsad, R. (2008). Gender factors associated with sexual abstinent behaviour of rural South African high school going youth in KwaZulu-Natal. *Health Education Research, 24,* 450–460.

Dunkle, K. L., Jewkes R. K., Brown, H. C., Gray, G. E., McIntyre, J. A., & Harlow, S. D. (2004). Gender-based violence, relationship power, and risk of HIV infection in women attending antenatal clinics in South Africa. *Lancet, 363*(9419), 1415–1421.

Harrison, A. (2010). Young people and HIV/AIDS in South Africa: Prevalence of infection, risk factors and social context. In S. S. Abdool Karim & Q. Abdool Karim (Eds.), *HIV/AIDS in South Africa* (2nd ed., pp. 305–328). Cape Town, South Africa: Cambridge University Press.

Harrison, A., Newell, M. L., Imrie, J., & Hoddinott, I. J. (2010). HIV prevention for South African youth. Which interventions work? Systematic review of current evidence. *BioMed Central Public Health, 10*(102), 1–12.

James, S., Reddy, P., Ruiter, R., Taylor, M., Jinabhai, C. C., & Van den Borne, B. (2005). The effects of a systematically developed photo-novella on knowledge, attitudes, communication and behavioural intentions with respect to sexually transmitted infections among secondary school learners in South Africa. *Health Promotion International, 20,* 147–155.

Jewkes, R., Morrell, R., & Christofides, N. (2009). Empowering teenagers to prevent pregnancy: Lessons from South Africa. *Culture, Health & Sexuality, 11,* 675–688.

Jewkes, R., Vundule, C., Maforah, F., & Jordaan, E. (2001). Relationship dynamics and teenage pregnancy in South Africa. *Social Science and Medicine, 52,* 733–744.

Kanku, T., & Mash, R. (2010). Attitudes, perceptions and understanding amongst teenagers regarding teenage pregnancy, sexuality and contraception in Taung. *South African Family Practice, 52,* 563–572.

Kirby, D. (2011). *The impact of sex education on the sexual behavior of young people*. Expert Paper No. 2011/12. New York, NY: United Nations Department of Economic and Social Affairs.

Makiwane, M., & Mokomane, Z. (2010). South Africa youths' higher-risk sexual behavior: An eco-developmental analysis. *African Journal of AIDS Research, 9*(1), 17–24.

Origanje, C., Meremikwu, M. M., Eko. E., Meremikwu, A., & Ehiri, J. E. (2009). Interventions for preventing unintended pregnancies among adolescents. *Cochrane Database Systematic Reviews, 4,* CD005215. doi:10.1002/14651858.CD005215.pub2.

Panday, S., Makiwane, M., Ranchod, C., & Lestoala, T. (2009). *Teenage pregnancy in South Africa with a specific focus on school-going learners*. Child, Youth, Family and Social Development, Human Sciences Research Council. Pretoria, South Africa: Department of Basic Education.

Pillay, Y. (2012, February). *PHC re-engineering in South Africa: Are we making progress?* Paper presented at the Public Health Association of South Africa (PHASA) Conference, Bloemfontein, South Africa.

Sathiparsad, R., & Taylor, M. (2005). Towards social work interventions in schools: Perceptions of educators. *Journal of Social Work, 41,* 265–275.

Sathiparsad, R., & Taylor, M. (2011). Making meaning of teenage pregnancy among school-going youth: The case of selected eThekwini Municipality secondary schools. *Agenda, 25*(3), 72–84. doi:10.1080/10130950.2011.621638

Statistics South Africa. (2013). *Quarterly Labour Force Survey*. Statistics South Africa. Retrieved from www.statssa.gov.za/publications/P0211/P02111stQuarter2013.pdf

Swartz, S., & Bhana, A. (2009). *Teenage tata: Voices of young fathers in South Africa*. Cape Town, South Africa: HSRC.

Taylor, M., Dlamini, N., Khanyile, Z., Mpanza, L., & Sathiparsad, R. (2012). Exploring the use of role play in a school-based programme to reduce teenage pregnancy. *South African Journal of Education, 32,* 441–448.

Taylor, M., Dlamini, S. B., Nyawo, N., Jinabhai, C. C., Huver, R., & de Vries, H. (2007). Reasons for inconsistent condom use by rural South African high school students. *Acta Paediatrica, 86,* 287–91.

Vundule, C., Maforah, F., Jewkes, R., & Jordaan, E. (2001). Risk factors for teenage pregnancy among sexually active Black adolescents in Cape Town. *South African Medical Journal, 91,* 73–80.

Willan, S. (2013). *A review of teenage pregnancy in South Africa—Experiences of schooling and knowledge and access to sexual and reproductive health services*. Durban, South Africa: Health Systems Trust.

Breast Cancer Screening Among Women of Child-Bearing Age

DAPHNE MUNYARADZI, JAMES JANUARY, and JULITA MARADZIKA

Department of Community Medicine, College of Health Sciences, University of Zimbabwe, Harare, Zimbabwe

We explored behavioral factors that contributed to late presentation of breast cancer. A cross-sectional survey of 120 women of child-bearing age was employed, and data were collected using interviewer-administered questionnaires addressing predisposing, enabling, and reinforcing factors associated with breast cancer screening. A total of 53.5% knew what breast cancer screening was; breast self-exam was the most commonly known form of screening, although only 7.5% practiced it. Lack of awareness (p = .004) and the knowledge of someone who previously had breast cancer (p = .0004) were prominent predictors for breast cancer screening, leading to either delay in or early presentation of the condition, respectively.

Screening for breast cancer is an imperative intervention in resource-limited settings such as Zimbabwe where the majority of women have little access to health care services. Although there are a lot of studies on breast cancer screening in other world regions, there still remains a paucity in research on breast cancer screening in Zimbabwe.

Cancer recently has been reported to be killing more people than HIV/AIDS, tuberculous (TB), and malaria combined, with almost 14 million people receiving cancer diagnosis and close to 8 million people dying from the condition worldwide every year (Centers for Disease Control and Prevention, 2014). More than 55% of new cancer cases and more than 60% of cancer deaths occur in less-developed regions of the world, with breast cancer being the second-most-diagnosed form of cancer globally (Ferlay et al., 2010).

The increase in cancer burden in Africa is partly due to the aging and growth of the population as well as the rising prevalence of risk factors associated with economic transition, including smoking, obesity, physical inactivity, and reproductive behaviors (Jemal et al., 2012). According to the Zimbabwe National Cancer Registry (2009), breast cancer accounts for 11.7% of total cancers, making it the second-most-common cancer in Zimbabwe. Although breast cancer incidence has been reported to be lower in sub-Saharan Africa as compared with Western nations, women with breast cancer in Africa have poorer survival rates than those in the developed world (Fregene & Newman, 2005). Due to inadequate resources and other pressing public health concerns such as HIV/AIDS, malaria, and TB (Jemal et al., 2012), the cancer burden in Africa still continues to receive relatively low public health priority. In addition, Zimbabwe and most developing countries lack clear health education programs on cancer awareness, and the absence of screening facilities in these resource-poor settings contributes to late presentation cancer cases (Anim, 1993). An understanding of women's perceptions on breast cancer is especially important in the development of preventive health programs in Zimbabwe and other resource-limited settings.

Our purpose for this study, therefore, was to assess the determinants of behaviors that hinder or promote the practice of breast cancer screening. We sought to explore the predisposing, enabling, and reinforcing factors associated with the practice of breast cancer screening among women of child-bearing age.

METHODS

Design and Sample

A cross-sectional descriptive study was used to describe and quantify the distribution of variables in our study population. In selecting the study design, we considered type of information to be obtained depending on the state of knowledge about the problem, resources available, and nature of the problem. Since knowledge of the situation and problem was superficial, this was deemed to be a suitable design as it was a small survey. We conveniently sampled a total of 120 women who were attending outpatient services at Marondera Provincial Hospital. This hospital was purposefully selected because it is the major referral hospital in the Mashonaland East province. The sample size was determined using the Dobson formula, which yielded a total sample size of 108, assuming a prevalence of breast cancer screening to be 7.6%. This was subsequently adjusted to 120 participants to increase the study's precision. The eligibility criteria for participation in the study included being a woman of child-bearing age (15 years to 49 years), being a resident of Marondera, and attending the outpatient department. Women were excluded from the study if they were seriously ill, had a psychiatric illness, or were non-Shona language speakers.

Data Collection

Interviewer-administered questionnaires with three sections—(a) demographics, (b) predisposing, and (c) enabling and reinforcing factors—which were used for data collection. The instrument was developed using constructs from phase four of the Precede–Proceed Model (Green & Kreuter, 2005). The tool was administered in the local Shona language by a native Shona speaker. We pretested the questionnaire at a local clinic with 10 randomly selected women. The clinic offered a relatively similar setup to the main hospital used in the study. The purpose of this exercise was to refine the questions in the questionnaire to suit the women in our study, which enhanced the validity of the data collection instrument. The study protocol was approved by the institutional review board of the University of Zimbabwe, College of Health Sciences. Women were recruited in the outpatient department of the hospital. The purpose of study was verbally explained to all the participants, confidentiality was assured, and written informed consent was obtained after which women responded to the items on the questionnaire. Each interview lasted an average of 60 minutes.

Data Analysis

After checking the collected data for completeness, we entered data into the Epi Info software package (version 3.5.3). Descriptive statistics including percentages, means, and standard deviations were calculated. Cross tabulations were performed to establish associations between demographic, predisposing, enabling, and reinforcing factors, with the utilization of breast cancer screening services. The chi-square and Fisher exact statistics were used to test for associations.

RESULTS

Demographics

A total of 120 women participated in the interviews at Marondera Provincial Hospital. The age range for the women was 16 years to 46 years (Mean = 28; $SD = 8.65$). Fisher's exact test was used to assess the significance of association between age and utilization of breast cancer screening services. Age was not found to be a predisposing factor for breast cancer screening.

Of the women interviewed, 3.3% were divorced, 14.2% were single, 2.5% were widows, and the majority of them were married (80%). The majority of the women were housewives (45%), 13.3% were students, 10% were nurses, 13.3% were nonmedical professionals, and the rest were general laborers. Women in the study who had reached secondary school level of education amounted to 70%, a fifth (20.8%) had tertiary education, with 9.2% having primary education only. Level of education predicted practice of breast cancer screening ($p = .001$).

A quarter of the respondents belonged to the apostolic sects, 34.2% were Pentecostal, 32.5% were either Catholic or Protestant, and 8.3% were Traditionalist. There was no association between knowledge of breast cancer screening and religion ($p = .58$); therefore, we learned that religion is not a significant predictor for breast cancer screening. In relation to participants' family income, a preponderance of the respondents (71.7%) considered their monthly income to be insufficient.

In all tests, p values <.05 were regarded as statistically significant. Sociodemographic characteristics such as place of residence ($p = .07$), employment status ($p = .096$), perceived income level ($p = .22$), and religion ($p = .17$) were found not to be potential determinants of breast cancer screening.

Predisposing Factors

Knowledge regarding breast cancer. A small percentage (36.7%) had good knowledge about breast cancer, whilst the rest had misconceptions about the condition. Regarding causes of breast cancer, 47.5% had no knowledge of its cause, 27.5% believed it is caused by abnormal cell division, 23.3% stressed it was caused by placing money in bra, and 1.7% declared it to have no known cause.

Table 1 shows what participants considered to be and not to be risk factors for breast cancer. An overall 77.1% in the rural and 74.6% in the urban setting believed placing money in the bra to be a risk factor for breast cancer. An average of 57% for both rural and urban women did not think size of the breasts was a risk factor for cancer. Amongst the rural population, 50% of the women gave incorrect responses about whether early menarche was a risk factor for breast cancer or not, while 35.4% did not have any idea. In urban settings, 45.1% of women gave incorrect responses, and another 45.1% of the women reported that they did not know that early menarche could be a risk factor for cancer. Comparing urban with rural settings, more urban participants (43.7%) were knowledgeable about the risk factors for breast cancer than their rural counterparts (31.3%). A preponderance of the participants (83.8%) believed breast cancer to be treatable, with 30.8% of the women reporting that it can be treated with surgery.

Knowledge regarding breast cancer screening. A total of 55.6% knew of breast cancer screening; 44.4% had no knowledge of it. Slightly more than half of the women (53.5%) knew that breast cancer screening is a way of detecting cancer, 5% thought it was a cure for breast cancer, while 40.6% did not know what it is, and 1% had different explanations for the concept. Although 55.6% knew of breast cancer screening, most women understood it in the form of breast self-examination. Breast self-examination was the most (50.8%) commonly known form of breast cancer screening mentioned by the women, followed by mammogram (15.8%), then ultrasound and other methods such as biopsy, each scoring 3.3%; clinical breast examination was cited by only 0.8%, and 38.3% did not know any form of breast cancer screening. An association was found between having heard of breast cancer screening and practicing it ($p = .0066$).

There were 48.7% females who correctly explained how to perform breast self-examination, 47.9% did not know, and 3.4% incorrectly explained the procedure. Only 12.6% reported that breast self-examination was to be done regularly after menstrual periods, with the rest being unaware of the time interval. An overall 7.5% practiced breast self-examination. Lack of awareness was found to be a significant predictor for breast cancer screening ($p = .004$).

Beliefs regarding breast cancer and breast cancer screening. Relatively more women (63.9%) believed early detection gives a better chance for effective treatment. Slightly more than half (52.9%) of the women in our study felt monthly self-breast exams were the best way to detect cancer. A number of participants (49.6%) believed that breast cancer screening saves lives and hence reduces the risk of mortality due to cancer. Close to half

TABLE 1 Risk Factors for Breast Cancer

	Rural ($n = 49$)			Urban ($n = 71$)		
Risk factors	Correct %	Incorrect %	Don't know %	Correct %	Incorrect %	Don't know %
Age 40$^+$ years	31.3	37.5	31.3	43.7	33.8	22.5
Family history of breast cancer	50	31.3	18.8	59.2	28.2	12.7
First child after 30 years	18.8	52.1	29.2	29.6	49.3	21.1
Placing money in bra	10.4	77.1	12.5	9.9	74.6	15.5
Being a woman	37.5	47.9	14.6	46.5	42.3	11.3
Never had children	18.8	62.5	18.8	12.7	64.8	22.5
Early menstruation	14.6	50	35.4	9.9	45.1	45.1
Having big breasts	60.4	12.5	27.1	73.2	8.5	18.3
Late menopause	10.4	45.8	43.8	14.1	45.1	40.8
Overweight	20.8	54.2	25	26.8	46.5	26.8
Having small breasts	68.8	8.3	22.9	45.8	10.4	43.8
Alcohol intake	45.8	29.2	25	41.4	35.7	22.9
Smoking	60.4	20.8	18.8	67.6	15.5	16.9
Unhealthy diet	43.8	25	31.3	50.7	21.1	28.2
Physical inactivity	27.1	50	22.9	31	33.8	35.2

(45.8%) of the women reported that breast injury may lead one to develop breast cancer. Other respondents (29%) felt that any lump on the breast signified the presence of cancer of the breast, with 50% reporting that a lump did not necessarily signify the presence of cancerous cells in the breast. Underwire bras were believed by a number of participants (42.5%) to cause breast cancer. The majority of women (84%) had no knowledge of whether or not mammogram predisposes an individual to breast cancer with time. Quite a large proportion of women did not know what a mammogram is (77.5%), and only 22.5% knew what a mammogram is. In addition to that, only 9.2% were knew the appropriate time interval between mammogram visits.

Perceptions regarding breast cancer and breast cancer screening. In this study we learnt that self-efficacy empowered the practice of breast self-examination ($p = .01$). A total of 47.1% perceived themselves as susceptible to breast cancer, 25.2% did not perceive themselves as susceptible to breast cancer, and the remaining 27.7% were neutral. A majority of women (70%) perceived breast cancer to be a very severe disease, 10.8% were neutral, and 19.2% did not recognize it to be a life-threatening condition. More than half (57.4%) of the women in our study perceived breast self-examination practice to be of benefit because they believed it avoids a lot of problems in the future. With regard to cost of breast cancer screening services being affordable, 72.5% were neutral. Perceived benefit, perceived susceptibility, and perceived severity, however, were not associated with the practice of breast self-examination: ($p = .13$), ($p = .56$), and ($p = .82$), respectively.

Enabling Factors

Women who at some time had utilized breast cancer screening services reiterated that availability and access to screening services, as well as examination by a male physician, were their top challenges. Those who had never utilized breast cancer screening services indicated lack of awareness, negative attitudes, and not knowing where to access services as the main reasons for not utilizing screening services.

Reinforcing Factors

We learned from the results of this study that a person who knew of someone who had breast cancer was more likely to practice breast cancer screening. There was a strong significant association between breast cancer screening practice and knowing someone who had/once had breast cancer ($p = .0004$). A third (34.7%) of the women knew someone who had breast cancer. Of the 12 women (10%) who utilized breast cancer screening services, 83.3% knew of someone who has or had breast cancer.

DISCUSSION

In planning for health promotion interventions aimed at effectively alleviating the burden of breast cancer in Zimbabwe and much of the developing world, there is a need to identify and target context-specific modifiable factors that are contributing to late presentation of cancer cases and lower survival rates. This study explored women of child-bearing age's views of breast cancer and breast cancer screening in response to the late presentation of the ailment. Results showed that in our sample of 120 Zimbabwean women of child-bearing age, several principles of breast cancer and breast cancer screening were not well understood or highly valued. Knowledge of aspects of breast cancer and breast cancer screening varied from mediocre familiarity and acceptance to near absence of understanding of the condition.

We present our findings to point out lack of awareness resulting in nonutilization of breast cancer screening services. The same was reported in a study in Angola in which scholars highlighted that apart from African women being susceptible to the more aggressive forms of breast cancer, the inexplicably greater mortality in contrast with first-world countries can be attributed to lack of awareness and delayed presentation, with 70%–90% of African women presenting with stage III/IV of the ailment (Sambanje & Mafuvadze, 2012).

Breast cancer screening is frequently done using a mammogram, and use of mammogram is restricted and inaccessible to most women in Africa, thus leaving breast self-examination as the most feasible and affordable alternative for African women (Sambanje & Mafuvadze, 2012). Our results, however, revealed that breast self-examination was practiced at a very low rate (7.5%) among women in our study sample. This is despite the fact that breast self-examination is the most commonly known form of breast cancer screening in Zimbabwe and a practical alternative in much of Africa. As reported in studies from other developing countries (e.g., Bello, Olugbenga-Bello, Oguntola, Adeoti, & Ojemakinde, 2011; Ermiah, Adballa, Buhmeida, Larbesh, & Collan, 2012; Hsieh, 2012; Noroozi, Jomand, & Tahmasebi, 2011), age was found to be an important predictor for breast cancer screening. Contrary to this, results from our study suggested that age is not a predictor for breast cancer screening. Possible reasons for the differences between our study and that of other countries may be due to differences in geographical locations, and another plausible explanation for these differences could be the small sample size utilized in our research.

Marital status has been cited as an important predictor for breast self-examination practice, with married women practicing breast self-examination more than single women (Noroozi et al., 2011). This is in contrast to our study's findings in which marital status was not associated with the practice of breast self-examination. The discrepancy between our study and that performed in Iran may be as a result of differences in marriage patterns and interactions in Zimbabwe and Iran, differences in religious practices, or all of these factors. Previous studies from Libya have indicated that higher levels of education were associated with breast self-examination practices with those women who performed monthly breast self-exams being more educated (Ermiah et al., 2012), which is consistent with results from our study. Only a third of the respondents in our study knew what breast cancer is, with the rest having misconceptions about cancer, which is in tandem with previous literature (Hsieh, 2012; Opoku, Benwell, & Yarney, 2012), where respondents displayed a lack of knowledge about the illness.

We established that women were aware of breast cancer and 47.4% were knowledgeable about breast cancer screening, conflicting with a study in Qatar (Donnelly et al., 2012), where the authors highlighted that there was a lack of awareness and knowledge of breast cancer screening. A possible explanation for such differences might be that in Zimbabwe women are sensitized about breast cancer screening during antenatal care. Sometimes clinical breast examinations are carried out during these antenatal care sessions, which may account for the high frequency in breast cancer screening knowledge among women in our study setting.

Perceived self-efficacy is a dominant and steady predictor for breast self-examination (Noroozi et al., 2011). Our study results also revealed the same, with a positive association existing between perceived self-efficacy and breast self-examination practice. Women who perceived more benefits of breast self-examination generally report more frequent breast self-examinations (Noroozi et al., 2011). Our study results revealed lack of awareness to be a significant predictor of nonutilization of breast cancer screening services. Contrary to our study's findings, studies from Nigeria and Taiwan demonstrated that low uptake of mammography was a direct result of the absence of national programs on breast cancer screening, minimum coverage of screening services, and high costs (Bello et al., 2011; Hsieh, 2012). A possible explanation for this difference between our study results and the two studies may be that the information dissemination strategies differ across countries.

More urban women were aware and knowledgeable about the risk factors for breast cancer than their rural counterparts. This can partly be due to media exposure differences between urban and rural populations in Zimbabwe, with the urban populace being more exposed to both electronic and print media. Regarding the sources where women obtained information on breast cancer and screening services, evidence from Nigeria revealed that most of the time women obtained their information from electronic media such as the radio (Bello et al., 2011). This, therefore, shows the importance of media in creating breast cancer awareness. Women of child-bearing age visit hospitals more frequently for different reasons and hence may be more exposed to health information. Participants had increased odds of having breast self-examination/clinical breast examination if they received information about breast cancer from a nurse or doctor, newspapers or magazines, or television or radio than those who did not (Donnelly et al., 2012). A study in Iran where women who received information through television and radio rather than from medical staff, however, perceived more barriers to breast self-examination (Noroozi et al., 2011). Health care centers were cited as the foremost source of information in our study setting, although there was no statistically significant association between health care centers as a source of information and the utilization of breast cancer screening services. Having a family or friend diagnosed with breast cancer was found to be associated with the likelihood of utilizing breast cancer screening, which is in tandem with studies by Hsieh (2012) and by Noroozi and colleagues (2011).

Study Limitations

Our study was hospital based, risking bias in the sense that people who utilize hospital services are different from those who do not. Possible interviewer effect may have influenced the subjects' responses. Resources for the study were limited, thereby limiting the scope of the study.

CONCLUSION

There is evidence that lack of awareness is answerable to nonutilization of breast cancer screening service. Low awareness levels of breast cancer screening in developing countries have been linked to high death rates compared with industrialized countries (Sambanje & Mafuvadze, 2012). The same authors found that most patients are diagnosed well after the breast cancer had advanced: 70%–90% of African women. We exposed an association between lack of awareness and utilization of breast cancer screening services, indicating that lack of awareness is a serious predictor for breast cancer screening. This seems to contribute to women not utilizing available breast cancer screening services, causing late detection, late presentation, and possibly high mortality related to breast cancer.

Breast cancer screening is regularly done using a mammogram in developed countries, whereas mammogram use is inaccessible and limited for most women in Africa, leaving breast self-examination as the only practiced form of breast cancer screening (Sambanje & Mafuvadze, 2012). In our study, however, breast self-examination was not common.

There is, therefore, a need to implement culturally relevant awareness programs, campaigns, and health education activities to enable people to become aware of breast cancer screening programs in line with the provisions of the Ottawa Charter of 1986.

REFERENCES

Anim, J. T. (1993). Breast cancer in sub-Saharan African women. *African Journal of Medicine and Medical Sciences, 22*(1), 5–10.

Bello, T., Olugbenga-Bello, A., Oguntola, A., Adeoti, M., & Ojemakinde, O. (2011). Knowledge and practice of breast cancer screening among female nurses and lay women in Osogbo, Nigeria. *West African Journal of Medicine, 30*(4), 296–300.

Centers for Disease Control and Prevention. (2014). *Cancer Prevention and Control. World Cancer Day.* Retrieved from http://www.cdc.gov/cancer/dcpc/resources/features/WorldCancerDay/

Donnelly, T., Al Khater, A., Al-Bader, S., Al Kuwari, M., Al-Meer, N., Malik, M., ... Chaudhry, S. (2012). Breast cancer screening among Arabic women living in the State of Qatar: Awareness, knowledge, and participation in screening activities. *Avicenna, 2012.* doi:10.5339/avi.2012.2

Ermiah, E., Adballa, F., Buhmeida, A., Larbesh, P., & Collan, Y. (2012). Diagnosis delay in Libyan female breast cancer. *BMC Research Notes, 5*(1), 452.

Ferlay, J., Shin, H.-R., Bray, F., Forman, D., Mathers, C., & Parkin, D. M. (2010). Estimates of worldwide burden of cancer in 2008: GLOBOCAN 2008. *International Journal of Cancer, 127*(12), 2893–2917. doi:10.1002/ijc.25516

Fregene, A., & Newman, L. A. (2005). Breast cancer in sub-Saharan Africa: How does it relate to breast cancer in African-American women? *Cancer, 103*(8), 1540–1550. doi:10.1002/cncr.20978

Green, L., & Kreuter, M. (2005). *Health program planning: An educational and ecological approach.* New York, NY: McGraw-Hill Education.

Hsieh, S. J. H. (2012). Understanding breast cancer screening practises in Taiwan: A country with universal health care. *Asian Pacific Journal of Cancer Prevention, 13*(9), 4289–4294.

Jemal, A., Bray, F., Forman, D., O'Brien, M., Ferlay, J., Center, M., & Parkin, D. M. (2012). Cancer burden in Africa and opportunities for prevention. *Cancer, 118*(18), 4372–4384. doi:10.1002/cncr.27410

Noroozi, A., Jomand, T., & Tahmasebi, R. (2011). Determinants of breast self-examination perfomance among Iranian women: An application of the health belief model. *Journal of Cancer Education, 26*(2), 365–374.

Opoku, S., Benwell, M., & Yarney, J. (2012). Knowledge, attitudes, beliefs, behaviour and breast cancer screening practices in Ghana, West Africa. *Pan African Medical Journal, 11*(1), 28.

Sambanje, N., & Mafuvadze, B. (2012). Breast cancer knowledge and awareness among university students in Angola. *Pan African Medical Journal, 11*(1), 70. doi:http://dx.doi.org/10.4314%2Fpamj.v11i1.

Zimbabwe National Cancer Registry. (2009). *Patterns of cancer in Zimbabwe.* Harare, Zimbabwe: Ministry of Health and Child Welfare, Government of Zimbabwe.

Cervical Cancer in Developing Countries: Effective Screening and Preventive Strategies With an Application in Rwanda

IMMACULEE MUKAKALISA, RUTH BINDLER, CAROL ALLEN, and JOANN DOTSON

College of Nursing, Washington State University, Spokane, Washington, USA

In this article we explore literature regarding cervical cancer screening methods available in developing countries. Cervical cancer is a preventable and curable disease, but it continues to threaten the lives of many women. Eighty-five percent of cases and the majority of deaths occur in developing countries. Cytology via Papinicolaou (Pap) smear is not generally a suitable method of screening in low-resource regions. Alternative methods include visual inspection by acetic acid (VIA), human papillomavirus–deoxyribonucleic acid (HPV–DNA), and careHPV–DNA. Education is needed for health care providers and women about preventive immunization and screening. A Rwandan project is described to demonstrate effective program planning and implementation.

Cervical cancer is the most common cancer among women in developing countries (Wright & Kuhn, 2012), and therefore it is an important international interdisciplinary topic. We examined cervical cancer screening methods currently used in developing countries, and we discuss effective alternative screening and preventive programs that are available, economically feasible, and culturally suitable for those countries. A specific program carried out in Rwanda is described as an exemplar of interest for health workers in developing countries.

BACKGROUND

According to the World Health Organization (WHO), in 2008 there were 529,000 new cases of cervical cancer, and more than 270,000 women die from this disease each year, 85% of them from developing countries (WHO, 2013a). Cervical cancer is preventable and often curable if the right interventions are made available to those who are at risk or develop cervical cancer. Researchers indicate that preventive strategies to reduce cervical cancer incidence should focus on preventing risk factors. Some of the human factors that have been shown to increase the likelihood of human papillomavirus (HPV) exposure and subsequent development of cervical cancer include the following: young age at first intercourse, high parity, and multiple sexual partners (Kachroo & Etzel, 2009). Girls in sub-Saharan Africa as young as 11–12 years old often engage in sexual and reproductive acts. Their male partners are usually older and often have multiple partners. Scholars have found that young girls have lower rates for practice of safe sex; therefore, such behavior increases the risk of cervical cancer and other sexually transmitted diseases (Louie, de Sanjose, & Mayaud, 2009). The practice of older men "initiating" young girls into sexual activity is prevalent in some communities in Africa and Asia, increasing the risk to young women who have little or no rights of refusal or ability to practice "safe sex." Screening and education about screening programs, therefore, play a vital role in cervical cancer prevention. The successful decrease in mortality from this disease in developed countries is attributable to effective screening and treatment (Sankaranarayanan, Budukh, & Rajkumar, 2001). In developing countries, however, the disease continues to cause thousands of premature deaths among women.

Cytology smears are the gold standard for cervical cancer screening. This method, however, has failed to achieve the same results in developing countries as in developed countries. In South American countries such as Chile, Colombia, and Costa Rica, where cytology screening programs have been available since the 1970s and 1980s, there was no decline in the incidence of cervical cancer reported or decrease in mortality rate until after the 1990s. Scholars contend that the failure of effective diagnosis in the 1970s and 1980s was attributable to low-quality cytology smears (Sankaranarayanan et al., 2001). Workers with inadequate knowledge and sample collection skills produced poor-quality specimen and cytology smears. Cervical cancer is preventable and curable if detected early; however, in order to minimize cervical screening barriers in low-resource settings, strategies should be socially and culturally appropriate, and health workers should be knowledgeable about correct procedures (Nene et al., 2007). Few women in developing countries have sufficient knowledge about cervical cancer and cervical cancer screening methods for effective diagnosis.

The Health Belief Model (HBM) is a conceptual framework that helps health care providers understand and influence behavioral factors that impact individual willingness to engage in specific health behaviors (Abotchie & Shokar, 2009). Researchers propose that the model is useful to determine the factors that might positively or negatively influence the uptake of cervical cancer screening. Proponents of the HBM assume that feeling vulnerable to a condition and claiming it as a serious health problem is a motivational factor that will increase people's action in taking preventive measures. Given acceptable screening methods, the challenge becomes how to help women in developing countries understand their risk of cervical cancer and that early detection of cervical cancer is not a death sentence. According to adherents of the HBM, a person's willingness to engage in a health-seeking behavior is influenced by perceived risks, perceived seriousness of the disease, perceived susceptibility, perceived benefits, and barriers to actions (Abotchie & Shokar, 2009).

The HBM can be applied to assess educational needs, and education is one key to preventing cervical cancer. Kachroo and Etzel (2009) indicated that low literacy and poverty are barriers to achieving preventive measures. Health literacy is essential for participation in health education. Understanding cervical cancer, the screening process, and preventive measures requires women to have a basic knowledge of their internal and external anatomy, as well as basic physiologic processes. Women also require education about cofactors of cervical cancer such as smoking tobacco. In addition, education is necessary to encourage seeking of screening and treatment at an earlier stage of the disease. Education can also address myths as well as cultural health beliefs associated with cervical cancer. Patients require explanations to be able to utilize the materials provided to educate about cancer (Kachroo & Etzel, 2009). Women's knowledge about cervical cancer and screening affects health behaviors. Qualitative interviews were carried out with 50 women in Kenya to explore awareness, attitudes, and behavior about cervical cancer and screening programs. The authors identified lack of knowledge about cervical cancer and the importance of early detection as significant barriers to effective programming (Ngugi, Boga, Muigai, Wanzala, & Mbithi, 2012).

Attempting to change health behaviors of any specific population group presents challenges. Once health policies and interventions are in place and address social and cultural characteristics, beliefs, and attitudes, however, the HBM can guide providers of many disciplines in raising community awareness of cervical cancer, availability of screening, and risks and benefits of screening through women's groups. Other health care barriers include lack of funds, nonavailability of insurance to access care, and health service inaccessibility. Many women in villages and rural areas have to walk long distances before they can attend a health facility. Sending teams of female providers into the countryside to perform testing on a regular basis might help overcome this barrier (Mupepi, Sampselle, & Johnson, 2011).

METHODS

We begin with a literature review to explore the methods of screening for cervical cancer. We then proceed to describe other methods of prevention and discuss conclusions of authors in review articles and, finally, to present work of researchers from more current literature not included in the reviews. Our search included journal articles from 2001 until 2013. Search terms included the following: *cervical cancer, screening, assessment prevention, HPV, sub-Saharan Africa, developing countries*. The search engine of CINAHL was used, and 81 articles were identified. After the review of identified articles, we found that only 25 met our search criteria, which were to address reports of cervical screening in developing countries as well as on prevention and supportive interventions for effective screening. We then applied the findings from these 25 articles to the planning and interpretation of a cancer screening program in Rwanda.

RESULTS

Methods of Screening for Cervical Cancer

Cytology or papinicolaou. Cytology or "Pap" smear is the most effective and common screening method. Cervical cytology consists of spreading and staining a smear of collected cervical cells and analyzing them under the microscope to detect lesions. The method enables professionals to accurately detect and stage high-grade lesions. This approach can contribute to early detection, thereby decreasing the incidence of advanced cervical cancer and associated mortality. Pap smears are challenging to perform in developing countries, however, because the process requires trained personnel and certified laboratories that are often unavailable (Maine, Hurlburt, & Greeson, 2011; WHO, 2013a).

Human papilloma virus–deoxyribonucleic acid (HPV–DNA) and careHPV. A common cause of cervical cancer is HPV. The HPV–DNA approach is a newer option for cervical cancer screening. The HPV–DNA testing consists of screening for high-risk strains of HPV. HPV testing has been shown to reduce mortality in high-grade lesions in advanced invasive cervical cancer and even in women with human immunodeficiency (HIV) disease (Louie et al., 2009). The HPV–DNA test has been shown to have promising results with high sensitivity and specificity to detect high-grade lesions, and therefore it is used as a primary screening test in women aged 30 years or older. Samples can be either self-collected or provider collected. There are some limitations, however, the test is expensive, it requires a laboratory, and the time needed to process the test is at least 7 hours. Although suitable for low-resource settings, it requires a sophisticated laboratory to read the samples. Unfortunately, most developing countries do not have reliable laboratory facilities (Maine et al., 2011).

In India, researchers found that HPV testing reduced cervical cancer incidence and mortality rate up to 50%. The testing is done either with cervical or vaginal samples collected with a brush by a trained provider in the case of cervical screening or by the woman herself in the case of the vaginal sample. The sensitivity of HPV–DNA testing ranged from 66% to 95% for all women tested, but researchers found a sensitivity of 85% among women 30 years old or greater (Sherris et al., 2009).

The alternative to HPV–DNA testing in low-resource-setting countries is *careHPV*. This moderated HPV test was developed for use in developing countries by Qiagen Gaithersburg Incorporated Laboratories in collaboration with the Bill and Melinda Gates Foundation and the nongovernment organization PATH. The test is simple and rapid; the results can be produced within 2.5 hours or less. A portable compact unit with a battery is operated by workers with minimal laboratory training. The test does not require a refrigerator, electricity, or running water. In the case of careHPV testing, HPV infection is detected with cervical or vaginal swabs, and the woman can collect the sample herself. The method was tried in China for the first time, and it showed reasonably promising results for the future (Louie et al., 2009; Wright & Kuhn, 2012).

The sensitivity of careHPV testing in China was 90% compared with visual inspection with acetic acid (VIA; described below) and Pap smear, at 41% and 85%, respectively (Gage et al., 2012). Unlike careHPV, the HPV–DNA test is more costly and requires more technology and time to process. Costs of testing vary by country; for example, for HPV–DNA, the price ranges from $26–$29 per person in India to $82 per person in South Africa (Goldie et al., 2005).

Visual inspection with acetic acid (VIA). VIA screening is the simplest method of screening with the lowest cost and greatest relative ease of use. The approach does not require high technology and has been demonstrated to reduce the deaths of women in developing countries (Wright & Kuhn, 2012). During VIA, 5% acetic acid or vinegar is applied to the cervical mucosa. Normal tissue is unaffected by vinegar wash, but abnormal cells, including dysplastic and cancerous cells, turn white. The screening method allows the practitioner to diagnose and treat abnormal cells almost immediately in a health center, typically using cryotherapy, which is the application of liquid nitrogen or carbon nitrogen to the dysplastic area. The process is also inexpensive; in a Chinese study, authors reported the cost estimate for VIA was $2.64 per test (Shi et al., 2012).

According to authors of a review article describing studies done in India comparing cytology, HPV, and VIA testing, VIA had the highest level of sensitivity, ranging from 50% to 96% (Maine et al., 2011). HPV–DNA was second, with sensitivity of 61%–90%, and cytology had a lower sensitivity of 31%–78%. High sensitivity can result in false positives with subsequent unnecessary treatment, but cryotherapy commonly used after VIA or visual inspection with Lugol's iodine (VILI) testing is a safe procedure with low incidence of tolerable side effects. In contrast with sensitivity, cytology was found to have the highest specificity at 91%–99%. The specificities for VIA and HPV–DNA testing were 44%–97% and 62%–94%, respectively (Maine

TABLE 1 Sensitivity and Specificity of Cervical Cancer Screening Methods in Several Studies

Methods of screening	Sensitivity	Specificity	Study location	Author and date
Cytology	53%–57%	99%	Latin American	Sherris et al. (2009)
	53%–57%		Sub-Saharan Africa	Wright and Kuhn (2012)
	31%–78%	91%–99%	India	Maine, Hurlburt, and Greeson (2011)
VIA	50%–96%	92%	India	Maine, Hurlburt, and Greeson (2011)
		94%–99%	India	Maine, Hurlburt, and Greeson (2011)
	77%	86%	India	Denny, Quinn, and Sankaranarayanan (2006)
	55%–73%		South Africa	Wright and Kuhn (2012)
	5%–58%	44%–97%	Kolkata and Mumbai, respectively (India)	Wright and Kuhn (2012)
		75%–77%	Jaipur and Congo, respectively	Wright and Kuhn (2012)
HPV–DNA	97%	86%	China	Louie, de Sanjose, and Mayaud (2009)
	61%–90%	62%–94%	India	Maine, Hurlburt, and Greeson (2011)
CareHPV–DNA	90%	84%	China	Louie, de Sanjose, and Mayaud (2009)

et al., 2011). See Table 1 for a comparative table on sensitivity and specificity of screening programs noted in scholarly publications.

Vaccination—Cervical cancer prevention method. Researchers indicate that preventive strategies to reduce cervical cancer incidence should focus on preventing risk factors. Another more recent preventive approach involves immunization. Women often become infected by HPV shortly after becoming sexually active. Eighty-seven percent of cases of cervical cancer are caused by seven types of the 40 HPV genotypes that infect the vaginal tract. Two types, HPV 16 and HPV 18, however, are responsible for 70% of all cases (Maine et al., 2011). Human papillomavirus (HPV), the acquired causative agent of most cervical cancer, is preventable by prophylactic vaccines (Louie et al., 2009). The HPV vaccine has been available since 2006 and can prevent 70% of HPV-caused cervical cancers if the three-dose vaccine series is completed. The series begins with one injection and is followed by a second 2 months later and a third at the end of 6 months. The available vaccines include Quadrivalent Gardasil, which prevents HPV 6, 11, 16, and 18; Bivalent Cervarix prevents only HPV 16 and 18. The cost for three doses of the Quadrivalent Gardisil vaccine is $360 in the United States. Cervarix costs $240 in Canada for the recommended three-dose regime (Canada

Free Press, 2010). Few governments and even fewer women in developing countries can afford either drug. In 2011, Mexico, Panama, and South Africa arranged to receive the Gardisil vaccine for U.S. $40 (Maine et al., 2011).

In 2011, Rwanda was the world's first low-income country to provide universal access coverage for the HPV vaccine. Rwanda received an offer from Merck & Co. Inc. for free 3-years' coverage of the HPV vaccine (Binagwaho et al., 2011). The Gardasil Access Program is managed by Axios Healthcare Development, which distributes free HPV vaccines to organizations and institutions within eligible low-income countries as long as they are capable of covering all other costs related to the vaccination program, including transportation, storage, community outreach, distribution of the vaccine, and data collection (Ladner et al., 2012). The achievement of over 93% coverage of three doses of the HPV vaccine in Rwanda was made possible through school-based vaccine clinics and community involvement in tracking and locating missing eligible enrolled and nonenrolled schoolgirls. The prophylactic HPV vaccine offers a new promise for primary prevention of cervical cancer. The HPV vaccine, however, does not replace cervical screening. Immunization can be ineffective due to missing follow-up doses and cost (Louie et al., 2009). It is clear that education and resources are key components to all cervical cancer screening and prevention programs.

Challenges to Cervical Cancer Screening in Developing Countries

The lack of screening and prevention for cervical cancer in developing countries has made it extremely challenging to decrease mortality rates. In developed countries where cytology-based cervical cancer screening is the standard of care, cervical intraepithelial neoplasia is often detected and treated before the development of invasive cancer. The failure to adopt and implement an effective screening program in low-resource countries is due to a complexity of multiple barriers, including cost, lack of quality-assured infrastructure, unavailable or untrained cytotechnologists or pathologists, and competing public health priorities such as communicable diseases.

Experiences With Various Screening Approaches

Based on international researchers' findings, the Alliance for Cervical Cancer Prevention (ACCP) was formed. The ACCP supported development of alternatives to cytology that were more appropriate for low-resource settings (ACCP, 2011). Resulting programs were suitable for developing countries and were found to be cost effective and have remarkably impacted the lives of many women (Sherris et al., 2009). The WHO has now provided specific guidelines for implementation of screening and treatment programs (WHO, 2013b).

The ACCP researchers conducted several studies examining VIA and HPV–DNA screening in developing countries including Africa, Asia, and Latin America. In India, 49,000 women aged 30–59 years were screened using the VIA approach over a 7-year period. Over the course of the study, the incidence and mortality of cancer declined by 25% for the whole cohort. For 30–39 year olds, the screening had a huge impact on women's lifetime cancer risks, reducing the incidence of cancer by 38% and mortality by 66%. The program was recognized as efficient and effective to detect and treat cervical cancer precursors in developing countries (Sherris et al., 2009).

The sensitivity of VIA testing has been assessed by researchers in India, Latin America, Africa, Thailand, and China. Sensitivity of the test ranged from 41% to 79%. When iodine was used instead of acetic acid, the sensitivity was higher, at 57% to 98% (Sherris et al., 2009). Visual inspection with acetic acid (VIA) has limitations in postmenopausal woman due to the cervical changes of this age group (Sherris et al., 2009).

Randomized control projects were implemented by researchers to determine factors associated with cervical cancer screening, treatment follow-up, efficacy, and cost effectiveness. Screening programs that worked for developed countries were not effective for developing countries where they existed, due in large part to barriers such as lack of knowledge about the disease, unfamiliarity with prevention concepts, economic inaccessibility of care, poor quality of services, and lack of family support, specifically from husbands (Nene et al., 2007).

To compare the effectiveness of three screening strategies (VIA, cytology, and HPV–DNA), researchers conducted a trial in rural areas of India, involving multicomponent strategies for service delivery. Community stakeholders, husbands, and health workers of both genders participated in the preventive activities, sensitization, education, and counseling (Nene et al., 2007). The project was a collaboration of Nargis Dutt Memorial Hospital (Barshi, India), the Tata Memorial Centre (Mumbai, India), and the International Agency for Research center (Lyon, France). The project included four subdistricts of the Osmanabad district in Maharashtra state; this was an underdeveloped rural region with a high prevalence of cervical cancer (27.4/100,000 women). The study was conducted between October 1999 and November 2003 at Nargis Dutt Memorial Hospital, a cancer hospital for diagnosis and treatment. Education and counseling were provided before and after screening and treatment. Proper hygiene, privacy, screening, and treatment were also provided at no cost. Female health workers offered education and counseling, while male health workers organized clinics and played the role of liaison with husbands and community leaders. Clinics were organized in villages, primary health centers, and schools. A total of 497 rural village women aged 30–59 years participated in a study that included a control group. Women in the VIA group with precancerous lesions had a colposcopy during the same session followed by a biopsy for those with abnormality; follow-up appointments for treatment at the central clinic were provided as needed. For the cytology and HPV screening, the specimens were collected and sent to the project's laboratories for analysis. The tests for both of these types of screening were performed by female nurses. The results of cytology and HPV were provided by a female health worker who at the same time arranged appointments for a colposcopy for those whose results were positive. Treatment options offered for women with positive cervical cancer included cryotherapy, a loop electrosurgical excision procedure, or conization. Those with low lesions were given options of follow-up or same-day treatment. Nene and colleagues (2007) indicated that the compliance with colposcopy among all women whose screening was positive differed by screening method. For visual inspection, compliance was 98.65%, cytology screening compliance for a colposcopy was 87.1%, and for HPV it was 88.1%. A colposcopy for visual inspection was carried out in the same clinic on the same day after the test. In the case of HPV and cytology screening, women were visited and received explanations about the test results and given appointments. According to the reported study results, having to contact women again and use an extra appointment for a colposcopy reduced compliance and increased loss to follow-up. Researchers concluded that the VIA method has the potential to reduce loss to follow-up and increase the coverage of those needing treatment (Nene et al., 2007).

Scholars from the ACCP reviewed studies that included reports of women's perspectives of cervical cancer screening and treatment approaches from developing countries including South Africa, Ghana, Thailand, India, Kenya, Peru, and El Salvador. Writers of the review concluded that women considered screening, regardless of type, performed by other women as highly acceptable. Also, women appeared to consider screening that was closely followed by treatment as very acceptable as well (Bradley et al., 2008). Scholars of the report also identified VIA, VIA Magnification (VIAM), and HPV–DNA as recommended alternatives to Pap smears in developing countries. The rationale for this recommendation is that Pap smears require the client to return to the clinic for a repeat smear or colposcopy and biopsy prior to treatment. Pap smears also require high-quality laboratories and qualified lab technicians, which may not be available in developing countries (Bradley et al., 2008). The HPV–DNA testing also involves some delays since the cervical cell samples are sent to the laboratory for reading (Bradley et al., 2008).

Recent guidelines from the WHO suggest that HPV is the test of choice in developing countries when feasible. The VIA is also acceptable, followed by cryotherapy to treat lesions. When both tests are available, VIA can follow HPV in order to verify the findings. The WHO guidelines will be helpful to identify the best screening and treatment options, depending on the particular resources that are accessible (WHO, 2013b).

Summary of Findings

The ACCP (2011) scholars concluded that HPV–DNA should become the standard test in developing countries because it is sensitive, requires little technology, and lengthens the interval between screenings. Where HPV–DNA screening is not available, however, VIA is preferred (WHO, 2013b).

Overall, women report satisfaction with VIA screening. As noted in the ACCP report, women in El Salvador reported approval of VIA screening, and their satisfaction was correlated with overall services, the confidence of the staff nurses, and technical ability during examination. In India, satisfaction was correlated with staff attitude, the service delivery strategies used, invitation process, health education, accessible clinics, and completing both screening and treatment in one visit in the primary health care facility. Most importantly, screening by female nurses rather than a male doctor was more comfortable for patients (Bradley et al., 2008). In Thailand, patients were very satisfied with the care they received from nurses (Bradley et al., 2008). In South Africa, the screening was done by female nurses from the same ethnic group and, according to the author, this was a key to overcoming barriers. Women in South Africa were more satisfied when screening was performed by female nurses. They did not feel frightened and ashamed related to challenges and societal objections to vaginal examinations (Bradley et al., 2008).

Early and effective screening programs can make a difference in decreasing cervical cancer. While a woman in the United States has a 70% chance of surviving cervical cancer due to relatively easy access to screening, only 58% of women in Thailand, 42% in India, and 21% in sub-Saharan Africa are likely to survive the disease (WHO, 2008). The uptake of screening remains low in developing countries due to lack of basic knowledge among women. Experts conducted a study on Ghanaian women's knowledge and beliefs about cervical cancer screening, and they found that the most important barriers to cervical cancer screening were lack of knowledge about screening and how to get screening services (Abotchie & Shokar, 2009).

There are obstacles to cervical cancer prevention and treatment in developing countries where screening is rarely available and almost unknown to many women. Obstacles include poverty, lack of effective screening, lack of women's knowledge of risks and treatment options, misunderstanding about prevention and early detection, lack of trained practitioners, financial constraints, and an efficient system of health care delivery (Ngugi et al., 2012; Salman, 2012). Even when screening is offered, women sometimes do not use the service. Winkler and colleagues found that, in Peru, attitudes and beliefs about screening, as well as lack of supportive systems, were major contributors to the lack of screening. In addition, lack of privacy in health centers, poor levels of staff courtesy, high cost, and women's fear of knowing that they indeed have cancer, all contributed to screening program failures in Peru, where cervical cancer had the highest incidence in the world (Winkler, Bingham, Coffey, & Handwerker, 2006).

An additional significant barrier to screening is lack of government efforts and planning, especially when there are competing health needs and diseases with high visibility and international attention that take priority over cancer screening (Egilman, Bird, Mora, & Druar, 2011). Lack of government investment in facilities and inadequate financial resources for training and services to enable successful screening programs are also significant barriers (Denny, Quinn, & Sankaranarayanan, 2006). The success of a screening program depends on it being not only affordable and acceptable, but also actively involving women and communities in program planning and implementation. Accessible referral sources upon diagnosis, treatment, and follow-up are necessary for a successful screening program (Louie et al., 2009).

DISCUSSION

Lessons From Screening Programs

In the majority of African communities, especially in rural areas, nurses assume doctors' roles. They are expected to integrate cervical screening into primary care settings. These nurses need special training programs and continuing education on the job in order to acquire necessary knowledge to inform their female clients and communities about cervical cancer and screening. Conclusions of researchers from studies in Uganda, Ghana, Tanzania, Nigeria, and Turkey indicated that health care professionals were often not updated with cervical cancer screening information. A study conducted in Uganda on 310 health workers (physicians, nurses, and others) was reported by researchers. A high survey response rate of 92% was achieved. Sixty- five percent of female health workers eligible for screening did not think they were susceptible to cervical cancer, and 81% had never been screened (Mutyaba, Mmiro, & Weiderpass, 2006). Female patients in that community did not get screened, not because they did not feel vulnerable, but because, according to the author, it was unlikely that medical workers could motivate them or advise them to get screened when nurses were lacking cervical cancer screenings themselves (Mutyaba et al., 2006). The new WHO guidelines are intended to address this gap and can be used by policymakers who consider the myriad influences and resources of individual communities in order to plan for the most effective screening and treatment measures (WHO, 2013b).

Researchers in Nigeria examined the knowledge level about cervical cancer among urban and rural women. Their results indicated that there was a need to make changes in education and establishment of effective screening control programs. Only 15.5% of the women who participated in the study were aware of availability of cervical screening. The poor knowledge of cervical cancer screening and prevention resulted in low attendance at cervical screening programs. As in Uganda, women in Nigeria did not believe that they were at risk for cervical cancer. Other authorities cited poor practices of nurses and doctors and indicated that they must not only be trained and retrained, but also that they have to change attitudes about cancer screening and improve their practice of cervical cancer screening (Nwankwo, Aniebue, Aguwa, Anarado, & Agunwah, 2011).

Our review of published research indicates that some women felt embarrassed to be physically exposed, especially when they see a male doctor, while some fear pain from the test. The role of nurses and other health care providers should be to address women's concern about privacy during and after the exam. Education should be provided in order to help overcome family and social belief barriers. Women need to know exactly what will happen during and after the test. In addition, every step of the test needs to be explained as it is done. Health care workers need to use whatever means they have to gain the trust of their female clients, whether they come to them for regular health services or they travel to their clients' communities to meet them. They also need to involve families, churches, and community leaders. Ndikom and Ofi (2011) indicate that prescreening counseling would help women in making informed choices about cervical cancer screening. Women empowered by education and advice from their nurses are more likely to make the wise decision to get screened as soon as they become eligible (Ndikom & Ofi, 2011).

African countries can benefit from examining findings in other developing nations. Turkish researchers explored knowledge, behaviors, and beliefs related to cervical cancer in Turkish women and revealed that the ineffective use of cervical cancer screening was due to poor knowledge and impractical behaviors of practitioners. Their work indicated that nurse practitioners should address cervical cancer screening, educate women and other health workers about attitudes, and explain the truths about cervical cancer screening (Reis et al., 2009).

In Thailand, patients were very satisfied with the care they received from nurses. In South Africa, cervical screening was done by the female nurses from the same ethnic group, and this was a key to overcoming barriers. Women in South Africa, who originally viewed screening as a service provided by men, were more satisfied when the screening was done by female nurses. They did not feel frightened or ashamed related to societal objections to vaginal examinations (Bradley et al., 2008). Female nurses recognize their acceptance by women and the important role that they play in providing cervical cancer screening.

Application in Rwanda

The first author, a native of Rwanda, traveled from the United States back to her home country in December 2010. Her mission was to pave the way for the American medical team that was providing medical care service in the areas of Ruhuha and Nyamata, in the district of Bugesera. In collaboration with "Health Development Initiative" (HDI), a local nongovernmental, nonprofit organization, the medical team from a city in the inland Pacific Northwest was able to conduct a pilot project for cervical cancer screening in 2011. Quality care for African women was a primary aim of the preventive and early treatment program. The team provided training to health care workers and cervical cancer screening. Doctors and nurses who attended the training learned how to screen for cervical cancer using the alternative method of VIA, chosen for its ease of administration in a setting such as Bugesera. The team provided cervical cancer screening to women who had not heard about cervical cancer, had never been screened, or were unable to afford medical care. Our literature review demonstrated the importance of this step of education in the screening program. The collaboration of the American medical team and the Rwandan health partners involved travel to some of the villages where women do not have access to health facilities. In low-income countries, traveling a long distance without transportation is a major barrier to screening. Having a native Rwandan knowledgeable about the culture, as well as being able to communicate with the representatives of health care in the local clinics, managers of the health centers, and members of the HDI and "Project Access," facilitated effective clarification and preparation for the work of this international health partnership. The team considered recommendations from researchers and experts, and then they discussed successful strategies to prepare for the cervical screening pilot project. The mobilization started with the involvement of the community, with involvement of health authorities, primary health workers, and community leaders. The announcement of the event was done over national radio, on church bulletins, and in health centers. The first author took on the role of facilitator and assisted in planning, preparation of brochures and flyers needed for the mobilization of women, and communication of the efforts and plans to the American team. As a result, 110 women were screened, 18% of whom had abnormal cervical cells; 23 women were treated at the site of the clinic.

CONCLUSION

The HBM can be applied to help health care providers tailor approaches to respond to both the need for acceptability of the program and the involvement of the community in program planning for cervical cancer screening.

In developing countries, nurses provide the majority of health care; they are the first responders and advocates for patients and therefore are critical to include in interprofessional teams. The HBM theoretical model can guide program planning to address women's perspectives about cervical cancer and their perceived risks and benefits of cervical cancer screening.

The project described in this article utilized and applied the findings of other cervical screening projects in developing countries, both in the type of screening method utilized and in the education provided for health workers and women. In addition, the unique approach of having a nurse who had lived in both Rwanda and the United States become a key person in planning the clinics, formulating informational approaches, and communicating with both African and American partners ensured success of this pilot project and paved the way for future partnerships.

In summary, multidisciplinary health care professionals play an important role in screening and prevention of cervical cancer in developing countries. Knowledge levels about the disease and its prevention should be a target of programs, and work within communities can focus on educating women and planning for effective approaches to screening and immunization. Barriers should be examined and eliminated so that women's programs can be implemented successfully. Experts have shown HPV–DNA testing in developing countries to be effective and reliable, with higher sensitivity than cytology and VIA. Promises are even greater with careHPV for cost effectiveness and simplicity in collecting samples. The HPV vaccine is now available in many developing countries and is believed to effectively reduce cervical cancer deaths. It should not automatically assume, however, to be more effective than screening and treatment. Rather, a combination of programs for immunization and screening would yield the greatest benefit.

REFERENCES

Abotchie, P. N., & Shokar, N. K. (2009). Cervical cancer screening among college students in Ghana: Knowledge and health beliefs. *International Journal of Gynecologic Cancer, 19*, 412–416.

Alliance for Cervical Cancer Prevention (ACCP). (2011). *Recent evidence on cervical cancer screening in low resource settings*. Retrieved from http://www.rho.org/files/ACCP_cxca_screening_2011.pdf

Binagwaho, A., Wagner, C., Gatera, M., Karema, C., Nutt, T. C., & Ngabo, F. (2011). Achieving high coverage in Rwanda national human papillomavirus vaccination program. *Bulletin of Health World Organization, 90*, 623–628

Bradley, J., Coffey, P., Arrossi, S., Agurto, I., Bingham, A., Dzuba, I.,...White, S. (2008). Women's perspectives on screening and treatment in developing countries: Experiences with new technologies and services delivery strategies. *Women's Health, 43*, 103–121.

Canada Free Press. (2010, October 25). GlaxoSmithKline Inc. drops the price of Cervarix. *Canada Free Press.* Retrieved from http://www.canadafreepress.com/index.php/article/29170

Denny, L., Quinn, M., & Sankaranarayanan, R. (2006). Screening for cervical cancer in developing countries. *ScienceDirect, 24,* 71–77. Retrieved from http://www.sciencedirect.com. doi: 10.1016/j.vaccine.2006.05.121

Egilman, D., Bird, T., Mora, F., & Druar, N. (2011). Get AIDS and survive? The "perverse" effects of aid. *International Journal of Occupational and Environmental Health, 17,* 364–382.

Gage, J. C., Ajenifuja, K. O., Wentzensen, N., Adepiti, A. C., Stoler, M., Eder, P. S. ... Schiffman, M. (2012). Effectiveness of a simple rapid human papillomavirus DNA test in rural Nigeria. *International Journal of Cancer, 131,* 2903–2909.

Goldie, J. S., Gaffikin, L., Goldhaber-Fiebert, J. D., Goldillo-Tobar, A., Levin, C., Mahe, C., ... Wright, T. C. (2005). Cost-effectiveness of cervical-cancer screening in five developing countries. *New England Journal of Medicine, 353,* 2158–2168.

Kachroo, S., & Etzel, C.J. (2009). Decreasing the cancer burden in developing countries: Concerns and recommendations. *European Journal of Cancer Care, 18,* 18–21.

Ladner, J., Besson, H. M., Hampshire, R., Tapert, L., Chirenje, M., & Saba, J. (2012). Assessment of eight HPV vaccination programs implemented in lowest income countries. *BioMed Central Public Health, 12,* 370.

Louie, S. K., de Sanjose, S., & Mayaud, P. (2009). Epidemiology and prevention of human papillomavirus and cervical cancer in sub-Saharan Africa: A comprehensive review. *Tropical Medicine and International Health, 14,* 1287–1302.

Maine, D., Hurlburt, S., & Greeson, D. (2011). Cervical cancer prevention in the 21st century: Cost is not the only issue. *American Journal of Public Health, 101,* 1549–1555.

Mupepi, S. C., Sampselle, C. M., & Johnson, T.R.B. (2011). Knowledge, attitudes, and demographic factors influencing cervical cancer screening behavior of Zimbabwean women. *Journal of Women's Health, 20,* 943–952.

Mutyaba, T., Mmiro, F., & Weiderpass, E. (2006). Knowledge, attitude and practices on cervical cancer screening among the medical workers of Mulago Hospital, Uganda. *BioMed Central Medical Education, 6,* 13.

Ndikom, C. M., & Ofi, B. A. (2011). Pre-screening counseling in cervical cancer prevention: Implications for nursing. *International Journal of Nursing and Midwifery, 3,* 158–164.

Nene, B., Jayant, K., Arrossi, S., Shastri, S., Budukh, A., Hingmire, S., ... Sankaranarayanan, R. (2007). Determinants of women's participation in cervical cancer screening trial, Maharashtra, India. *Bulletin of the World Health Organization, 85,* 264–272.

Ngugi, C. W., Boga, H., Muigai, A. W. T., Wanzala, P., & Mbithi, J. N. (2012). Factors affecting uptake of cervical cancer early detection measures among women in Thika, Kenya. *Health Care for Women International, 33,* 595–613.

Nwankwo, K. C., Aniebue, U. U., Aguwa, E. N., Anarado, A. N., & Agunwah, E. (2011). Knowledge attitudes and practice of cervical cancer screening among urban and rural Nigerian women: A call for education and mass screening. *European Journal of Cancer Care, 20*, 362–367.

Reis, N., Babis, H., Kose, S., Sis, A., Engin, R., & Yavan, T. (2012). Knowledge, behavior and beliefs related to cervical cancer and screening among Turkish women. *Asian Pacific Journal of Cancer Prevention, 13*, 1463–1470.

Salman, K. F. (2012). Health beliefs and practices related to cancer screening among Arab Muslim women in an urban community. *Health Care for Women International, 33*, 45–74.

Sankaranarayanan, R., Budukh, A. M., & Rajkumar, R. (2001). Effective screening programs for cervical cancer in low- and middle-income developing countries. *Bulletin of the World Health Organization, 79*, 954–962.

Sherris, J., Wittet, S., Kleine, A., Sellors, J., Luciani, S., Sakaranarayana, R., . . . Barone, M. (2009). Evidence-based, alternative cervical cancer screening, approach in low resource settings. *International Perspectives on Sexual and Reproductive Health, 35*, 3.

Shi, J., Chen, J., Canfell, K., Feng, X., Ma, J., Yong, Z., . . . Qiao, Y. (2012). Estimation of the costs of cervical cancer screening, diagnosis, and treatment in rural Shanxi, Province, China: A micro-costing study. *BioMed Central Health Services Research*. doi:10.1186/1472-6963-12–123

Winkler, J., Bingham, A., Coffey, P., & Handwerker, W. P. (2006). Women's participation in a cervical cancer screening program in northern Peru. *Oxford Journal of Medicine, 23*(1), 10–24.

World Health Organization (WHO). (2008). High papillomavirus vaccine delivery strategies that achieved coverage in low and middle income countries. *Bulletin of the World Organization, 89*, 821–830B. doi:10247/BLT.11.089.862

World Health Organization (WHO). (2013a). *Cancer: Fact sheet no. 297.* Retrieved from http://www.who.int/mediacentre/factsheets/fs297/en/

World Health Organization (WHO). (2013b). *WHO guidelines for screening and treatment of precancerous lesions for cervical cancer prevention.* Geneva, Switzerland: Author.

Wright, T., & Kuhn, L. (2012). Alternative approaches to cervical cancer screening for developing countries. *Best Practice & Research Clinical Obstetrics and Gynecology, 26*, 197–208.

South African Mothers' Coping With an Unplanned Caesarean Section

SAMANTHA VAN REENEN and ESMÉ VAN RENSBURG

Faculty of Health Sciences, Department of Psychology, North-West University, Potchefstroom, South Africa

In this study, researchers explored mothers' coping strategies in dealing with birth by unplanned Caesarean section. Mothers' experiences of a traumatic birth could be influenced by perceived strengths when coping with the stress related to the incident. Coping strategies resulted in reassessment of the birth process and were associated with a more positive and memorable experience. In-depth interviews with 10 women explored their lived experiences of childbirth. Data were analyzed thematically. Phenomenological theory served as a framework for the structuring, organizing, and categorizing of data. Mothers described several factors and coping strategies that they perceived to be effective in reducing the impact of their traumatic birth experiences.

Researchers suggest that Caesarean deliveries have increased substantially in recent years (Hamilton, Martin, & Ventura, 2007). In South Africa, Caesarean sections account for as many as 72% of deliveries in the private sector (Fokazi, 2011). Childbearing is acknowledged as a significant developmental transition for women, especially for first-time mothers (Darvill, Skirton, & Farrand, 2008). Birth by unplanned Caesarean section, however, has been identified as a traumatic experience for women; one that has the potential to disrupt this transition to motherhood (Roux & van Rensburg, 2011; Ryding, Wiren, Johansson, Ceder, & Dahlstrom, 2004). Given the alarming statistics of Caesarean sections performed in South Africa's private sector, the exploration of the impact of Caesarean deliveries on these women's well-being becomes significant (Roux & van Rensburg, 2011).

According to Gibbons and Thomson (2001), there is a correlation between women's experiences of birth, their expectations, and their perceived abilities to cope with the process. The processes occurring during a traumatic birth experience, such as during an unplanned Caesarean section, could affect a woman's emotional and psychological state and could be influenced by perceived strengths when coping with the stress related to the incident (Singer et al., 2010). Coping strategies could thus result in reassessment of the birth process, and be associated with a more positive, acceptable, and memorable experience (Escott, Slade, Spiby, & Fraser, 2005).

In this study, the researchers aimed to develop a comprehensive and insightful understanding of the factors relevant to South African women's experiences of birth by unplanned Caesarean section. Specifically, the objective of this article is to explore and describe these mothers' subsequent coping strategies.

BACKGROUND AND MOTIVATION

The impact of a Caesarean birth on women has begun receiving more attention in recent years. For a woman desiring a natural birth, a birth culminating in an unplanned Caesarean section may color and complicate her labor experience (Roux & van Rensburg, 2011). In existing literature on the topic, researchers persistently document negative psychological and emotional responses to Caesarean delivery among women (Gamble & Creedy, 2009; Ryding, Wijma, & Wijma, 1998; Stadlmayr et al., 2006; Weiss, Fawcett, & Aber, 2009; Yokote, 2008). Despite this, not all women who deliver their babies by Caesarean section experience negative psychological outcomes (Ryding et al., 2004). Although there are women who feel devastated by their Caesarean birth experiences and have long-term negative psychological outcomes, there are women whose post-Caesarean psychological profile and birth appraisal is relatively positive (Clement, 2001).

Individual responses to threats and challenges are embedded in a complex web of contents, including the event's characteristics; genetics; physical conditions; life stage, and family, social, and cultural factors. These factors influence how an individual perceives, frames, evaluates, interprets, and is affected by an event (Strumpfer, 2005). For new mothers, this may account for some of the individual variation in post-Caesarean psychological outcomes (Baston, Rijnders, Green, & Buitendijk, 2008; Clement, 2001). A woman's attitude toward birth, her expectations, and her personal and subjective attributed meaning to giving birth could affect her feelings of satisfaction, strength, esteem, and achievement (Gibbons & Thomson, 2001). Psychological vulnerability, cultural factors, and aspects of care received also appear to influence the psychological effects of caesarean delivery (Clement, 2001). Furthermore, coping strategies may moderate the impact of women's stressful labor experiences, and effect more positive appraisal outcomes (Aldwin & Werner, 2007).

Coping refers to the cognitive, behavioral, and belief strategies that are intentionally employed in order to manage internal and external demands (Hamilton & Lobel, 2008; Lazarus & Folkman, 1984). These demands are experienced as being challenging and exceeding perceived personal resources required for intervention. Coping strategies are not concerned with an objective evaluation of a successful outcome, but rather a subjective experience of an attempt to effect or manage a perceived stressful event (Lazarus & Folkman, 1984). Both situational and intrapersonal factors including available resources, competing demands, and the perceived controllability of a situation influence how an individual copes with stress (Hamilton & Lobel, 2008; Lobel, Yali, Zhu, De Vincent, & Meyer, 2002; Moos & Holahan, 2003). Furthermore, there is an active interplay between past experiences, current perceptions, and the perceived results of the mechanisms employed, resulting in reevaluation of the experience (Thoits, 1995).

Successful coping is linked with resilience resources (Tugade, Fredrikson, & Feldman Barrett, 2004). *Resiliency* is a pattern of psychological actions consisting of a drive to be tough in the face of unwarranted demands, the goal-directed behavior of coping and rebounding, and of supplementary emotions and cognitions (Strumpfer, 2002). Although coping and resilience are related constructs, they are distinct in that coping refers to a wide set of skills and purposeful responses to stress, whereas resilience refers to positive adaptation in response to serious adversity (Rosen, Glennie, Dalton, Lennon, & Bozick, 2010). Through specifying mothers' achievement of positive adjustment in the face of traumatic or negative birth experiences, resilience encapsulates the view that adaptation to significant adverse birth experiences can occur through coping trajectories (Luthar, Cicchetti, & Becker, 2000).

A number of possible coping responses have been identified and examined by researchers in literature (Avero, Corace, Endler, & Calvo, 2007; Carver, Scheier, & Weintraub, 1989; Endler & Parker, 1990, 1999; Lazarus & Folkman, 1984). Updegraff and Taylor (2000) group these strategies into three general categories: active coping, acceptance and positive reinterpretation, and avoidance coping. Active coping refers to strategies that are directed at problem solving, and it entails taking direct action to confront the stressor and reduce its effects (Carver et al., 1989). Acceptance and positive reinterpretation refer to acceptance of a stressor as real and unavoidable, as well as attempts to focus on the positive aspects of a situation (Updegraff & Taylor, 2000). Avoidance coping refers to primarily emotion-focused strategies, which may reduce the distress associated with a stressful event by denial or withdrawal from the situation, without reducing the noxious aspects of the situation itself (Endler & Parker, 1990, 1999).

Variations in coping strategies are associated with variations in adaptive and maladaptive emotional adjustment (Avero et al., 2007). Active coping can lead to adjustment and improvement by both reducing the distress and the impact of a traumatic event, as well as by contributing to perceptions of stress-related growth. Acceptance and positive reinterpretation coping may be most adaptive in situations that are not controllable by direct action. In contrast, an avoidant coping style appears to be a less adaptive response to a stressful life event and can ultimately lead to greater long-term distress and disruptive cycles of intrusion and avoidance (Updegraff & Taylor, 2000).

An unplanned Caesarean section has been described as a distressing, difficult, and disappointing experience, one that confronted women with considerable adjustment difficulties (Roux & van Rensburg, 2011). In some instances, this can have significant and far-reaching consequences for their psychological well-being (Fenwick, Gamble, & Hauck, 2007; Porreco & Thorp, 1996; Ryding et al., 1998). Thus, exploration and understanding of how women respond to and cope with an unplanned Caesarean section has important implications for therapeutic intervention. Despite this, phenomenological research on how women cope with an unplanned Caesarean section is virtually nonexistent, both internationally and in South Africa. The researchers in this study therefore aimed at exploring and understanding how a group of South African women coped with their experiences of an unplanned Caesarean section.

RESEARCH DESIGN

An exploratory, descriptive, qualitative research design was used to explore and describe women's subjective experiences of an unplanned Caesarean section. Qualitative research examines the lived experience in an effort to describe, explain, understand, and give meaning to peoples' experiences, behaviors, interactions, and social contexts (Fossey, Harvey, McDermott, & Davidson, 2002; Strauss & Corbin, 1998). Within qualitative research, phenomenology refers to the individual's personal construction of the meaning of a phenomenon (Mertens, 2009). Original data are comprised of "naive" descriptions obtained through open-ended questions and dialogue, and the researcher describes the structure of the experience based on reflection and interpretation of the research participant's story (Moustakas, 1994). Such an approach places this study within the interpretive phenomenological perspective (Roux & van Rensburg, 2011). The researchers explored in detail how mothers made sense of their unplanned Caesarean experiences with the intention of understanding their meaning, while simultaneously interpreting how themes of meaning are structured.

RESEARCH METHODS

The research began with ensuring ethically sound research, followed by data collection and analysis.

Ethical Considerations

Several measures were taken to ensure the ethicality of this research. This was in accordance with the Ethical Code of Professional Conduct of the Health Professions Council of South Africa (HPCSA, Professional Board for Psychology, 2004). First, the research protocol was approved by the relevant ethics committee. Thereafter, prospective participants were informed of the background to the study and the voluntary nature of participation in the study. Interviews proceeded once participants had given verbal and written consent. The researcher was fully aware of the sensitive and emotional nature of exploratory inquiry, and the rights and needs of the individual were therefore considered at all times. Furthermore, the participants were assured of confidentiality. Finally, participants were debriefed at the resolution of the interview process to resolve any questions or unease.

Population and Sampling

Phenomenology uses purposive, nonprobability sampling procedures, where participants are included because they have a specific knowledge of the phenomena (Baker, Wuest, & Stern, 1992). For the purposes of this study, an *unplanned Caesarean section* referred to a surgical, Caesarean delivery, despite the mother's desire to deliver her baby naturally. Such a delivery may have occurred after labor had begun due to unexpected maternal or fetal conditions, or prior to labor, as is the case in an emergency Caesarean delivery. Thus, in this study, the population of interest was comprised of mothers who had wanted to deliver their babies naturally, but who had instead had to deliver their babies by Caesarean section. Within the population of interest, participants had to comply with the following criteria:

- married women,
- mothers aged 25–30 years,
- birth of each woman's first-born child culminated in a Caesarean delivery,
- a period of 2 to 4 years had elapsed since each woman's unplanned Caesarean delivery,
- no previous miscarriages had been experienced, and
- for Caucasian women: Cultural beliefs about and values associated with childbearing touch all aspects of social life in any given culture. Such beliefs and values could lend different perspectives to the meaning of childbirth to the childbearing woman (Callister, 2006).

Selection of participants included snowball sampling, as discussed by Babbie (2007), where women nominated acquaintances whom they thought may be willing to participate in the research. The sample comprised 10 women, with a mean age of 28 years, who volunteered for in-depth phenomenological semistructured interviews. Interviews were not limited to a certain number but continued until data saturation had taken place in order to deepen, enrich, and complete categories, themes, and concepts (Brink & Wood, 2001). Saturation was determined when data became repetitive, and further concepts or themes were no longer emerging.

Data Collection

Various aspects were explored in in-depth phenomenological interviews, allowing the researcher to probe certain aspects offered by participants in order to understand and explore their contributions in as much depth as possible. A semistructured, open-ended approach allowed for the exploration of relevant opinions, perceptions, feelings, and comments in relation to the women's experiences.

Data Analysis

Thematic content analysis allows for detailed analysis of data (Nystedt, Hogberg, & Lundman, 2008). When it comes to analysis, phenomenological researchers engage in active and sustained reflection as they "dwell" with the data and interrogate the content. By applying the analytical method as suggested by Wertz (1983) and Giorgi (1985), analysis involved systematic readings of the transcripts and field notes by first dwelling on the phenomenon (through empathetic immersion and reflection), and then describing emergent psychological structures (i.e., constituents and recurrent themes). Analysis continued with a cross-category search to identify recurring regularities expressed as themes that were seen at an interpretive level as underlying threads of meaning running through condensed meaning units, codes, or categories (Graneheim & Lundman, 2004). Themes were then categorized so that data could be synthesized and comparisons could take place.

Measures to Ensure Trustworthiness

To ensure validity of results, Lincoln and Guba's model (1985) of trustworthi-ness of qualitative research was applied to this study. The model identifies five aspects of enhanced trustworthi-ness of a study, namely, credibility, transferability, confirmability, dependability, and authenticity.

To enhance credibility, the researcher engaged in active and sustained reflection during data interpretation to ensure quality, and to highlight the complexity of participants' experiences (Marshall & Rossman, 1995). The researcher aimed to suspend previous assumptions in order to be open to the phenomenon as it appeared, and to generate a sense of reality and a personal recognition of the phenomenon through precise and rich description. This refers to the extent to which the findings are a function solely of the research participants and conditions of the research, with no biases, motivations, and researchers' perceptions (Krefting, 1991).

Transferability was achieved through thorough description of the research context and the assumptions that were central to the research. The criteria applied were made explicit, according to the purpose and orientation of the study (Patton, 2002).

To ensure confirmability in this study, the researcher and an external auditor, a psychology professor with extensive experience in qualitative research, reached agreement that the findings, conclusions, and recommendations made by the researcher were supported by the data and that the researcher's interpretation of the data was meaningful and relevant.

Dependability was achieved through clear and thorough description of methods used in gathering, analyzing, and interpreting data, as well as in the precise and comprehensive reporting of data. Documentation was such that other researchers would be able to follow the investigative process and reach similar conclusions given the researcher's data, perspective, and situation (Marshall & Rossman, 1995).

FINDINGS

Through thematic content analysis, researchers identified themes relevant to exploring how women coped with their experiences of birth by unplanned Caesarean section. These themes include *information, control, support,* and *time.* The data held within these themes were then analyzed into discrete parts, concepts relevant in the exploration of mothers' coping with unplanned Caesarean section. The categories are named and explained below, indicating and discussing the concepts that have been connected/grouped within each category.

Information

Information received was acknowledged by mothers as important in their experienced sense of inclusion, choice, and control. Women described the significance of communication and information in relation to perceived levels of *preparedness* and *having questions answered.*

Preparation.   Once the decision to perform an emergency Caesarean section had been made, six of the women described the ensuing events as "complete and utter chaos" (*Mom #8*). For some women, this contributed to a sense of bewilderment: "It just felt like everything was just going so fast, all rushing past me so quickly. And there was nothing I could do to stop it. I was just lost in it" (*Mom #10*). Although anxiety provoking, however, the pandemonium was less distressing for those women who had been prepared during pregnancy for the possibility of having a Caesarean section: "[My doctor] said he would try to give me a natural birth, but he also said that we must see what happens" (*Mom #1*). As Mom #2 described, "I obviously really wanted to give natural birth, but I also knew that sometimes it does go wrong, it wouldn't be the absolute end of the world, and so I was aware of that." This was important for the expectant mothers in that "I knew what to expect, I knew what would happen, I knew about the recovery process" (*Mom #3*). Thus, having developed knowledge of the Caesarean procedure prior to labor contributed to a greater sense of surety and security in terms of levels of predictability, controllability, and expectancies. Thus, mothers were able to cope with their Caesarean section experiences as previous preparation helped to decrease subsequent feelings of disappointment to a certain degree.

Having questions answered. In the commotion that accompanied a Caesarean delivery, women were left feeling disorientated, uncertain, and insecure. As Mom #6 explained, "I couldn't really comprehend what was happening and why it was happening." Thus, post-Caesarean, women spoke of the need to have their questions answered, and to be able to talk about their Caesarean section with caregivers to try to appreciate the circumstances surrounding their labor experiences. The explanation by doctors as to the reasons behind why the Caesarean had to be performed helped to reassure mothers that it was the right thing to do, as well as to calm their anxieties about their own and their babies' well-being: "The doctor came and explained everything that happened and everything that she had to do. It made a difference, you know. It just kind of reassures you that everything is ok, you're going to be ok, and that the baby is going to be ok" (*Mom #9*). This was comforting for women, in that "It makes you feel better, because you know exactly why it happened. I think a lot of women actually wonder, 'Did I do something wrong? Was it my fault?' At least if you get that explained, you know why" (*Mom #9*). This was important for women in that they "knew it wasn't anything [they] had done" (*Mom #3*), and that it didn't "make [them] bad mother[s]" (*Mom #1*). Understanding gained through such discussion, therefore, determined the level of acceptance of the procedure and the degree of satisfaction with the birth experience.

Control

For all of the women in this study, an unplanned Caesarean section was associated with a loss of control. Loss of control was described in relation to a loss of physical or emotional control, and it was primarily related to unmet expectations. Nevertheless, mothers were able to achieve some sense of control over isolated aspects of their Caesarean deliveries, and this was acknowledged as significant in determining more positive birth appraisals. Control was effected in *decision making* and *inclusion in the process*.

Involvement in decision making. The extent to which mothers felt that they had been involved in decision making determined their feelings of confidence and satisfaction. Mothers who felt that they had not been included in decision making described feeling ignored, intimidated, and pressuried by staff and doctors. For these women, a sense of being undermined during labor contributed to more negative birth appraisals. Conversely, mothers who felt that they had played a role in decision making felt respected and valued, and they were more accepting of consequent events. As Mom #1 said, "My gyne was amazing; he asked me, he listened, and I wasn't pushed into it. I knew that my rights and my wishes were being respected. I had wanted a natural and I had tried, and when it had to happen then, well it had to."

Inclusion in the process. The desire to have a natural birth was often associated with a conscious and active process of birthing. Nine of the mothers aspired to work with their bodies to deliver their babies themselves. The passivity of a Caesarean section, therefore, left mothers feeling disengaged and removed from the birth of their child and that the active and physical experience of childbirth had been lost. Therefore, being informed and aware of what was happening during labor and birth was an important variable in determining how women experienced and coped with the birth:

> My [gynecologist] talked me through it and, before he did anything, he told me what he was going to do, and [he] did everything so I could see it. Even in surgery, I could see all the instruments, which helped. I guess it kind of helped to connect me with my body a bit, (*Mom #1*)

Inclusion in the Caesarean procedure thus helped contribute to a sense of control by promoting sustained participation and contribution.

Support

Support was identified as a significant mediator in women's birth and labor experiences, as it served a protective and encouraging role. Mothers in this study recognized several sources of support, including *doctors, midwives, and medical staff*; their *husbands*; *family and friends*; and their *religion*.

Doctors, midwives, and medical staff. Characteristic qualities and attributes of doctors, midwives, and staff played a significant role in reducing the stress experienced by mothers during birth. A soothing personality style was a source of reassurance and comfort for mothers, and helped to lower anxious responses. As Mom #6 described, "[The doctor] is a very calm sort of person. You know, the way he talks to you, he just has a way of making you feel at ease." Furthermore, throughout the entire birth process, the level of care received from staff was perceived to be of significant value. Sympathetic, attentive, and supportive assistance from staff, especially during the initial period after the surgery, played a significant role in mothers' experiences of the Caesarean delivery. Encouraging, placating, and accommodating staff members were "wonderful in helping to accept what was happening" (*Mom #3*). Their support helped mothers to feel "a lot more comfortable, it helps to take off the edge, and it just made it so much easier" (*Mom #8*). Women valued having professional caregivers who appeared to care about them as individuals, and were more positive about their Caesarean experience.

Husband. A husband's presence was of remarkable significance in women's labor and birth experiences. The shared experience of their babies' births represented an intimate connection between husbands and wives, and it "was exciting going through it together" (*Mom #3*). Furthermore, it was symbolic of the transformation into a family unit. These women described that "as a family, [it was] the ultimate connection" (*Mom #1*). Additionally, affection and support from their husbands was a source of reassurance and consolation to women. Husbands were identified as a considerable source of comfort, providing women with a sense of familiarity in the unknown, anxiety-provoking Caesarean environment: "I don't know how I would've done it without him. Having the person you love and trust the most there, it kind of eases all the rest of it" (*Mom #2*). Thus, having their husbands present helped to neutralize or counteract women's feelings of uncertainty and anxiety.

Family and friends. Family members and friends were regarded by mothers as other significant sources of environmental support

> My Mom and my sister were at my house for 7 weeks straight after [my daughter] was born, and I didn't have to lift a finger or anything. We just used to sit and we'd just talk. And that's how we kind of got through it, (*Mom #10*).

As Mom #7 said, "It was difficult, but I called my mother-in-law and sister-in-law, and they were just amazing. .... Their support was incredible." Family and friends served to reassure mothers, assist them in self-care tasks, and calm their anxieties. Difficult feelings and physical limitations that followed the Caesarean section were thus experienced as more manageable with the care and assistance of others.

Religion. For six women, religion appeared to influence their coping processes and outcomes through tenets and attitudes. During labor and surgery, prayer for safety and well-being was described as a way in which mothers were able to achieve a sense of comfort: "I wasn't alone, I had [God's] hand on me, I knew it would always be alright" (*Mom #1*). Post-Caesarean, mothers described their faith as having contributed to an acceptance of the process as the way it had to be: "God had other plans for me" (*Mom #3*). Thus, a trust in a higher being helped to calm mothers' anxieties and encourage peace of mind. Furthermore, mothers described an appreciative approach to the birth outcomes: "There [my baby] was, and no matter how it happened, here was a beautiful miracle" (*Mom #3*). As Mom 1 described, "I just kept reminding myself that God had blessed with me with this baby, and knowing that I was given the ability to love him just made it easier" (*Mom #1*). Prayer groups were also identified as a source of support: "I remember everybody sitting with me and they were praying for me, for strength and for calm. It was so powerfully reassuring and soothing" (*Mom #3*). Thus, mothers' religious beliefs helped in relieving stress, retaining a sense of control, and maintaining hope and a sense of meaning and purpose.

Attitudinal and Emotional Response

Postpartum responses to unplanned Caesarean section varied amongst women. For some women, the initial postpartum period was characterized by *positive emotional reaction*. For others, it reflected *disengagement*.

Positive emotional reaction. Despite the trauma associated with unplanned Caesarean section, five of the mothers experienced the emotional adjustment during the postpartum period as relatively uncomplicated. Affectionate recollections of mother–infant bonding, family union, and maternal role acquisition illustrated positive post-Caesarean experiences: "All thoughts of the process disappear and you're so aware of this little life. ... I just stopped focusing on myself, and let myself think about him" (*Mom #1*). Mom 3 said, "I loved him no matter what; he was still my baby and [the Caesarean] wouldn't change how I felt about him." For some mothers, having a positive attitude involved a conscious decision. Mom #4 described how "the whole was just so exhausting. It was so hard. But I couldn't dwell on it, it wasn't about me, it was about [my baby]. I had to pick myself up and move on." Regardless of whether mothers experienced a natural positive reaction or had to consciously regulate their responses, time spent between mother and infant was described by these women as "an amazing, special, bonding time" (*Mom #1*).

Disengagement. For five of the women, the experience of early motherhood was marred by emotional disturbance. These mothers reported a variety of traumatic stress reactions, depressive symptoms, and grief responses. For these women, addressing and dealing with their negative birth experiences was challenging. Four of the women reported that during this time, they had resisted interpersonal interaction: "I didn't want to see anybody. ... I refused for them to come and see me. I didn't even want to see the baby" (*Mom #5*). Mom #10 explained, "I just really needed time on my own, to just deal with stuff, to get through it." Other mothers enjoyed fantasies about getting out of the situation: "I wanted to run away; it was all I could think about" (*Mom #8*). Other functional distractions included "TV, reading, listening to music, computer games, washing dishes, making food, anything routine that stopped my world from completely being absorbed by this thing that happened" (*Mom #7*). Thus, disengagement served to help mothers "get out of our heads for a while" (*Mom #8*).

Time

For seven mothers, coming to terms with their labor experiences was a longitudinal course. Mom #5 said, "That initial period was crazy; I battled for a long time after [the Caesarean]." In the months following the birth, mothers described a gradual process of acceptance: "It took a while for me to take it all in, and process it all" (*Mom #8*). Increasingly, "It got easier. It was slow, but it did get easier" (*Mom #3*). For these women, passage of time promoted both an emotional engagement with the experience and an increased sense of appreciation for circumstances surrounding the experience. Ultimately, positive adjustment to their negative birth experiences was dependent on women's on-going coping strategies.

DISCUSSION

Becoming a mother is a life-changing event and a status passage, particularly for first-time mothers (Fenwick, Holloway, & Alexander, 2009). Many women enter labor with particular anticipations of the birth, and it has been shown that whether or not expectations are met, women still consider them to be important after delivery (Lavender, Walkinshaw, & Walton, 1999; Roux & van Rensburg, 2011). It has been suggested that forming a positive appraisal of birth depends on how well events have lived up to expectations; studies have shown that when such expectations are fulfilled, women report higher levels of satisfaction (Baston et al., 2008; Hauck, Fenwick, Downie, & Butt, 2007; Tulman & Fawcett, 2003). Roux and van Rensburg (2011) found that an unplanned Caesarean section was described as a distressing, difficult, and disappointing experience for women, one that confronted mothers with considerable adjustment difficulties. Despite unfulfilled expectations and negative experiences, however, mothers described several strategies, resources, and factors that promoted adaptation, coping, and adjustment.

For the women in this study, the provision of clear and realistic information prior to birth enhanced feelings of preparedness and enhanced emotional well-being after the Caesarean surgery. Furthermore, women emphasized the need to discuss the circumstances surrounding their birth experiences afterwards and to have their questions answered. This is consistent with research that indicates that communication by the health care professionals is an important factor in promoting women's understanding of the indications for an operative birth (MacMillan, 2010), in determining the degree to which women accept their Caesarean delivery as having been necessary

(Clement, 2001), and in whether women have positive or negative memories of the event (Fenwick et al., 2009; Murphy, Pope, Frost, & Liebling, 2003). Thus, information and knowledge received prior to childbirth about the Caesarean process appears to reduce post-Caesarean psychological distress (Jay, 2008; Nilsson & Lundgren, 2009), and increase women's confidence in their ability to cope with the experience (Ip, Tang, & Goggins, 2009).

Another key aspect of communication that was identified as an important dimension of care was the extent to which women felt informed about or involved in decision making. Being informed and contributing to what is happening during labor and birth has been identified as an important variable in determining how women experienced the birth (Howarth, Swain, & Treharne, 2011; Melender, 2002), by contributing to a sense of inclusion and respect in the process (Lyberg & Severinsson, 2010). Decision making may involve aspects about labor and the actual Caesarean section, hospital admission, medication and pain relief, and treatment of the baby immediately after delivery (Clement, 2001; McDonald, Amir, & Davey, 2011). In this study, women who felt that they had been informed and involved in decision making felt respected and valued, and they were more accepting of consequent events. Furthermore, they were more positive about having relinquished control to caregivers.

The degree to which women felt prepared, informed, and involved in decision-making seemed to have a positive effect on their sense of self, and it was identified as a significant contributor to women's sense of control over the experience. Research (Gibbins & Thomson, 2001; Lobel & DeLuca, 2007) consistently suggests that a perceived sense of control may enhance psychological outcomes, adjustment, and satisfaction with the experience, even if expectations differ from reality (Al-Nuaim, 2004; Gibbins & Thomson, 2001; Updegraff & Taylor, 2000). Maintaining a sense of control has been linked with establishing purpose and fulfillment, and therefore with more desirable delivery outcomes (Fenwick at al., 2009; Olde, van der Hart, Kleber, & van Son, 2006).

Mothers' social networks were identified as a remarkable source of support for women. Many studies have identified the contribution of supportive care to a positive evaluation of the birth (Baston et al., 2008; Hauck et al., 2007; Waldenström, 2004). The most important source of support and encouragement for women came from their husbands. The familiarity and company of their partners provided a sense of comfort and security throughout the birth experience. These findings are supported by other studies, which describe partners as valuable in providing support, encouragement, and reassurance, and in helping a woman to maintain control and acting as her advocate (Gibbons & Thomson, 2001; Hodnett, Gates, Hofmeyr, & Sakala, 2011; Lavender et al., 1999).

Support from family and friends was identified as an important resource, especially post-Caesarean. Social support may be in the form of emotional assistance, aid, information, validation, or affirmation (Cacciatore, Schnebly, & Froen, 2009; Melender, 2002). For many women, the unfamiliar territory of pregnancy and early motherhood created a need for others to help guide them through the transition. Aside from professional advice and counseling, Darvill and colleagues (2008) explain, informal "mentorship" from friends and relatives serves as a valuable source of support for women, as it affords some positive feedback to them to normalize their feelings and experiences, and in so doing support their individual self-concept.

In this study, caregiving by health care professionals contributed significantly to women's perceptions of childbirth. Research on women's experiences of Caesarean childbirth consistently suggests that the perceived quality of care received has an important influence on the psychological impact of a Caesarean section (Clement, 2001; Parratt, 2002; Waldenström, 2004). Attentive, considerate, and sympathetic caregiving was reported to affect mothers' experiences of birth by unplanned Caesarean section positively, by contributing to a sense of support (Roux & van Rensburg, 2011). Novick (2009) explains that women value working with professionals who appear to care about them as individuals.

Notably, religion was identified as significant in predicting more positive birth experiences. The relationship between religion or spirituality and mental health and coping has been receiving more attention in recent years (Miller & Thoresen, 2003). Religious involvement appears to buffer individuals against the negative effects of a traumatic experience (Halama & Bakosova, 2009; Kendler, Gardner, & Prescott, 1997; Krumrei & Pargament, 2008). It may help in bolstering feelings of (secondary) control, increasing women's confidence in their ability to manage their experiences, and in enhancing self-concept (Ellison & Levin, 1998). Through prayer and other intrapsychic religious coping efforts, primary appraisals of the birth may be altered, leading mothers to reassess the meaning of the birth experience as an opportunity for spiritual growth (Graham, Furr, Flowers, & Burke, 2001; Koenig & Larson, 2001).

The women in this study described different emotional reactions to their Caesarean experiences. Attitudes toward childbirth have been identified to influence how likely a woman is to experience an adverse psychological outcome after a caesarean (Clement, 2001), as well as how she will cope with the experience (Hamilton & Lobel, 2008). This is because of the significance of emotion-regulation coping strategies (Reisenzein & Weber, 2009). Emotional and attitudinal responses to traumatic experiences represent varying cognitive adaptations and schemas, and are determinant of adaptive versus maladaptive appraisals and coping patterns (Lobel, Hamilton, & Cannella, 2008).

Last, time appeared to play a role in women's coping with their traumatic labour experiences. Research suggests that coping strategies often change over time (Aldwin & Werner, 2007; Strumpfer 2005). Waldenström (2004) explains that as time passes, positive affect for one's role as a mother may favorably color a woman's feelings about her birthing experience. Thus, it is possible that, despite the initial trauma and negative feelings associated with the Caesarean section, the effect of childbirth may have changed over time as mothers' attention and focus shifted.

From women's descriptions, several coping styles and strategies in relation to managing traumatic birth experiences were identified. The new mothers highlighted the significance of receiving social support. Literature identifies the seeking of social support as an active coping strategy (Prati & Pietrantoni, 2009). Seeking social support for emotional reasons includes attaining moral support, sympathy, and understanding (Updegraff & Taylor, 2000). Seeking social support may also be for instrumental reasons, such as in seeking advice or assistance (John & Gross, 2007). Information seeking, another active coping response, appears to be effective in reducing the impact of a traumatic event by focusing on confronting and resolving certain aspects of a stressful experience (Updegraff & Taylor, 2000). Additionally, such information may promote acceptance and positive reinterpretation of an event through improved understanding of circumstances surrounding a traumatic event, as well by contributing to an increased sense of mastery and control over the experience (Fenwick et al., 2009; John & Gross, 2007).

For the women in this study, religion as a source of emotional support encouraged reconsideration of the circumstances surrounding their traumatic birth experiences. This reflects a process of acceptance and reinterpretation of the experience. Acceptance and reinterpretation, an emotion-focused aspect of resiliency, is the tendency to manage distress emotions, rather than deal with the experience per se (Lazarus & Folkman, 1984). As a traumatic experience gradually becomes construed in more positive terms, a person is intrinsically able to continue active, problem-focused coping strategies (Carver et al. 1989). This has been acknowledged as a significant determinant of stress-related growth (Updegraff & Taylor, 2000). Thus, with passage of time, women's initial negative appraisals of the birth experience developed into more positive ones. Although this reflects a measured acceptance and reappraisal, however, it also reveals an initial avoidance of addressing and coping with the experience (Carver et al., 1989).

Avoidance coping, which refers to primarily emotion-focused coping strategies, has been identified as reducing the distress associated with a stressful event by denial or withdrawal from the situation, without reducing the noxious aspects of the situation itself (Endler & Parker, 1990, 1999). The women in this study reported varying forms of behavioral and mental disengagement, which served to distract and delay them from thinking about and dealing with their experiences. These coping responses are generally acknowledged as less helpful in that they often impede adaptive coping. In terms of resiliency, however, avoidance coping may be useful in reducing short-term distress, and it may be an effective strategy for dealing with a short-term stressor such as a traumatic labor experience (Melender, 2002; Updegraff & Taylor, 2000).

CONCLUSIONS AND LIMITATIONS

The recent proliferation of research on coping shows evidence of the recognition of the prospective and potential of this construct. Facilitating adaptive coping may represent effective means to alleviate stress during the postpartum period and reduce its undesirable effects on women and their offspring (Veloso, 2007). Further exploration of such an aspect of competence may provide insight into the ability of new mothers to continue to thrive and function despite their high-risk status, and it may lead to increased empirical efforts to understand individual variations in response to adverse childbirth experiences. This, in turn, could contribute to the development and expansion of theory and research in the field, as well as the designing of appropriate prevention and intervention strategies (Luthar et al., 2000).

Several methodological limitations may underestimate or misrepresent the impact of the present study. The small sample may limit the generalizability of results. The researchers did not discriminate between planned versus unplanned pregnancies. This distinction could have important implications for the levels of preparedness, anxiety, and adaptation experienced. Furthermore, this research did not control for the use of instruments (e.g., forceps) or other interventions (e.g., labor induction) that may obscure subjective experiences. The women who participated in this study were all Caucasian. Within the South African context, there are women from other racial groups who experience unplanned Caesarean sections. These women live in communities that hold different cultural values and it is important that their perspectives be explored to investigate how different cultural backgrounds influence women's experiences and coping of unplanned Caesarean sections. The study did not control for individual characteristics, which may have influenced subjective responses and reactions to stress. It is also possible that the effect of childbirth may have changed over time. As time passes, positive affect for one's role as a mother may favorably color a woman's feelings about her birthing experience (Waldenström, 2004). Last, additional reviewers and their interpretations of the data could have added reliability and validity to the research findings.

REFERENCES

Al-Nuaim, L. A. (2004). Views of women towards cesarean section. *Saudi Medical Journal, 25,* 707–710.

Aldwin, C. M., & Werner, E. E. (2007). *Stress, coping and development: An integrative perspective* (2nd ed.). New York, NY: Guilford.

Avero, P., Corace, K. M., Endler, N. S., & Calvo, M. G. (2007). Coping styles and threat processing. *Personality and Individual Differences, 35*, 843–861.

Babbie, E. R. (2007). *The basics of social research* (4th ed.). Belmont, CA: Thomas Wadsworth.

Baker, C., Wuest, J., & Stern, P. N. (1992). Method slurring: The grounded theory/phenomenology example. *Journal of Advanced Nursing, 17*, 1355–1360.

Baston, H., Rijnders, M., Green, J. M., & Buitendijk, S. (2008). Looking back on birth three years later: Factors associated with a negative appraisal in England and in the Netherlands. *Journal of Reproductive and Infant Psychology, 26*, 323–339.

Brink, P. J., & Wood, M. J. (2001). *Basic steps in planning nursing research: From question to proposal.* Sudbury, MA: Jones and Bartlett Publishers.

Cacciatore, J., Schnebly, S., & Froen, F. (2009). The effects of social support on maternal anxiety and depression after stillbirth. *Health & Social Care in the Community, 17*, 167–176.

Callister, L. C. (2006). Cultural meanings of childbirth. *Journal of Obstetric, Gynecologic & Neonatal Nursing, 24*, 327–334.

Carver, C. S., Scheier, M. F., & Weintraub, J. K. (1989). Assessing coping strategies: A theoretically based approach. *Journal of Personality and Social Psychology, 56*, 267–283.

Clement, S. (2001). Psychological aspects of caesarean section. *Best Practice Research, Clinical Obstetrics & Gynaecology, 15*(1), 109–126.

Darvill, R., Skirton, H., & Farrand, P. (2008). Psychological factors that impact on women's experiences of first-time motherhood: A qualitative study of the transition. *Midwifery, 26*, 357–366.

Ellison, C. G., & Levin, J. S. (1998). The religion-health connection: Evidence, theory, and future directions. *Health Education & Behaviour, 25*, 700–720.

Endler, N. S., & Parker, J. D. A. (1990). Multidimensional assessment of coping: A critical evaluation. *Journal of Personality and Social Psychology, 58*, 844–854.

Endler, N. S., & Parker, J. D. A. (1999). *Coping inventory for stressful situations (CISS): Manual* (2nd ed.). Toronto, Ontario: Multi-Health Systems.

Escott, D., Slade, P., Spiby, H., & Fraser, R. B. (2005). Preliminary evaluation of a coping strategy enhancement method of preparation for labour. *Midwifery, 21*, 278–229.

Fenwick, J., Gamble, J., & Hauck, Y. (2007). Believing in birth—Choosing VBAC: The childbirth expectations of a self-selected cohort of Australian women. *Journal of Clinical Nursing, 16*, 1561–1570.

Fenwick, S., Holloway, I., & Alexander, J. (2009). Achieving normality: The key to status passage to motherhood after a caesarean section. *Midwifery, 25*, 554–563.

Fokazi, S. (2011). *Experts call for cut in C-section birth rates.* Received from http://www.iol.co.za/lifestyle/family/birth/experts-call-for-cut-in-c-section-birth-rates-1.1029667

Fossey, E., Harvey, C., McDermott, F., & Davidson, L. (2002). Understanding and evaluating qualitative research. *Australian and New Zealand Journal of Psychiatry, 36*, 717–732.

Gamble, J., & Creedy, D. K. (2009). An exploratory study of mothers' experiences and perceptions of an unplanned caesarean section. *Midwifery, 25*, 21–30.

Gibbons, J., & Thomson, A. M. (2001). Women's expectations and experiences of childbirth. *Midwifery, 17*, 302–313.

Giorgi, A. (1985). Sketch of a psychological phenomenological method. In A. Giorgi (Ed.), *Phenomenology and psychological research* (pp. 8–22). Pittsburgh, PA: Duquesne University Press.

Graham, S., Furr, S., Flowers, C., & Burke, M. T. (2001). Religion and spirituality in coping with stress. *Counseling and Values, 46*(1), 2–13.

Graneheim, U. H., & Lundman, B. (2004). Qualitative content analysis in nursing research: Concepts, procedures and measures to achieve trustworthiness. *Nurse Education Today, 24*, 105–112.

Halama, P., & Bakosova, K. (2009). Meaning in life as a moderator of the relationship between perceived stress and coping. *Studia Psychologica, 51*, 142–148.

Hamilton, B. E., Martin, J. A., & Ventura, S. J. (2007). Births: Preliminary data for 2006. *National vital statistics reports* (vol. 56, no 7). Hyattsville, MD: National Center for Health Statistics.

Hamilton, J. G., & Lobel, M. (2008). Types, patterns, and predictors of coping with stress during pregnancy: Examination of the Revised Prenatal Coping Inventory in a diverse sample. *Journal of Psychosomatic Obstetrics & Gynecology, 29*, 97–104.

Hauck, Y., Fenwick, J., Downie, J., & Butt, J. (2007). The influence of childbirth expectations on Western Australian women's perceptions of their birth experience. *Midwifery, 23*, 235–247.

Health Professions Council of South Africa (HPCSA), Professional Board for Psychology. (2004). *Ethical Code of Professional Conduct Health Professions Act, 1974: 1974, Generic, Annexure 1-2, Annexure 11-12, form 223.* Retrieved from http://www.hpcsa.co.za/downloads/ethical_rules/ethical_rules_of_conduct_2011.pdf

Hodnett, E. D., Gates, S., Hofmeyr, J., & Sakala, C. (2011). Continuous support for women during childbirth. *Cochrane Database Systematic of Reviews, 2.* Retrieved from http://onlinelibrary.wiley.com/doi/10.1002/14651858.CD003766.pub3/abstract

Howarth, A. M., Swain, N., & Treharne, G. J. (2011). Taking personal responsibility for well-being increases birth satisfaction of first time mothers. *Journal of Health Psychology, 16*, 1221–1230.

Ip, W., Tang, C. S. K., & Goggins, W. B. (2009). An educational intervention to improve women's ability to cope with childbirth. *Journal of Clinical Nursing, 18*, 2125–2135.

Jay, A. (2008). Effective postnatal care. In I. Peate & C. Hamilton (Eds.), *Becoming a midwife in the 21st century* (pp. 174–208). Chichester, UK: John Wiley & Sons, LTD.

John, O. P., & Gross, J. J. (2007). Individual differences in emotional regulation. In J. J. Gross (Ed.), *Handbook of emotion regulation* (pp. 351–372). New York, NY: Guilford.

Kendler, K. S., Gardner, C. O., & Prescott, C. A. (1997). Religion, psychopathology, and substance use and abuse: A multimeasure, genetic-epidemiologic study. *American Journal of Psychiatry, 154*, 322–329.

Koenig, H. G., & Larson, D. B. (2001). Religion and mental health: Evidence for an association. *International Review of Psychiatry, 13*, 67–78.

Krefting, L. (1991). Rigour in qualitative research: The assessment of trustworthiness. *American Journal of Occupational Therapy, 45*, 214–222.

Krumrei, E. J., & Pargament, K. I. (2008). Are gratitude and spirituality protective factors against psychopathology? *International Journal of Existential Psychology and Psychotherapy, 3*(1), 1–5.

Lavender, T., Walkinshaw, S. A., & Walton, I. (1999). A prospective study of women's views of factors contributing to a positive birth experience. *Midwifery, 15*(1), 40–46.

Lazarus, R. S., & Folkman, S. (1984). *Stress, appraisal and coping.* New York, NY: Springer.

Lincoln, Y. S., & Guba, E. G. (1985). *Naturalistic inquiry.* Beverley Hills, CA: Sage.

Lobel, M., & DeLuca, R. S. (2007). Psychosocial sequelae of cesarean delivery: Review and analysis of their causes and implications. *Social Science & Medicine, 64,* 2272–2284.

Lobel, M., Hamilton, J. G., & Cannella, D. T. (2008). Psychosocial perspectives on pregnancy: Prenatal maternal stress and coping. *Social and Personality Psychology Compass, 2,* 1600–1623.

Lobel, M., Yali, A. M., Zhu, W., De Vincent, C. J., & Meyer, B. A. (2002). Beneficial associations between optimistic disposition and emotional distress in high-risk pregnancy. *Psychology and Health, 17*(1), 77–96.

Luthar, S. S., Cicchetti, D., & Becker, B. (2000). The construct of resilience: A critical evaluation and guidelines for future work. *Child Development, 71,* 543–562.

Lyberg, A., & Severinsson, E. (2010). Fear of childbirth: Mothers' experiences of team-midwifery care: A follow-up study. *Journal of Nursing Management, 18,* 383–390.

MacMillan, D. T. (2010). Understanding the health beliefs of first time mothers who request an elective cesarean versus mothers who request a vaginal delivery. *Nursing Dissertations,* paper 14. Retrieved from http://digitalarchive.gsu.edu/nursing_diss/14

Marshall, C., & Rossman, G. B. (1995). *Designing qualitative research* (2nd ed.). Thousand Oaks, CA: Sage.

McDonald, K., Amir, L. H., & Davey, M. (2011). Maternal bodies and medicines: A commentary on risk and decision-making of pregnant and breast-feeding women and health professionals. *BMC Public Health, 11*(5). Retrieved from http://www.biomedcentral.com/1471-2458/11/S5/S5

Melender, H. (2002). Fears and coping strategies associated with pregnancy and childbirth in Finland. *Journal of Midwifery and Women's Health, 47,* 256–263.

Mertens, D. M. (2009). *Research and evaluation in education and psychology: Integrating diversity with quantitative, qualitative, and mixed methods* (3rd ed.). London, England: Sage.

Miller, W. R., & Thoresen, C. E. (2003). Spirituality, religion, and health: An emerging research field. *American Psychologist, 58*(1), 24–35.

Moos, R. H., & Holahan, C. J. (2003). Dispositional and contextual perspectives on coping: Toward an integrative framework. *Journal of Clinical Psychology, 59,* 1387–1403.

Moustakas, C. E. (1994). *Phenomenological research methods.* Thousand Oaks, CA: Sage.

Murphy, D. J., Pope, C., Frost, J., & Liebling, R. E. (2003). Women's views on the impact of operative delivery in the second stage of labour: Qualitative interview study. *British Medical Journal, 327*(7424), 1132–1136.

Nilsson, C., & Lundgren, I. (2009). Women's lived experience of fear of childbirth. *Midwifery*, *25*(2), 1–9.

Novick, G. (2009). Women's experience of prenatal care: An integrative review. *Journal of Midwifery & Women's Health*, *54*, 226–237.

Nystedt, A., Hogberg, U., & Lundman, B. (2008). Women's experiences of becoming a mother after prolonged labour. *Journal of Advanced Nursing*, *63*, 250–258.

Olde, E., van der Hart, O., Kleber, R., & van Son, M. (2006). Posttraumatic stress following childbirth: A review. *Clinical Psychology Review*, *26*(1), 1–16.

Parratt, J. (2002). The impact of childbirth experiences on women's sense of self: A review of the literature. *Australian Journal of Midwifery*, *15*(4), 10–16.

Patton, M. Q. (2002). *Qualitative research and evaluation methods*. Thousand Oaks, CA: Sage.

Porreco, R., & Thorp, J. A. (1996). The cesarean birth epidemic: Trends, causes, and solutions. *American Journal of Obstetric Gynaecology*, *175*, 369–374.

Prati, G., & Pietrantoni, L. (2009). Optimism, social support, and coping strategies as factors contributing to posttraumatic growth: A meta-analysis. *Journal of Loss and Trauma*, *14*, 364–388.

Reisenzein, R., & Weber, H. (2009). Personality and emotion. In P. J. Corr & G. Matthews (Eds.), *The Cambridge handbook of personality psychology* (pp. 54–71). Cambridge, England: Cambridge University Press.

Rosen, J. A., Glennie, E. J., Dalton, B. W., Lennon, J. M., & Bozick, R. N. (2010). *Non-cognitive skills in the classroom: New perspectives on educational research*. Research Triangle Park, NC: Research Triangle Institute International.

Roux, S. L., & van Rensburg, E. (2011). South African mothers' perceptions and experiences of an unplanned Caesarean section. *Journal of Psychology in Africa*, *21*, 429–438.

Ryding, E. L., Wijma, K., & Wijma, B. (1998). Experiences of emergency Cesarean section: A phenomenological study of 53 women. *Birth*, *25*, 246–251.

Ryding, E. L., Wiren, E., Johansson, G., Ceder, B., & Dahlstrom, A. (2004). Group counselling for mothers after emergency caesarean section: A randomized controlled trial of intervention. *Birth*, *31*, 247–253.

Singer, L. T., Fulton, S., Kirchner, L., Eisengart, S., Lewis, B., Short, E., ... Baley, J. E. (2010). Longitudinal predictors of maternal stress and coping after very low-birth-weight birth. *Archives of Paediatric & Adolescent Medicine*, *164*, 518–524.

Stadlmayr, W., Amsler, F., Lemola, S., Stein, S., Alt, M., & Burgin, D., ... Bitzer, J. (2006). Memory of childbirth in the second year: The long-term affect of a negative birth experience and its modulation by the perceived intranatal relationship with caregivers. *Journal of Psychosomatic Obstetrics & Gynecology*, *27*, 211–224.

Strauss, A. L., & Corbin, J. M. (1998). *Basics of qualitative research: Techniques and procedures for developing grounded theory* (2nd ed.). Thousand Oaks, CA: Sage.

Strumpfer, D. J. W. (2002). *Psychofortology: Review of a new paradigm marching on*. Retrieved from http://general.rau.ac/psychq

Strumpfer, D. J. W. (2005). The strengths perspective: Fortigenesis in adult life. *Social Indicators Research*, *77*, 11–36.

Thoits, P. A. (1995). Stress, coping, and social support processes: Where are we? What next? *Journal of Health and Social Behaviour*, *35*(Suppl.), 53–79.

Tugade, M. M., Fredrickson, B. L., & Feldman Barrett, L. (2004). Psychological resilience and positive emotional granularity: Examining the benefits of positive emotions on coping and health. *Journal of Personality, 72,* 1161–1190.

Tulman, L., & Fawcett, J. (2003). Recovery from childbirth: Looking back 6 months after delivery. *Health Care for Women International, 12,* 341–350.

Updegraff, J. A., & Taylor, S. E. (2000). From vulnerability to growth: Positive and negative effects of stressful life events. In J. Harvey & E. Miller (Eds.), *Loss and trauma: General and close relationship perspectives* (pp. 3–28). Philadelphia, PA: Brunner-Routledge.

Veloso, C. M. (2007). Medication use of childbirth and unplannedCesarean sections: Associations with stress and coping. *Dissertation Abstracts International: Section B: The Sciences and Engineering, 68,* 674.

Waldenström, U. (2004). Why do some women change their opinion about childbirth over time? *Birth, 31*(2), 102–107.

Weiss, M., Fawcett, J., & Aber, C. (2009). Adaptation, postpartum concerns, and learning needs in the first two weeks after caesarean birth. *Journal of Clinical Nursing, 18,* 2938–2948.

Wertz, F. J. (1983). From everyday to psychological description: Analyzing the moments of a qualitative data analysis. *Journal of Phenomenological Psychology, 14,* 197–241.

Yokote, N. (2008). Women's experiences of labour, surgery and first postnatal week by an emergency caesarean section. *Journal of Japan Academy of Midwifery, 22*(1), 37–48.

"I May Not Say We Really Have a Method, It Is Gambling Work": Knowledge and Acceptability of Safer Conception Methods Among Providers and HIV Clients in Uganda

SARAH FINOCCHARIO-KESSLER

Department of Family Medicine, University of Kansas Medical Center, Kansas City, Kansas, USA

RHODA WANYENZE

Department of Disease Control and Environmental Health, Makerere University School of Public Health, Kampala, Uganda

DEBORAH MINDRY

Center for Culture and Health, University of California, Los Angeles, Los Angeles, California, USA

JOLLY BEYEZA-KASHESYA

Department of Obstetrics and Gynaecology, Mulago Hospital, Makerere University College of Health Sciences, Kampala, Uganda

KATHY GOGGIN

Health Services and Outcomes Research, Children's Mercy Hospitals and Clinics; and Schools of Medicine and Pharmacy, University of Missouri-Kansas City, Kansas City, Missouri, USA

CHRISTINE NABIRYO

The AIDS Support Organization, Kampala, Uganda

GLENN WAGNER

RAND Corporation, Santa Monica, California, USA

In this qualitative study, researchers assessed knowledge, acceptability, and feasibility of safer conception methods (SCM; timed unprotected intercourse [TUI], manual self-insemination, and sperm washing) among various health care providers (n = 33) and 48 HIV clients with recent or current childbearing intentions in Uganda.

While several clients and providers had heard of SCM (especially TUI), few fully understood how to use the methods. All provider types expressed a desire to incorporate SCM into their practice; however, this will require training and counseling protocols, sensitization to overcome cultural norms that pose obstacles to these methods, and partner engagement (particularly by men) in safer conception counseling.

In this article, researchers have integrated perspectives from both providers (HIV, family planning and traditional health) and HIV patients regarding knowledge and acceptability of three safer conception methods (timed unprotected intercourse [TUI], manual self-insemination, and sperm washing). We describe current efforts in the absence of clear guidelines, training, or adequate resources. These findings are relevant for an interdisciplinary international audience given the intersecting domains of HIV prevention and treatment, sexual and reproductive health, health policy, and human rights in the context of culturally sensitive behaviors, stigma, poverty, and gender inequality. This topic of safer conception is both timely and relevant given challenges faced in many African countries to balance the strong value placed on childbearing and the risks of HIV acquisition or transmission.

The childbearing desires and intentions among women and men living with HIV, and the multitude of factors that influence reproductive decision making, have been well summarized in recent review articles (Hoyt, Storm, Aaron, & Anderson, 2012; Nattabi, Thompson, Orach, & Earnest, 2009). Researchers in Uganda indicate that between 28% and 59% of people living with HIV (PLHIV) want to have a child in the future (Beyeza-Kashesya et al., 2010; Kakaire, Osinde, & Kaye, 2010; Wagner, Kityo, & Mugyenyi, 2012). The cultural value of children, the role of parent as integral to one's adult identity, and relationship dynamics present strong motivators for childbearing (Nattabi et al., 2009). Expanded coverage of antiretroviral therapy (ART) for treatment and prophylaxis during pregnancy has led to a decline in mother-to-child transmission from 31% in 2009 to 21% in 2011 in Uganda (UNICEF, 2012), but the risk of horizontal transmission in the context of conception remains prominent. With approximately half of PLHIV in serodiscordant partnerships (Uganda Ministry of Health [MOH] and ICF International, 2012), most new infections occur in the context of stable relationships (Allen et al., 2003). High pregnancy rates among PLHIV (Uganda Bureau of Statistics [UBOS] and ICF International, 2012) indicate the need for effective contraception and safer conception methods (SCMs) that can play a critical role in reducing new HIV infections (Hoyt et al., 2012; Matthews, Smit, Cu-Uvin, & Cohan, 2012).

Methods to reduce HIV transmission to uninfected partners during attempts to conceive, or SCM, range greatly in the level of technology and financial resources required (Matthews et al., 2012; Matthews & Mukherjee, 2009). High-resource options such as sperm washing (female uninfected) plus insemination or in vitro fertilization (Sauer et al., 2009) are not yet a realistic option for most serodiscordant couples in sub-Saharan Africa. Low-cost behavioral methods include TUI limited to peak fertility days (male or female uninfected), and manual self-insemination with partner's sperm (male uninfected), each of which has demonstrated reduced risk of acquisition and transmission of HIV (Barreiro, Castilla, Labarga, & Soriano, 2007; Mmeje, Cohen, & Cohan, 2012).

There are also several methods that are not specific to the context of conception but that greatly reduce sexual transmission risk. Antiretroviral therapy (ART; and a resultant undetectable viral load more specifically) has been shown to reduce infections in serodiscordant couples by 96% (Cohen et al., 2011), and medical male circumcision decreases the risk of transmission among men by 51% (Gray et al., 2007); both of these methods, used alone or in combination with any of the above described methods, can substantially reduce transmission during conception. In addition, preexposure antiretroviral prophylaxis (PrEP) for the uninfected partner may reduce risk during conception attempts (Vernazza, Graf, Sonnenberg-Schwan, Geit, & Meurer, 2011, Thigpen et al., 2012), but its efficacy in this context has not been established, nor is it widely available in Uganda or other sub-Saharan African countries at the present time. While these methods, and ART in particular, can greatly reduce transmission risk during conception, some level of risk for transmission remains and therefore the use of these methods in combination with SCMs has real value for HIV prevention.

While feasible SCMs are available, successful utilization of these methods requires that providers and clients have adequate knowledge and self-efficacy to either counsel clients or apply these strategies with their partner. Unfortunately, HIV client counseling on the use of these methods is not currently being implemented in sub-Saharan Africa, or any other part of the world, as part of standard care. Researchers demonstrate an unmet need for reproductive counseling among HIV clients in Uganda (Wagner et al., 2012; Wanyenze, Wagner, Tumwesigye, Nannyonga, Wabwire-Mangen, & Kamya, 2013), South Africa (Schwartz et al., 2012), Brazil (Finocchario-Kessler et al., 2012), and the United States (Mindry et al., 2013) to facilitate safer conception and childbearing, as clients who want to have children typically have no communication with their providers about how to reduce risk during conception. Furthermore, whether or not specific strategies are culturally acceptable to clients, and whether or not providers are motivated to engage clients in safer conception counseling, is largely unknown. We are unaware of any study that has evaluated the knowledge and attitudes of sub-Saharan African HIV providers and their clients regarding specific SCMs.

Various types of providers are positioned to inform the childbearing decisions of HIV clients. HIV providers (physicians, nurses, counselors) have ongoing periodic interactions with clients of reproductive age, while family planning (FP) providers care for referred clients (mostly female) with contraception needs. Traditional health (TH) provider, in this context herbalist and traditional birth attendants, are also a common source of health services in Uganda, including services related to fertility and childbearing (Ssali et al., 2005). In this study, researchers examine the perspectives of a range of providers (HIV, FP, and TH) and PLHIV regarding their current level of knowledge and perceived cultural acceptability and feasibility of implementing targeted low-resource methods specific to safer conception in Uganda.

METHODS

Study Setting

Researchers conducted the study between July and September of 2012 at The AIDS Support Organization (TASO) HIV care and treatment sites in the capital city of Kampala and Jinja, which is a periurban center about 50 km from Kampala. TASO is a non-governmental organization founded in 1987 to provide care and support for HIV/AIDS infected and affected people in Uganda. The Kampala site is located next to the Mulago National Referral Hospital and has over 6,700 active clients. The Jinja site is located within the Jinja Regional Referral Hospital, and it provides HIV care to over 8,000 clients. In addition to ART and counseling services, TASO provides FP and contraception services at its clinics, but it refers clients to FP clinics located within the same hospital complex (Jinja Regional and Mulago National Referral Hospitals) for more specialized services. In comparison to public health clinics, TASO clinics have greater resources and more diversified staff, which allows for the provision of a wider array of services. The clientele served by TASO as well as public health clinics, however, tend to be of lower socioeconomic status, as middle- to high-income earners typically go to private clinics.

Sample

We enrolled HIV, FP, and TH providers and HIV clients to examine their perspectives on the knowledge, acceptability, and feasibility of various SCM and other factors influencing provision of support for safer childbearing among HIV clients. We interviewed a mix of nurses, medical or clinical officers, counselors, and "expert clients" from the participating HIV clinics. Expert clients are PLHIV who have been trained to provide support and information to fellow PLHIV, and also serve as liaisons between providers and clients. Family planning (FP) providers were identified from the hospital settings in which the HIV clinics are housed, and the TH providers were identified from the communities surrounding the clinics. We stratified client recruitment by gender, and eligibility criteria included being (a) age 18 years or older, (b) in a heterosexual relationship, and (c) recently conceived (in past year) or have the intention to conceive a child in the near future (e.g., within the next year). Clients were identified through provider and self-referrals (following announcements made in the waiting room of the clinic) on a few select days designated for recruitment. Clients received 15,000 Ush (approximately U.S. $6.00) for completing the interview; providers received 20,000 Ush (approximately U.S. $8.00). All participants provided informed verbal consent. The study protocol was reviewed and approved by the Institutional Review Boards at the RAND Corporation, University of Missouri-Kansas City, and Makerere University.

Instrument

We used separate semistructured interview guides with open-ended questions and semistructured follow-up questions and probes to elicit themes and determine their frequency and salience among providers and clients. The interviews covered several areas related to the childbearing needs of HIV clients and the support services available to meet these needs. This analysis focuses specifically on content related to SCM to limit risk of HIV transmission to sexual partners. All respondent were asked similar questions to assess their knowledge of any SCM and perceived acceptability and feasibility of the following three specific SCMs: (a) timed unprotected intercourse (TUI), (b) manual self-insemination for couples where the man is HIV-negative and the woman is HIV-positive; and (c) sperm washing for couples where the man is HIV-positive and the woman is HIV-negative. Since some of the SCMs are relevant to couples depending on the HIV status of specific members of the couple, client participants were asked to respond to the questions hypothetically rather than with regard to their relationship with their current partner. Highly trained, master's degree level interviewers conducted client and TH provider interviews in Luganda. HIV and FP provider interviews were conducted in English by senior study investigators. Interviews generally took 30–45 minutes to administer, with client interviews conducted at the clinic and provider interviews conducted at the respondent's workplace.

Analysis

We used descriptive statistics to characterize the sample population and quantify provider and client knowledge of SCMs. Interviews were digitally recorded, translated into English (when conducted in Luganda), and transcribed verbatim. We conducted content analysis to identify themes, using a staged technique described by Bernard and Ryan (2010). We used *ATLAS.ti* (2004) software to mark contiguous blocks of transcript text that pertained to the major topical domains of interest. We then pulled out all text associated with a particular domain and created subthemes within each primary code or domain. Two team members each coded all content within 10 interviews to assess whether both were coding the content equivalently and to reach consensus where there was any disagreement (Bernard, 2009); the remaining interviews were divided between the two team members and coded.

RESULTS

The sample included 33 providers, consisting of 18 HIV (four medical or clinical officers, three nurses, seven counselors, four expert clients), 10 FP (seven midwives, one nurse, and two doctors), and five TH providers (three herbalists, two traditional birth attendants). Eight of the providers were male, and all but five had been providing care for at least 4 years. Forty-eight clients participated; half ($n = 24$) were male, mean age was 37 years, 33 (69%) were on ART, and 38% reported their partner's serostatus was discordant or unknown (see Table 1).

Knowledge of Safer Conception Methods

When prompted with specific types of SCMs, the majority of providers reported that they had heard of one or more of the methods highlighted in this study (TUI, manual self-insemination, and sperm washing). Providers who claimed some knowledge of any SCM were most familiar with TUI followed by artificial insemination (even though the question was about manual self-insemination); however, only 15% ($n = 5$) could describe any

TABLE 1 Characteristics of Provider ($n = 33$) and Client ($n = 47$) Participants

	FP ($n = 10$)	HIV ($n = 18$)	TH ($n = 5$)	Total ($n = 33$)
Mean age (SD)	46.2 (9)	37.8 (7)	62.6 (13)	44.1 (12)
Female	9 (90%)	11 (61%)	4 (80%)	24 (73%)
Kampala	6 (60%)	9 (50%)	2 (40%)	15 (456%)
Jinja	4 (40%)	9 (50%)	3 (60%)	18 (54%)

	Kampala ($n = 23$)	Jinja ($n = 24$)	Total ($n = 47$)
Mean age (SD)	34.5 (6)	38.5 (9)	36.6 (8%)
Female	13 (57%)	11 (46)	24 (51%)
Have 1+ children	23 (100%)	23 (96%)	46 (98%)
Mean number of children (SD; range)	3.4 (2.3; 1–9)	4.9 (3.7; 0–17)	4.1 (3.2; 0–17)
Some secondary education	11 (48%)	7 (29%)	18 (38%)
On ART	19 (83%)	18 (75%)	37 (79%)
Partner HIV status: Negative/unknown	9 (39%)	11 (46%)	20 (43%)
Wants another child	21 (91%)	19 (79%)	40 (85%)

TABLE 2 Comparing Providers and Clients' Level of Knowledge of Each Safer Conception Method

	Timed unprotected intercourse			Manual self-insemination			Sperm washing		
	None	Aware	Know	None	Aware	Know	None	Aware	Know
Providers									
HIV $n = 18$	1(6)	17(95)	10(56)	12(67)	6(33)	2(11)	6(33)	12(67)	1(6)
FP $n = 10$	4(40)	6(60)	3(30)	4(40)	6(60)	1(10)	8(80)	2(20)	1(10)
TP $n = 5$	4(80)	1(20)	0	3(60)	2(40)	0	5(100)	0	0
Patients									
Female $n = 24$	10(42)	14(58)	7(29)	19(79)	5(21)	2(8)	19(79)	5(21)	2(8)
Male $n = 24$	9(38)	15(62)	11(46)	16(67)	8(33)	2(8)	17(71)	6(25)	2(8)

None = have no knowledge of the method; Aware = have heard of the method (includes those who also have knowledge); Know = can provide at least a partial explanation of the method.

method other than TUI in any detail. Among clients, 61% ($n = 29$) had heard of one or more methods to reduce risk during conception, with 37% ($n = 18$) able to describe any of the methods. Clients were most familiar with the concept of TUI as a method they had been counseled on or had employed, while awareness of either artificial or manual self-insemination was largely attributed to radio advertisements and communication with other clients. We highlight below qualitative data reflecting providers' and clients' level of knowledge of each of the targeted SCMs. Quantitative summaries of SCM knowledge are presented in Table 2.

Timed Unprotected Intercourse

Provider knowledge of TUI. Among HIV providers, 95% (17/18) were aware of the method of strategically limiting unprotected intercourse to the few days each month that the woman is ovulating and thus most fertile to maximize the likelihood of conception, while minimizing the risk of HIV transmission, and 56% (10/18) could describe key elements of the method. Descriptions of how providers counsel clients on the use of this method did not always explicitly emphasize consistent condom use outside of this ovulation window:

> I may not say we really have a method, but it is gambling work.... I take them through their menstrual period ... to discover their ovulation time and maybe that is where they will concentrate, on that time, rather than having to hit many times with open sex (without condom) and they don't succeed. (*HIV#20, female, age 46*)

Moon beads (color-coded beads in the shape of a necklace) are an existing innovative method used for tracking ovulation that was referenced by both HIV and FP providers. Six of 10 FP providers illustrated their familiarity with the concept of tracking ovulation for TUI; however, their training was oriented to targeting the fertile days to avoid sex and prevent pregnancy. Consequently, some FP providers referred to the peak ovulation days of highest conception potential as "unsafe," given the historic application of this method as contraception, while the HIV providers referred to these days as "safe," given their focus on preventing transmission:

> The one we usually tell them about, we use the moon beads. So they can time the days when the madam is unsafe. That is why they have to control the number of [times of] intercourse. (*FP#26, female, age 56*)

> We generally use condoms, and if you are set and want a baby, you know the safe days. Since you don't need a whole month to make a baby, we teach them about the safe days, with moon beads … then other days use a condom. (*HIV#13, female, age 55*)

Only one of the five traditional providers demonstrated familiarity with the concept of TUI.

Client knowledge of TUI. Most clients ($n = 29$; 60%) had heard about TUI as a strategy to reduce the risk of HIV transmission, and several could describe aspects of the method. The consensus among informed clients was that unprotected sex should be limited to a woman's most fertile days, and condoms should be used in all other instances. What appeared less clear to these respondents was the length of the window period for unprotected sex, and how to consistently identify ovulation. While the first quote describes a conservative fertility window of one day, the second quote illustrates a much looser interpretation of continual unprotected sex until a child is conceived:

> He (doctor) told me that when a woman gets to the time of getting pregnant, you stop using condoms for those days [when woman is ovulating] and after doing it for only one day, you again use condoms because I have a different virus [viral strain of HIV] than my wife. This [method] is what I used the last time to get the child that I have. (*C#21, male, age 50*)

> You have to be aware that with a wife, you do not use a condom when you want to have a child, since you lack the knowledge of when she will conceive. (*C#13, male, age 53*)

Knowledge of how to calculate a woman's ovulation to determine when unprotected sex should occur varied among clients. Some female clients identified the importance of this knowledge and the need for training: "Sometimes we forget to know when you began [to have your period] and how to count days [until ovulation]. I also think if one is trained, it would help" (*C#22, female, age 35*). Clients also noted that increased physical arousal indicated ovulation: "You feel like you want to 'meet' with your loved one. That is what I know, and if you go and 'meet' him, you can get pregnant" (*C#2, female client, age 38*). Interestingly, some of the male clients provided more specific explanations of how to track ovulation: "After 5 days of menstruating, you then have to count like 7 days and it should also be before 14 days because if she goes beyond 14 days she can't get pregnant" (*C#23, male, age 35*).

Many clients described counselors as the primary source for information about safer conception, and described the process and various considerations raised by the counselor regarding the plan to have a child:

> I first come to my counselor whom I inform about my intentions. She inquires of whether the man is ready to take care of me. Has he got money? Is he in need of a child? So she encourages me to come along with my husband on a given date. We go to her office and discuss it. Where he mentions that he is ready to have a baby, then I go back and have my CD4 count. In the past, once you were about 500 [CD4 count] you begin to plan to get pregnant. (*C#17, female, age 37*)

Maintaining a high CD4 cell count prior to conception attempts was repeatedly reported to providers as important in terms of assessing the woman's health status:

> The counselor tells us ... when the CD4 is high, you can have unpro-tected sex when the woman is ovulating and the woman can conceive. After conception, you then go back to using condoms. But you can only do this after they check the CD4 for you and your wife to ensure that you move along as a couple. (*C#49, female, age 39*)

While the importance of maintaining a high CD4 count was raised by providers as a sign of good maternal health status and lowering risks to the mother with regard to childbirth, clients talked about it specifically in the context of safer conception and transmission risk, suggesting a misconcep-tion as to value of a higher CD4 in this context:

> Because when the CD4 level is low, the chance of infecting your partner is high. When the CD4 is low, the health care provider can advise you to hold on [wait until CD4 count rises before attempting to conceive]. (*C#43, male, age 42*)

Manual Self-Insemination

Provider knowledge of manual self-insemination. Although we asked specifically about manual self-insemination, many providers responded with remarks about artificial insemination, providing a general description of its process, and indicating it occurred in specialty fertility centers in Kampala. Some were familiar with the concept of insemination given its local use for animal husbandry. After clarification that we were asking about manual self-insemination, 42% ($n = 14$) of all providers (six HIV, six FP, and two TH) mentioned having heard of self-insemination that could be accomplished at home, but only two HIV and one FP provider could actually provide any level of description. One provider shared a success story from a serodiscordant couple for whom he cared:

> There is a very nice model couple. The man is negative, the woman is positive, but somehow they agreed and used a very local method of getting a sterile syringe and getting semen from the condom and the woman injected herself. And as we talk, she's pregnant. (*HIV#17, female, age 35*)

Other providers acknowledged that this method is not included in guidelines or part of standardized care, and that it was questions from their clients that often prompted their awareness of this option. Several commented on the lack of data regarding the effectiveness of the method to prevent transmission or achieve pregnancy, resulting in their reluctance to inform their clients of the method:

> Actually we are getting those testimonies from them [clients]. But we don't know how perfect it is ... but they always want to inquire from us if that is the right thing to do ... we don't have the correct answer to tell them. They may read on the Internet, so they come and tell us this is what we found out, so we are going to practice that. We don't know how effective it is. I've never got anyone telling me the results of using a syringe. I think it fails. (*HIV#4, female, age 37*)

> We don't know how safe it is. Yeah, we rarely talk about it.... talk about things we are not sure of. So we just know that that kind of thing is there. Maybe some of them [patients] know, but we don't bring it up during our sessions. (*HIV#5, female, age 30*)

One provider (*HIV provider, HIV#2, female, age 46*) expressed concern that the use of the syringe might damage the sperm and result in birth defects and malformations.

Client knowledge of manual self-insemination. Similar to providers, many clients had heard of artificial insemination or were familiar with the concept from radio advertisements, the Internet, communication with other patients, or due to its application in animal husbandry. But few clients ($n = 13$, 27%) were aware that manual insemination could be performed at home by the couple:

> I have heard about that method, but I didn't know whether it's applicable in such a way [performed by couple at home]. I know it's done in specialized hospitals or anywhere else where they can get your sperm. (*C#24, male, age 28*)

Only four clients were able to demonstrate some knowledge of the method, and one client actually described how self-insemination works, that it applies to couples where the man is uninfected, and talked about the training she received from counselors at a nearby research unit within the larger hospital complex:

> They [counselors at research project] taught us, after having sex, and the man has ejaculated in the condom. He pours his semen into the woman. If you use that, you can conceive, and that is when he is not positive. (*C#7, female, age 30*)

Sperm Washing

Provider knowledge of sperm washing. While some HIV (67%) and FP (20%) providers had heard of the term "sperm washing," most could not describe in any detail what the procedure entailed, and none of the TH providers had heard of the procedure. One provider referred to a new fertility center in Kampala, and he described his understanding of sperm washing:

> I heard that men who have weak sperms in contaminated semen can have them washed, energized, given nutrients, and injected in the woman. (*HIV#6, male, age 44*)

The most precise description was as follows:

> I just heard about it, I have not confirmed that it's really very true or possible. They say it can be done medically where they just pick out the sperm and then do artificial insemination, because the virus is not in the sperm, but it is in the semen. (*HIV#8, female, age 35*)

Client knowledge of sperm washing. Few clients (*n* = 11; 23%) had heard about sperm washing, and those who had reported fellow clients, the radio, and newspapers as sources of information. Only four respondents could provide at least a partial description of the process. Several clients described the process of taking sperm from the man that would be inserted in the woman (insemination), but only two made clear the distinction of washing or treating the sperm first, showing evidence of misunderstanding the process:

They can put medicine on them [sperm]; and later the woman can have them. I think that can also help to reduce the HIV infection. (*C#17, female, age 37*)

According to the small knowledge I have, it might be effective because I think sperms are not concentrated with HIV. If they are withdrawn and given to an HIV negative woman, it's a sure deal that she will remain negative. (*C#51, male, age 24*)

One client expressed concern that sperm washing could negatively impact birth outcomes or result in deformities (*C#11, female, age 33*).

Other Safer Conception Strategies Mentioned by Clients

Some male and female clients mentioned misconceptions about the benefits of avoiding rough sex that might bruise or wound the partner, and talked about "romancing" their partner before intercourse to facilitate natural lubrication to reduce entry points for HIV transmission. These themes were reportedly included in counseling sessions and workshops for discordant partners:

The method is to avoid forced sex. You have to agree and ensure that you don't have any wound and this can help to prevent reinfections. (*C#34, male, age 35*)

It is what I meant about carefully romancing your wife before sex. It can help both the woman and man not get infected. (*C#26, male, age 34*)

Male circumcision was mentioned as a way to further reduce transmission to uninfected male partners: "Circumcised men rarely get HIV, and I think if they use this method [TUI] they can prevent being infected" (*C#4, female, age 34*).

One client suggested the use of postexposure prophylaxis (PEP) for an uninfected partner in a serodiscordant relationship after timed unprotected sex to conceive a child. Another patient talked about the use of PrEP, mentioning the medication by name:

If one partner has been on drugs for a longer period, there is a drug called TRUVADA that a [HIV] negative person takes to prevent infection. (*C#23, female, age 36*)

Both providers and clients mentioned the need for training to increase their knowledge of SCMs and practical guidance on how to implement them at both the clinic and community levels:

I like the way you are telling me about these new things. I don't know if you have recorded them like on a CD, like really what happens when you use the syringe, so that people look at how it is done. So I don't know if these things are there, but I want some reading materials. (*HIV#2, female, age 46*)

It would really help if you go into the communities and train people about it [SCM]. (*C#37, male, age 37*)

Perceived Acceptability and Feasibility of Safer Conception Methods

Most providers and clients felt TUI was feasible because it draws on the existing practice of tracking ovulation, can be accomplished in the privacy of one's home, and does not cost money. Once the distinction between manual self-insemination (at home) versus artificial insemination (provider-facilitated at a clinic) was made clear, there was increased support for this method. Manual self-insemination was perceived as far more feasible for couples given the low cost of materials (syringe) and the ability to implement this at home. Thus, TUI and manual self-insemination were considered feasible options *if* providers and couples have appropriate training and support. All participants aware of sperm washing and artificial insemination discussed the cost as a significant barrier for the majority of Ugandans and nearly all clients at TASO.

While options that allow clients to protect their partners and conceive a child were welcomed by nearly all participants, cultural and religious objections to alternative (and thus seen as abnormal) conception strategies reduce the acceptability of these methods for some. This section is organized by common concerns regarding the acceptability and feasibility of SCMs expressed by providers and clients that may apply to one or more of the discussed methods.

Securing Partner Support

Partner support and couple cooperation were seen as integral to the success of these methods by both providers and clients. This begins with the initial step of coming for counseling together as a couple to facilitate open communication and planning for safer conception: "The counselor has to seat the two of you; because if I only tell one of the couple, the other person will not have received the adequate information about what should or shouldn't be done" (*C#44, female, age 32*).

Open communication about sex and planning pregnancy among couples is not common, yet will be necessary to effectively implement SCM: "Let me say 70% [of couples] lack communication, yet when you and the woman do communicate, you can discuss this method and it can work for you" (*C#15, male, age 33*). The level of commitment between serodiscordant partners influenced willingness to pursue SCM rather than abandoning the relationship:

> It also depends on the kind of relationship that exists—you need to understand and love each other. Then, it also depends how long you have lived together. Otherwise if you have just met, you just have to separate [instead of use that method]. (*C#29, female, age 32*)

Recognizing the cultural context and challenge for women to insist on SCMs without support of their partners, providers and clients discussed the difficulty for women to regulate and limit which days of the month they have unprotected sex:

> The problem [is] their husbands. Unless they come with their husband here to be told and they know what to do. Since they [husbands] are the head of the house, they don't want to go on women's commands. But I think if men are cooperative, you bring those men, we talk to them. I think they can do. (*FP#3, female, age 48*)

> I think the method is good, but the challenge is men who are not consistent with condoms. He can use it today and the next time refuse to use it. This puts you in danger of reinfection, you see. (*C#22, female, age 35*)

Some women expressed the fear of losing their partner if they refused unprotected sex and pressed their partner to use a SCM:

> I can accept it if I want to have a child, but you can't convince the men [to ejaculate into a cup].... The man can decide to get another partner of unknown status who they can have children with. If he sees that you don't want to have unprotected sex with him, he would go. (*C#4, female, age 34*)

As one client noted, "The cause of most family violence is due to disagreements about when they [couple] should and should not have sex" (*C#9, male, age 49*). Thus it is important to emphasize the need to engage male partners in counseling and to empower women without increasing their risk of violence. While these methods may challenge some cultural norms about sexual decision making, there are men interested in using these methods:

> For a man who has an upright thinking, a man who is not interested in passing on the virus to his wife, I believe they will also welcome it, because there are men who are interested in having children, but their fear is how to do it [safely]. (*HIV#3, male, 38*)

Non-Traditional Conception

Client responses validated providers' concerns that sperm washing plus artificial insemination deviated too far from normal conception practices, and thus were unacceptable to some:

> Although it prevents infection, there is no enjoyment like the natural way of a man ejaculating directly into the vagina when you are all still hot. When you use that method [sperm washing plus artificial insemination], the sperm is inserted into you when it's cold, and that is not good. Then also I think the child who is born using this method is not like a real child. (*C#31, female, age 23*)

Questions regarding paternity were also raised as a potential challenge with clinic-based methods to achieve conception. The strong preference for conceiving the traditional or "natural" way was also expressed:

> You know, depending on our cultures, for a woman to go and have artificial insemination, later the man may not accept that is actually HIS child. He might think that in the laboratory they changed and put another man's sperm into his wife. Catholics believe so much in doing things the religious way, the Godly way. The natural way. (*FP#7, female, age 34*)

Careful efforts to ensure confidence in the clinic-based processes will be important to ensure the trust of clients: "It would be very important that they do it when both of us are present as a couple, [rather] than drawing my sperms and leaving it in the hospital and then my wife goes to get it, because the doctor can accidentally get someone else's sperm" (*P#30, male, age 58*).

Participants expressed concern that masturbation or assisted ejaculation may pose a challenge, as it is not frequently part of sexual relationships; however, they felt education and sensitizing people could help change social norms regarding masturbation for the purpose of safer conception:

> Perhaps it [manual self-insemination] can help, but how do you tell a man to withdraw and ejaculate into a cup [*laughs*]? Because there are men who can't really be convinced. I really see it's hard. (*C#4, female, age 34*)

> I don't even know how many men can even accept masturbation. You know with everything that has a cultural connotation around it, it really begins with sensitization. If you begin to sensitize the people, with time, it can take off. (*C#7, female, age 34*)

Accurately Tracking Ovulation

The ability to accurately and consistently track ovulation (required for TUI and manual self-insemination) was noted by providers and clients; however, most providers felt this challenge could be overcome with adequate training:

> The literate easily understand and they are able, but for those who are not literate you would have to devise another method, maybe like using moon beads that could tell them the unsafe [fertile] days. (*HIV#10, female, age 30*)

> Actually clients are very intelligent. If you tell a woman to follow her menstrual secretions, she is able. Many women know about these changes, it is about you directing them to what this kind of discharge stands for—many can understand. But the temperature thing [to detect ovulation] is really difficult in our setting. (*FP#7, female, age 34*)

Some clients echoed the importance of training for ovulation tracking:

> It needs a lot of calculations and … we may not know how the cycle moves. We don't observe the inner organs so as to know the period. I told you that it's too scientific. (*C#51, male, age 24*)

Other situations that would make accurate ovulation tracking difficult were also raised, such as irregular menstrual periods or the absence of menstruation among lactating women, which were raised by one FP provider. An HIV counselor talked about the added challenges posed by people living in extreme poverty:

> When you're needy, even those choices and luxuries of having to study your body, to know when you're on or not on [ovulating], when you're surviving, struggling to survive, that one becomes not an issue. Some people have to squat to see the kind of secretions coming out. So, it needs a very good environment—where you don't have to go outside. (*HIV#17, female, age 35*)

Risk of HIV Transmission

Recognizing TUI is a harm reduction strategy that only minimizes risk of HIV transmission, one HIV provider articulated her discomfort with this risk, while another explained why many patients were willing to take this risk:

> They [serodiscordant couple] might say, "You told us only once, we might not get HIV, but now I'm positive." You'll carry the blame. So, anything that has a big risk, I don't think I would sell that information. Because

the chances are not 100% guaranteed that only once you can't get [HIV].
(HIV# *17, female, age 35*)

Other Concerns Related to the Feasibility of Safer Conception Methods

One man described the frustration associated with and the patience needed to accept the delayed conception process that can result from following guidance for TUI:

> The challenge I have met is thinking that she got pregnant while using timely intercourse when actually she did not get it [pregnancy] and when we wait for the next time she can get pregnant you may find that she is sick and you have to wait for yet another time. (*P#23, male, age 35*)

Other concerns were raised about the implementation of manual self-insemination by male clients who were uncertain how effectively or quickly they could collect and transfer the sperm to ensure its quality:

> It needs knowing the time the sperms can last because you can delay and the sperms expire. Also not every sperm can create a human being, so you can insert unproductive sperms into your wife. (*C#33, male, age 56*)

While costs and cultural preferences may limit the feasibility of sperm washing and artificial insemination, when asked about the expense as a barrier, one male client said, "That won't deter them. A person can give all they have in order to have a child" (*C#13, male, age 53*).

DISCUSSION

Despite increased recognition of the reproductive rights of PLHIV (Barroso & Sippel, 2011), and several studies documenting childbearing desires among PLHIV and their partners (Nattabi et al., 2009), this is one of the first studies to examine the knowledge, acceptability, and feasibility of SCM from the perspectives of both providers and clients. We present our findings to reveal that providers and clients often have some knowledge of TUI as a safer conception method, as this strategy is often used as part of family planning and pregnancy prevention. In comparison, relatively little was known about manual self-insemination or sperm washing among providers or clients. Male and female clients expressed motivation to use safer conception strategies to protect their partner; both for the sake of the partner and so they can stay healthy to care for the client and their children. Several clients also expressed the importance of such methods for young people in serodiscordant relationships who have not yet had children.

We observed variation in the level of knowledge of SCM between the different types of providers. HIV providers had the most knowledge, particularly with regard to TUI and sperm washing, compared with both FP and TH providers. While one might expect FP providers to be at least as knowledgeable about TUI, a common FP method for timing pregnancy, it is not surprising that HIV providers had greater knowledge of sperm washing, as the nature of the procedure has specific application to couples living with HIV. Although clients in this setting seek help from TH providers when they have challenges with conception (Kyomuhendo, 2003), TH providers had the least amount of knowledge of each of the SCMs, perhaps because of the absence of formal medical training or limited access to published findings. Similar to the HIV and FP providers, however, the TH providers expressed an openness and desire to learn more about these methods so that they could properly counsel and inform their clients.

Participants revealed several gaps in terms of the knowledge, practice, and policy guidance in relation to SCMs among the clients and providers. Several clients and providers had heard about some of the SCMs (especially timed unprotected intercourse), but they could not provide a comprehensive description of how they are implemented, and the clients who reported using the methods exhibited partial understanding. This partial knowledge could limit the success of their attempts to conceive (e.g., failure to time or recognize the fertile period) and ultimately undermine providers' and clients' confidence in these methods. The partial knowledge could also increase risk of HIV transmission to uninfected partners due to extended unprotected sex beyond the fertile window.

Timed unprotected intercourse and manual self-insemination were generally well received by both providers and clients as feasible options for widespread use, largely because they require little to no money and can be implemented by the couple at home. Yet even these methods pose challenges regarding the need for effective training of both providers and clients. Structured protocols need to be developed for provision of evidence-based training on SCMs to empower providers to effectively guide and support their clients. Sensitization is required to overcome cultural norms that may pose obstacles to specific components of the SCM (e.g., masturbation; alternatives to "natural" routes of conception; uncertainties regarding paternity; couple communication and planning of pregnancies) as well as avoidance of judgmental or value laden counseling.

Both providers and clients (mostly female, but male clients as well) spoke to the need to engage partners in the process of safer conception counseling as a prerequisite to couples being able to successfully implement SCMs. Gender disparities with regard to power dynamics and decision making within couples can greatly influence the success of implementing health strategies that require the involvement of both partners (Pulerwitz, Michaelis, Verma, & Weiss, 2010). Men have not traditionally been involved in family planning and reproductive health service delivery, but research with HIV-affected couples has shown that the desire for children is just as strong among the men in these relationships as it is among their female partners (Wagner & Wanyenze, 2013). Participation of men, and involvement of both partners as a couple, requires disclosure of HIV status, which can be a major barrier to implementation of any SCM. In fact, providers will likely need to assist clients with safe disclosure to their partners prior to being able to begin any couples-based safer conception counseling.

The uncertainty regarding the risk of transmission, even when SCMs are correctly implemented, remains an impediment to provision of safer conception counseling for some providers. When correctly implemented, many of the SCMs carry no risk of transmission. Timed unprotected intercourse (TUI) will always involve some risk, however, and research is needed to more clearly establish the levels of risk involved with this method under specific scenarios, including whether or not the infected partner is on ART. As ART access in Africa increases, concurrent use of ART and SCMs will further reduce transmission risk and may increase provider confidence in addressing safer conception support. Policy recommendations and guidelines from appropriate authorities, including Ministries of Health, will also reassure and encourage providers to offer safer conception counseling. Current sexual and reproductive health and prevention of mother-to-child transmission guidelines in Uganda and other countries do not address safer conception of HIV infected individuals who desire to have children (Uganda Ministry of Health, 2011; Uganda AIDS Commission, 2011). The only safer conception counseling guidelines that have been developed for PLHIV in sub-Saharan Africa are those published by the South African Association of HIV Providers in 2012 (Bekker et al., 2011), but these guidelines have not yet translated into routine provision of safer conception counseling in South Africa or elsewhere in the region.

This study is limited in its generalizability to nonclinic-based populations and its ability to explore nondisclosure as a barrier, because nearly all enrolled clients had disclosed their HIV status to their partner. We present useful insights into the acceptance and existing knowledge gaps and concerns about SCMs among providers and clients. Systematic quantitative data are needed to substantiate these qualitative findings and further elucidate the factors related to knowledge, attitudes, and practices regarding use of SCMs. Quantitative data illustrated in Table 2 are intended to facilitate comparisons, but they should be interpreted in light of the small sample size. Accordingly, we have begun the second phase of our research which will prospectively follow a cohort of male and female HIV clients in Uganda with intentions to conceive, together with their HIV, FP, and TH providers, to assess how knowledge, attitudes, and practices evolve in this developing component of HIV care. In the future we plan to use data from this mixed methods study to develop and evaluate the implementation of a safer conception counseling protocol for PLHIV.

In conclusion, we found low in-depth understanding of SCMs, but both providers and clients generally express a belief that low cost SCMs are feasible and could be acceptable in Uganda. Implementation of these strategies in Uganda and elsewhere will require standardized guidelines and culturally appropriate training as well as sensitization to address concerns among clients and providers. As safer conception needs of PLHIV become increasingly apparent, and clinics begin to engage in efforts to inform their clients of existing options, research will be needed to examine the prevalence of and barriers to utilization of specific SCM so as to inform the development of effective training and counseling programs.

ACKNOWLEDGMENTS

We acknowledge the extraordinary efforts of the providers, interviewers (Joseph Kyebuzibwa and Jacque Nakitende), and all of our colleagues at TASO Jinja and TASO Mulago who assisted in this study.

FUNDING

This study was supported by R01 HD072633.

REFERENCES

Allen, S., Meinzen-Derr, J., Kautzman, M., Zulu, I., Trask, S., Fideli, U., ... Haworth, A. (2003). Sexual behavior of HIV discordant couples after HIV counseling and testing. *AIDS, 17*, 733–740.

Barreiro, P., Castilla, J. A., Labarga, P., & Soriano, V. (2007). Is natural conception a valid option for HIV-serodiscordant couples? *Human Reproduction, 22*, 2353–2358.

Barroso, C., & Sippel, S. (2011). Sexual and reproductive health and rights: Integration as a holistic and rights-based response to HIV/AIDS. *Women's Health Issues, 21*(6), S250–S254.

Bekker, L. G., Myer, L., Rees, H., Cooper, D., Mall, S., Mnyami, C., ... Schwartz, S. (2011). Guidelines on safer conception in fertile HIV-infected individuals and couples. *Southern African Journal of Medicine, 12*, 31–44.

Bernard, H. R., & Ryan, G. W. (2010). *Analyzing qualitative data: Systematic approaches*. Thousand Oaks, CA: Sage.

Beyeza-Kashesya, J., Ekstrom, A. M., Kaharuza, F., Mirembe, F., Neema, S., & Kulane, A. (2010). My partner wants a child: A cross-sectional study of the determinants of the desire for children among mutually disclosed sero-discordant couples receiving care in Uganda. *BMC Public Health, 10*, 247.

Cohen, M. S., Chen, Y. Q., McCauley, M., Gamble, T., Hosseinipour, M. C., Kumarasamy, N., ... Fleming, T. R. (2011). Prevention of HIV-1 infection with early antiretroviral therapy. *New England Journal of Medicine, 365,* 493–505.

Finocchario-Kessler, S., Bastos, F. I., Malta, M., Anderson, J., Goggin, K., Sweat, M., ... Kerrigan, D. (2012). Discussing childbearing with HIV-infected women of reproductive age in clinical care: A comparison of Brazil and the US. *AIDS and Behavior, 16,* 99–107.

Gray, R. H., Kigozi, G., Serwadda, D., Makumbi, F., Watya, S., Nalugoda F., ... Wawer, M. J. (2007). Male circumcision for HIV prevention in men in Rakai, Uganda: A randomised trial. *Lancet, 369,* 657–666.

Hoyt, M. J., Storm, D. S., Aaron, E., & Anderson, J. (2012). Preconception and contraceptive care for women living with HIV. *Infectious Diseases in Obstetrics and Gynecology, 2012,* 604183. doi:10.1155/2012/604183

Kakaire, O., Osinde, M. O., & Kaye, D. K. (2010). Factors that predict fertility desires for people living with HIV infection at a support and treatment centre in Kabale, Uganda. *Reproductive Health, 7,* 27.

Kyomuhendo, G. B. (2003). Low use of rural maternity services in Uganda: Impact of women's status, traditional beliefs and limited resources. *Reproductive Health Matters, 11,* 16–26.

Matthews, L. T., & Mukherjee, J. S. (2009). Strategies for harm reduction among HIV-affected couples who want to conceive. *AIDS and Behavior, 13*(Suppl. 1), 5–11.

Matthews, L. T., Smit, J. A., Cu-Uvin, S., & Cohan, D. (2012). Antiretrovirals and safer conception for HIV-serodiscordant couples. *Current Opinion HIV AIDS, 7,* 569–578.

Mindry, D., Wagner, G., Lake, J., Smith, A., Linnemayr, S., Quinn, M., & Hoffman, R. (2013). Fertility desires among HIV-infected men and women in Los Angeles County: Client needs and provider perspectives. *Maternal and Child Health Journal, 17,* 593–600.

Mmeje, O., Cohen, C. R., & Cohan, D. (2012). Evaluating safer conception options for HIV-serodiscordant couples (HIV-infected female/HIV-uninfected male): A closer look at vaginal insemination. *Infectious Diseases in Obstetrics and Gynecology, 2012,* 1–7. doi:10.1155/2012/587651

Muhr T. (2004). ATLAS.ti. [Software]. Berlin, Germany: ATLAS ti Scientific Software Development.

Nattabi, B., Li, J., Thompson, S. C., Orach, C. G., & Earnest, J. (2009). A systematic review of factors influencing fertility desires and intentions among people living with HIV/AIDS: Implications for policy and service delivery. *AIDS and Behavior, 13,* 949–968.

Pulerwitz, J., Michaelis, A., Verma, R., & Weiss, E. (2010). Addressing gender dynamics and engaging men in HIV programs: Lessons learned from Horizons research. *Public Health Reports, 125,* 282–292.

Sauer, M. V., Wang, J. G., Douglas, N. C., Nakhuda, G. S., Vardhana, P., Jovanovic, V., & Guarnaccia, M. M. (2009). Providing fertility care to men seropositive for human immunodeficiency virus: Reviewing 10 years of experience and 420 consecutive cycles of in vitro fertilization and intracytoplasmic sperm injection. *Fertility and Sterility, 91,* 2455–2460.

Schwartz, S. R., Mehta, S. H., Taha, T. E., Rees, H. V., Venter, F., & Black, V. (2012). High pregnancy intentions and missed opportunities for patient-provider communication about fertility in a South African cohort of HIV-positive women on antiretroviral therapy. *AIDS and Behavior, 16*, 69–78.

Ssali, A., Butler, L. M., Kabatesi, D., King, R., Namugenyi, A., Kamya, M. R., ... McFarland, W. (2005). Traditional healers for HIV/AIDS prevention and family planning, Kiboga District, Uganda: Evaluation of a program to improve practices. *AIDS and Behavior, 9*, 485–493.

Thigpen, M. C., Kebaabetswe, P. M., Paxton, L. A., Smith, D. K., Rose, C. E., Segolodi, T. M., ... Henderson, F. L. (2012). Antiretroviral preexposure prophylaxis for heterosexual HIV transmission in Botswana. *The New England Journal of Medicine, 367*, 423–434.

Uganda AIDS Commission. (2011). *National Strategic Plan 2011/12– 2014/15*. Kampala, Uganda: Author.

Uganda Bureau of Statistics (UBOS) and ICF International. (2012). *Uganda Demographic and Health Survey 2011*. Kampala, Uganda: UBOS; and Calverton, MD: ICF International.

Uganda Ministry of Health (MOH). (2011). *The integrated national guidelines on antiretroviral therapy, prevention of mother to child transmission of HIV and infant & young child feeding*. Kampala, Uganda: Author. Retrieved from http://www.emtct-iatt.org/wp-content/uploads/2014/05/GL_Integrated-National-Guidelines-on-ART-PMTCT-and-IYCF-June-2011-MOH-Uganda_0.pdf

Uganda Ministry of Health (MOH) and ICF International. (2012) *2011 Uganda AIDS Indicator Survey: Key Findings*. Calverton, MD: MOH and ICF International. Retrieved from http://health.go.ug/docs/UAIS_2011_REPORT.pdf

United Nations Chilren's Fund (UNICEF). (2012). *Count down to zero: Elimination of new HIV infections among children by 2015 and keeping their mothers alive, Uganda*. Retrieved from http://www.unicef.org/french/aids/files/hiv_pmtctfactsheetUganda.pdf

Vernazza, P. L., Graf, I., Sonnenberg-Schwan, U., Geit, M., & Meurer, A. (2011). Pre-exposure prophylaxis and timed intercourse for HIV-discordant couples willing to conceive a child. *AIDS, 25*, 2005–2008.

Wagner G, L. S., Kityo C., & Mugyenyi, P. (2012). Factors associated with intention to conceive and its communication to providers among HIV clients in Uganda. *Maternal and Child Health Journal, 16*, 510–518.

Wanyenze, R. K., Wagner, G. J., Tumwesigye, N. M., Nannyonga, M., Wabwire-Mangen, F., & Kamya, M. R. (2013). Fertility and contraceptive decision-making and support for HIV infected individuals: Client and provider experiences and perceptions at two HIV clinics in Uganda. *BMC Public Health, 13*, 98.

"Abortion—It Is My Own Body": Women's Narratives About Influences on Their Abortion Decisions in Ghana

GEORGINA YAA ODURO

Department of Sociology and Anthropology, University of Cape Coast, Central Region, Cape Coast, Ghana

MERCY NANA AKUA OTSIN

Department of Population and Health, University of Cape Coast, Central Region, Cape Coast, Ghana

Globally, abortion has emerged as a critical determinant of maternal morbidity and mortality. The Ghana government amended the country's abortion law in 1985 to promote safe abortion. This article discusses the findings of a qualitative study that explored the decision-making experiences of 28 female abortion seekers aged between 15 and 30 years in Ghana. Key findings from the study are that individuals claimed autonomy in their abortion decisions; underlying the abortion decisions were pragmatic concerns such as economic difficulties, child spacing, and fear of parental reaction. In conclusion, we examine the health implications of Ghanaian women's abortion decisions.

Issues relating to abortion have become critical in global discourses on maternal and child health. While in some Western cultures abortion is backed by legal provisions within the context of human rights, some cultures in Africa tend to frown upon abortion basically due to religious and sociocultural beliefs and values. Thus abortion is a sensitive issue that permeates the cultural, social, moral, religious, and legal dimensions. In view of the sensitive nature of the phenomenon, abortion continues to attract research interests from various academic disciplines such as sociology, medicine, cultural studies, and gender studies among others. Drawing on the findings of a study that explored Ghanaian women's knowledge and interpretation of abortion laws and their implications for safe abortion services, we conclude that women's abortion decisions are influenced by myriad complex factors. It is therefore important that stakeholders become more sensitive to these complex factors when making and enforcing policies and thereby contribute toward improving women's health.

Abortion, whether induced or spontaneous, is the termination of a pregnancy before the fetus is capable of extrauterine life (World Health Organization [WHO], 2008). Induced abortion, which is the focus of this article, though often bordered by cultural, social, religious, moral, and legal prohibitions, has been practiced by human society from time immemorial. The work of Devereux (1976) points to its frequency across time and culture. In fact, induced abortion has been and is still a vital reproductive option for many women (Shah & Ahman, 2010). Approximately 50% of women worldwide have experienced abortion at a point in their life (Population Reference Bureau, 2012). Although the actual incidence of abortion is difficult to define, varied estimations have been suggested by different bodies.

Marie Stopes International (2007), for example, estimated that there is the probability of every one in three women between the ages of 16 and 45 inducing an abortion. This implies that most women at a point in their lives will experience an unwanted pregnancy and might resort to induced abortion (Puri, Ingham, & Matthews, 2007). Although abortion is performed on women, to what extent are they involved in or in charge of the decision to terminate a pregnancy? How do communal demands intersect with personal values in a society like Ghana where a child does not only belong to the parents but also to the extended family and community at large (Bleek, 1978; Mbiti, 1969; Nukunya, 1992; Oduyoye, 1995)?

In this article, we examine the reasons that inform the decision of some Ghanaian women to terminate pregnancy. The role of the extent of knowledge about Ghana's legal position on abortion and its influence on their abortion decision, choice of abortion facilities, and conduct of safe or unsafe[1] abortions are also explored. We examine the players involved in women's abortion decisions and the implications on women's health. We begin with an examination of abortion trends from the global, African, and Ghanaian contexts, followed by a presentation of the theoretical framework and research methods that guided our study. Next, we present our data concluding with a discussion of the implications for women's health.

Trends in Abortion: The Global and Local Contexts

Women the world over become pregnant unintentionally, due to varying reasons such as unplanned sexual activities, a lack of or inadequate access to birth control services, contraceptive failure, and sexual assault (Crane &

Hord-Smith, 2006; Patel & Johns, 2009). While some of these women try to terminate their pregnancies through safe means, others terminate their pregnancies by whatever means are available to them, even if it is against the law, unsafe, and might result in complications. This shows the extent to which a woman would go to terminate an unwanted pregnancy even at the peril of her health and life (Crane & Hord-Smith, 2006; Henshaw et al., 1998).

Globally, it is estimated that out of 210 million pregnancies occurring annually, 40 to 50 million of them end in induced abortions (WHO, 2008). Other estimates purport that out of every five pregnancies occurring world-wide, one ends in an abortion (Sedgh, Singh, Henshaw, Åhman, & Shah, 2007). Kumar, Hessini, and Mitchell (2009) in a more vivid description report that as many as 81 women experience abortion around the world every minute.

On the African continent, although most of its 54 countries have restrictive abortion laws in operation, current estimates show a rise in the annual incidence of abortions from 5.6 million in 2003 to 6.4 million in 2008 (Guttmacher Institute, 2012; Singh et al., 2009). Legality of abortion in Africa is classified into six different categories within which abortion is permitted. These range from total prohibition to partial permission based on reasons such as to save a woman's life, preserve her physical and mental health, and on abortion permitted on socioeconomic grounds, to abortion without any restrictions as pertains in South Africa (Guttmacher Institute, 2012). Ghana's legal position on abortion is partial; thus, abortion is permitted under certain conditions. The lack of clarity and knowledge about the abortion laws in many African countries, coupled with poor access to health services, however, often result in many women using clandestine, risky, unorthodox, and unsafe means to induce abortion, thereby significantly increasing their risk of dying through complications (Svanemyr & Sundby, 2007). For example, out of the 6.4 million abortions that occurred in 2008 in Africa, it is estimated that only 3% were performed under safe conditions (Guttmacher Institute, 2012). This raises a lot of concerns since the literature suggests that the majority of morbidity and mortality cases are from unsafe abortions (Grimes, 2003).

In Ghana, abortion is frowned upon, and whenever issues about abortion come up for discussion in the public domain, people are often very judgmental. Senah (2003) attributes the controversy associated with abortion to religious, cultural, and moral factors in view of the value and importance placed on life. According to Lithur (2004), the combination of social perceptions, traditional and cultural values, religious teachings, and the laws governing abortions have reinforced people's negative attitudes toward abortion. She reiterated further that a community may shun and give a woman derogatory names if it becomes public knowledge that she has terminated a pregnancy. The stigma of abortion is so pervasive that sometimes in women's desire to avoid it, they resort to clandestine abortions that often end in complications. The social stigma further impedes adequate medical care through women's desire to keep their abortions secret. For example, participants in a study on abortion in Cameroon identified the social stigma attached to abortions as hindering their ability to seek medical care in the event of abortion complications (Guttmacher Institute, 2009; Johnson-Hanks, 2002; Kumar, Hessini, & Mitchell 2009; Schuster, 2005). Ghana's maternal mortality rate currently stands at 451 maternal deaths per 100,000 live births of which abortion stigma has been identified as a contributor (Guttmacher Institute, 2010).

In a bid to end the needless deaths of women, the law governing abortions in Ghana was amended in 1985, thereby permitting abortions on most physical and psychological grounds. The current law states that an abortion performed by a qualified medical practitioner is legal if the pregnancy is the result of rape, incest, or the defilement of a mentally challenged or retarded woman; if the continuation of the pregnancy would risk the life of the pregnant woman or threaten her physical or mental health; or where there is a substantial risk that the child born may suffer from or later develop a serious physical abnormality or disease (Morhee & Morhee, 2006). Yet, not much progress has been made since the liberalization of the abortion law in 1985; unsafe abortions still remain a major public health problem in the country and are currently the second most important contributors to maternal mortality in Ghana (Ghana Statistical Service, Ghana Health Service, & Macro International Inc., 2009; Guttmacher Institute, 2010).

Other researchers suggest that abortion complications rank high in cases handled at the gynecological and obstetrics wards of various hospitals in Ghana (Srofenyoh & Lassey, 2003; Yeboah & Kom, 2003), which is a situation that some observers blame on the fact that the translation of the law into effective services has been limited. Even in health institutions where the laws on abortion are expected to be operational, it is not so. In a recent study, it was identified that fewer than one in seven health facilities admitted offering abortion services (Ghana Statistical Service, Ghana Health Service, & Macro International Inc., 2009). In another claim, among women within the reproductive ages, only 4% think abortion is legal in Ghana and in this category 17% do not know the circumstances under which abortion is legally permissible (Ghana Statistical Service et al., 2009).

Notwithstanding the current context surrounding abortions in Ghana, the participants in this study braved all odds and sought a safe avenue, specifically a nongovernmental organization (NGO) clinic to terminate their unwanted pregnancies. From the literature, the article is framed by the following assumptions:

- Abortion seekers in Ghana are generally not aware of the laws governing abortion.
- The abortion decision is often made by only the woman and her partner.

Framing the Study: The Social Ecological Model

The existing literature suggests that persons intending to terminate their pregnancies are more often than not influenced by complex interplay and several divergent factors (Bankole, Singh, & Haas, 1998; Trent & Hoskin, 1999). Therefore, in wanting a theoretical framework that succinctly reflect these influences, we found the social ecological model valuable. The social ecological model, also known as the social ecological perspective, is a comprehensive theoretical framework that has been employed in the explanation of human behavior in diverse fields such as public health, education, disability, violence prevention, and child development (Dahlberg & Krug, 2002; Swartz, 2007). Social ecology focuses on the study of people in an environment and the influences they have on one another. Feltson and Carlson (2001) defined it as the nested arrangement of family, school, community, and public policy on behavior. In 1979, in response to the focus of most theorists on a dichotomous perspective of behavioral change that is either from an individual or a societal-level perspective, Bronfenbrenner argues that these two levels interact continuously and evolve into various interrelated components and influences (Bronfenbrenner, 1979).

It was adapted and modified by Dahlberg and Krug (2002), however, to reflect the interplay of influences on people at the individual, relationship, community, and societal levels as represented in Figure 1.

At the individual level, the model focuses on individual characteristics such as knowledge, attitude, beliefs, skills, age, and educational background in influencing behavior and decisions. The second factor is the relationship level, and it considers the importance of relationships with family, intimate partners, and peers and the role of the immediate social circle of an individual on his or her decisions. At the community level, the model explores the influences of settings in which social relationships occur like schools, workplaces, and neighborhoods, and on an individual level. Last, societal-level factors focus on broad societal factors that either create or inhibit an individual from undertaking certain behaviors. These factors

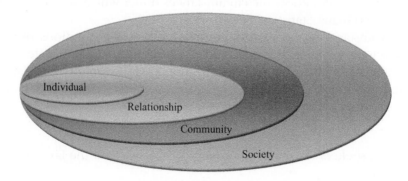

FIGURE 1 Social ecological model (Dahlberg & Krug, 2002).

include the influence of social norms, public policies, and religious and cultural belief systems on behavior and decisions (Dahlberg & Krug, 2002).

In our study, we considered influences from all the four levels of the ecological theory on study participants' abortion decisions. At the individual level the study examined the role of the participant in terminating pregnancy; here consideration was made of how participants' background and characteristics may have affected their decision. At the relationship level, the influence of intimate partners, family, friends, and health workers on the abortion decision-making process was examined; at the community level, the location of the facility in the neighborhood and accessibility were considered in participants' decision to terminate their pregnancy; while public policy, specifically the influence of Ghana's abortion laws on pregnancy termination, was considered at the societal level.

METHODOLOGY

We collected women's voices about their decisions and experiences on abortion through the qualitative approach, specifically narratives. Narrative inquiry is based on the premise that human beings come to understand and give meaning to their lives through stories (Andrews, Squire, & Tambokou, 2008). For deeper understanding of what the abortion experiences and decision-making processes meant for the participants, a total of 28 women between ages 15 and 30 years who had had elective pregnancy terminations participated in the study. The purposive sampling technique was used to recruit members. Purposive sampling focuses on specific characteristics, which in this case was an NGO clinic that performs abortions and women who had experienced induced abortions. Participation was, however, voluntary.

Data were collected through participant interviews over a period of 3 weeks in 2011. All the interviews were conducted by the researchers at the health facility after the participants had been discharged. At the clinic, clients were taken through counseling sessions prior to the abortion, and the researchers sat through the counseling sessions. Explanations were given to the clients by the health workers for the presence of the researchers, and clients were asked for their voluntary participation in the research. Through that approach, 28 people between the ages of 15 and 30 years were recruited for the study.

The purpose and the objectives of the study were explained to participants prior to the start of each interview. They were also assured of anonymity and confidentiality, and their informed verbal and written consents were obtained. In addition, permission was sought from them to record the interviews. Upon hearing about the use of tape recorders, some of the participants expressed misgivings and wanted assurance that their interviews would not be aired on the radio. Their apprehension was calmed with reassurance that the information solicited was solely for academic purposes.

On average, each of the interviews lasted between 35 minutes and 1 hour. The 28-item interview guide focused on participants' background characteristics, their sexual relationships, and abortion experiences as well as the influences on their abortion decisions. Pseudonyms were used for each participant, and participants were debriefed after each interview in order to reduce any possible anxieties that might have occurred during the course of the interview. Interviews were conducted in the local language (Twi) and transcribed verbatim. Ethical approval for the study was granted by the University of Cape Coast after a proposal outlining the aims and the objectives of the study had been presented. In addition, permission was sought and granted by the country director, clinical services manager, and center manager of the NGO clinic where the fieldwork took place. Miles and Huberman's (1994) framework for analyzing qualitative data served as a guide to uncovering the experiences of the participants.

The stigma and shame surrounding abortion in Ghana is so pervasive that efforts by us to recruit participants from public health facilities proved futile, hence our decision to recruit participants from an NGO clinic. This is not surprising, however, for Gammeltoft (2003) reports that even in Vietnam—a country that at one time had the world's highest abortion rate and currently has relatively easy access to abortion services—had persons who induced abortions experiencing stigma and feelings of regret that lead to keeping their abortions a secret. Koster (2003) reports similar experiences in Nigeria, where there is huge shame, fear of ridicule, and taboos associated with abortion.

RESULTS

Demographic Characteristics of the Study Participants

Sixty percent of the 28 women involved in the study were between ages 20 and 29 years old, findings which contrast with other studies by Ghana Statistical Service and others (2009) that reports that women under 20 years old have the highest probability of inducing abortions. Six of the participants were younger than 20 years old, with five women aged 30. In terms of the residential pattern, 89% of the participants lived in the community where the NGO clinic was located, thus emphasizing the benefits of locating health facilities within communities. The ease of access to the abortion clinic may be explained by the third element of the social ecological theory whereby settings and neighborhood influences tend to have an impact on people's decisions. Regarding religion, 22 of the 28 participants identified themselves as Christians, with the remaining six being Muslims.

The educational level of the participants was generally low. Eighteen of the 28 participants did not study beyond primary school, two attained vocational school education, while five had some level of secondary school education, one had no formal education, and only two participants were able to complete secondary school. The marital statuses of the 28 participants was that 16 of them were not married, which is not surprising since more single people tend to engage in abortion compared with married people; also, Ghanaian culture frowns on out-of-wedlock birth (Nukunya, 1992; Oduyoye, 1995). Seven were married and five were in cohabiting relationships. The majority of the participants (18) were self-employed, four worked for others, while two were students, two were in vocational training, and two others were unemployed.

Abortion Law and the Abortion Decision: It's Just My Body That Is Involved

The first assumption guiding this study was that abortion seekers in Ghana are not generally aware of the abortion law. In this regard, we explored the relationship between participants' knowledge of Ghana's abortion law and its influence on their abortion decision. Out of the total sample, only two participants, with secondary school education, demonstrated some knowledge about the abortion legislation in Ghana. This is what they said:

> The law allows it if the pregnancy resulted from rape, incest or if it can lead to the woman's death. (*Monica, 22 years*)

> Abortion is a criminal offense and when caught you can be imprisoned. But if it is done in a health facility by someone who has been trained, then it is okay. (*May, 24 years*)

When asked where they got their information, sources such as books, radio, friends, school, and television were mentioned. Sixteen out of the 28 participants mentioned that they did not know anything about the abortion legislation, which reflects the value of higher formal education in knowledge acquisition, particularly knowledge of laws and policies. The lack of knowledge and misinterpretation of the law by the 16 participants reflected in their responses as shown here:

> I don't know that such a law exist in Ghana. (*Nina, 24 years*)

> What I know about the law in Ghana concerning abortion is that if you give birth and you put it in a polythene bag and you are caught, you will be put in prison. *But if you have your own body* and you use it for abortion, I do not believe the Ghanaian law will do you anything. (*Paulina, 24 years*)

Thirty-year-old Mansa also rationalized her behavior:

> Abortion is illegal. But this one, *it is my own body,* and I alone understand what I am going through. I don't want any problems with anyone. That is why I have come here to terminate it, I know I cannot kill a child, but now, the pregnancy is not yet a child. (*Mansa, 30 years*)

Rukiyatu corroborated the above assertions as follows:

> I know abortion is illegal, but I think since *it is my own body* there is nothing wrong with it in my opinion; the police can arrest me only if I give birth and throw it away. (*Rukiyatu, 19 years*)

Although Ghana's abortion law was amended in 1985 to permit termination on certain grounds, it is clear from the aforementioned narratives that many of the participants view Ghana's position on abortion as totally illegal. Some participants therefore felt it was safer to terminate a pregnancy than to have the child and dispose of it, which could result in their arrest. They further explained that it was better to terminate a pregnancy they were not ready to carry since it involved just their lives, while giving birth and manhandling or killing the child could involve another life. To them, abortion does not carry any prosecution, but killing a child could attract punishment. Irrespective of the position and interpretation of the law on abortion in Ghana, of interest to this article is the strong notion of the body, self, autonomy, and personal values projected by participants in a communally entrenched African society like Ghana. Another interesting finding is participants' interpretation of not being murderers so far as the fetus is not yet a child. So how and where did participants acquire such notions? Could it be the result of advocacy and human right education?

Betrayed By My Body

Another theme that emerged from the participants related to what they called betrayals and disappointments by their bodies. Seventy-one percent of participants lamented about contraceptive failures. Three of the seven married participants resorted to abortion as a birth-spacing method in view of the young ages of their children. A twenty-one-year-old young mother, Joyce, for example, observed the following:

> If you give birth in quick succession, your body will soon become like an "abrewa" (old woman). My child is still young, she is just 11 months, I want her to grow a little before giving birth again. I thought I was in my safe period and yet look at my situation. (*Joyce, 21 years*)

Joyce was further worried about the devastating effect of rapid delivery on her female body.

For 15-year-old Lydia, she rationalized her abortion in terms of her body being immature as well as the challenge of her young age in carrying through the demands of a growing child:

> I think my body is too young to carry a baby. I am still in school and want to do something meaningful with my life. If I become a mother right now, I cannot have any good future. Actually, the pregnancy was a mistake. I never thought such a thing could happen to me, it was my first sex. (*Lydia, 15 years*)

In addition to the challenge of pregnancy for her young body were the pragmatic reasons of her education and securing a future. For another participant, the decision to terminate the pregnancy was a form of self-empowerment; apart from the pregnancy interfering with her career, it would also make her financially dependent on a man. She argued:

> I am doing this because of my job. If I keep the pregnancy, I cannot do the job and I will lose it. If I lose the job, how will I survive? I don't want to be dependent on any man so that he can control me. We have been using condoms and I can't fathom how this happened. (*Mariama, 23 years*)

In Mariama's view, becoming dependent on a man would disempower her. Thirty-year-old Sophia, the only participant to have cited health concerns underlying her abortion decision, said the following:

> Pregnancy really makes me suffer. I will be sick throughout and I cannot eat. Even this one, since it happened I am not able to eat normally. All that I am able to take is porridge, and even the little porridge I buy, I can't drink all. (*Sophia, 30 years*)

Two other participants who felt betrayed by their bodies had the additional headache of fear of their parents' and guardians' reactions. Juanita was a single girl and an orphan who resided with her grandmother, while Sandra, also single, lived with her parents. They both resorted to the abortion to avoid negative reactions from their guardians for fear of disappointing them with out-of-wedlock pregnancies, as Juanita said:

> I do not want my grandmother to find out; she will be angry with me. (*Juanita, 17 years*)

While Sandra an apprentice seamstress said related her concern:

> If I do not remove it and my mother finds out, she will virtually kill me. (*Sandra, 18 years*)

Other researchers have confirmed that fear of parents' retaliation causes children to resort to abortion (Bankole et al., 1998; Svanemyr & Sundy, 2007). One dramatic case was a young girl who was dragged to the abortion clinic by her disappointed aunt for her pregnancy to be aborted. She explained that the girl's biological parents were abroad and she was afraid of their reaction, should they discover the pregnancy. The fear of parental reactions to the discovery of pregnancies of children and wards is an important factor in the abortion decisions of participants. It reflects the community and relationship factors in the social ecological theory.

Although the participants felt betrayed in different ways by their bodies and contraceptives, they also had varied reasons for the abortion. The reasons ranged from social, cultural, perceived parental reactions, medical, career, and educational ambitions. Financial reasons also emerged as an issue as reflected in the case of 30-year-old Naomi, who observed, "I already have two children that I am struggling to take care of, it is not easy, so I can't have another child." The narratives further help to explain how the individual-level influences in the ecological theory in terms of participants' circumstances such as age, educational level and ambitions, attitudes, and so on informed their abortion decisions. Of interest is Mariama's desire to avoid dependency on men thereby working toward her empowerment and so resorting to abortion to help her actualize her dream to secure a better future.

The Self and Abortion Decision: "I Control My Body"

Another theme related to the body and derived from the narratives was the issue of control over the body. As we earlier mentioned, in Ghana, like in most other African countries, people's identity tends to be more communally inclined rather than individual (Assimeng, 1999; Mbiti, 1969; Nukunya, 1992). Whereas some of the partners of these women wanted them to keep their pregnancies, the women acted otherwise. Twenty-year-old Fuseina was among the 16 women who had strong views on the self and allowed personal ideas to inform her abortion decision. According to her, her partner wanted her to keep the pregnancy, but she felt she should have the final say in what happens to her body:

> He said that I should keep it; when he asks about it, I will tell him I miscarried it. It is my own body and I think I should have the right to decide when to carry a child. (*Fuseina, 20 years*)

Matilda, on the other hand, was reported by her partner to her mother for wanting to terminate the pregnancy. She was supported by her mother, however, with the claim that the partner does not have any control over her body since their relationship was not formalized by marriage:

The man wanted me to give birth, but I told him that I want to remove it. . . . He told my mother that I was pregnant and want to remove it . . . . and my mother said, yes, I should remove it . . . after all, he has not asked for my hand in marriage and therefore does not have any control over my body. (*Matilda, 29 years*)

Asked her reason for the abortion, Memuna also explained her situation:

The father of my son is traveled overseas and will be returning soon; it will not be good if he comes to see me carrying another man's child. (*Memuna, 20 years*)

Five of the participants mentioned making the final decision to terminate the pregnancy because of differences between them and their partners. Some attributed their actions to their partner's indifference, economic difficulties, nonreadiness for motherhood, and irresponsibility. Elizabeth and Patricia, for example, mentioned that after discussing with their partners aboutwhat to do about the pregnancy, the indifference shown by them influenced their decision to abort:

I took the final decision alone. When I told him about it, he wasn't very happy and we quarreled. Though we are still together, he has not asked anything about it. (*Elizabeth, 22 years*)

I decided alone, he knows that I am pregnant but he has not said anything about it. (*Patricia, 21 years*)

Two other participants showed their determination and autonomy in their decisions by going against their partner's advice. Maame Esi, for example observed the following:

He said that I should keep it and that God will help us take care of it, but I said, "No, we already have two children and we should use our resources in taking very good care of them." Although he stood his grounds, I removed it. (*Maame Esi, 29 years*)

Nineteen-year-old Mavis also exhibited some level of autonomy in her abortion decision. Instead of informing and consulting her partner about her pregnancy, she asked a friend for advice and acted upon it without the knowledge or involvement of her partner. This is her voice:

I decided with only the friend who brought me here. She is my best friend and I trust her. I did not tell the man who impregnated me, I know he would not have allowed the abortion. (*Mavis, 19 years*)

Mavis's choice of a friend over her partner regarding the pregnancy and abortion is also worth noting. This reflects the living out of the title of the paper and the notion that "it is her own body." She therefore actualized her intentions with the termination without the partner's knowledge or involvement.

DISCUSSION

The first theme of the article focused on participants' knowledge of Ghana's abortion law in relation to their abortion decisions. Although the study did not use a large sample size to enable generalization, it is clear from 57% of the participants that there was generally a low level of knowledge and interpretation of the abortion law. The laws governing abortion in Ghana articulate that abortion is not an offense if the pregnancy is the result of rape, incest, or the defilement of a mentally challenged or retarded woman; when continuation of the pregnancy would risk the life of the pregnant woman or be injurious to her physical or mental health; or where there is a substantial risk that if the pregnancy is carried to term, the child would suffer from or later develop a serious physical abnormality or disease (Morhee & Morhee, 2006). This is information that is not widely known. The low level of knowledge about the law could be attributed to the lack of education on the law as well as lack of general discussions on abortion due to its sensitivity in the Ghanaian society. The ignorance has huge implications for women's health because if women find the law prohibitive, there is the tendency for them to resort to unsafe abortion procedures.

Koster (2003) has argued that a woman's ability to obtain safe abortion services is affected not just by the law in a particular country but also by how these laws are interpreted and enforced and the attitude of the medical community toward abortion. Although the legalization of abortion does not totally obliterate a woman's recourse to abortion, it is an essential prerequisite for making it safe, because when abortions are legal it usually reduces a woman's chance of resorting to unsafe abortions (Berer, 2000). Additionally, the legalization of abortion is a necessary but insufficient step toward widespread access to safe abortion services and that for women to have access to safe abortion services there is a need for them to know, interpret, and understand the laws pertaining to abortions in their countries (Grimes et al., 2006; Hord & Wolf, 2004; Sai, 2004). The abortion law also falls in Dahlberg and Krug's (2002) fourth level of the social ecological theory, specifically, the societal level. Thus, it helps to explain the implications of the policy for women's health.

The second theme captioned by what the women narrated as "betrayed by my body" reveals a high level of individual influence in study participants' abortion decisions. It reflects the first level of the social ecological theory. The narratives also show that underlying the notion of the self and autonomy in women's abortion decisions were economic reasons, health issues, desire to further one's studies, the challenge of young age, job insecurity, and desire for empowerment. The third theme of "I control my body" also reflects similar studies where women had abortions to protect their moral integrity just like 20-year-old Memuna who resorted to abortion to protect her relationship with her son's father who was due to return from overseas. This scenario corroborates findings by Bleek (1981), Agadjania (1998), Schuster (2005), and Lie, Robson, and May, (2008) where women resorted to abortions in cases of pregnancies resulting from premarital and extramarital sexual encounters.

The foregoing findings are corroborated by other studies in which researchers report instances where the fear of parental reaction to pregnancy and force and threat by parents cause their children to abort their pregnancies or risk being sanctioned by them. The likely interference of pregnancy in career and educational ambitions also have led to abortions (Agadjania, 1998; Guttmacher Institute, 2009; Lie et al., 2008). Such scenarios reflect the influence of relationship and community factors in the social ecological theory that frames this study.

In the last assumption framing the study, we examined the players involved in women's abortion decisions. Zeleny (1979) explains decision making as an act of selecting the most desirable alternative. Some people believe that because a woman bears the greatest burden in pregnancy, it is her sole prerogative to decide what to do about it. Yet from a sociological point of view, this notion might be misleading since there are various stakeholders involved in the pregnancy and the abortion decision-making process. Some of the players involved in the abortion decision may not be overt but implied. Some participants reported that the attitude of their partners influenced their abortion decision. Twenty-four-year-old Nina, though married, shared her story: "My husband was very angry with me when I told him I was pregnant. He told me I should have protected myself and started behaving cold towards me, I therefore realized the child was unwanted." Such situations question the extent to which decision making is individually enacted or influenced by other factors.

Puri, Ingham, and Matthews (2007) and Johnson-Hanks (2002) in different studies reported the influences of one's social network in the abortion decision-making process. Similarly, Lee, Klienbach, Hu, Peng, and Chen (1996) have indicated that even the national culture of an individual plays a role in abortion decision making. Their comparative research, which studied the attitudes of Chinese and American youths on abortion, discovered that the Chinese youth had a favorable attitude toward abortion compared with their American counterparts. The study revealed the drastic cultural differences in the orientations of the Americans, who saw fetuses as sacred, compared with their Chinese counterparts.

In another study on abortion decision making, Trent and Hoskin (1999) reported aboutthe influence of religious orientation on the process. Fielding and Schaff's (2004) study in the United States of America involving women with unwanted pregnancies found out that those whom the women spoke to before an abortion was important in shaping their decisions. Although pregnancy is the result of sexual act between a man and a woman, women tend to bear the brunt of the result of the sexual act. Two of the participants reported how their male partners shied away from their responsibilities and deserted them during the pregnancy. Thus, the article reveals some gender dynamics reflected in violence and societal attitude to unfaithfulness by women. Whereas Elizabeth was violently beaten by the very man who impregnated her, Memuna reported terminating her pregnancy because she was impregnated by someone other than her regular partner who was outside the country. Memuna's actions might have been influenced by the fact that, in the African and the Ghanaian society, although it is culturally acceptable for a man to be unfaithful to his partner, it is highly stigmatized and unacceptable among women. As reiterated by Oduyoye (1995), while society approves of multiple and extramarital relations for men, the same is not expected of women. Thus, the sociocultural factors of gender, religion, and culture seem at play in the experiences of the study participants.

Social and psychological theories of control may be useful in explaining the behavior of the participants. Hirschi (1969) argues that humans are selfish beings who make decisions based on the choices that give them the greatest satisfaction in meeting their needs and wants. Containment theory as developed by Walter Reckless (1967), states that behavior is not caused by outside stimuli or outer container, but also by what a person wants most at any given time, which is the strong influence of the inner container (Jensen, 1973). According to the theory, weak social systems result in deviant behavior. The theory observes that people act rationally, but if they were given the chance to act like a deviant, they would. So, basically, if one has strong social bonds to positive influences, deviant behavior is less likely than for someone who has no such ties. In women's abortion decisions, therefore, other forces of control in addition to personal values and autonomy could be seen.

Implications and Conclusion

Myriad complex factors tend to explain why women terminate their pregnancies. Relating the study to the social ecological model, it could be argued that participants were affected by a broad range of intrapersonal-, interpersonal-, and societal-level influences with multiple implications, particularly for their health. Although participants in this study had the option of a safe NGO-run abortion clinic and benefited from safe abortion procedures, for many women, the available option is illegal[1] and unsafe abortions. Unfortunately, the devastating effects of unsafe abortions are numerous. Estimates indicate that unsafe abortions claim the lives of approximately

80,000 women yearly, 95% of whom are in the less industrialized world (Guttmacher Institute, 2009; WHO, 2008). The estimates further revealed that every hour, seven women, mostly from the less industrialized world, die from the complications of unsafe abortions (WHO, 2008).

In addition to the above issues, the lack of knowledge concerning the legality of abortions may be a barrier to treatment in the event of abortion complications. Because of ignorance, in the event of abortion complications, some women do not go to health facilities for treatment because of fear of prosecution by the law enforcement agencies (Banerjee & Clark, 2009). Studies in Cameroun, Ghana, Uganda, and Zambia cited the fear of legal consequences and stigma as hindering women from seeking care (Guttmacher Institute, 2009).

In this article, we reveal unmet contraceptive needs for some of the women as well as lack of sufficient knowledge and education on the use of contraceptives, because many of them reported contraceptive failure as responsible for the abortion. We also believe that insufficient sex education for Ghanaian women is a contributory factor because effective sex education has been identified as an antidote to unplanned pregnancy (Awusabo-Asare, Abane, & Kumi-Kyereme, 2004; Kirby, 2002).

We conclude by recommending the intensification of sex education, making it available for women and creating easy access to contraceptives. In spite of the sensitivity about abortion in Ghana and many other African contexts, education about abortion, its legal position in different countries, as well as the opportunity for citizens to understand and interpret the abortion law may change women's current unfortunate situation. Implementation of these suggestions will go a long way to help women to avoid or reduce unwanted pregnancies. In the event of such pregnancies, they may be in a better position to make informed decisions regarding how to handle the pregnancy since the fetus resides in women's bodies. Although abortion is an extremely sensitive subject in the Ghanaian context, we find the presence of the NGO clinic and the services being provided by them are very positive in saving women from many complications and deaths. In sum, the Ministry of Health and allied bodies should intensify education on the abortion law, so that women would be in position to access proper and legal services due to them in cases of unwanted pregnancies because the 1985 abortion law in Ghana permits abortion under certain conditions.

NOTE

1. Legal abortion is an abortion performed by a licensed physician or someone acting under the supervision of a licensed physician. Illegal abortion is the practice that is either self-induced or induced by someone who is not a physician or not acting under the supervision of a physician. Abortion is said to be illegal, even if it is induced by a physician but violates the laws of the state governing abortions (WHO, 2008).

REFERENCES

Agadjania, V. (1998). Quasi-legal abortion services in sub-Saharan setting: Users' profile and motivations. *International Family Planning Perspectives, 28*(3), 111–116.

Assimeng, J. M. (1999). *Social structure of Ghana: A study of persistence and change.* Tema, Ghana: Ghana Publishing Corporation.

Awusabo-Asare, K., Abane, A. M., & Kumi-Kyereme, A. (2004). *Adolescent sexual and reproductive health in Ghana: A synthesis of research evidence* (Occasional Report No. 13). New York, NY: Alan Guttmacher Institute.

Banerjee, S. K., & Clark, K. A. (2009). Exploring the pathways of unsafe abortion. *A prospective study of abortion clients in selected hospitals of Madya Pradesh, India.* New Delhi, India: Ipas.

Bankole, A., Singh, S., & Haas, T. (1998). Reasons why women have induced abortions: Evidence from 27 countries. *International Family Planning Perspective, 24*(3), 127–128. Retrieved from http://www.guttmacher.org/pubs/journals/2411798.html

Berer, M. (2000). Making abortions safe: A matter of good public health policy and practice. *Bulletin of the World Health Organization, 2000, 78*(5), 580–592.

Bleek, W. (1978). Induced abortion in a Ghanaian family. *African Studies Review, 2*(1), 103–120.

Bleek, W. (1981). Avoiding shame: The ethical context of abortion in Ghana. *Anthropological Quarterly, 54*(4), 203–209.

Bronfenbrenner, U. (1979). *The ecology of human development.* Cambridge, MA: Harvard University Press.

Crane, B., & Hord-Smith, C. (2006). *Safe abortion: An essential strategy for achieving the millennium development goals to improve maternal health, promote gender equality and reduce poverty.* Retrieved from http://www.unmillennuimproject.org/documents/Crane_and_Hord-Smith-final.pdf.

Dahlberg, L. L., & Krug, E. (2002). Violence: A global public health problem. In E. Krug, L. L. Dahlberg, A. B. Zwi, & R. Lozano (Eds.), *World report on violence and health* (pp. 54–56). Geneva, Switzerland: World Health Organization.

Devereux, G. (1976). *A study of abortion in primitive societies.* New York, NY: International Universities Press.

Felton, E., & Carlson, M. (2001). The social ecology of child health and wellbeing. *Annual Review of Health, 22,* 143–166.

Fielding, S. L., & Schaff, E. A. (2004). Social context and the experience of a sample of U.S. women taking RU-486 (Mifepristone) for early abortion. *Qualitative Health Research, 14*(5), 300–302.

Gammeltoft, T. (2003). The ritualisation of abortion in contemporary Vietnam. *Australian Journal of Anthropology, 14*(2), 129–143.

Ghana Statistical Service, Ghana Health Service, & Macro International Inc. (2009). *Ghana Maternal Health Survey, 2007.* Calverton, MD: Macro International.

Grimes, A. D. (2003). Unsafe abortion: The silent scourge. *British Medical Bulletin, 67,* 99–101.

Grimes, A. D., Benson, J., Singh, S., Romero, M., Ganatra, B., Okonofua, F. E., & Shah, I. H. (2006). Unsafe abortion: The preventable pandemic. *The Lancet, 368*(9550), 1908–1919.

Guttmacher Institute. (2009). *Facts on abortion and unintended pregnancy in Africa.* Retrieved from http://www.guttmacher.org

Henshaw, S. A., Singh, S., Oye-Adeniran, B., Adewole, I., Iwere, N., & Cuca, Y. P. (1998). *The incidence of abortion in Nigeria.* New York, NY: Guttmacher Institute.

Hord, C., & Wolf, M. (2004). Breaking the cycle of unsafe abortions in Africa. *African Journal of Reproductive Health, 8*(1), 29–34.

Jensen, G. F. (1973). Inner containment and delinquency. *Journal of Criminal Law and Criminology, 64,* 464.

Johnson-Hanks, J. (2002). "The lesser shame": Adolescent abortion in Cameroon. *Social Science and Medicine, 55*(8), 1337–1349.

Kirby, D. (2002). Do abstinence-only programs delay the initiation of sex among young people and reduce teenage pregnancy? Retrieved from http://www.thenationalcampaign.org/resources/reports.aspx

Koster, W. (2003). *Secret strategies: Women and abortion in Yoruba society, Nigeria.* Retrieved from http://www.googlebooks.com

Kumar, A., Hessini, L., & Mitchell, E.M.H. (2009). Conceptualising abortion stigma. *Culture Health and Sexuality, 11*(6), 625–639.

Lee, Y. T., Klienbach, R., Hu, P. C., Peng, Z. Z., & Chen, X. Y. (1996). Cross cultural research on abortion and euthanasia. *Journal of Social Issues, 52*(12), 138–142.

Lie, M. S., Robson, S. C., & May, C. R. (2008). *Experiences of abortion: A narrative review of qualitative studies.* Retrieved from http://www.biomedcentral.com

Lithur, N. O. (2004). Destigmatising abortion: Expanding community awareness of abortion as a reproductive health issue in Ghana. *African Journal of Reproductive Health, 8*(1), 70–74.

Marie Stopes International. (2007). *Safe abortion: Life saving intervention and human right.* Retrieved from http://www.mariestopes.org.uk

Mbiti, J. S. (1969). *African religions and philosophy.* London, England: Heinemann.

Miles, M. B., & Huberman, M. A. (1994). *Qualitative data analysis.* London, England: Sage.

Morhee, R., & Morhee, E. (2006). Overview of the law and the availability of abortion services in Ghana. *Ghana Medical Journal, 40*(3), 80–86.

Nukunya, G. K. (1992). *Tradition and change in Ghana: An introduction to sociology.* Accra, Ghana: Ghana Universities Press.

Oduyoye, M. A. (1995). *Daughters of Anowa: African women and patriarchy.* New York, NY: Orbis Books.

Patel, C. J., & Johns, L. (2009). Gender attitudes and attitudes to abortion: Are there gender differences? *The Social Science Journal, 46*(3), 493–505.

Population Reference Bureau. (2012). *Unsafe abortion facts and figures.* Retrieved from http://www.prb.org

Puri, M., Ingham, R., & Matthews, Z. (2007). Factors affecting abortion decisions among young couples in Nepal. *Journal of Adolescent Health, 40*(6), 535–542.

Sai, F. (2004). International commitments and guidance on unsafe abortion. *African Journal of Reproductive Health, 8*(1), 16–18.

Schuster, S. (2005). Abortion in the moral world of the Cameroon grass fields. *Reproductive Health Matters, 13*(26), 130–138.

Sedgh, G., Singh, S., Henshaw, S., Åhman, E., & Shah, I. H. (2007). Induced abortion: The global reality and avoidable risks. *The Lancet, 370*, 1338–1345.

Senah, K. (2003). Maternal mortality in Ghana: The other side. *Institute of African Studies Research Review, 19*(1), 50–52.

Shah, I., & Ahman, E. (2010). Unsafe abortion in 2008: Global and regional levels and trends. *Reproductive Health Matter, 18*(36), 90–101.

Singh, S., Wulf, D., Hussain, R., Bankole, A., & Sedgh, G. (2009). *Abortion worldwide: A decade of uneven progress.* New York, NY: Guttmacher Institute.

Srofenyoh, E. K., & Lassey, A. T. (2003). Abortion care in a teaching hospital in Ghana. *International Journal of Obstetrics and Gynaecology, 82*(1), 77–78.

Svanemyr, J., & Sundby, J. (2007). The social context of induced abortions among young couples in Cote d'Ivoire. *African Journal of Reproductive Health, 11*(2), 13–17.

Swartz, S. (2009). *The moral ecology of South Africa's township youth.* New York, NY: Palgrave Macmillan.

Trent, K., & Hoskin, A. W. (1999). Structural determinants of the abortion rate: Across sectional analysis. *Social Biology, 46*(1), 62–82.

World Health Organization (WHO). 2008. *Education material for teachers of midwifery: Midwifery education modules (2nd ed.)—Managing Incomplete Abortion, Module 6.* Geneva, Switzerland: Author.

Yeboah, R. W. N., & Kom, M. (2003). Abortion: The case of Chenard Ward Korle Bu from 2000 to 2001. *Institute of African Studies Research Review, 19*(1), 57–59.

Zeleny, M. (1979). *Multiple criteria decision making.* New York, NY: McGraw Hill.

"He Doesn't Love Me Less. He Loves Me More": Perceptions of Women Living With HIV/AIDS of Partner Support in Childbearing Decision-Making

YEWANDE SOFOLAHAN-OLADEINDE

Pharmaceutical Health Services Research Department, School of Pharmacy, University of Maryland, Baltimore, Maryland, USA

COLLINS O. AIRHIHENBUWA

Department of Biobehavioral Health, Pennsylvania State University, University Park, Pennsylvania, USA

Our purpose in this study was to understand the importance of male partner support in the childbearing decision-making processes of women living with HIV/AIDS (WLHA) by exploring their perceptions of support after disclosure, prepartum, and postpartum. We conducted in-depth interviews with 15 WLHA who were receiving clinical HIV care at a teaching hospital in Lagos. Results show that all male partners were consistently supportive, except the partner of the only unmarried participant. Other subthemes that emerged include the following: emotional support and reassurance; partnership and faith; and tangible support. We reveal important implications for HIV treatment and care programs.

Much of the research on the sexual and reproductive desires/intentions of people living with HIV has focused on women and largely excluded their male partners. A review of the existing literature reveals that the role and support of male partners is a key factor considered by women living with HIV/AIDS (WLHA) when making childbearing (CB) decisions (Beyeza-Kashesya et al., 2010; MacCarthy, Rasanathan, Ferguson, & Gruskin, 2012; Ujiji, Ekström, Ilako, Indalo, & Rubenson, 2010). The overall health and well-being of women and children improves when male partners are involved in

CB decision-making, voluntary counseling, and testing services (Conkling et al., 2010; Farquhar et al., 2004; MacCarthy et al., 2012; Ramirez-Ferrero & Lusti-Narasimhan, 2012). For the purposes of this article, CB decisions are limited to decisions made during pregnancy and postpartum. We expand the literature by exploring WLHA perceptions of male partner support in the CB decision-making process after disclosure, during pregnancy, and after childbirth. In particular, we explore whether male partners were supportive and how this support was shown to their female partners living with HIV. Since male partner support is critical to a family's health and well-being, we argue that HIV programs designed for women and children, such as prevention of mother-to-child transmission (PMTCT) services, should involve men.

According to the World Health Organization (WHO), 50% of women and their partners attending antenatal care (ANC) clinics in sub-Saharan Africa are in serodiscordant relationships (i.e., one partner is HIV positive and one is not). Indeed, most new HIV infections occur within these heterosexual serodiscordant relationships since many people living with HIV/AIDS (PLWHA) may not have initially disclosed their status to their partners (Ramirez-Ferrero & Lusti-Narasimhan, 2012), and they may not have been aware of their partner's status initially (WHO, 2012). Reports from several researchers indicate that men resist seeking HIV testing and counseling, even after discovering their partner's status. They usually assume that their own HIV status is the same as their HIV-positive partner's (or will eventually become the same), which contributes to them engaging in risky sexual behaviors (Crankshaw et al., 2012; MacCarthy et al., 2012; Ramirez-Ferrero & Lusti-Narasimhan, 2012; Rujumba et al., 2012). Thus, it is important that we consider the role of male partners in the CB decision-making processes of WLHA regardless of whether they are involved in serodiscordant (+/−) or seroconcordant (+/+) relationships.

Many women Believe that a woman's identity is affirmed by her motherhood status (Airhihenbuwa, 2007; Nduna & Farlane, 2009; Smith & Mbakwem, 2007). Accordingly, WLHA in Nigeria and many African countries sometimes plan to have children with partners whose HIV statuses are unknown (Sofolahan & Airhihenbuwa 2012). Chen, and colleagues (2001) reported that knowledge of a partner's HIV status influenced CB desires and expectations of WLHA. Women in serodiscordant relationships who wish to have children risk the possibility of transmitting HIV to their uninfected partners in the process of fulfilling their CB desires, while those in seroconcordant relationships risk reinfection with a different strain of HIV or with other sexually transmitted diseases (STDs) when trying to conceive (Cooper et al., 2007; Matthews et al., 2011).

Our review of the available literature exposed important gaps in knowledge that we seek to fill. First, many scholars who study sexual and reproductive health and PMTCT in sub-Saharan Africa have reported findings that mostly portray male partners as being unsupportive of their female partners, for example, by abandoning them when they disclose their HIV-positive status or abusing them physically, emotionally, or both (Iwuagwu, 2009; Nduna & Farlane, 2009; Smith & Mbakwem, 2007, 2010). Second, scholars have not assessed WLHA's perceptions of male partner support within the context of CB decisions, and how WLHA may inadvertently make their partners vulnerable to HIV infection (Oladapo et al., 2005; Smith & Mbakwem, 2007, 2010).

In this article, we expand on the current literature by exploring the WLHA perceptions of male partner support in the CB decision-making process after disclosure, during pregnancy, and after childbirth. In particular, we explore whether male partners were supportive, and how this support was shown to their female partners living with HIV. We contribute by offering preliminary insights into WLHA's perceptions of male partner support of their CB decisions and delineating different forms of partner support. Since male partner support is critical to a family's health and well-being, it is important to involve men in HIV programs designed for women and children, such as prevention of PMTCT services.

THEORETICAL FRAMEWORK

The PEN-3 cultural model was the overall organizational framework that guided the study. PEN-3 was used to develop the interview guide and for data analysis. The model was developed by Collins Airhihenbuwa to aid in understanding the role of culture in addressing Africans' health behaviors and decisions (Airhihenbuwa, 1995, 2007; Airhihenbuwa & Webster, 2004). The PEN-3 model enables researchers to emphasize cultural factors outside of the individual that collectively influence decision-making. PEN-3 has three domains, and each domain has three dimensions (see Figure 1). The three interconnected domains are cultural empowerment (CE), relationships and expectations (RE), and cultural identity (CI). Cultural empowerment

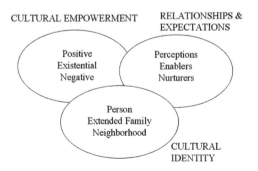

FIGURE 1 The PEN-3 Model.

considers the positive, existential (unique), and negative cultural values that are factored into health behaviors and decisions. Relationships and expectations consider factors such as perceptions, enablers, and nurturers that influence health behaviors and decisions. Cultural identity determines the appropriate level of focus for interventions—the person, the extended family, or the neighborhood—by addressing how one's identity plays a critical role in influencing health decisions (Airhihenbuwa, 2007; Airhihenbuwa & Webster, 2004).

The domain of interest in this study is relationships and expectations. Thus, we explore the perceptions, enablers, and nurturers of male partner support that are factored into the CB decisions of WLHA. Perceptions include the values and beliefs that may promote or hinder health behaviors when factored into CB decisions of WLHA. Enablers are the institutional (health care) support services that may influence CB decisions of WLHA. Nurturers are partners and significant others who may support or discourage CB among WLHA. In this article, we focus on WLHA perceptions of the role of male partners in CB decision-making.

METHOD

Study Site

The study was conducted between July and August 2012 at a teaching hospital located in southwestern Nigeria. With a population of about 9 million, a total fertility rate of 5.4%, and a mix of Nigerians from different ethnic groups, Lagos is the second most populous state in Nigeria (National Bureau of Statistics [NBS], 2006; National Population Commission [NPC], 2006).

Partnering with the physicians at the pediatric clinic, we were able to identify and recruit WLHA when they brought their infants to the clinic. This was ideal, because HIV-exposed and infected infants were seen on two designated days of the week at the pediatric ward of the hospital. In order to reduce the stigma associated with HIV, and because the clinicians attended to patients with HIV and other blood-related diseases, the section of the hospital where HIV patients were seen was referred to as the hematology clinic.

Study Design

We collected the data for this study as part of a larger study aimed at examining the sexual and reproductive health care needs of WLHA and related impacts on their CB decisions. The main focus of the study was to examine the different contextual factors that contribute to the CB experiences of

WLHA within their families and in health care settings. Using a qualitative research design methodology, we conducted in-depth interviews over a 2-month period with 15 WLHA. According to qualitative research standards, the number of interviews required to reach saturation should be about 30 (Cresswell, 1998). We reached saturation, however, after interviewing 15 WLHA; due to logistical reasons such as time and resource constraints, we felt it was not feasible (or necessary) to conduct 30 interviews. We developed a semistructured interview guide to explore the past CB experiences of WLHA, future CB plans, husband/partner feelings about current and previous pregnancies, and the role of partners after disclosure of HIV status and during pregnancy. We interviewed participants individually in a private room at the clinic, and we obtained verbal informed consent from participants prior to recording. Interviews lasted between 30 and 45 minutes each and were conducted in either English or Pidgin English. All interviews were audiorecorded, translated, transcribed, and analyzed. The participants were given 1,000 Naira (U.S.$7) as an incentive to cover their transportation costs. Ethical approval was obtained from the Institutional Review Boards of Penn State University and the teaching hospital.

Recruitment

Six women whom we previously interviewed in 2011 when they were pregnant had given us approval to contact them via telephone during the year after they gave birth. Given that we wanted a broad representation of WLHA in order to capture their recent CB experiences, in addition to these six, we purposively recruited nine more women with varied childbirth experiences who also had given birth within the year. To be eligible for the study, participants had to be between the ages of 18 and 43 years, and have a child less than 1 year old.

Interview Guide

The interview guide we used did not include direct questions about the partner's role in decisions to get pregnant and remain pregnant. Some of the additional probes that were used during the interviews to elicit WLHA's perspectives on the partner's role during pregnancy, in future pregnancies, and postpartum behavior include the following: (a) How did your husband/partner feel during your last pregnancy? Does your partner still want more children? (b) Has your partner (husband) been supportive during your pregnancy? Has your partner (husband) been supportive after your pregnancy? Probe: In what way has he been supportive? In what way has he been unsupportive?

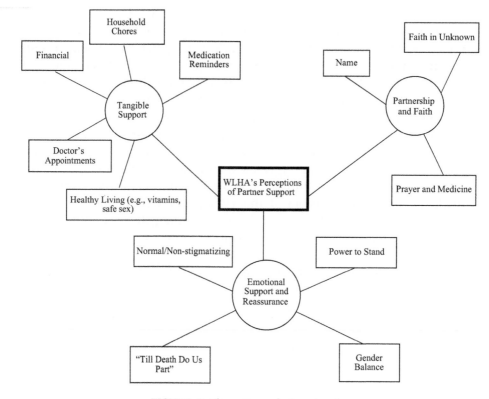

FIGURE 2 Thematic analysis network.

Data Analysis

The first author thoroughly read all interview transcripts to become immersed in the data, and loaded them into NVivo 9 to aid in organization and data management. We then subjected the interview data to thematic analysis following the Attride-Stirling protocol (Attride-Stirling, 2001). We conducted a within-case analysis (Creswell, 1998), and we developed a coding framework based on commonly occurring themes in the text (step 1). We coded data until saturation was reached. Next, we conducted a cross-case analysis to identify "basic themes" from the coded text (step 2). Finally, we clustered the basic themes into "organizing themes," which we further refined into "global themes," and then organized into a "thematic network" shown in Figure 2. The PEN-3 model was used to organize and identify the three major areas under which the themes were clustered. These follow: (a) emotional support and reassurance, (b) partnership and faith, and (c) tangible support (see Figure 2). We describe each theme in the results that follow. To ensure intercoder reliability, the second author read the transcripts and confirmed the global themes identified by the first author.

RESULTS

Participant demographic information is summarized in Table 1.

Based on the participants' responses, the level of male partner support was consistent both after disclosure of HIV positive status and after childbirth. Words used by participants to describe how their partner supported them included "being there," "backing up," "standing behind," and "encouraging with his words." The themes presented in Figure 2 are based on the responses of all of the 14 married WLHA who had delivered a baby in the past year and who reported being supported by their male partners. Three major themes follow: (a) emotional support and reassurance, (b) partnership and faith, and (c) tangible support. All of the married WLHA who participated in the study reported that their partners were supportive of their CB goals. The only participant who reported having an unsupportive partner was the one unmarried participant. This woman reported that the father of her child had not been involved in the life of her daughter, and he often ignored her requests for financial support.

Emotional Support and Reassurance: "He Doesn't Push Me Away Because I Have HIV"

Emotional support came in different forms, from partners "being there," to "backing up," "standing behind," "encouraging with his words," and encouraging them to have more children in order to balance the gender distribution in their families. Partners reassured WLHA that they were going to be there for them and reaffirmed the marriage vow "till death do us part," by treating them in nonstigmatizing ways (i.e., denying their female partner's HIV status) and by providing the encouragement necessary to withstand the stress of living with HIV.

Some of the phrases used to describe partner support included the following: "He assures me that he will stay with me and that he is not going anywhere"; "It is as if I don't have it [HIV]. He doesn't push me away because I have HIV"; "He doesn't look at me like I have this condition and he has to stay away"; and "He gives me the power to stand knowing that nothing will happen to me" among many others.

Participant narratives revealed the positive effects of partner support, as one participant described:

> He advises me, calms me down and makes me happy. Anytime I look at my back I see him there standing by me. I met someone here that was telling me her husband does not know about her status and she said that if he knows, "I am going back home to my father's house straight." I told her that my husband knows and I am still at home.

TABLE 1 Characteristics of the Study Population

Characteristic	Number ($N = 15$)
Participant age	
26–30 years	5
31–35 years	9
36–40 years	1
Mean (range)	31.9 (28–38 years)
Child age	
0–5 months	7
6–10 months	7
11–12 months	1
Mean (range)	6.3 months (3 weeks–12 months)
Education	
Primary	1
Secondary	9
Higher	5
Employment status	
None	9
Self-employed	4
Employed	2
Ethnicity	
Yoruba	2
Ibo	9
Ishan	2
Delta Ibo	2
Relationship status	
Married	14
Single	1
Religion	
Christianity	15
Mean # years since diagnosis (range)	4.4 years (1 month–14 years)
Currently on ARVs	
Yes	13
No	2
Partner status	
Negative	9
Positive	3
Unknown/untested	3
Child status	
Negative	11
Positive	1
Unknown/untested	3
Mode of delivery	
Vaginal birth	10
Cesarean section	5
Breastfeeding	
Yes	5
No	10
Currently living children	
1	5
2	5
≥ 3	5

Learning of one's HIV positive status can be devastating, especially if there is no support system. Partner support helps buffer some of the stress associated with being infected with HIV:

> He has been very, very supportive in all aspects as if I don't have it. He helps me a lot and he takes care of me. ... I almost killed myself when I found out [HIV positive]. If not for him and my doctor friend, I am sure I would be gone [dead] now. The only thing [that is different] is that I come to the clinic and I take drugs. Even with that he doesn't love me less. He loves me more.

One of the participants revealed how, unbeknownst to her husband, she secretly went for family planning shortly after the birth of her first child. After expressing concerns about her health to her husband, she was surprised by his willingness to limit the number of future children he wanted:

> I did family planning after Kemi without telling my husband. If not, I would have taken in [gotten pregnant] sooner than that. I told him I wanted Kemi to grow and for my tissues to heal very well, because of the CS [cesarean section] before taking in again. My husband has even said he would like to have four or five children, but because of this thing [HIV] he would reason with me. [What is important is] that it is about my life first and the life of the children. After we have one more to make three, [he agreed] that it is okay so I will go for family planning.

Participants also identified another type of emotional support provided by male partners: relating to them in a nonstigmatizing manner. This support manifested as the male partner's denial of WLHA status, and this provided many of them with some reassurance that their male partners were not going to abandon them because they were HIV positive. Some of the women reported that their partners showed support by continuing to see them as normal, not believing they were infected with HIV, and relating to them just as they had done before disclosure, as one woman explained:

> He supported me because I told him everything. Even up till now, he doesn't believe that I even have HIV, because before I did not take drugs, but due to the baby I started taking the drugs. Maybe now that I am taking drugs, he will believe somehow. He doesn't push me away that because I have HIV ... the only problem now is [convincing] him to come and know his status.

This type of support manifested as denial of a partner's HIV status has potentially negative consequences, since such partners tend to neglect necessary protective measures to prevent disease transmission. Another participant noted how the fact that her husband did not believe that she was infected with HIV served as a barrier against her taking necessary protective and preventive measures:

> My husband does not even believe that I have this disease. He still sees me as normal. He doesn't believe in anything HIV, so even when I force him he refused to use condoms. Even when I told him, he told me to remove my mind from it and I should not think about it [HIV]. Right from the first day, I don't think about it at all and forget there is something like this in me because of his support.

Many male partners were involved in the CB decision-making process. A desire to balance the genders among their children was one of the determining factors in CB decisions, as one participant stated:

> I don't want to have any more children, but I have to because I have only girls. Assuming I have a boy, then maybe I won't. If I just have a male child, that means I don't have any problem. I need a boy in my family. My husband wanted me to get pregnant to try and see if it will be a boy. He was very happy when I got pregnant and the scan showed it was a boy.

Even with the desire to balance the genders among their children, women who reported experiencing stressful pregnancies or difficult deliveries wanted to wait before having more children, regardless of what their male partners wanted, as one participant stated:

> My husband still wants us to have more children, because we are looking for a baby girl since I have four boys. Even though I want to born [give birth], I will stay like 4 years because of this problem of HIV. When I was pregnant the last time, the stress was too much on my body. This thing is not easy and it is not encouraging me to have another baby now. If at all I will ever try, not now.

Partnership and Faith: "My Husband Joined Me in Prayers and Faith"

Participants referred to the spiritual support male partners provided WLHA when they shared similar values of their faith. Most of the women interviewed stated that their husbands felt very happy about their most recent pregnancy, especially when it was planned and expected. Couples who were pregnant with their first children, however, were afraid of infecting their unborn children with HIV. To conquer this fear of pediatric HIV, many women relied on prayer while accessing PMTCT services at the hospital:

I won't do anything different the next time I get pregnant, because my first child is okay. So I will still follow the same thing—come to the hospital and follow what they tell me to do. My husband was very happy, because the time I was pregnant, two of us used to pray for our baby to be negative and God answered us.

Husbands supported their wives in their faith through the naming of their children. The meaning of their children's names also reflected the circumstances surrounding their birth, as one participant explained:

When I was pregnant, my husband and I held hands and did a prayer of agreement with faith for 10 minutes that we want this baby to be a boy since God has blessed us with a girl. We believed, even before we did scan that the baby I am carrying is a boy. That is why we chose the name *Kamsiyochukwu* that means Samuel from the Bible. I asked from the Lord and He gave him to me.

Further supporting this point, another participant stated the following:

With my prayer and Christianity it helped me a lot and everything with my pregnancy went normally. That's why we named her *Amarachukwu*. It means the miracle of God, the grace of God. Before we were able to get pregnant, it was by God's grace; that I was able to carry this pregnancy, God made it to be so. Delivery was even the same thing. It was by God's grace that I did everything and so that was why we gave my baby Amarachukwu.... My husband joined me in prayers. I had to have faith. My life is in God's hand.

Tangible Support: "Somebody Doing 5% Before, Now He Does 10% More"

Tangible support refers to the physical support provided by male partners. For WLHA, this tangible support may take the form of assistance with household chores, financial assistance, medication reminders, and being accompanied to their doctor's appointments. One participant described tangible support as, "somebody doing 5% before, now he does 10% more for me not to think." The participants also stated that tangible support is particularly strong during pregnancy and immediately after childbirth.

Many women expressed that their partners were very supportive by helping with household chores such as cooking, cleaning, fetching water; providing transportation money for hospital appointments; reminding them to take their medications at certain times; using condoms even when they prefer sex "flesh-to-flesh"; and purchasing vitamins, fruits, and vegetables. These women further expressed the importance of having this tangible form of partner support especially when pregnant, because "there are some jobs [household chores] a pregnant woman cannot do."

Husbands also showed support for their wives by fully supporting their delivery and infant feeding decisions. Whether it had to do with delivery location or mode of delivery, breastfeeding or formula feeding, all women stated that their husbands were supportive of whatever decisions they made. One participant explained about her mode of delivery:

> My husband was having faith that I will be able to deliver normally, but he had given me part payment for the cesarean section of 50,000 Naira (U.S.350), just in case, which I had deposited at Ifako. During antenatal care... they just saw that I had given birth before with CS, so they advised that once I have been cut, I should forget about delivery pack [for normal delivery]. It's my husband that was even cleaning and dressing the stitches for me.

When deciding where to deliver her baby, one participant explained:

> I told my husband that I want to deliver at the redemption camp and he agreed. Even if I was living far from the camp, I will still prefer to deliver at camp, because I waited for 6 years before I conceived and there are some spiritual challenges I passed through, so I believe it is only through prayer I was able to deliver safely.

Another participant stated how her husband supported her on making the best decision for their family on infant feeding:

> When I told him that I wanted to breastfeed since they said it is [a] 50/50 [chance of infection], he said no, that he doesn't want anything bad to happen so he is going to provide the formula and that I should not worry. Sometimes if I feel bad about it [not breastfeeding] he will say that I should not worry. Even when the [extended] family was pressurizing me that I should breastfeed, he was angry with them and they were quarreling. With my first child, the battle was too much about breastfeeding and my husband really backed me up.

Only the partner of a single mother was described as being unsupportive:

> He did not support me at all when I was pregnant. I would call his phone and it would be switched off or even when it is not, he will not pick his calls. . . . After I gave birth to the baby in February, he called to ask how the baby and I were doing. He came that weekend to see the baby. Since then, I have not set my eyes on him. The day she saw him she was so happy and that was the very first time I saw my baby laugh. Last week I tried to call him to tell him that the baby is sick and running temperature. I called his number throughout that day he didn't pick up. After that I

turned off my phone. I cannot kill myself. I will just keep on managing to take care of this child.

DISCUSSION AND CONCLUSION

Our aim was to illustrate the ways in which the different forms of male partner support influenced the CB decisions of WLHA who attended an outpatient clinic at a teaching hospital in Lagos, Nigeria. We identified three key types of male partner support in the context of CB decisions of WLHA: emotional support and reassurance, partnership and faith, and tangible support. These findings expand on previous work by highlighting the complex nature of CB decisions and contributing factors, which are deeply rooted in personal beliefs and support from significant others, especially male partners (Kanniappan, Jeyapaul, & Kalyanwala, 2008; Matthews et al., 2011; Ujiji et al., 2010). This is important, because CB is deemed a necessary part of a successful marriage in traditional African society, and also because the success of HIV prevention and treatment programs geared toward women and children depends on the support they receive from male partners and significant others (Beyeza-Kashesya et al., 2009; MacCarthy et al., 2012; Ramirez-Ferrero & Lusti-Narasimhan, 2012).

Historically, most sexual and reproductive health programs have been linked to women's health and have largely excluded men (Ramirez-Ferrero & Lusti-Narasimhan, 2012). This has proved to be detrimental to the sexual health of both men and women, especially when it comes to efforts aimed at HIV prevention and treatment. Our findings suggest that the CB decisions of WLHA were not always influenced by their partners' desires for children; the desire to balance the gender distribution among their children was a greater determining factor in WLHA CB decisions. For example, for some participants who already had a female child, the desire to have a male child or vice versa usually served as the driving force behind their CB decisions.

CB decisions usually involve women and their partners, and they include decisions related to getting pregnant, remaining pregnant, supporting the pregnancy (such as ANC attendance, healthy diet, emotional support), delivery options, and postpartum behaviors (e.g., infant feeding, family planning). Furthermore, decision-making is a process that may change over time based on several factors (Beyeza-Kashesya et al., 2009). One factor that played a role in the participants' CB decision-making was their prior CB experiences. Although WLHA and their male partners may decide to have a certain number of children, that number may change based on their CB experiences. Women who reported experiencing stressful pregnancies or difficult deliveries wanted to wait longer before having more children or they no longer wanted to have more children, regardless of what their male partners wanted. This finding is similar to findings from other studies report-ing that WLHA feared getting pregnant and worsening their health (Chen et al., 2001; Cooper et al., 2007; Nduna & Farlane, 2009). None of the partici-pants interviewed expressed fear of being abandoned by their partners or of experiencing intimate partner violence based on disclosure of HIV-positive status or CB decisions. This is contrary to findings reported in previous lit-erature on the nonsupportive role of partners of WLHA (Iwuagwu, 2009; Nduna & Farlane, 2009; Smith & Mbakwem, 2007, 2010). Although the defi-nition and degree of partner support varied, most participants reported that their husbands and partners were supportive, except for the only unmarried mother.

Support in the form of males treating their female HIV-positive partners in a nonstigmatizing way, while at the same time denying their HIV-positive status, is an unexpected yet important finding. While this form of support may have some protective effects on the emotional and psychological state of WLHA, it has potentially negative consequences since such partners tend to neglect necessary protective measures to prevent disease transmission. The finding was unexpected because it deviates from what has been reported in previous studies about male partners being unsupportive and stigmatizing their female partners living with HIV. Also, as public health professionals we would only consider this denial of HIV status as leading to potentially risky sexual behavior, but the WLHA in this study considered it to be a manifestation of their partner's support.

Extended family members such as in-laws also are involved in the CB decision-making process. This can create an additional source of stress on WLHA, especially when their male partners are not supportive of their CB decisions. Some of the participants reported that their husband's support influenced relationships with extended family, especially in-laws, to cre-ate an environment conducive to certain practices such as formula feed-ing, alternative delivery options such as cesarean section, contraceptive use, HIV treatment (e.g., PMTCT, ARV use), and keeping clinic appointments (Ramirez-Ferrero & Lusti-Narasimhan, 2012). Smith and Mbakwem (2007, 2010) noted that male partners and husbands supported their wives so much that they became coconspirators in hiding their wives' HIV status from family members.

This study has some limitations that may affect its generalizability to the population of all WLHA in Lagos and in Nigeria. We interviewed WLHA to as-sess their perceptions of male partner support in CB decision-making. Since we do not have data from their partners to back this up, their responses may not truly reflect the male partners' views. In addition, social desirability bias may have played a role in how participants portrayed their partner's sup-port to the researchers. Future research should include participants' spouses or male partners. The findings from this study are biased toward WLHA who had access to health care at the particular teaching hospital where the participants were recruited. Given that this hospital is considered one of the best in Lagos state when it comes to care of PLWHA, it may not be representative of other outpatient clinics providing PMTCT, HIV treatment, and care services. Last, due to logistical issues, limited resources, and time constraints, we were not able to further explore the case of the one unmarried mother who reported that her partner was being unsupportive. Therefore, we cannot say if her marital status played a role in the lack of support or if other factors were responsible. This is an area for exploration in the future.

Despite the limitations, this study has several strengths. The teaching hospital where we conducted the study provides high-quality care to PLWHA at a highly subsidized rate, which enables WLHA from diverse backgrounds to access care. This allowed for the recruitment of WLHA with diverse views on the topic to be interviewed. Second, the follow up postpartum with six of the participants enhanced credibility since they revealed more to the researchers over time as trust was established.

Notwithstanding the limitations, the results of this study have implications for HIV treatment and care programs geared toward improving the health of men, women, and children. If the UNAIDS vision of getting to zero (i.e., zero new infections, zero AIDS-related deaths, and zero discrimination) is to become a reality by 2015, we cannot exclude men from the conversation. Policies must be created that include men in sexual and reproductive health and maternal and child health discussions.

ACKNOWLEDGMENTS

The authors thank the participants who contributed to this study and the staff of the hematology clinic, especially Chief Nursing Officer Sabiyi, Adedoyin Dosunmu, and all the resident physicians for their support. In addition, the authors would like to thank Diane Cooper and colleagues at the Women's Health Research Unit, University of Cape Town, for granting the authors permission to adapt their interview guide for this study.

FUNDING

This study was funded by the Penn State Africana Research Center and the Hintz Graduate Education Enhancement Fellowship awards.

REFERENCES

Airhihenbuwa, C. O. (1995). *Health and culture beyond the Western paradigm.* Thousand Oaks, CA: Sage.

Airhihenbuwa, C. O. (2007). *Healing our differences: The crisis of global health and the politics of identity.* Lanham, MD: Rowman & Littlefield.

Airhihenbuwa, C. O., & Webster, J. D. W. (2004). Culture and African contexts of HIV/AIDS prevention, care and support. *SAHARA-J: Journal of Social Aspects of HIV/AIDS*, *1*(1), 4–13.

Attride-Stirling, J. (2001). Thematic networks: An analytic tool for qualitative research. *Qualitative Research*, *1*(3), 385–405.

Awiti Ujiji, O., Ekström, A. M., Ilako, F., Indalo, D., & Rubenson, B. (2010). "I will not let my HIV status stand in the way." Decisions on motherhood among women on ART in a slum in Kenya—A qualitative study. *BioMed Central Women's Health*, *10*(1), 1–10.

Beyeza-Kashesya, J., Ekstrom, A. M., Kaharuza, F., Mirembe, F., Neema, S., & Kulane, A. (2010). My partner wants a child: A cross-sectional study of the determinants of the desire for children among mutually disclosed sero-discordant couples receiving care in Uganda. *BioMed Central Public Health*, *10*(1), 247–257.

Beyeza-Kashesya, J., Kaharuza, F., Mirembe, F., Neema, S., Ekstrom, A. M., & Kulane, A. S. (2009). The dilemma of safe sex and having children: Challenges facing HIV sero-discordant couples in Uganda. *African Health Sciences*, *9*(1), 2–12.

Chen, J. L., Phillips, K. A., Kanouse, D. E., Collins, R. L., & Miu, A. (2001). Fertility desires and intentions of HIV-positive men and women. *Family Planning Perspectives*, *33*(4), 144–165.

Conkling, M., Shutes, E. L., Karita, E., Chomba, E., Tichacek, A., Sinkala, M., . . . Allen, S. A. (2010). Couples' voluntary counselling and testing and nevirapine use in antenatal clinics in two African capitals: A prospective cohort study. *Journal of the International AIDS Society*, *13*(1), 1–10.

Cooper, D., Harries, J., Myer, L., Orner, P., Bracken, H., & Zweigenthal, V. (2007). "Life is still going on": Reproductive intentions among HIV-positive women and men in South Africa. *Social Science & Medicine*, *65*(2), 274–283.

Crankshaw, T. L., Matthews, L. T., Giddy, J., Kaida, A., Ware, N. C., Smit, J. A., & Bangsberg, D. R. (2012). A conceptual framework for understanding HIV risk behavior in the context of supporting fertility goals among HIV-serodiscordant couples. *Reproductive Health Matters*, *20*(39), 50–60.

Cresswell, J. W. (1998). *Qualitative inquiry and research design. Choosing among five traditions*. Thousand Oaks, CA: Sage.

Farquhar, C., Kiarie, J. N., Richardson, B. A., Kabura, M. N., John, F. N., Nduati, R. W., . . . John-Stewart, G. C. (2004). Antenatal couple counseling increases uptake of interventions to prevent HIV-1 transmission. *Journal of Acquired Immune Deficiency Syndromes (1999)*, *37*(5), 1620–1626.

Iwuagwu, S. C. (2009). *Sexual and reproductive decisions and experiences of women living with HIV/AIDS in Abuja, Nigeria* (Doctoral dissertation). Retrieved from http://opensiuc.lib.siu.edu/cgi/viewcontent.cgi?article=1001&context=dissertat ions

Kanniappan, S., Jeyapaul, M. J., & Kalyanwala, S. (2008). Desire for motherhood: Exploring HIV-positive women's desires, intentions and decision-making in attaining motherhood. *AIDS Care*, *20*(6), 625–630.

MacCarthy, S., Rasanathan, J. J. K., Ferguson, L., & Gruskin, S. (2012). The pregnancy decisions of HIV-positive women: The state of knowledge and way forward. *Reproductive Health Matters*, *20*(39), 119–140.

Matthews, L. T., Crankshaw, T., Giddy, J., Kaida, A., Smit, J. A., Ware, N. C., & Bangsberg, D. R. (2011). Reproductive decision-making and periconception practices among HIV-positive men and women attending HIV services in Durban, South Africa. *AIDS and Behavior, 17*(2), 461–470.

National Bureau of Statistics (NBS). (2006). *Federal Republic of Nigeria population census.* Retrieved from http://www.nigerianstat.gov.ng/nbsapps/ Connections/Pop2006.pdf

National Population Commission (NPC). (2006). *Population and housing census of the Federal Republic of Nigeria.* Retrieved from http://www. population.gov.ng/images/Priority%20Tables% 20Volume%20I-update.pdf

Nduna, M., & Farlane, L. (2009). Women living with HIV in South Africa and their concerns about fertility. *AIDS and Behavior, 13*(1), 62–65.

Oladapo, O., Daniel, O., Odusoga, O., & Sotubo, O. (2005). Fertility desires and intentions of HIV-positive patients at a suburban specialist center. *Journal of the National Medical Association, 97*(12), 1672–1680.

Ramirez-Ferrero, E., & Lusti-Narasimhan, M. (2012). The role of men as partners and fathers in the prevention of mother-to-child transmission of HIV and in the promotion of sexual and reproductive health. *Reproductive Health Matters, 20*(39), 103–109.

Rujumba, J., Neema, S., Byamugisha, R., Tylleskär, T., Tumwine, J. K., & Heggenhougen, H. K. (2012). "Telling my husband I have HIV is too heavy to come out of my mouth": Pregnant women's disclosure experiences and support needs following antenatal HIV testing in eastern Uganda. *Journal of the International AIDS Society, 15*(2), 1–10.

Smith, D. J., & Mbakwem, B. C. (2007). Life projects and therapeutic itineraries: Marriage, fertility, and antiretroviral therapy in Nigeria. *AIDS, 21*, S37–S41.

Smith, D. J., & Mbakwem, B. C. (2010). Antiretroviral therapy and reproductive life projects: Mitigating the stigma of AIDS in Nigeria. *Social Science & Medicine, 71*(2), 345–352.

Sofolahan, Y. A., & Airhihenbuwa, C. O. (2012). Childbearing decision-making: A qualitative study of women living with HIV/AIDS in Southwest Nigeria. *AIDS Research and Treatment.* doi:10.1155/2012/478065

World Health Organization (WHO). (2012). *Guidance on couples HIV testing and counselling including antiretroviral therapy for treatment and prevention in serodiscordant couples: Recommendations for a public health approach.* Retrieved from http://www.who.int/hiv/pub/guidelines/97892415 01972/en/index.html

"Our Hands Are Tied Up": Current State of Safer Conception Services Suggests the Need for an Integrated Care Model

KATHY GOGGIN

Health Services and Outcomes Research, Children's Mercy Hospitals and Clinics; and Schools of Medicine and Pharmacy, University of Missouri-Kansas City, Kansas City, Missouri, USA

DEBORAH MINDRY

Center for Culture and Health, University of California, Los Angeles, Los Angeles, California, USA

JOLLY BEYEZA-KASHESYA

Department of Obstetrics and Gynaecology, Mulago Hospital, Makerere University College of Health Sciences, Kampala, Uganda

SARAH FINOCCHARIO-KESSLER

Department of Family Medicine, University of Kansas Medical Center, Kansas City, Kansas, USA

RHODA WANYENZE

Department of Disease Control and Environmental Health, Makerere University School of Public Health, Kampala, Uganda

CHRISTINE NABIRYO

The AIDS Support Organization, Kampala, Uganda

GLENN WAGNER

RAND Corporation, Santa Monica, California, USA

We conducted in-depth interviews with a variety of health care providers (n = 33) in Uganda to identify current services that could support and act as barriers to the provision of safer conception counseling (SCC). Consistent with their training and expertise, providers of all types reported provision of services for people living with a diagnosis of HIV or AIDS who desire a child. Important barriers, including a lack of service integration, poor communication between stakeholders, and the absence of policy guidelines, were identified. Drawing on these data, we propose a model of integrated care that includes both SCC services and prevention of unplanned pregnancies.

Researchers have identified the lack of safer conception counseling (SCC) as a glaring gap in the current state of services for people living with HIV/AIDS (PLHIV) across Africa. The lack of accessible supportive services negatively impacts HIV-infected women's ability to make informed reproductive health decisions and reduces the likelihood that HIV-infected men will employ risk reduction methods with their uninfected female partners. It also leads to delays and thereby reduces the efficacy of preventing mother-to-child transmission of HIV. In this article, we provide data on what services Ugandan providers are currently offering and what barriers they encounter for the provision of SCC. We present data on the complicated dynamics of providing these services as well as the drivers of regular provision and uptake of safer conception methods. Our findings have the potential to inform both service- and policy-level efforts to bring these services to the people who need them. Drawing on our rich data from a variety of providers, we offer a new model of integrated care that addresses the most critical barriers for PLHIV and providers of all types. We believe that our findings will be of use to a wide variety of professionals who are engaged in improving service provision and international health policy.

The availability of antiretroviral therapy (ART) has significantly improved the health and lives of PLHIV and led to an increase in desires to bear children (Nattabi, Li, Thompson, Orach, & Earnest, 2009; Finocchario-Kessler et al., 2012). Recently, researchers in sub-Saharan Africa have found that 28%–73% of PLHIV express a desire to have a child (Heys, Kipp, Jhangri, Alibhai, & Rubaale, 2009; Snow, Mutumba, Resnicow, & Mugyenyi, 2013; Wanyenze et al., 2011). Fertility desires are greatest among young PLHIV (15–24 years; Beyeza-Kashesya et al., 2011), likely reflecting cultural norms to have a family and the likelihood that they had not yet begun or completed their family when they acquired HIV. Data from Ugandan studies corroborate these findings and indicate growth in the number of Ugandan PLHIV who desire to have children from a low of 7% in early 2003 (Homsy et al., 2009) to 30%–59% in 2009 (Beyeza-Kashesya et al., 2010; Kakaire, Osinde, & Kaye, 2010). PLHIV are acting on these desires, with 30% of discordant couples reporting that they have had a child after they knew of their discordant status (Beyeza-Kashesya et al., 2010) and one-third of women who initiated ART becoming pregnant during a 4-year follow-up period (Myer et al., 2010). Given that 90% of newly infected Ugandans are of reproductive age (Wabwire-Mangen, Odiit, Kirungi, Kaweesa Kisitu, & Okara Wanyama, 2009), these trends are likely to continue. Left unassisted, the quest of PLHIV for childbearing has the potential to increase the rate of HIV transmission not only to unborn children, but also to uninfected partners. As such, effective safer conception services for those who wish to conceive are urgently needed.

Innovations in the prevention of vertical or mother-to-child-transmission (MTCT) have reduced rates of MTCT from a high of 30% with no intervention to around 1%–2% if timely antiretroviral prophylaxis and replacement feeding are provided (UNAIDS, 2009). Similarly, horizontal transmission to uninfected partners can be significantly reduced through the use of established safer conception methods (SCMs; Matthews & Mukherjee, 2009). Methods include timed unprotected intercourse during the female's fertile period, manual insemination if the male partner is negative, and assisted reproductive technology such as sperm washing for HIV-infected male clients, although this latter option is not accessible or affordable in most low-resource settings (Matthews, Smit, Cu-Uvin, & Cohan, 2012). There are also several methods that are not specific to the context of conception but that greatly reduce sexual transmission risk. ART (and a resultant undetectable viral load more specifically) has been shown to reduce infections in serodiscordant couples by 96% (Cohen et al., 2011), diagnosis and treatment of STIs greatly reduces risk (Gray et al., 2001), and medical male circumcision decreases the risk of transmission among men by 51% (Gray et al., 2007). In addition, preexposure antiretroviral prophylaxis (PrEP) for the uninfected partner may reduce risk during conception attempts (Thigpen et al., 2012; Vernazza et al., 2011), but its efficacy in this context has not been established, nor is it widely available in Uganda or other sub-Saharan countries at the present time. Unfortunately, persistent barriers prevent most couples from receiving SCC where they could learn about and receive assistance to employ these prevention strategies.

Researchers (Finocchario-Kessler et al., in press; Schwartz et al., 2012; Wagner, Linnemayr, Kityo, & Mugyenyi, 2012) have noted numerous client- and provider-level barriers for the regular provision of SCC. Client barriers include the following: cultural norms impacting the acceptability of SCC methods, clients' low health literacy, and lack of male partner involvement. Provider barriers to the provision of SCC include their longstanding focus on prevention of pregnancy, which makes providers uncomfortable with suggesting any form of unprotected sex to clients and results in negative attitudes toward PLHIV having children (Beyeza-Kashesya et al., 2010). Another important barrier for both clients and providers is HIV stigma, which interacts with preexisting stigma associated with sexuality, gender, race, and poverty, and has a negative impact on care (Banteyerga et al., 2005; Feyissa, LakewAbebe, Girma, & Woldie, 2012). In fact, the judgmental attitudes of some providers about their clients' fertility desires was a contributing factor to the widespread stigmatization of childbearing among PLHIV (Agadjanian & Hayford, 2009; Cooper et al., 2009; Myer, Morroni, & Cooper, 2006; Steiner, Finocchario-Kessler, & Dariotis, 2013; Wagner et al., 2012). Ironically, instead of reducing births among PLHIV, this stigmatization has paradoxically been associated with increasing the likelihood that HIV-infected women will continue to have children (Aka-Dago-Akribi, Du Loû, Msellati, Dossou, & Welffens-Ekra, 1999; Cooper, Harries, Myer, Orner, & Bracken, 2007; Craft, Delaney, Bautista, & Serovich, 2007). While provider attitudes have begun to change in light of improved client health outcomes and the recognition that significant proportions of PLHIV continue to have children and have a right to make their own fertility decisions (e.g., Barroso & Sippel, 2011; Baryamutuma & Baingana, 2011; World Health Organization [WHO], United Nations Population Fund [UNFPA], International Planned Parenthood Federation [IPPF], UNAIDS), residual concerns persist and manifest themselves in mixed messages that undermine any support that providers may offer clients. Just as these attitudes inhibit providers' behavior, clients have also internalized this stigma (Cooper et al., 2009; Nduna & Farlane, 2009; Wagner & Wanyenze, 2013), increasing their reluctance to communicate with providers about their childbearing desires. These delays prevent the opportunity to benefit from SCC and hamper early initiation of prevention of mother-to-child transmission (PMTCT).

These client-and-provider-level barriers are important considerations for the development of effective interventions; however, to date few inquiries have examined the issue from a systems-level perspective. As such, we know little about what is currently being done that could support or hamper efforts to make SCC available to those who could benefit from it. To address this gap, we draw on the perspective of HIV, family planning (FP), and traditional health (TH) providers to examine the following: (a) what services are currently being offered by different provider types that could support SCC and (b) what individual- and system-level barriers will need to be addressed. Drawing on these data, we propose a model of integrated care that includes both prevention of unplanned pregnancies and SCC services for those who desire pregnancy.

METHODS

Study Setting

This study was conducted in collaboration with The AIDS Support Organization (TASO) sites in Kampala and Jinja, Uganda, between July and September of 2012. Founded in 1987, TASO is now one of the largest indigenous nongovernmental organizations in Uganda providing comprehensive HIV prevention, care, and support services for over 100,000 HIV infected and affected Ugandans annually.

The Kampala TASO site is located next to the Mulago National Referral Hospital Complex and is the main and oldest branch, which serves over 6,700 active HIV-infected patients. The Jinja TASO site is located 45 miles east of Kampala within the Jinja Regional Referral Hospital and provides HIV primary care to over 8000 clients. In addition to ART and counseling services, TASO provides FP and contraception services.

Sample

We conducted in-depth, semistructured individual interviews with HIV care providers (i.e., medical/clinical officers, nurses, counselors, and expert clients), FP counselors, and TH providers, to explore the following: (a) what services they are currently providing related to safer conception among HIV-infected clients, (b) what additional trainings they desire related to safer conception, and (c) barriers they perceive for the regular provision of support for safer childbearing among HIV clients. We sought to interview a varied group of providers from the participating HIV and FP clinics and within the community. Providers were identified from the hospital settings in which the HIV clinics are housed, and the TH providers were identified from the communities surrounding the clinics. Providers were approached by a member of the study team and asked if they would be willing to share their thoughts and experiences with treating HIV-infected clients who are interested in having a child. Interviews averaged 30–45 minutes and, consistent with local norms, all providers were offered 20,000 Ush (U.S. $8) for participating. All providers gave verbal informed consent, at which time we stressed that their responses were not linked to payment and would not be shared with their employer. The study protocol was reviewed and approved by the appropriate Institutional Review Boards at each participating site.

Instrument

We used semistructured interviews to elicit themes as well as to determine how common or salient these themes were among an array of respondents. An interview guide was developed for providers that included mostly open-ended questions, but also semistructured follow-up questions and probes. After eliciting basic demographic and background-related information, the interview covered several areas related to the childbearing needs of HIV-infected clients and the support services available to meet these needs; however, our analysis here focused specifically on the portion of the interviews related to what providers were currently doing related to SCM, what additional training they desired, and what barriers they saw for provision of these services going forward.

Study interviewers had a master's degree in social sciences, experience conducting qualitative interviews, received specific training for this study, and were native Luganda speakers. Providers were asked to choose which language (Luganda or English) they preferred for the interview. Luganda interviews were conducted by the study interviewers, and English interviews were conducted by the senior investigators of the study.

Analysis

Interviews were digitally recorded, translated into English (when conducted in Luganda), and transcribed verbatim. Data were entered in Atlas.ti. The initial coding scheme was developed by three team members using a grounded theory approach, which informed the development of a thematically organized codebook. Thereafter, coding was conducted by two team members with review by the third team member, an anthropologist with extensive experience in qualitative data coding. Where there was disagreement, a secondary review achieved consensus, and changes to the coding were made accordingly (Bernard & Ryan, 2010). Topical codes were used to index provider interviews in order to compare their perspectives and experiences. Results were aggregated to identify common themes, patterns, and key factors related to provider experiences addressing client fertility needs and knowledge and use of SCM. Key themes for this analysis included: client–provider interactions, provider attitudes, provider concerns, SCM, current services provided, and structural challenges.

RESULTS

Sample Description

The sample included 33 providers (17 from Kampala and 16 from Jinja), including 18 HIV (four medical/clinical officers, three nurses, seven counselors, four expert clients), 10 FP (seven midwives, one nurse, and two doctors), and five TH (three herbalists, two traditional birth attendants) providers. Nine of the providers were male, and all but five had been providing client care for at least 4 years.

What Services Do Providers Currently Offer for HIV Clients Who Want a Child?

When asked to describe their consultations with HIV-infected clients who want to have a child, all providers reported focusing on the clients' health first, stressing the importance of ensuring optimal health and getting CD4 cell counts (a key measure of immune functioning) above 400 before attempting pregnancy. All providers, including TH providers, encouraged clients who want to conceive to engage in health behaviors such as adherence to allopathic treatment, regular blood work, antenatal care, PMTCT, good nutrition and clean water, planning for delivering in a qualified health facility, and consistent use of condoms until ready to conceive. While there was considerable overlap in what different providers encouraged clients to do, they offered unique services consistent with their training and expertise (see Table 1). For example, providing screening and treatment for sexual

TABLE 1 Unique Services Currently Offered to Clients Who Want to Have a Child

HIV care provider	Family planning provider	Traditional provider (herbalist or birth attendant)
HIV primary care	Diagnosis/treat STIs	Infertility counseling
Blood work	Fertility counseling	Herbs for:
ART	*Safer conception counseling*	Infertility
Diagnosis/treat STIs	Educate about PMTCT	Symptoms/side effects
PMTCT	Postnatal care	Increase in CD4s
Antenatal care		Healthy pregnancy

Note: Services in italics were mentioned but not routinely offered. ART = antiretroviral therapy. PMTCT = prevention of mother-to child transmission.

transmitted infections (STIs) were routinely reported by qualified HIV and FP providers. One nurse related her experience:

> So for those ones [who want children] we always teach, educate them, when [is] the proper time to have a child. We advise them, we teach them, about their CD4 counts and viral load. Then if both, if the husband and the wife, are accessing care with us, we start treating them as a couple. Because we have to treat for any STI, anything, especially that by the time they conceive, everything is as normal as we want it. And we tell them once you conceive, we want you to use condoms throughout because we don't want our baby to get the virus. So most of them understand. (*Female, HIV nurse, rural*)

Some HIV and FP providers reported offering fertility counseling including teaching clients to use the SCM of timed unprotected intercourse. Three providers described assisting clients to use manual self-insemination. One FP provider reported that she had heard of another provider using PrEP with a serodiscordant couple:

> This, I didn't do it myself but G did it and it worked. There is a discordant couple where the lady is HIV negative and the man is positive, so when the lady was exposed she was given PrEP and then she conceived. She gave them some fertility drugs which the lady swallowed and she conceived while she took the PrEP for 1 month. She has a 7 month old baby boy now. We monitored her until she gave birth. (*Female, FP nurse, rural*)

Consistent with their belief system, TH providers offered counseling and herbs they felt would address infertility, HIV symptoms, and ART side effects, boost CD4 cell counts, and promote a healthy pregnancy, but nearly all reported urging clients to seek allopathic care as well:

When an HIV positive person comes here in need of treatment, I always counsel and encourage the person that whereas I am going to give my medicine, the immune booster, I ask you to first go for check-up from the biomedical doctors or in big hospitals like Mulago, Rubaga, Nsambya, Kibuli, Namirembe—those big hospitals or go to the counselor. I let them first take a blood test to confirm whether they are HIV positive or negative. After confirming that he/she is positive, I start counseling him/her to go and get drugs called ARVs from the biomedical hospitals because it does [not] cost anything there unlike our herbal medicine that we charge....I encourage them to go and get ARVs as well as more counseling from the experienced medical doctors so as to receive full treatment. (*Female, herbalist, urban*)

Challenges to Providing Safer Conception Services

Beyond challenges noted in prior research, providers highlighted important individual- and system-level barriers to the provision of SCC including a lack of service integration, poor communication between all stakeholders, and the absence of policy guidelines.

Lack of service integration. A major structural barrier that came up in varied ways for different HIV and FP providers were challenges associated with the lack of integration of reproductive health, including SCC, and HIV care. An FP provider noted the following:

We actually need to work under one roof. We really need to integrate all these together [safer conception, PMTCT, FP, ART care] because they are all very important. And sometimes you see a client comes to clinic and then has another appointment to come to family planning, and then has another appointment to go to another clinic. It's not nice. If we make everything in one day and then we provide all the services, even if they spend a longer time in the hospital but they will have gone home with all the services, the better. (*Female, FP nurse, rural*)

Providers also noted that a lack of time, adequate private space in FP clinics, administrative support, and a systematic way to know if clients follow through with referrals and get needed services were barriers to provision of SCC, as an HIV counselor at the rural site noted:

We are not providing a holistic maternal health package, because we are lacking the antenatal care and even when we refer, there are challenges of follow-up. Like, you may not know that a mother has gone and actually, even when we refer [for care], there is no feedback....Sometimes they don't reach the other service center where we sent them; they come back for 6-month regular [visit], but they have not started the [PMTCT] process. (*Male, HIV counselor, rural*)

Poor communication between all stakeholders: Providers and clients. Most providers indicated that infrequent discussion with clients about childbearing prior to pregnancy was the norm. Some providers noted this is in part due to a generalized reluctance in the culture to discuss matters regarding sex. As one HIV provider put it, "Eeh, sex here is still taboo" (female, HIV counselor, urban). When such communication occurred, two-thirds of providers indicated that it was the client who usually initiated discussions about their childbearing desires, whereas only a third of providers reported they routinely initiated these discussions. Most providers reported female clients were more likely to raise the subject of childbearing with providers than were male clients, and these discussions most often occurred after a client was already pregnant. Most of these clients told providers they became pregnant "by mistake" and most had not previously discussed childbearing desires with their provider or partners:

> Some they just find themselves pregnant. So once we detect that someone is pregnant, then we enroll them into our PMTCT services. But others, they inquire first. But those are the minorities. Majority are like they just find themselves pregnant. (*Female, HIV nurse, urban*)

Half of the sample reported that clients now felt "free" to discuss childbearing with their providers, speculating this was because some providers who used to tell clients not to have children are now saying it is okay if they are in good health. Nevertheless, the other half of the sample believed clients were still apprehensive to inquire about planning a pregnancy because some providers told them they already had enough children, communicated their disapproval by speaking harshly, or simply anticipated a negative response from their provider who was always urging condom use and pregnancy prevention:

> There is a group that is well informed that having children is okay. What you need to do as a medical worker is to see this lady is healthy and you support her. But there is a group that is lagging behind due to lack of evidence-based information and they discriminate against these women and still see it as so bad. And this is a group that forces women out of the clinics. They get pregnant and stay out without coming for care, and even for PMTCT. (*Female, FP doctor, urban*)

Providers frequently referred to clients' reproductive rights to make their own childbearing decisions and described their role as providing the necessary information for their clients to make informed decisions:

> According to what I see, the availability of PMTCT programs coupled with if the woman and her husband are ready and prepared to care for

the child, they have a right to have a child. (*Female, HIV expert client, rural*)

Nevertheless, many providers' descriptions of what they thought about HIV-infected clients having children and what they say to clients revealed considerable ambivalence about supporting clients' desires to have children. Citing the cultural importance of having children, many providers expressed support for clients without children to have at least one child. However, providers' description of what they usually say to clients revealed that two-thirds generally discouraged clients from having children, and most were less likely to support clients' desires to have children when clients already had "enough" children:

> If they already have children, I advise them not to have more children. If they have no children, I advise them to have a child. (*Female, traditional herbalist, urban*)

Many providers revealed attitudes that highlighted the real conflict they find themselves in between supporting HIV-infected clients' desires to have children and the risk of new HIV transmissions that it presents. Not surprisingly, many of these providers would prefer that clients not have children:

> Actually, you tell them about the risk for transmitting HIV, which is first and foremost, because you, like, may never know; maybe this one time you're going to try to have the child is when you're going to contract the virus. And you may not stop them because if they really are determined to have the child, they will go ahead anyway.... So you give them the information; then the decision is entirely theirs and really when it's at the end of the day if they have a safe—if HIV is not transmitted at that time, then that is very good. If the HIV is transmitted at that very moment when they are trying to get their baby, you will not be the one to blame. They will have themselves. They take responsibility; it's not like we did not tell them, like—we were told about it, so we went into it knowing the consequences, so like that, because you cannot make these clients feel they have the right to have their child as they need. (*Female, HIV counselor, rural*)

Allopathic providers and traditional health providers. TH providers reported treating clients who cannot afford or do not want to attend allopathic clinics and those who have had or fear negative reactions from allopathic providers (e.g., those who have been raped, are single parents, or are HIV-infected and pregnant). Given their reach to clients who do not always access allopathic care, TH providers felt that integrating allopathic services with traditional services would be useful to facilitate better communication and improved client care:

This [interaction between providers] prevents being suspicious of each other and wishing bad for each other.... It helps in mutual communication and consultations because now the medical doctor can't come to consult me and when I go to consult him he doesn't want to tell me. (*Female, traditional birth attendant, urban*)

Lack of policy guidelines addressing safer conception counseling.   Several HIV and FP providers explained that the lack of a clear policy from the Ministry of Health encouraging the provision of safer conception services and clarifying ART treatment guidelines for clients who want to conceive was another significant barrier:

The only way it can be really modified, it is maybe by the Ministry [of Health] to come up with a policy in relation to HIV specifically. That's when the service providers will have [their] blessing to make sure they get the information to break the cultural barriers. But otherwise, without a policy . . . our hands are tied up. (*Male, HP doctor, urban*)

DISCUSSION

Consistent with their training and expertise, providers of all types reported provision of some form of services for PLHIV who desire a child. Given providers' unique skills and varied cultural prominence, this study provides important data to inform the development of an effective model of safer conception service provision that integrates all providers and addresses multiple barriers to care. This focus on provider- and system-level opportunities and barriers responds to calls to advance implementation science for HIV and safer preconception counseling (Steiner, Dariotis, Anderson, & Finocchario-Kessler, 2013).

We present our findings to offer further evidence that most providers have shifted away from strong prohibition of childbearing among PLHIV (Agadjanian & Hayford, 2009; Cooper et al., 2009; Nduna & Farlane, 2009) to accepting the validity of PLHIV desiring to bear children. Despite this shift, providers and their clients rarely communicate about childbearing desires prior to pregnancy. This is in part due to providers' residual concerns about transmission risks associated with childbearing and inadequate training that diminishes their self-efficacy. Contributing to providers' reluctance to explore their clients' fertility desires is a lack of basic knowledge (Finocchario-Kessler et al., in press) and confidence in their ability to impart useful information about SCM to their clients. Providers in our study uniformly reported the desire for more training in SCC skills for use with clients and their partners. Expert clients and TH providers also desired additional training covering basic HIV disease management and prevention information. Many HIV and FP providers also pointed out the need for clear policy guidance from the Ministry of Health. Widespread training tailored to providers' individual expertise, scope of practice, and client population would clearly increase the provision of quality SCC and likely enhance PMTCT and other important health practice as well. Equally as important as the provision of these types of basic educational trainings is the need to assist providers in exploring their own thoughts and biases about SCC.

Addressing Provider Ambivalence

Assisting providers to develop counseling skills that include holding their biases in check as they work with clients would reduce the associated stigma and encourage clients to be forthcoming about their fertility desires. Unfortunately, many of the providers we interviewed seemed unaware that their own negative beliefs about PLHIV having children were obvious in their descriptions of how they counseled clients. This lack of insight is likely a product of providers' SCC knowledge deficits, historic singular focus on preventing new infections, low perceived self-efficacy for their ability to effectively assist clients with SCC, coupled with feeling external pressure to support clients' fertility desires. Not surprisingly, many feel obligated to outwardly express support for their clients' desires to have a child while harboring personal reservations about their role in actually supporting their clients to have children. Educational trainings alone will not adequately address these issues. Provider trainings will need to go beyond simple education and employ strategies to assist providers in not only developing empathy but a full understanding of the perspectives of PLHIV who want to have children (Logie & Gadalla, 2009; Weiss, Ramakrishna, & Somma, 2006).

Grounding the provision of SCC in a harm reduction framework that encourages and supports the provider's role in ensuring PLHIV have children in a manner that reduces both horizontal and vertical transmission risk will likely enhance providers' ability to embrace a supportive stance. Helping providers to shift from feeling responsible for the potentially negative outcomes of SCC (i.e., horizontal transmission, vertical transmission, inability to care for the child long term) to focusing on their responsibility to arm their clients with the best information so clients can make an informed decision is the goal. Similar framing is routine for issues like breastfeeding in HIV care (WHO, 2013). Developing a cadre of providers with expertise in providing in-depth SCC and on-going support to which providers can refer interested clients will also likely enhance providers' buy-in. Ultimately, if providers develop the knowledge and requisite empathy, and embrace the role of experts assisting PLHIV to make an informed decision, better outcomes and reduced stigma will follow. On-going booster trainings for providers should include the sharing of successful SCC stories to further reduce stigma and reinforce the importance of providers' role in appropriate SCC. Careful selection of stories that highlight the couple's ability to overcome barriers that providers have cited (e.g., male partner involvement, couple's ability to practice safer sex outside of fertile window, successful use of manual insemination, etc.) will continue to reinforce the important role that providers can play in SCC.

Bridging HIV Prevention Efforts Among Providers

Significant differences in underlying belief systems about the nature of health and disease as well as health care provision have produced a longstanding cultural divide between allopathically trained and TH providers that also contributes to poor SCC provision. This divide manifests itself in poor communication between HIV/FP and TH providers and a lack of recognition by many allopathic providers of the role that TH providers already play in the health care system. Vastly outnumbering doctors and residing in the same communities as clients, TH providers are far more accessible for many. Accordingly, four of five Ugandans seek care from a TH provider each year (Aboo, 2011). TH providers also welcome clients who cannot afford or do not want to attend allopathic clinics because they have had or fear negative reactions from providers. Clients learn not to tell either type of provider that they are receiving services from the other, which can have devastating health effects (e.g., toxic interactions between some traditional herbal treatments and antiretrovirals; Mills et al., 2005). There is a need to view TH providers as being able to play a complementary role to allopathic care. Results of this study indicate that many TH providers encourage clients to seek allopathic care and provide services to HIV-infected clients who are trying to get pregnant. As such, TH providers should be included in a comprehensive model of SCC provision. TH providers desire and will need education and training, but they could play a vital role in encouraging their HIV-infected clients to access SCC prior to getting pregnant.

Integrated Model of HIV Safer Conception Counseling

Based on the findings of this study, existing literature, and international policy guidelines (Bekker et al., 2011), we propose an integrated model for SCC provision. Our hope is that this model will stimulate future research to evaluate its impact on clients and providers. As depicted in Figure 1, in this new model of integrated care all provider types make meaningful contributions consistent with their expertise and the types of clients they treat. Critical to the success of this model will be enhancing linkages between services provided to PLHIV and communication across provider categories as well

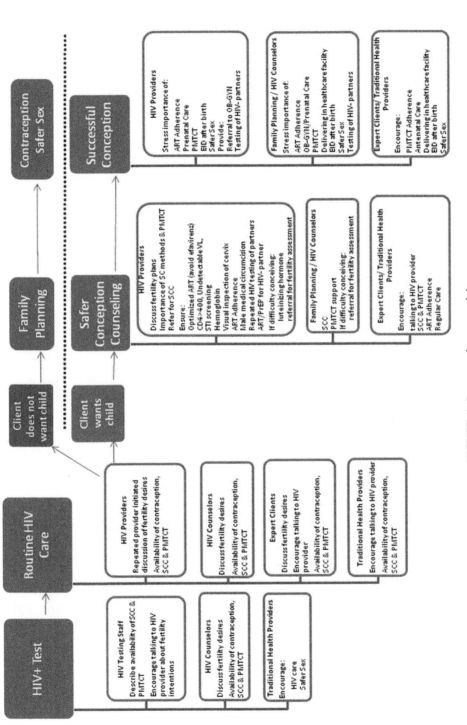

FIGURE 1 Integrated care model.

as communication between providers and clients. As such, we urge starting as early as possible by introducing the existence of FP and SCC services during HIV counseling and testing. While this is an extremely stressful time when clients have much to think about, informing clients that support exists to start/continue their family or ensure that conception is prevented may assist clients in accepting and proactively dealing with their new diagnosis. In most settings, newly diagnosed clients will be assigned an HIV counselor who can play an important role in normalizing clients' fertility desires and questions and reinforcing the existence of FP and SCC services. TH providers who treat newly diagnosed clients can play an important role by encouraging their clients to seek allopathic care and practice safer sex until they have talked with their providers about their fertility desires.

Once clients have initiated care, HIV providers should repeatedly initiate discussions about clients' fertility desires and stress the availability of FP services, SCM, and PMTCT. Starting this conversation early and having it repeatedly will significantly reduce stigma and encourage clients to openly discuss their fertility goals. In most settings, HIV counselors and expert clients will have significant contact with clients during routine care. As such, they can play a key role in normalizing fertility desires, reducing stigma, increasing awareness of SCM, and encouraging clients to share their fertility intentions with their providers. TH providers can do the same and should really stress the importance of talking to HIV providers when HIV-infected clients contact them for help with infertility. Encouraging and facilitating repeated conversations with a host of different providers will reduce stigma and allow clients to make their best decision. As the literature indicates, not talking about it leads to stigma that drives clients out of care, but it does not prevent pregnancies. These conversations will sometimes result in clients deciding that they do not wish to conceive, and providers should refer them to well-established FP services that can assist them in their goal. When clients decide that they do wish to conceive, providers need to work with clients to ensure that their health is sufficient to support their conception desires and stress the importance of SCM. They should refer to other providers who have the expertise and time to work with clients and their partners to provide high-quality SCC.

HIV counselors would be ideal for providing SCC because they already assist clients with difficult issues, have sufficient time to spend educating clients, have training in related and necessary matters like disclosure, and are most often colocated with HIV primary care providers so care can be integrated. FP providers are also ideal candidates for provision of SCC because they have considerable expertise in providing reproductive health counseling for HIV-infected clients including teaching women about their monthly cycles and how to identify their peek ovulation period. FP providers are also comfortable with discussing sex with clients and have educational tools to assist in client education. Engaging FP providers in SCC, however, would require a significant shift in orientation from their current singular goal of preventing pregnancies to adoption of a harm reduction model where clients are urged to limit risk as much as possible. Most importantly, FP providers are not often colocated in HIV clinic settings and would therefore require clients to travel to another setting to receive services. This would reduce the likelihood that SCC could be fully integrated into routine HIV care where it would have its largest positive impact. In the end, the determination of which provider will offer in-depth SCC should be determined by what will make it easiest for clients to access services.

TH providers could play a key role in reaching clients that might not otherwise engage allopathic care until they are already pregnant. They could also help to spread the word that there are safer conception options available and play an important role throughout care by encouraging their clients to: seek allopathic care, talk to their providers about their fertility desires, practice safer sex until they have a plan for conceiving that has been informed by SCC, and adhere to regular care, ART, PMTCT, and safer conception strategies.

Once clients conceive, HIV providers can facilitate and encourage clients to take care of their health (e.g., ART adherence, regular visits), their baby's health (e.g., prenatal care, PMTCT, early infant diagnosis), and their partners' health (e.g., revert to practicing safer sex all of the time, HIV testing for partners). Ensuring that clients are referred and make it to appropriate OB-GYN prenatal care is also critical. HIV counselors and FP providers can also reinforce the importance of maintaining everyone's health.

Limitations

This study it is not without its limitations, including a relatively small sample of providers, particularly with regard to the number and type of TH providers. Allopathic care providers were drawn from two different sites within the same nongovernmental organization, so their perspectives and service provision may be different from other providers. Further, as an organization, TASO has already embraced a progressive view of PLHIV fertility rights and inculcated that into their internal policies and service provision models. Nevertheless, providers in this study still evidenced ambivalence, misconceptions, low self-efficacy, and the desire for more training that would likely be echoed by non-TASO providers. Finally, while we have demonstrated the need for an integrative model for the provision of safer conception services, we have not yet tested the proposed model.

CONCLUSION

We provide novel data on the types of services offered by different types of providers in regards to PLHIV fertility desires and the system-level barriers to implementation of SCC. Progress has been made in shifting providers' perspective from a nearly uniformly negative appraisal of PLHIV having children to a more open and accepting stance. Nevertheless, providers of all types still harbor concerns that interfere with their ability to effectively counsel their clients. Additional training and behavioral intervention to addresses providers' lingering reservations will greatly enhance the provision of SCC. Insights gained in this study were used to propose a new integrated model of care that enlists all providers in the support for and provision of SCC. Future studies exploring the utility of many of the observations, service provision suggestions, and the proposed model are needed.

ACKNOWLEDGMENTS

We acknowledge the extraordinary efforts of the providers, interviewers (Joseph Kyebuzibwa and Jacque Nakitende), and all of our colleagues at TASO Jinja and TASO Mulago who assisted in this study.

FUNDING

This study was supported by R01 HD072633.

REFERENCES

Aboo, C. (2011). Profiles and outcomes of traditional healing practices for severe mental illnesses in two districts of Eastern Uganda. *Global Health Action*, 4(7), 7117–7131. doi:10.3402/gha.v4i0.7117

Agadjanian, V., & Hayford, S. R. (2009). PMTCT, HAART, and childbearing in Mozambique: An institutional perspective. *AIDS and Behavior*, 13(1), S103–S112. doi:10.1007/s10461-009-9535-0

Aka-Dago-Akribi, H., Du Loû, A. D., Msellati, P., Dossou, R., & Welffens-Ekra, C. (1999). Issues surrounding reproductive choice for women lying with HIV in Abidjan, Côte d'Ivoire. *Reproductive Health Matters*, 7(13), 20–29.

Banteyerga, H., Kidanu, A., Abebe, F., Alemayehu, M., Fiseha, B., Asazenew, A., . . . Shibru, A. (2005). *Perceived stigmatization and discrimination by healthcare providers towards persons with HIV/AIDS*. Addis Ababa, Ethiopia: Intra Health International, USAIDS. Retrieved from http://www.hrhresourcecenter.org/node/5

Barroso, C., & Sippel, S. (2011). Sexual and reproductive health and rights: Integration as a holistic and rights-based response to HIV/AIDS. *Women's Health Issues*, 21(6), S250–S254. doi:10.1016/j.whi.2011.07.002

Baryamutuma, R., & Baingana, F. (2011). Sexual, reproductive health needs and rights of young people with perinatally acquired HIV in Uganda. *African Health Sciences*, 11(2), 211–218.

Bekker, L. G., Black, V., Myer, L., Rees, H., Cooper, D., Mall, S., & Schwartz, S. (2011). Guideline on safer conception in fertile HIV-infected individuals and couples. *The Southern African Journal of HIV Medicine*, *12*(2), 31–44.

Bernard, H. R., & Ryan, G. W. (2010). *Analyzing qualitative data: Systematic approaches*. Thousand Oaks, CA: Sage.

Beyeza-Kashesya, J., Ekstrom, A. M., Kaharuza, F., Mirembe, F., Neema, S., & Kulane, A. (2010). My partner wants a child: A cross-sectional study of the determinants of the desire for children among mutually disclosed sero-discordant couples receiving care in Uganda. *BMC Public Health*, *10*(247). doi:10.1186/1471-2458-10-247

Beyeza-Kashesya, J., Kaharuza, F., Ekström, A. M., Neema, S., Kulane, A., & Mirembe, F. (2011). To use or not to use a condom: A prospective cohort study comparing contraceptive practices among HIV-infected and HIV-negative youth in Uganda. *BMC Infectious Diseases*, *11*, 144. doi:10.1186/1471-2334-11-144

Cohen, M. S., Chen, Y. Q., McCauley, M., Gamble, T., Hosseinipour, M. C., Kumarasamy, N., . . . HPTN 052 Study Team. (2011). Prevention of HIV-1 infection with early antiretroviral therapy. *New England Journal of Medicine*, *365*, 493–505. doi:10.1056/NEJMoa1105243

Cooper, D., Harries, J., Myer, L., Orner, P., & Bracken, H. (2007). "Life is still going on": Reproductive intentions among HIV-positive women and men in South Africa. *Social Science & Medicine*, *65*(2), 274–283.

Cooper, D., Moodley, J., Zweigenthal, V., Bekker, L. G., Shah, I., & Myer, L. (2009). Fertility intentions and reproductive health care needs of people living with HIV in Cape Town, South Africa: Implications for integrating reproductive health and HIV care services. *AIDS and Behavior*, *13*, 38–46. doi:10.1007/s10461-009-9550-1

Craft, S. M., Delaney, R. O., Bautista, D. T., & Serovich, J. M. (2007). Pregnancy decisions among women with HIV. *AIDS and Behavior*, *11*(6), 927–935.

Feyissa, G. T., LakewAbebe, L., Girma, E., & Woldie, M. (2012). Stigma and discrimination against people living with HIV by healthcare providers, Southwest Ethiopia. *BMC Public Health*, *12*, 522. doi:10.1186/1471-2458-12-522

Finocchario-Kessler, S., Bastos, F. I., Malta, M., Anderson, J., Goggin, K., Sweat, M., . . . Rio Colloboritive Group. (2012). Discussing childbearing with HIV-infected women of reproductive age in clinical care: A comparison of Brazil and the US. *AIDS and Behavior*, *16*, 99–107. doi:10.1007/s10461-011-9906-1

Finocchario-Kessler, S., Wanyenze, R., Mindry, D., Beyeza-Kashesya, J., Goggin, K., Nabiryo, C., & Wagner, G. (In press). "I may not say we really have a method, it is gambling work": Knowledge and acceptability of safer conception methods among providers and HIV clients in Uganda. *Health Care for Women International*.

Gray, R. H., Kigozi, G., Serwadda, D., Makumbi, F., Watya, S., Nalugoda, F., . . . Wawer, M. J. (2007). Male circumcision for HIV prevention in men in Rakai, Uganda: A randomised trial. *Lancet*, *369*(9562), 657–666.

Gray, R. H., Wawer, M. J., Brookmeyer, R., Sewankambo, N. K., Serwadda, D., Wabwire-Mangen, F., . . . The Rakai Project Team. (2001). Probability of HIV-1 transmission per coital act in monogamous, heterosexual, HIV-1-discordant couples in Rakai, Uganda. *Lancet*, *357*(9263), 1149–1153.

Heys, J., Kipp, W., Jhangri, G. S., Alibhai, A., & Rubaale, T. (2009). Fertility desires and infection with the HIV: Results from a survey in rural Uganda. *AIDS, 23*(1), S37–S45. doi:10.1097/01.aids.0000363776.76129.fd

Homsy, J., Bunnell, R., Moore, D., King, R., Malamba, S., Nakityo, R., . . . Mermin, J. (2009). Reproductive intentions and outcomes among women on antiretroviral therapy in rural Uganda: A prospective cohort study. *PLoS One, 4*(1), e4149. doi:10.1371/journal.pone.0004149

Kakaire, O., Osinde, M. O., & Kaye, D. K. (2010). Factors that predict fertility desires for people living with HIV infection at a support and treatment centre in Kabale, Uganda. *Reproductive Health, 7*, 27. doi:10.1186/1742-4755-7-27

Logie, C., & Gadalla, T. M. (2009). Meta-analysis of health and demographic correlates of stigma towards people living with HIV. *AIDS Care, 21*, 742–753. doi:10.1080/09540120802511877

Matthews, L. T., & Mukherjee, J. S. (2009). Strategies for harm reduction among HIV-affected couples who want to conceive. *AIDS Behavior, 13*(1), 5–11. doi:10.1007/s10461-009-9551-0

Matthews, L. T., Smit, J. A., Cu-Uvin, S., & Cohan, D. (2012). Antiretrovirals and safer conception for HIV-serodiscordant couples. *Current Opinion in HIV and AIDS, 7*(6), 569–578. doi:10.1097/COH.0b013e328358bac9

Mills, E., Foster, B. C., Van Heeswijk, R., Phillips, E., Wilson, K., Leonard, B., . . . Kanfer, I. (2005). Impact of African herbal medicines on antiretroviral metabolism. *AIDS, 19*(1), 95–97.

Myer, L., Carter, R. J., Katyal, M., Toro, P., El-Sadr, W. M., & Abrams, E. J. (2010). Impact of antiretroviral therapy on incidence of pregnancy among HIV-infected women in sub-Saharan Africa: A cohort study. *PLOS Medicine, 7*(2): e1000229. doi:10.1371/journal.pmed.1000229

Myer, L., Morroni, C., & Cooper, D. (2006). Community attitudes towards sexual activity and childbearing by HIV-positive people in South Africa. *AIDS Care, 18*(7), 772–776.

Nattabi, B., Li, J., Thompson, S. C., Orach, C. G., & Earnest, J. (2009). A systematic review of factors influencing fertility desires and intentions among people living with HIV/AIDS: Implications for policy and service delivery. *AIDS and Behavior, 13*(5), 949–968. doi:10.1007/s10461-009-9537

Nduna, M., & Farlane, L. (2009). Women living with HIV in South Africa and their concerns about fertility. *AIDS and Behavior, 13*(1), S62–S65. doi:10.1007/s10461-009-9545-y

Schwartz, S. R., Mehta, S. H., Taha, T. E., Rees, H. V., Venter, F., & Black, V. (2012). High pregnancy intentions and missed opportunities for patient-provider communication about fertility in a South African cohort of HIV-positive women on antiretroviral therapy. *AIDS and Behavior, 16*(1), 69–78. doi:10.1007/s10461-011-9981-3

Snow, R. C., Mutumba, M., Resnicow, K., & Mugyenyi, G. (2013). The social legacy of AIDS: Fertility aspirations among HIV-affected women in Uganda. *American Journal of Public Health, 103*(2), 278–285. doi:10.2105/AJPH.2012.300892

Steiner, R. J., Dariotis, J. K., Anderson, J. R., & Finocchario-Kessler, S. (2013). Preconception care for people living with HIV: Recommendations for advancing implementation. *AIDS, 27*(1), S113–S119. doi:10.1097/QAD.0000000000000059

Steiner, R., Finocchario-Kessler, S., & Dariotis, J. K. (2013). The time has come to engage HIV providers in conversations with their reproductive age clients about fertility desires and intentions: A historical review of the HIV epidemic in the United States. *American Journal of Public Health*, *103*(8), 1357–1366. doi:10.2105/AJPH.2013.301265

Thigpen, M. C., Kebaabetswe, P. M., Paxton, L. A., Smith, D. K., Rose, C. E., Segolodi, T. M., . . . TDF2 Study Group. (2012). Antiretroviral preexposure prophylaxis for heterosexual HIV transmission in Botswana. *New England Journal of Medicine*, *367*(5), 423–434. doi:10.1056/NEJMoa1110711

UNAIDS. (2009, November). *AIDS epidemic update*. Geneva, Switzerland: Joint United Nations Programme on HIV/AIDS (UNAIDS) and World Health Organization (WHO). Retrieved from http://www.unaids.org/en/dataanalysis/knowyourepidemic/epidemiologypublications/2009aidsepidemicupdate/

Vernazza, P. L., Graf, I., Sonnenberg-Schwan, U., Geit, M., & Meurer, A. (2011). Preexposure prophylaxis and timed intercourse for HIV-discordant couples willing to conceive a child. *AIDS*, *25*(16), 2005–2008. doi:10.1097/QAD.0b013e32834a36d0

Wabwire-Mangen, F., Odiit, M., Kirungi, W., Kaweesa Kisitu, D., & Okara Wanyama, J. (2009). *Uganda HIV prevention response and modes of transmission analysis*. Kampala, Uganda: Uganda National AIDS Commission. Retrieved from http://siteresources.worldbank.org/INTHIVAIDS/Resources/375798-1103037153392/UgandaMoTCountrySynthesisReport7April09.pdf

Wagner, G. J., Linnemayr, S., Kityo, C., & Mugyenyi, P. (2012). Factors associated with intention to conceive and its communication to providers among HIV clients in Uganda. *Maternal and Child Health Journal*, *16*(2), 510–518. doi:10.1007/s10995-011-0761-5

Wagner, G. J., & Wanyenze, R. K. (2013). Fertility desires and intentions and the relationship to consistent condom use and provider communication regarding childbearing among HIV clients in Uganda. *ISRN Infectious Diseases*. Retrieved from http://dx.doi.org/10.5402/2013/478192

Wanyenze, R. K., Tumwesigye, N. M., Kindyomunda, R., Beyeza-Kashesya, J., Atuyambe, L., Kansiime, A., . . . Mirembe, F. (2011). Uptake of family planning methods and unplanned pregnancies among HIV-infected individuals: A cross-sectional survey among clients at HIV clinics in Uganda. *Journal of the International AIDS Society*, *14*(1). doi:10.1186/1758-2652-14-35

Weiss, M. G., Ramakrishna, J., & Somma, D. (2006). Health-related stigma: Rethinking concepts and interventions. *Psychology Health and Medicine*, *11*(3), 277–287.

World Health Organization (WHO). (2013). *Infant and young child feeding*. Fact Sheet No. 342. Retrieved from http://www.who.int/mediacentre/factsheets/fs342/en/

World Health Organization (WHO), United Nations Population Fund (UNFPA), International Planned Parenthood Federation (IPPF), & UNAIDS. (2011). *Sexual and reproductive health and HIV/AIDS: A framework for priority linkages*. Retrieved from http://www.who.int/reproductive-health/stis/framework.html

"My Legs Affect Me a Lot. . . . I Can No Longer Walk to the Forest to Fetch Firewood": Challenges Related to Health and the Performance of Daily Tasks for Older Women in a High HIV Context

ENID SCHATZ

Department of Health Sciences; and Department of Women's & Gender Studies, University of Missouri, Columbia, Missouri, USA; Institute of Behavioral Science, University of Colorado-Boulder, Boulder, Colorado, USA; and MRC/Wits Rural Public Health and Health Transitions Research Unit, School of Public Health, Faculty of Health Sciences, University of the Witwatersrand, Johannesburg, South Africa

LEAH GILBERT

Department of Sociology, University of the Witwatersrand, Johannesburg, South Africa

Compromised health negatively impacts older persons' ability to participate in expected social roles. Researchers have published little empirical work, however, to explore these issues in HIV endemic African settings. Qualitative interviews with 30 women, aged 60-plus, in rural South Africa, provide insight into the relationship between health and daily activities, with attention to the fulfillment of social roles. In this poor HIV endemic context, older women make connections between their compromised health and their (lack of) capacity to perform the daily tasks that they view as expected of them. By expanding the conceptualization of health to include the capacity to achieve the expectations and perform the tasks expected of one, we better understand how and why health and performance of daily activities are so intricately linked in the minds of respondents. This also provides a starting point for thinking about the social and structural support needed by older persons in these settings, especially as HIV erodes familial supports.

In this article we explore older women's health in the context of their expected roles and performance of daily activities. We focus on how the socio-cultural context in rural South Africa in an era of HIV shapes these women's daily activities and impacts on their health and well-being. The findings we present are from the larger Agincourt Gogo [Grandmother] Project, which included in-depth interviews with older women (50-plus) in rural South Africa, about their health, roles and responsibilities, and relationships with kin (Ogunmefun, Gilbert, & Schatz, 2011; Schatz, 2007; Schatz & Ogunmefun, 2007). We further explain the findings using a wide reconceptualized notion of the meaning of health and well-being. To provide a vivid picture of the lives of older women in this setting, Lerato's[1] story sheds light on the context of this article and the issues it raises.

Lerato is a 61-year-old woman living with one of her daughters, a fostered granddaughter whose mother is working and living with a new partner in Johannesburg, and three orphaned grandchildren left by her eldest son who died of AIDS. Lerato has high blood pressure, which she believes was caused by the distress of losing her son, who had been the primary income earner in the household. She must travel 6 kilometers each month to collect her blood pressure medicine. In addition, she continues to worry about her grandchildren. She finds it stressful to maintain her household on her pension and a few child grants. She also worries about the "promiscuity of youth today" that puts her teenage grandchildren at risk of becoming infected with HIV. Her days consist of domestic chores and keeping her household functioning; she gets some assistance, but she acts as the household manager. With a yard tap but no piped water in the house, her daughter fills the water storage barrels used for cooking and bathing. She often has to nag her grandchildren to collect firewood needed for cooking and heating bath water. Thus, she sometimes resorts to paying for a truckload of wood or going to collect it herself. Lerato keeps a small garden near her house where she grows spinach, onions, tomatoes, and some maize. Because what she grows is insufficient for subsistence, she buys most of her groceries at local shops or during trips to nearby towns. Lerato laments how little of her time is spent visiting with neighbors, weaving grass mats, and being taken care of by her children and grandchildren, as older people "should be." Instead, Lerato's time, energy, and pension largely are spent taking care of others.

BACKGROUND

In developed countries meaningful activity is considered a crucial component of overall health and well-being (Bryant, Corbett, & Kutner, 2001; Forhan,

---

[1] Lerato is a composite representing the lives of many of our HIV-*affected* respondents. It highlights contextual factors, as well as connections among health, well-being and performance of daily activities.

Law, Vrkljan, & Taylor, 2010). This has not been widely researched in less developed countries, however, despite the growing research on health and well-being in these aging populations (Johnson & Climo, 2000; Kowal et al., 2010, 2012). For this reason, more empirical work exploring this issue in developing country settings like southern Africa is needed. Individuals' conception of and participation in daily activities are likely to impact and be impacted by individuals' perceptions and experiences of health (Akinsola & Popovich, 2002; Bohman, Vasuthevan, van Wyk, & Ekman, 2007). Given the centrality of meaning and perceptions, capturing contextual and cultural specificity of daily activities and perceived roles and responsibilities is essential (Hopkins, Kwachka, Lardon, & Mohatt, 2007; Kowal, Gunthorpe, & Bailie, 2007). Personal beliefs and attitudes, as well as cultural and societal values, shape the meaning of older persons' lives (Doble & Santha, 2008). Further, culture can influence the person, environment, *and* participation in daily tasks (Beagan & Etowa, 2009).

In HIV endemic contexts like rural South Africa, older women's health and their social environment frame their daily lives. Distinguishing features of postapartheid rural South Africa, the setting for this study, include endemic poverty, high temporary labor migration rates, an emerging noncommunicable disease epidemic, and high HIV prevalence (Collinson, 2009; May, 2003; Mayosi et al., 2009; National Department of Health, 2013). Few local employment opportunities contribute to increasing migration out of the rural areas; these migrants often leave children behind to be raised by their own parents (Collinson, 2009; Madhavan, 2004; Posel, 2001).

At the same time, elderly South Africans are increasingly plagued by noncommunicable diseases—hypertension, high blood pressure, diabetes, and stroke (Kahn, 2006; Mayosi et al., 2009; National Department of Health, 2013; Westaway, 2010). In addition, they are asked to care for ailing children and HIV-infected and orphaned grandchildren (Munthree & Maharaj, 2010; Ogunmefun et al., 2011; Schatz & Gilbert, 2012). Older poor South Africans are aided by government-sponsored noncontributory pensions. The pension is an important economic asset to households; the cash transfer often serves as a household rather than individual benefit (Ardington et al., 2010; Case & Deaton, 1998; Case & Menendez, 2007; Ogunmefun et al., 2011).

While multigenerational households predate HIV in South Africa (Madhavan, 2004; Møller, 1998), in the current environment multigenerational households facilitate older persons becoming primary caretakers of the sick, of children of the sick, and of the orphaned (Akintola, 2004; Bohman, van Wyk, & Ekman, 2011; Ogunmefun et al., 2011). The younger generation that should take on the roles of older persons' caregivers are becoming sick, leaving the older generation to *provide care* instead of being *cared for* (Burman, 1996; Kautz, Bendavid, Bhattacharya, & Miller, 2010; Mudege & Ezeh, 2009; Schatz & Gilbert, 2012). In addition, older persons and their households must cope with the loss of income and support previously provided by the sick or those lost to AIDS (Schatz, Madhavan, & Williams, 2011; Williams & Tumwekwase, 2001). Increased AIDS-related morbidity and mortality in older persons' households and social networks affect their mental and physical health and daily activities (Mudege & Ezeh, 2009; Munthree & Maharaj, 2010; Schatz & Gilbert, 2012; Westaway, 2010).

In the South African context, older women are the ones to carry most of the burden associated with this scenario, and therefore we focus on women aged 60 and over. Older women are more likely to be caretakers of those infected and affected by HIV than older men (Munthree & Maharaj, 2010). Feeling overwhelmed and worried about family members can negatively impact relationships with kin and the ability to complete expected tasks such as household chores (Mudege & Ezeh, 2009; Schatz, 2007). Older women in these settings generally report worse physical and mental health, and poorer overall quality of life, than their male counterparts (Gómez-Olivé, Thorogood, Clark, Kahn, & Tollman, 2010; Ice, Yogo, Heh, & Juma, 2010). Declining physical health due to aging—including hypertension, chronic pain, and decreased movement—can lead to decreased performance of domestic duties (Mudege & Ezeh, 2009).

Using data from qualitative interviews with 30 South African women, aged 60-plus, we describe their daily activities and their perceptions of how their social reality, the environment, health, and well-being impact their daily lives. In the sections that follow we provide details about the Agincourt research context and methods, summarize physical and mental health complaints, and outline the ways respondents describe activities in their daily lives, and then analyze connections between health and performance of these activities. We conclude with a discussion of how understanding interrelationships between older women's perceptions of health, their social environments, and their daily roles and responsibilities provides a strong starting point for policy and programmatic interventions that will concretely address older women's needs in such and similar HIV endemic settings.

DATA AND METHODS

The data for this article come from the Gogo [Grandmother] Project, which was conducted in the South African Medical Research Council/University of Witwatersrand Rural Public Health and Health Transitions Research Unit (Agincourt) study site. The Agincourt site, named for the rural administrative subdistrict in which the 25 participating villages are located, is home to a health and sociodemographic surveillance site (Kahn et al., 2007). In 1992 the Agincourt research team began conducting a yearly census of all households in the site to track births, deaths, migration, and household relationships.

The rural Agincourt subdistrict, near the South Africa—Mozambique border, is arid, has few industries or employment opportunities, and the land is unsuitable for subsistence agriculture. Extremely high local unemployment rates push nearly half of adult men and over a third of adult women to migrate temporarily to towns and urban areas in search of employment (Collinson, 2009). Due to underemployment and the irregularity of remittances, old-age pensions, a government sponsored noncontributory benefit for those aged 60 and over, are an important household resource (Ardington et al., 2010; May, 2003; Schatz & Ogunmefun, 2007). Mpumalanga Province, where Agincourt is situated, has one of the highest antenatal HIV-prevalence rates in South Africa of 36.7% in the latest national survey (National Department of Health, 2012).

Significant growth in the population over age 60 in the field site has occurred alongside changes in age and cause-specific mortality (Madhavan & Schatz, 2007). Significant increases in mortality among children under 5 and prime-aged adults are largely attributable to AIDS-related illnesses (Byass et al., 2011). Among women in the 50–64 age group, women in older age groups, and to a lesser extent among men, stroke, diabetes, and hypertension top the list of leading causes of death (Gómez-Olivé et al., 2010; Kahn, 2006; Mayosi et al., 2009). This double burden of disease highlights changes in the morbidity and mortality profiles, but it says little about the effects on older persons, their households, or the ways that health and disease impact gendered and generational dynamics—a theme we chose to highlight in this article.

The data for this article come from the larger Gogo Project, which used Agincourt census data to generate a stratified random sample of 90 women aged 50–75, with whom semistructured interviews were conducted. While the study was stratified to compare households with and without recent deaths from AIDS-related causes, virtually all of the women interviewed had been impacted by HIV in some way—whether they had an adult child who had died elsewhere, were currently taking care of a sick adult child, or were caring for fostered or orphaned children (Schatz & Ogunmefun, 2007; Schatz, 2007). The project interview guides focused on older women's roles, responsibilities, and relationships, with a focus on caregiving and pension use in sustaining and maintaining households. Three local female interviewers made up the study staff. They conducted and recorded all interviews in Shangaan (the local language). They then translated and transcribed each interview into English, which were closely reviewed by the principal investigator; corrections to translation and content were made in consultation with the interviewers.

In this article we focus on interviews with 30 South African women aged 60–75 (from Phase I of the Gogo Project). Table 1 provides basic demographic details of these 30 Gogo Project respondents. As the table shows, the majority of the sample were widowed or divorced, over two-thirds lived in households with at least four other household members, and all but five lived in households that include children under the age of 15.

TABLE 1 Demographics of the Gogo Project Sample

Item	No.
Marital status[a]	
Never married	1
Married	5
Divorced	3
Widowed	21
Household size[b]	
Lives alone	2
2–4 household members	5
5–8 household members	11
9–12 household members	4
13+ household members	3
Average household size	6.8
Children in household[b]	
Number of children	
None	5
1–2	12
3–5	9
6+	4
Average number of children	2.6
At least 1 fostered child in household	14
At least 1 orphaned child in household	7
Wealth[a]	
Above average	7
Average	10
Poor	13
N	30

[a]Information collected by/ranked by Gogo Project interviewers.
[b]Data from 2003 Agincourt census for individuals in sample.

The average household size was about seven members, two to three of whom were children. Nearly half had at least one fostered child in the household, and a little less than one-third had an orphaned child in the household. Using designations made by the interviewers, there were just seven households deemed above average in terms of wealth, with one-third viewed as average, and 13 households ranked as poor.

Analyses of the 30 narratives began with open coding for emergent themes. In addition to the primary coder, two additional coders open and close coded the data. Intercoder reliability was checked, and discrepancies were discussed in a group format in order to make decisions about what to include and why. Four main themes emerged related to health, well-being and performance of daily activity: (a) older women's discussions of physical health (*gogo* health), (b) emotional and psychological health (mental health), (c) tasks and daily activities (daily life), and (d) assistance with health issues and performance of daily activities (assistance).

In this article we summarize the first two themes and focus on the third and fourth. We compiled, explored, and tallied coded segments of each theme for patterns, commonalities, and differences across individuals. In order to assess how health and performance of daily activities intersect and impact one another, we used the constant comparative method (Glaser, 1965). We read individuals' narratives against one another to identify patterns of relationships among the themes, as well as differences in the ways the respondents connected their health and well-being to functioning in their daily lives. In the sections below we analyze older women's explanations of the performance of their daily tasks and activities and how their health connects to their participation in those activities and what they perceived as expected roles and responsibilities within their social and environmental context.

ANALYSIS OF FINDINGS

To make sense of our data, we found it useful to rely on a reconceptualization of the meaning of "health" as linked to three fundamental ideas about health, which are most relevant to this article:

1. Health is a capacity, a relative ability to perform.
2. Health is the use of that capacity to achieve expectations defined in terms of values, tasks, and individual fulfillment.
3. Individual capacities and expectations operate to negotiate the demands of the social and physical environment. (Tarlov, 1992, p. 724)

These ideas have provided the conceptual framework for our analysis of the findings that follows.

Reporting on Their Daily Activities

The lives of older women in the study revolved around caring for their homes and families. One of the primary daily activities in which older women we interviewed participated is the surrogate parenting of their grandchildren due to the specific circumstances posed by the HIV epidemic and the associated loss of the "middle generation" (Ogunmefun et al., 2011; Schatz, 2007). Other activities discussed include making grass mats or traditional beer to sell, cooking, cleaning, collecting water and firewood, ploughing, pounding maize, and caring for the sick (if there is a sick relative). For example, Anna described her daily activities in this way:

> When I get up in the morning, I greet my children. I clean my yard, wash my children, and do everything in my home. I go to cut wood. If it is [the season for] ploughing, I plant maize in order to get food. Finally, I cook for my children.

Many of these activities entail rigorous or extended exertion; the majority of the study respondents (24 out of 30), when asked about their daily physical well-being, however, reported ailments and symptoms related to fair or poor health. Compromised physical health was largely associated with common aging complaints like general body pain and fatigue; additionally, a third of the respondents reported having high blood pressure (Schatz & Gilbert, 2012). Poor mental health or social well-being was also prominent—23 of the 30 respondents complained about symptoms or conditions related to stress or depression. The respondents reported that the loss of kin to AIDS, financial concerns about making ends meet, a lack of respect from kin, and fears related to caregiving for the sick led them to "worry a lot" and "think too much" (Schatz & Gilbert, 2012). Respondents also made connections between their physical health and social well-being, arguing that worry *caused* their high blood pressure, or their poor physical health lead to feelings of worry and depression, primarily because they lamented about who would take care of their families if they could not (Schatz & Gilbert, 2012).

Given the reported poor physical and mental health, it was somewhat surprising that about half (16 out of 30) of the respondents said that they participate in daily activities without much trouble; only seven explicitly mentioned having trouble due to their health or age. Four respondents alluded to being capable of household tasks, but they reported that they did not need to participate in such tasks every day or in some cases at all because they live with adult children or grandchildren who provide them with substantial support. For example, Nyeleti helps around the house, but her family members do most chores. This allows her to participate in potentially income-producing activities:

> I wake up in the morning. I prepare the grass that is used to weave mats. Then I help my child to wash dishes, clean the yard, or sometimes also sweep the yard. But I'm not forced to work; I'm just helping my child. The job that I do is to weave grass mats and hoeing. My children and my grandchildren [fetch water].

Pearl, on the other hand, had trouble completing daily tasks. She explained her situation in this way:

> I am old and partially disabled, so I can't do anything at home. It's only my daughter-in-law who cooks, washes, and cleans the house. And my grandchild goes to fetch firewood and water using a wheelbarrow.

Respondents made clear connections between activities and perceived roles and responsibilities within their households and networks. Comparing the narratives of those women who claimed to have little trouble completing tasks with those who needed to ask for assistance, the latter category seemed more troubled about their role in their household. For example, Thandiwe fits in the former category:

> I do cook for myself when my grandchildren and also children are not at home. I can go and fetch water, sweep the house, the yard and go to a shop to buy something. But I'm not forced to do this because I do have children and grandchildren who can do this for me. My favorite work here at home is to weave grass mats and making *marula* peanuts for my children.

Although poor and living in a large household, Thandiwe seems content with her participation in daily tasks and activities, but she also is pleased that her family often completes these tasks so that she can participate in other activities that she loves.

In cases where older women, despite remaining capable, were able to "relax" because their children and grandchildren took over tasks, respondents expressed a sense of pride in being able to spend time on self-defined meaningful occupations, like weaving grass mats. On the other hand, not being physically capable of participating in activities—even those that primarily served others—seemed to be viewed negatively mainly because being limited in this way made them feel that they were not performing according to cultural–societal expectations. Most of the respondents, however, seemed to believe that many of the household duties (e.g., collecting water and firewood, cooking, cleaning) in which they had participated for most of their lives should be passed on to the next generation, and that their time should instead be spent on leisure and "enjoyable" activities. Due to high HIV prevalence among the productive age group, however, this "imagined" or expected reality has eluded most of them.

Connecting Health and Performance in a Specific Cultural Context

While assigning codes to older South African women's reports of health and activities was fairly straightforward, understanding the connections among the well-being of the individual, the context in which they live, and the meaning of their participation in daily tasks and activities is more complex. Many respondents made reference to ways in which their mental or physical health impacted their participation in daily tasks and activities, or vice versa; since these are cross-sectional data, however, the direction of causality remains unclear. We are less concerned with causality than highlighting connections among these areas to provide insights for policymakers interested in addressing not just the individual, but also the individual within the social environment in which she lives.

There were respondents who complained about how their poor health negatively impacts their participation in daily tasks, thus drawing our attention to the conceptualization of health as capacity and a relative ability to perform (Tarlov, 1992). This was the case with Grace, who complained about "painful legs" from working on a citrus farm in her younger years:

> [My legs] affect me a lot because I can no longer walk long distances to visit relatives. And I am no longer able to go to the forest to fetch firewood. ... I have been to many doctors and even visited the Zion church so that they can pray for me, but none of these helped.

Similarly, Tebogo complained of pain interrupting the performance of her daily tasks; she lamented that she lacked help:

> Even when I try to cook, I even feel the pain because no one will help me to do my jobs every day, like cooking and fetching water. I don't have a girl to help me. If I had a girl, some of the jobs she would do.

This quote is also worth noting for its reflection of gendered expectations in the division of household labor—only a "girl" is useful in this context of daily domestic tasks. This was the common cultural understanding accepted among our participants and as such has a bearing on the "social reality" in which older women find themselves since the available men—young or old—do not easily or naturally avail themselves to be of help in the performance of these tasks (Akintola, 2004; Munthree & Maharaj, 2010; Oppong, 2006).

Two accounts further emphasize the links between health and performance of daily activities. Sinah, a moderately well-off widow, when compared with other respondents, reported that she had become ill recently. She had no power, no appetite, and was not feeling well. She went to the clinic, but the nurses could not diagnose her ailment and did not give her any medicine to help. She would have liked to go to the hospital, but she said she did not have money for transport. In addition to these physical health problems, she also complained of being emotionally troubled:

> Yes [I have a lot of worries and cry a lot]. My husband died. My parents died. Even my children have died. If I remember them, I cry. I am taking care of my grandchildren and I can't afford to. No one is helping me. Today I am sick and I don't have money to see a doctor, [or] even to go the hospital. Now when I want to do jobs like washing clothes for myself, I fail.

Impairments in Sinah's emotional and physical health have led her to feel that she is "failing" in the performance of her daily tasks and therefore not conforming with familial and societal expectations.

Having to complete additional caregiving or other related activities may lead to respondents' experiencing, or at least recognizing, emotional or physical health problems as an impediment. Sister, a widow who lives in a poor household with 13 other members, discussed how health and daily responsibilities interact in her life. She had gone to the doctor to get tablets for body pains, which she claimed helped but did not cure her pains. She had also asked her local pastor to pray for her health. When asked what her daily life is like, she responded in this way:

> I used to wake up in the morning and help my grandchildren to wash themselves when they go to school. And sometimes help by washing their clothes and cooking for them. [But this affects me] because sometimes I am thinking too much and I can't fall asleep at night. ... I went to a doctor and the doctor said that I have high blood, so I must not think too much, then he gave me some treatment.

For Sister, her activities led her to worrying too much, which led her to visiting the doctor and being diagnosed with high blood pressure. Although it is not likely that these tasks were the direct cause of her high blood pressure, she clearly draws a connection between these burdens, her emotional well-being, and, in the end, also with her physical health. It further illustrates how her help-seeking behavior is embedded in this social and cultural milieu as shown in other studies (Gilbert, Selikow, & Walker, 2010; Schatz & Gilbert, 2012).

In addition to the cultural and social context discussed, the social reality of the HIV endemic setting, as described earlier, can be linked to older women's perceptions of their health and well-being. Mumsy, relates her worries:

> Yes, I worry a lot. As I have said that I have grandchildren, they might become infected [with HIV/AIDS]. Myself, I know that the disease [has] no one who cures it. If you see your child become sick and you are waiting for her to die, every day when you look at her, she feels pain and you don't help. And the day of dying, you don't know.

There is no doubt that the HIV epidemic dominates older women's worries and expands their roles as demonstrated in other studies. At the same time, however, it presents these women with new challenges and a necessity to adjust their expectations and daily performance based on their limited capacity (Tarlov, 1992).

DISCUSSION AND CONCLUSION

Rural South African older women's responsibilities often involve caring for their sick children and grandchildren, broadening their roles without adding structural and social support. A challenging environment, like that of high

HIV prevalence, endemic poverty and high unemployment, the sense of a lack of control over one's own environment, and of limited capacity due to ill health, can prevent individuals from choosing activities that have meaning and worth to them, and it may hinder access to resources needed to engage in such activities (Connor Schisler, & Polatajko, 2002; Hammell, 2008). As the middle generation is lost to AIDS, despite their own declining health, older South African women in particular are required to perform tasks that otherwise their children would have completed (Munthree & Maharaj, 2010; Ogunmefun et al., 2011), while simultaneously losing their own caregivers (Kautz et al., 2010).

While grandmothers have traditionally played a role in extended family care in rural South Africa (Madhavan, 2004), as evidenced in the above narratives, the loss of adult children appears to have increased the weight of dependence on them. "Secondary role strain" can occur when caregiver responsibilities conflict with women's other roles (Ice et al., 2010). Rather than living out their lives as respected and cared-for elders, which is expected in this cultural milieu, the women in this study are financially and socially responsible for many of their grandchildren. Financial worries in particular may be amplified when an income earner dies, putting further demands and pressures on older persons' resources, including pensions (Ogunmefun et al., 2011). The need to cover expenses related to one's own health and the health of family members exacerbates negative impacts on older persons' health and well-being. Social connections seem to play a key role for older women, particularly female household heads (Schatz et al., 2011), yet needing to beg assistance and borrow from friends and neighbors to support their caregiver role may lead to feeling overwhelmed and helpless (Munthree & Maharaj, 2010). The high primary and secondary stigma associated with the care for a member of the family living (or dying) with AIDS shaped the nature of support (or lack thereof) from friends and neighbors and contributed to their feeling of "ill health" (Gilbert & Walker, 2010; Ogunmefun et al., 2011).

In other studies, older African women reported being "physically and emotionally exhausted" and "overworked" due to constant domestic and caregiving responsibilities (Munthree & Maharaj, 2010). While in our study ill health was not directly connected to caregiving, it was connected to the emotional strains that caring and loss create as well as to their limited capacity to perform their roles as expected, and in a number of cases may be related to the associated stigma of caring for someone with HIV.

Caregiving responsibilities can be stressful, resulting in poor health, which may be why caregivers in Kenya report more health problems, more health visits, and poorer self-assessed health than noncaregivers (Ice et al., 2010). As found in the Kenyan study, however, caregiving did not significantly decrease mental health, suggesting that the role may give parents/grandparents a sense of love and fulfillment, reducing negative feelings (Ice et al., 2010). This sense of love and fulfillment was not as evident in the passages outlined here, but the feeling of being bound to family and the profound sense of love and obligation do come through in other work from this study (Schatz, 2007).

Similar to the findings in our study, the researchers in another study of caregivers in Kenya, who were mostly women, highlighted complaints about physical ailments—poor eyesight, joint pains, and dizziness—and how these reduced the caregivers' participation in everyday activities and provision of care (Muga & Onyango-Ouma, 2009). These caregivers relied on their children to complete tasks that their health prevented them from doing, making it difficult to live independently or to support others. Importantly, this growing body of work shows the multidirectional pathways among health, well-being, and participation in daily tasks. It also sheds some light on the links between health and general performance in a specific cultural and social context and how these shape utilization of health care (Gilbert et al., 2010).

Although the experiences of older men are not captured in the current study, significant gender differences in the manifestation of health, well-being and activity in this and similar settings are likely (Gómez-Olivé et al., 2010; Westaway, Olorunju, & Rai, 2007). Women traditionally have taken on the role of the primary domestic worker, while men have sought employment and had limited domestic responsibilities related to childcare, cleaning, cooking, and caring for the sick (Mudege & Ezeh, 2009). Thus, women's roles are more likely to include medicating, washing, feeding, and giving emotional support to those sick with AIDS (Lindsey, Hirschfeld, & Tlou, 2003; Mudege & Ezeh, 2009; Munthree & Maharaj, 2010). Thus, explorations of the nature of carework and the intersections of health, well-being, and performance need to be interrogated through a gendered lens.

As indicated earlier, the cross-sectional data we analyzed do not provide information on causation. Understanding associations between health and capacity to participate in meaningful activities, however, remain crucial to older South Africans' aging more successfully. In this article we begin to examine the interrelationship of individual well-being, the social environment, and capacity to participate in and perform daily activities. A policy and programmatic focus on older person's mental and physical health may improve older persons' well-being and their ability to continue to contribute to the well-being of their households and communities. Community-based programs that entail minimal travel, but provide social and medical support for common mental and physical ailments of aging, would greatly benefit this population. Programs should address *both* mental and physical health, *and* highlight their interconnections. It is also essential that programs acknowledge older persons' increasing financial, emotional, and physical challenges related to the ways AIDS impacts their lives and those of their families—as shown in this article, this pertains to women in particular. These programs should assist in reassessing and realigning older persons' roles and obligations so that self-care, work, and leisure contribute to health and well-being in positive ways (Forhan et al., 2010).

The HIV endemic context germinates stressful situations—for example, trying to make ends meet, caring for ill adult children in a stigmatizing environment, raising grandchildren, and losing those who should be one's own caregiver in old age—that mediate individuals' health and their ability to participate in daily activities. As women in these settings deal with growing physical limitations, it is essential to continue to unpack the complex meaning of health and well-being among older women in rural South Africa. In this article we provide a starting point for policy and programmatic interventions that will concretely address some of older women's needs in HIV endemic settings—for example, stronger, cheaper, and more proximate health care for their physical *and* mental health needs. Future studies must continue to explore how older women (and men) in HIV endemic settings view their health and the ways health, capacity, and performance of daily activities influence and shape one another.

ACKNOWLEDGMENTS

We owe thanks to the South African Medical Research Council/University of the Witwatersrand Rural Public Health and Health Transitions Research Unit (supported by the Wellcome Trust [085477/Z/08/Z]) for providing study site access, sample selection assistance, and support throughout the data collection and analysis. The authors are indebted to Catherine Ogunmefun, fieldwork manager, and to Asnath Mdaka, Florence Mnisi, and Joyce Nkuna, the three interviewers who collected the data. We thank Allison Kabel, Diane Smith, and the anonymous reviewers for comments on earlier drafts.

FUNDING

This research has benefited from the NICHD-funded University of Colorado Population Center (grant R21 HD51146) and grants from the Andrew Mellon Foundation through the University of Kwa-Zulu Natal HIV/AIDS Node.

REFERENCES

Akinsola, H. A., & Popovich, J. M. (2002). The quality of life of families of female-headed households in Botswana: A secondary analysis of case studies. *Health Care for Women International, 23*, 761–772. doi:10.1080/07399330290107502

Akintola, O. (2004). *A gendered analysis of the burden of care on family and volunteer caregivers in Uganda and South Africa* (No. Health Economics and HIV/AIDS Research Division). Durban, South Africa: University of Kwa–Zulu Natal.

Ardington, C., Case, A., Islam, M., Lam, D., Leibbrandt, M., Menendez, A., & Olgiati, A. (2010). The impact of AIDS on intergenerational support in South Africa: Evidence from the Cape Area Panel Study. *Research on Aging*, *32*(1), 97–121. doi:10.1177/0164027509348143

Beagan, B., & Etowa, J. (2009). The impact of everyday racism on the occupations of African Canadian women. *Canadian Journal of Occupational Therapy*, *76*, 285–293.

Bohman, D. M., van Wyk, N. C., & Ekman, S. L. (2011). South Africans' experiences of being old and of care and caring in a transitional period. *International Journal of Older People Nursing*, *6*, 187–195. doi:10.1111/j.1748-3743.2010.00225.x

Bohman, D. M., Vasuthevan, S., van Wyk, N. C., & Ekman, S. (2007). "We clean our homes, prepare for weddings and go to funerals": Daily lives of elderly Africans in Majaneng, South Africa. *Journal of Cross-Cultural Gerontology*, *22*, 323–337.

Bryant, L. L., Corbett, K. K., & Kutner, J. S. (2001). In their own words: A model of healthy aging. *Social Science & Medicine*, *53*, 927–941. doi:10.1016/S0277-9536(00)00392-0

Burman, S. (1996). Intergenerational family care: Legacy of the past, implications for the future. *Journal of Southern African Studies*, *22*, 585–598. doi:10.1080/03057079608708513

Byass, P., Kahn, K., Fottrell, E., Mee, P., Collinson, M. A., & Tollman, S. M. (2011). Using verbal autopsy to track epidemic dynamics: The case of HIV-related mortality in South Africa. *Population Health Metrics*, *9*(1), 46–52. doi:10.1186/1478-7954-9-46

Case, A., & Deaton, A. (1998). Large cash transfers to the elderly in South Africa. *The Economic Journal*, *108*, 1330–1361.

Case, A., & Menendez, A. (2007). Does money empower the elderly? Evidence from the Agincourt demographic surveillance site, South Africa. *Scandinavian Journal of Public Health*, *35*(69 Suppl.), 157–164. doi:10.1080/14034950701355445

Collinson, M. A. (2009). *Striving against adversity: The dynamics of migration, health and poverty in rural South Africa*. (Medical Dissertation). Epidemiology and Public Health Sciences, Department of Public Health and Clinical Medicine, Umeå University, Umeå, Sweden.

Connor Schisler, A. M., & Polatajko, H. J. (2002). The individual as a mediator of the person-occupation-environment interaction: Learning from the experience of refugees. *Journal of Occupational Science*, *9*(2), 82–92.

Doble, S., & Santha, J. (2008). Occupational well-being: Rethinking occupational therapy outcomes. *Canadian Journal of Occupational Therapy*, *75*, 184–190.

Forhan, M., Law, M. C., Vrkljan, B. H., & Taylor, V. (2010). The experience of participation in everyday occupations for adults with obesity. *Canadian Journal of Occupational Therapy*, *77*, 210–218.

Gilbert, L., Selikow, T.-A., & Walker, L. (2010). *Society, health and disease in a time of HIV/AIDS*. Johannesburg, South Africa: Macmillian.

Gilbert, L., & Walker, L. (2010). "My biggest fear was that people would reject me once they knew my status. . .": Stigma as experienced by patients in an HIV/AIDS clinic in Johannesburg, South Africa. *Health & Social Care in the Community*, *18*, 139–146. doi:10.1111/j.1365-2524.2009.00881.x

Glaser, B. G. (1965). The constant comparative method of qualitative analysis. *Social Problems*, *12*, 436–445.

Gómez-Olivé, F. X., Thorogood, M., Clark, B., Kahn, K., & Tollman, S. (2010). Assessing health and well-being among older people in rural South Africa. *Global Health Action, 3*(Suppl. 2), 23–35. doi: 10.3402/gha.v3i0.2126

Hammell, K. W. (2008). Reflections on well-being and occupational rights. *Canadian Journal of Occupational Therapy, 75*(1), 61–64.

Hopkins, S. E., Kwachka, P., Lardon, C., & Mohatt, G. V. (2007). Keeping busy: A Yup'ik/Cup'ik perspective on health and aging. *International Journal of Circumpolar Health, 66*(1), 42–50.

Ice, G. H., Yogo, J., Heh, V., & Juma, E. (2010). The impact of caregiving on the health and well-being of Kenyan Luo grandparents. *Research on Aging, 32*(1), 40–66. doi:10.1177/0164027509348128

Johnson, N. E., & Climo, J. J. (2000). Aging and eldercare in lesser developed countries. *Journal of Family Issues, 21*, 683–691. doi:10.1177/019251300021006001

Kahn, K. (2006). *Dying to make a fresh start: Mortality and health transition in a new South Africa.* (Medical Dissertation). Epidemiology and Public Health Sciences, Department of Public Health and Clinical Medicine, Umeå University, Umeå, Sweden.

Kahn, K., Tollman, S. M., Collinson, M. A., Clark, S. J., Twine, R., Clark, B. D., ... Garenne, M. L. (2007). Research into health, population and social transitions in rural South Africa: Data and methods of the Agincourt Health and Demographic Surveillance System. *Scandinavian Journal of Public Health, 35*(69 Suppl.), 8–20. doi:10.1080/14034950701505031

Kautz, T., Bendavid, E., Bhattacharya, J., & Miller, G. (2010). AIDS and declining support for dependent elderly people in Africa: Retrospective analysis using demographic and health surveys. *British Medical Journal, 340*, c2841. Retrieved from http://www.bmj.com/content/340/bmj.c2841

Kowal, E., Gunthorpe, W., & Bailie, R. S. (2007). Measuring emotional and social wellbeing in Aboriginal and Torres Strait Islander populations: An analysis of a Negative Life Events Scale. *International Journal for Equity in Health, 6*(18). doi:10.1186/1475-9276-6-18

Kowal, P., Chatterji, S., Naidoo, N., Biritwum, R., Fan, W., Lopez Ridaura, R., ... Boerma, J. T. (2012). Data Resource Profile: The World Health Organization Study on global AGEing and adult health (SAGE). *International Journal of Epidemiology, 41*, 1639–1649. doi:10.1093/ije/dys210

Kowal, P., Kahn, K., Ng, N., Naidoo, N., Abdullah, S., Bawah, A., ... Tollman, S. M. (2010). Ageing and adult health status in eight lower-income countries: The INDEPTH WHO-SAGE collaboration. *Global Health Action, 3*(Suppl. 2), 11–22. doi:10.3402/gha.v3i0.5302

Lindsey, E., Hirschfeld, M., & Tlou, S. (2003). Home-based care in Botswana: Experiences older women and young girls. *Health Care for Women International, 24*, 486–501.

Madhavan, S. (2004). Fosterage patterns in the age of AIDS: Continuity and change. *Social Science & Medicine, 58*, 1443–1454. doi:10.1016/S0277-9536(03)00341-1

Madhavan, S., & Schatz, E. (2007). Coping with change: Household structural and composition in rural South Africa, 1992–2003. *Scandinavian Journal of Public Health, 35*(Suppl. 69), 85–93.

May, J. (2003). *Chronic poverty and older people in South Africa*. Chronic Poverty Research Centre Working paper 25. Durban, South Africa: School of Development Studies, University of Natal.

Mayosi, B. M., Flisher, A. J., Lalloo, U. G., Sitas, F., Tollman, S. M., & Bradshaw, D. (2009). The burden of non-communicable diseases in South Africa. *The Lancet*, *374*(9693), 934–947. doi:10.1016/S0140-6736(09)61087-4

Møller, V. (1998). Innovations to promote an intergenerational society for South Africa to promote the well-being of the black African elderly. *Society in Transition*, *29*(1–2), 1–12.

Mudege, N. N., & Ezeh, A. C. (2009). Gender, aging, poverty and health: Survival strategies of older men and women in Nairobi slums. *Journal of Aging Studies*, *23*, 245–257. doi:10.1016/j.jaging.2007.12.021

Muga, G. O., & Onyango-Ouma, W. (2009). Changing household composition and food security among the elderly caretakers in rural western Kenya. *Journal of Cross-Cultural Gerontology*, *24*, 259–272. doi:10.1007/s10823-008-9090-6

Munthree, C., & Maharaj, P. (2010). Growing old in the era of a high prevalence of HIV/AIDS: The impact of AIDS on older men and women in KwaZulu-Natal, South Africa. *Research on Aging*, *32*, 155–174. doi:10.1177/0164027510361829

National Department of Health. (2012). *The 2011 national antenatal sentinel HIV & syphilis prevalence survey in South Africa*. Pretoria, South Africa: Author.

National Department of Health. (2013). *Strategic plan for the prevention and control of non-communicable diseases 2013–17*. Pretoria, South Africa: Author.

Ogunmefun, C., Gilbert, L., & Schatz, E. (2011). Older female caregivers and HIV/AIDS–related secondary stigma in rural South Africa. *Journal of Cross-Cultural Gerontology*, *26*(1), 85–102. doi:10.1007/s10823-010-9129-3

Oppong, C. (2006). Familial roles and social transformations: Older men and women in sub-Saharan Africa. *Research on Aging*, *28*, 654–668. doi:10.1177/0164027506291744

Posel, D. R. (2001). Who are the heads of household, what do they do, and is the concept of headship useful? An analysis of headship in South Africa. *Development Southern Africa*, *18*, 651–670.

Schatz, E. (2007). "Taking care of my own blood": Older women's relationships to their households in rural South Africa. *Scandinavian Journal of Public Health*, *35*(Suppl. 69), 147–154.

Schatz, E., & Gilbert, L. (2012). "My heart is very painful": Physical, mental and social wellbeing of older women at the times of HIV/AIDS in rural South Africa. *Journal of Aging Studies*, *26*(1), 16–25. doi:10.1016/j.jaging.2011.05.003

Schatz, E., Madhavan, S., & Williams, J. (2011). Female-headed households contending with HIV/AIDS-related hardship in rural South Africa. *Health & Place*, *17*, 598–605. doi:10.1016/j.healthplace.2010.12.017

Schatz, E., & Ogunmefun, C. (2007). Caring and contributing: The role of older women in multi-generational households in the HIV/AIDS era. *World Development*, *35*, 1390–1403.

Tarlov, A. R. (1992). The coming influence of a social sciences perspective on medical education. *Academic Medicine*, *67*, 724–731.

Westaway, M. S. (2010). The impact of chronic diseases on the health and well-being of South Africans in early and later old age. *Archives of Gerontology and Geriatrics, 50*, 213–221. doi:10.1016/j.archger.2009.03.012

Westaway, M. S., Olorunju, S. A. S., & Rai, L. J. (2007). Which personal quality of life domains affect the happiness of older South Africans? *Quality of Life Research, 16*, 1425–1438. doi: 10.1007/s11136-007-9245-x

Williams, A., & Tumwekwase, G. (2001). Multiple impacts of the HIV/AIDS epidemic on the aged in rural Uganda. *Journal of Cross-Cultural Gerontology, 16*, 221–236.

Grandparents Fostering Orphans: Influences of Protective Factors on Their Health and Well-Being

MAGEN MHAKA-MUTEPFA and ROBERT CUMMING

School of Public Health, University of Sydney, Sydney, New South Wales, Australia

ELIAS MPOFU

Department of Rehabilitation, University of Sydney, Sydney, New South Wales, Australia

In this study the authors explore the impact of protective factors on the health and well-being of grandmothers who are primary care-givers. Although researchers in Africa have studied grandparents who assume primary caregiving responsibilities, it is rare that they do so from a strength perspective, hence the need to examine the utility of personal, social, and environmental assets on caregiving. Grandmothers are the primary caregivers of orphaned children due to HIV and AIDS deaths; thus it becomes pertinent to establish how they are coping without the provision of social security. The results of this study will be beneficial to all stakeholders interested in the welfare of elders with similar responsibilities. Knowledge about the health and well-being of grandmothers who are caregivers will assist public service and private sectors to formulate viable poli-cies concerning elderly carers who foster orphans, particularly in countries with high HIV prevalence.

Grandparents may have full custody of their grandchildren, particularly after the death of the parent carers (Nyasani, Sterberg, & Smith, 2009). This is especially true in the sub-Saharan African context given the high mortality from the HIV pandemic among younger or child-bearing par-ents. In Zimbabwe alone, there were 1,943,845 orphans by 2007. About 1,008,480 children became orphans in Zimbabwe due to HIV and worsening macroeconomic conditions (UNAIDS, 2011). A grandmother as a caregiver is not a new phenomenon (Nyasani et al., 2009), particularly part-time care, and with cultural and moral obligation to take up orphan care (Nyambedha, Wandibba, & Aagaard-Hansen, 2003a; Nyasani et al., 2009). Healthy grandparenting makes for quality child outcomes such as good behavior, social competence, good communication, and coping skills (Gupta & Simonsen, 2007). Caregiving presents both opportunities and costs to the health and well-being of grandmother carers.

Health and well-being does not just mean the absence of disease, but living a satisfying quality of life (World Health Organization [WHO], 2001). Well-being was defined according to four criteria: (a) absence of psychopathology; (b) healthy patterns of behavior; (c) adequate role functioning at home, work, or both; and (d) high quality of life (Norris, Stevens, Pfefferbaum, Wyche, & Pfefferbaum, 2008). Well-being is one of the most important outcomes in health care, yet it is rarely studied within the context of caregiving. Benefits may arise from being actively involved with carer tasks activities rather than being indolent or inactive. An active lifestyle is associated with health and well-being across the developmental span (Chen & Feeley, 2012; Hughes, Waite, LaPierre, & Luo, 2007). Grandparenting, though mostly not voluntary, may lead to self-fulfillment and positive affirmation to primary caregivers (Hughes et al., 2007; Poehlmann, 2003). Costs may arise from associated stressors from time and energy pressures and workload from carer roles (Degeneffe, Chan, Dunlap, Man, & Sung, 2011; Kamya & Poindexter, 2009). The day-to-day care of children, especially very young children, is physically taxing and can involve loss of sleep and exposure to infections (Kamya & Poindexter, 2009). These physical demands may increase if grandchild care coincides with the onset of physical aging (Hughes et al., 2007). The assets for grandparents to flourish in carer roles are in need of study because they are protective of the carers' health and well-being.

Well-being can also be inflenced by group social participation in that the participants develop a sense of belonging, personal freedom, and self-esteem and gain new knowledge and enjoy life to the fullest (Diener & Ryan, 2009). Grandparents who live in more accepting social environments (people who understand and value them) experience more well-being.

Protective Factors

A protective factor refers to resources that prevent or reduce vulnerability for the development of a psychological disorder. The protective factors protect grandmothers against vulnerabilities and difficulties they encounter in the primary carer roles. The factors promote mental health and well-being. A previous study classified protective factors into four groups: personal resources (e.g., optimism, safety), social resources (e.g., companionship), object resources (e.g., housing), and energy (e.g., money, free time; Hobfoll, Neria, Gross, Marshall, & Susser, 2006). In the current study protective factors encompassed personal assets (e.g., self-concept and overall coping skills), social assets (e.g., access to health services, religiosity, and social networks), and environmental assets (e.g., healthy physical environment, leisure, and available finances). For instance, the level of psychoeducation and financial stability positively influences well-being (Diener, Oishi, & Lucas, 2003; Michalos, 2008) and health. Protective capacities also enable coping despite the impediments encountered in life (Killian, 2004). The extent to which grandchild care affects health depends on the balance between the demands of caregiving and the resources available to the grandparent (Hughes et al., 2007; Hughes & Waite, 2002).

Certain people have high self-esteem, internal locus of control, and problem-solving capabilities (Rutter, 2011), which we call personal assets. These traits make people believe they can influence or control their life direction and behavior. They usually are highly successful people and lead happy lives. When mastery is lacking, however, self-efficacy is reduced and a challenging event becomes maladaptive and results in helplessness (Craig, 2012). The positive personality traits together with other protective factors bolster health and well-being through perceptions and positive appraisal of the carer roles and enacted support (Bigbee, Boegh, Prengaman, & Shaklee, 2011; Degeneffe et al., 2011; Gerard, Landry-Meyer, & Roe, 2006; Ice, Sadruddin, Vagedes, Yogo, & Juma, 2012; Kipp, Tindyebwa, Karamagi, & Rubaale, 2007; Kuhn, Fulton, & Edelman, 2003). These traits are multicultural and would apply better in African cultures because of the emotional support Africans render one another. The connection a grandparent has with his/her inner self influences well-being (self-concept) as in any relationship. In addition, not allowing past negative social experiences to influence present and future decision making also heightens well-being.

Appraisal in caregiving is seen as how a person perceives the role of caring for others. Some carers view caregiving as their responsibility. For example, if a grandparent carer accepts caregiving as his/her responsibility, he/she is likely to cope with carer roles. According to Ross and Aday (2006) and Ice and colleagues (2011), positive appraisal is negatively correlated with stress. In the context of caregiving, personal assets help to buffer stressors by enabling the carers to cope with their role. The resources have the potential to modify, cushion, or alter a person from the negative consequences of difficulties (Craig, 2012; Ice, Heh, Yogo, & Juma, 2011). For instance, carers who felt a moral obligation to foster orphans had higher emotional well-being and superior health (Gaudine, Gien, Thuan, & Dung, 2010; Ogunmefun, Gilbert, & Schatz, 2011; Schatz & Ogunmefun, 2007).

Lower personal asset resources are associated with poor health and well-being. Personal assets can give grandparents more energy, keep them healthier, and can be a source of pride and self-respect (Hughes et al.,

2007; Waldrop & Weber, 2001). On the other hand, internal perception of grandparental roles as a sacrifice and a burden may make carers give up and succumb to all the negative trends that come with caregiving (e.g., poor health, emotional distress, lower well-being, and inability to seek assistance). The main problem with primary caregiving is that the grandparents may not be prepared for this role.

Accurate perceptions of the self, the world, and the future are essential for mental health (Craig, 2012; Norris et al., 2008). Considerable research evidence suggests that positive self-evaluations, perceptions of control or mastery, and optimism are characteristics of human thoughts (Craig, 2012; Degeneffe et al., 2011; Fergus & Zimmerman, 2005; Killian, 2004) and benefit grandmother carers.

Social assets refer to support groups, respite care, access to services, and spirituality as forms of social supports that grandmother carers could access in an African context. Previous research reported that grandmother carers who sought formal assistance from professionals had lower psychosocial adjustment problems than those who did not (Hayslip & Shore, 2000). As social support, extended families and spouses (family social capital) assist grandmothers by providing instrumental forms of care (such as emotional well-being and behavioral management and overall role satisfaction). Support operates as a protective factor because it reduces the negative risks that may confront the carer (Nyambedha et al., 2003a; Oburu & Palmerus, 2005; Poehlmann et al., 2008). Typical formal social protection programs include pensions, unemployment benefits, housing benefits, self-help groups, home-based care groups, and social-security benefits (Stockstrom, 2008). Appraisal of low social support by grandparent carers can affect well-being (Gerard et al., 2006) and health.

Involvement in grandparenting carer roles may be gendered in some settings, with more grandmother carers than grandfathers (Hayslip & Kaminski, 2005; Howard et al., 2006; Nyambedha, Wandibba, & Aagaard-Hansen, 2003b). This would be the case in patriarchal societies such as in Africa and other developing world settings. The gendered grandparenting roles mean grandmothers with resources may have better health and well-being.

Grandmothers may also participate in social gatherings as a form of socialization. If the grandparent participates in activities in the community, she socializes with others and may develop better well-being. Poor relationships among grandparents and the community may impact carer participation in community activities; for instance, the grandmothers might not train as home-based carers or other training activities. Spirituality is also a form of social gathering. Spirituality was used by grandmother carers as a way of coping with carer roles (Kipp et al., 2007; Neele-Barnes, 2010; Ross & Aday, 2006) hence better health and well-being. Church members were said to be the best form of support as they had all the qualities of trust, fulfilling relationships, and the ability to empathize.

Environmental assets refer to a supportive environment, a positive emotional climate, and the availability of supports and resources within the family and the community that can serve a protective function (Hayslip & Kaminski, 2005; Hobfoll et al., 2006 ; Killian, 2004). Most previous research findings suggest that family resources (i.e., financial status, caregiver education, perceived availability of instrumental and emotional support) relative to risks (i.e., impoverished status, role restrictions) affect carers' well-being (Brintnall-Peterson, Poehlmann, Morgan, & Shlafer, 2009; Minkler & Fuller-Thomson, 2005). Environmental assets that bolster carers' health and well-being include employment opportunities, access to basic needs, and recreation.

Study Goals

In this study researchers address the knowledge gap on influences of personal, social, and environmental factors as protective factors on the health and well-being of grandmothers with child carer responsibilities in Zimbabwe. The following research question guided the study: How do grandmother carers' personal, social, and environmental assets influence their health and well-being as carers of orphaned children?

The study focuses on assets as protective factors. Findings may assist public service and private sectors to formulate viable policies concerning caregivers.

METHOD

A cross-sectional survey design was used for the study. The cross-sectional survey is appropriate for collecting data at a single point in time to measure associations between the different outcomes (health and well-being) and predictor variables (personal, social, and environmental assets).

Procedure

The University of Sydney Human Research Ethics Committee and the Medical Research Council of Zimbabwe approved the project. Three geographic areas were chosen for the study: one low-density (high socioeconomic status [SES]) suburb, one high-density (low SES) suburb, and a rural district. Grandparents provided individual written consent. They were recruited through the schools their grandchildren attended. Probability proportionate to size method was used to select 18 schools. Children fostered by grandparents were chosen from social registers, and systematic sampling was used to select the children's grandparents for the study. An average of 16 children was selected from each of the low-density ($n = 6$) schools, an average of 25 children from each of the high-density schools ($n = 4$), and 25 children from each of the rural schools ($n = 8$). A few of the grandparents ($n = 10$) sampled in the low-density schools resided in high-density suburbs.

The grandmothers were assured of confidentiality in writing and verbally and of the right to withdraw their participation at any time without penalties. Identification numbers were used to maintain anonymity of participants. Data were collected in family homes or at grandmothers' workplaces by the first listed author.

Measures

Data on health and well-being were collected using the World Health Organization Quality of Life Questionnaire (WHOQOL-BREF; WHO, 1996), and a global statement rating. In addition, data on participant characteristics were also collected (age, marital status, residence, level of education, monthly income, and whether the carer was fostering orphans or nonorphans). Income earned is a proxy for higher SES and was associated with better health.

The WHOQOL-BREF is a 26-item measure of health (mental and physical) and well-being (social relations and environment) and other areas of life. This scale has four categories or domains: physical health (7 items), psychological health (6 items), social relationships (3 items), and environment (8 items). Domains are not scored where 20% or more of items are missing, and they are unacceptable where two or more items are missing (or one item in the three-item social domain; Skevington & O'Connell, 2004). Items inquire "how much," "how completely," "how often," "how good," or "how satisfied" the respondent felt in the last 2 weeks; different response scales are distributed across the domains (Skevington & O'Connell, 2004). The first two domains are made up of physical and psychological health. Health included facets of activities of daily living, dependence on medicines, energy and fatigue, work capacity, self-esteem, personal beliefs, and others. Results of the WHOQOL-BREF were summed to get an overall score, which was then transformed to a 0–100 scale, called the Total Quality of Life, with higher scores indicating a better quality of life and other areas of life. Reliability of scores from the measure with the current sample was .83.

In addition, participants self-rated for health on a 5-point scale ranging from 1 (*very bad*) to 5 (*very good*). Well-being included facets on personal relationships, social support, sexual activity, physical safety, home and physical environment, financial resources, and others. A statement such as "How often do you have negative feelings such as blue mood, despair, anxiety, depression?" was ranked from 1 (*never*) to 5 (*always*). Quality of life was also measured on a 5-point scale from 1 (*very poor*) to 5 (*very good*).

Data Analysis

Hierarchical regression analysis (Mertler & Vannatta, 2005) was used to estimate the strengths of the relationships between the predictor protective factors and the criterion variables health and well-being controlling for demographics. Separate models were developed for physical and mental health. All protective effects were examined while controlling for age, marital status, education, and income earned; residence (rural, low-density urban, and high-density urban); and whether the children fostered were orphans or nonorphans. The informants' education and residence were used as measures of SES and were treated as nominal measures. The analysis included blocks of variables categorized as personal, social, and environmental assets to determine whether each block increased the variance accounted for after taking into account the previous blocks. This was accomplished by utilizing the increment R^2 test.

Altogether, four hierarchical regression analyses were conducted to examine the association among protective factors and the two criterion variables. The variance inflation factor for the variables was less than 10; thus there was no collinearity. The three assumptions of linearity, constant variance, and normality were met.

RESULTS

Participants were 241 grandmothers (mean age = 61.1; SD = 10.9, age ranges = 36–100). The participation rate was 93%. Eighty-one percent of the grandmothers had primary or no education, while the rest had completed high school, had a college certificate, or had a university degree. Half the sample resided in a rural area and the other half resided in urban areas (low and high density). Sixty-two percent of the grandmothers earned an average of U.S. $300 per month. Twenty-seven percent of grandmothers were fostering orphans only, 36% were fostering both orphans and nonorphans, and 38% were fostering nonorphans. Fifty-four percent of the carers were widowed, 34% were married, 10% were divorced, and the rest never married. Forty-five percent of caregivers lived in skipped-generation households. Twenty-eight percent of the carers rated their health as bad, 45% as moderate, and 27% as good. Grandmothers rated their quality of life as poor (48%), neither poor nor good (35%), and good (17%).

Thirteen percent of the grandmothers in the current sample revealed that they were living with HIV and AIDs and were on antiretroviral drugs. Forty percent of the children's parents had died of HIV-related illnesses, and 17% of children's parents had died from other causes. Thirty-six percent of the grandchildren were reported by their carers to have tested HIV positive. There were 969 grandchildren (see Table 1 for children's characteristics) being fostered, and the children's ages ranged from 4 months to 18 years. Of the children who were not attending school, 24% could not afford school fees, and the rest were still too young to be in school.

In Table 2 we present the descriptive statistics, alphas, and correlation coefficients of the predictor variables (age, income, personal assets, social

TABLE 1 Grandchildren Characteristics

Variable	$n = 969$	%
Type of grandchildren		
Maternal	455	46.5
Paternal	242	25.1
Both	275	28.4
Children's health		
Sick	130	16.1
Not sick	676	83.9
Type of illness		
Acute	85	63.7
Chronic	45	36.3
Children who attend school		
No	347	35.8
Yes	622	89.4
No. of children fostered		
Orphans	418	43.1
Nonorphans	551	56.9

assets, and environmental assets) and outcome variables (health—physical and psychological health—and well-being—social relations and environment). Results revealed that caregivers had favorable personal assets in problem-solving skills and meaningful life (see Table 2). The mean scores were lowest in availability of finances (1.8) and leisure (0.23). Correlations with the highest coefficients were income and environment (0.58) and mental health and environment (0.54).

Predicting Physical Health From Protective Factors

Results of the regressions predicting the physical and mental health scores are presented in Table 3. Findings suggest personal assets of caregivers accounted for a significant amount of variance above and beyond the variance accounted for by demographics, $\Delta R^2 = .167$, $p < .001$. The addition of social assets was also significant and accounted for a significant amount of additional variance, $\Delta R^2 = .069$, $p < .001$. Social assets accounted for a significant amount of variance above and beyond the variance accounted for by personal assets. The addition of environmental assets, although still significant, did not account for a significant amount of additional variance, $\Delta R^2 = .004$, $p < .001$. In the final model, age ($\beta = -1.9$ $p = .01$), residence (urban high; $\beta = 11.2$, $p = .01$), self-esteem ($\beta = 1.4$, $p = .01$), mastery ($\beta = 2.2$, $p = .000$), social networks ($\beta = 4.7$, $p = .01$), and access to health services ($\beta = 10$, $p < .001$) were significantly associated with physical health. The four steps accounted for statistically significant increments in the amount of variance accounted for by physical health. Older age was associated with lower physical health.

TABLE 2 Correlation Matrix, Means, *SD*, and Cronbach Alphas of the Study Variables

Item	Age	Income	Physical health	Mental heath	Social relation	Enviro-nment	Mastery	Self-esteem	Problem solving	Meaningful	Self-efficacy	Physic enviro.	Available finance	Cronbach's alpha	Mean (*SD*)
Demographics															
Age	1														61.1 (11)
Income	−.262**	1													1.21 (1.3)
Outcome variables															
Physical health	−.327**	.368**	1											0.87	53.9 (22.7)
Mental health	−.256*	.379**	.608**	1										0.88	60.9 (17.7)
Social relations	−.225**	.387**	.358**	.436**	1									0.85	46.7 (20.8)
Environment	−.152*	.583**	.441**	.540**	.388**	1								0.91	47.7 (16.9)
Personal assets															
Mastery	−.318**	.428**	.569**	.474**	.260**	.350**	1								4.10 (1.96)
Self-esteem	.101	.389**	.207**	.319**	.225**	.399**	.202**	1							4.51 (1.77)
Problem solving	−.172*	.271**	.274**	.377**	.220**	.288**	.461**	.296**	1						5.31 (1.53)
Meaningful	−.091	.346**	.228**	.491**	.310**	.385**	.332**	.321**	.390**	1					5.0 (1.83)
Self-efficacy	−.297**	.434**	.525**	.474**	.248**	.394**	.504**	.269**	.388**	.326**	1				4.49 (1.49)
Environmental assets															
Physic environment	−.217**	.255**	.184**	.230**	.162*	.578**	.118	.220**	.105	.264**	.150*	1			3.14 (1.30)
Available finances	−.104	.636**	.364**	.419**	.342**	.644**	.337**	.381**	.304**	.329**	.423**	.217**	1		1.76 (1.01)
Leisure	−.057	.139*	.245**	.339**	.197**	.411**	.146*	.027	.112	.023	.310**	.062	.264**		0.23 (0.42)

*$p < .05$; **$p < .01$.

TABLE 3 β Coefficients for Demographics, Personal, Social, and Environmental Assets Associated With Health ($n = 241$)

Measures	Physical health				Mental health			
	Model 1	Model 2	Model 3	Model 4	Model 1	Model 2	Model 3	Model 4
Demographics								
Age	−3.18**	−2.45*	−1.92*	−1.93*	−2.27**	−1.53*	−1.39*	−1.43*
Marital status	4.39	3.63	3.37	3.03	1.51	.80	1.55	1.06
Income earned	12.47*	1.35	.35	−1.59	11.72*	2.10	.12	−2.60
Education	−1.47	−1.65	−1.68	−1.75	2.86	2.36	2.41	2.32
Carer for orphans	−5.01	−4.63	−4.46	−4.00	−2.34	−1.95	−1.92	−1.27
Rural	−5.13	−3.46	−3.25	−4.82	−8.23*	−6.46*	−6.8**	−9.07**
Urban high	3.99	9.8*	9.27*	11.22*	0.96	6.46*	6.56*	9.29*
Personal assets								
Coping skills		3.14	2.94	2.47		4.19*	4.13*	3.47*
Self-esteem		2.17**	1.56**	1.43*		1.61*	1.43*	1.26*
Mastery		2.21**	2.24**	2.21**		2.19**	1.93**	1.90**
Social assets								
Social network			4.79*	4.74*			2.50	2.43
Religiosity			−2.59	−3.10			3.80	3.09
Access to health			−10.1**	−10**			−2.907	−2.69
Enviro assets								
Healthy env.				1.34				1.87*
ΔR^2	.167	.177	.069	.004	.195	.257	.027	.019
R^2		.344	.413	.417		.452	.479	.498

*$p < .05$; **$p < .01$.

Note. Physical health standardized β are presented in Table 2: Model 1, $\Delta F(7, 233) = 7.9$, $p < .001$; Model 2, $\Delta F(10, 230) = 7.7$, $p < .001$; Model 3, $\Delta F(13, 227) = 0.4$, $p < .001$; Model 4, $\Delta F(14, 226) = 0.7$, $p < .001$. Mental health standardized β are presented in Table 2: Model 1, $\Delta F(7, 233) = 8.1$, $p < .001$; Model 2, $\Delta F(10, 230) = 10.8$, $p < .001$; Model 3, $\Delta F(13, 227) = 2.9$, $p < .001$; Model 4, $\Delta F(14, 226) = 0$, $p < .001$.

Predicting Mental Health From Protective Factors

Personal assets of caregivers accounted for a significant amount of variance above and beyond the variance accounted for by demographics, $\Delta R^2 = .257$, $p < .001$ (see Table 4). The addition of social assets was also significant and accounted for a significant amount of additional variance, $\Delta R^2 = .027$, $p < .001$. The social assets of caregivers accounted for a significant amount of variance above and beyond the variance accounted for by personal assets. The addition of environmental assets accounted for a significant amount of additional variance, $\Delta R^2 = .019$, $p < .001$. In the final model, age ($\beta = −1.4$ $p = .01$), residence: urban high ($\beta = 9.3$, $p = .01$), rural ($\beta = −9.1$, $p < .001$), self-esteem ($\beta = 1.3$, $p = .004$), overall coping ($\beta = 3.5$, $p = .03$), mastery ($\beta = 1.9$, $p < .001$), and healthy physical environment ($\beta = 19$, $p = .003$) were significantly associated with mental health.

TABLE 4 β Coefficients for Demographics, Personal, Social, and Environmental Assets Associated With Well-Being ($n = 241$)

Measures	Well-being			
	Model 1	Model 2	Model 3	Model 4
Demographics				
Age	−.76*	−.48	−.38	−.44
Marital status	5.03	4.79	6.00*	5.11*
Income earned	13.42**	9.05*	5.76	.76
Education	−2.87	−3.13	−2.98	−3.15
Carer for orphans	−2.01	−1.70	−1.73	−.54
Rural residence	−1.47	−.76	−1.77	−5.81*
Urban high	−5.78	−3.46	−2.94	2.05
Personal assets				
Coping skills		2.72	2.49	1.28
Self-esteem		.83	.68	.36
Mastery		.79*	.46	.39
Social assets				
Social network			3.76	3.63
Religiosity			5.28**	3.98*
Access to health			−.87	−.47
Environmental assets				
Healthy env.				3.44**
ΔR^2	.282	.045	.049	.082
R^2		.327	.376	.458

**$p < .001$; *$p < .05$.

Note: *Well-being standardized β are presented: Model 1, $\Delta F(7, 233) = 17.5$, $p = .000$; Model 2, $\Delta F(10, 230) = 1.3$, $p = .000$; Model 3, $\Delta F(13, 227) = 0.8$, $p = .000$; Model 4, $\Delta F(14, 226) = 3.7$, $p = .000$.

Predicting Well-Being From Protective Factors

Personal assets accounted for a significant amount of variance above and beyond the variance accounted for by demographics, $\Delta R^2 = .045$, $p < .001$. In step 3, addition of social assets accounted for a significant amount of additional variance, $\Delta R^2 = .049$, $p < .001$. The addition of environmental assets accounted for a significant amount of variance above and beyond the variance accounted for by social assets, $\Delta R^2 = .082$, $p < .001$. In the final model, caregiver marital status ($\beta = 5.1$, $p = .002$), residing in rural areas ($\beta = −5.8$, $p = .003$), religiosity ($\beta = 4.0$, $p = .01$), and a healthy physical environment ($\beta = 3.4$, $p < .001$) were significantly associated with well-being. Residing in rural areas was associated with lower well-being than residing in urban areas.

DISCUSSION

Researchers explored the impact of protective factors on health and well-being of grandmother carers fostering orphans and nonorphans. Resources (personal, social, and environmental) were found to play a major role in caregiving.

The Impact of Protective Factors on Grandmothers' Health

Personal assets seemed to be the most significant factor in health. Mastery and high self-esteem were associated with physical health. Coping skills, mastery, and high self-esteem were associated with mental health. Personal assets are important in that they assist grandparents in the way they perceive caregiving roles. Grandparents with a positive attitude toward life are likely to see caregiving as a challenge rather than a burden. Previous studies postulated that caregiving had a positive impact on health and well-being whether it was caring for an orphan or nonorphan (Brintnall-Petersen, 2009; Gerard et al., 2006; Degeneffe et al., 2011; Hughes et al., 2007; Sands et al., 2005;). This depends on how the caregiver appraises the situation and the availability of protective factors. Based on our results, we agree that perception of one's life as meaningful, high self-esteem, mastery, and coping skills had a positive impact on caregiving.

Previous research has revealed that most full-time carers (custodial carers) report less satisfaction with grandchildren care than part-time carers (traditional carers; Bigbee, Musil, & Kenski, 2011; Ross & Aday, 2006), which is inconsistent with our findings. These previous researchers did not look at the confounding effect of resources as this may not have been an issue especially in high-income countries. This is further supported by the fact that in the current study grandmothers with high SES background had better mental health. This could be explained by availability of resources that assist carers to provide for their grandchildren without stressing.

The extent to which grandchild care affects health depends on the balance between the demands of caregiving and the resources available to the grandparent (Hughes et al., 2007; Hughes & Waite, 2002; Ross & Aday, 2006; U.S. Census Bureau, 2012). Whether carers lived in skipped-generation households, were part time or full time, married or single proved insignificant; as long as resources were available, then grandmothers would cope with caregiving. There was evidence of association between health and type of residential area. Grandmothers residing in urban suburbs had better health than those residing in rural areas. Grandmothers in rural areas lived long distances from clinics and could not afford to commute unlike their urban counterparts. This finding is similar to a previous study done for WHO Study on Global AGEing and Adult Health (SAGE) countries (U.S. Census Bureau, 2012).

The Impact of Protective Factors on Carers' Well-Being

There was very strong evidence of association between well-being and support (family social capital and spirituality). This is consistent with previous studies that found that support from spouses, relatives, friends, and other children led to increased well-being and overall role satisfaction (Davidson, DiGiacomo, & McGrath, 2011; Hayslip (Jr.) & Kaminski, 2005; Mhaka-Mutepfa, Phasha, Mpofu, Tchombe, Mwamwenda, Kizito & Jere-Folotiya, 2008; Nyasani et al., 2009; Ogunmefun et al., 2011) and that spiritual support also led to increased well-being (Chen & Feeley, 2012; Hodge & Horvath, 2011; Kamya & Poindexter, 2009; Ross & Aday, 2006). Grandparents enjoyed social networking with members of their congregations and received emotional support. In our study, support from neighbors, government, and nongovernmental oganizations (NGOs) was provided on a very small scale.

When environmental assets were added to the model, a healthy physical environment accounted for a significant amount of variance above and beyond the variance accounted for by social assets. Luo and colleagues (2012) emphasized the benefit of having a good environment in caregiving, suggesting that grandmothers should live in a healthy physical environment to achieve well-being. Grandmothers who resided in rural areas had lower well-being than those who resided in urban areas. Residents of urban areas got resources from doing menial jobs, rental income, and support from their surviving children. There were differences from previous research findings that suggest that family resources (i.e., support) relative to risks affect carers' well-being (Brintnall-Peterson et al., 2009; Minkler & Fuller-Thomson, 2005). Social networks were not associated with well-being. Social networks in the current study included attending gatherings. Grandmothers in our study stated that they were coerced to attend political gatherings and this could have masked the positive effect of social networking.

Previous scholars who have looked at carer support have also demonstrated the benefits and utility of support in caregiving (Ice et al., 2012; Kipp et al., 2007; Nyasani et al., 2009; Schatz & Ogunmefun, 2007). In these studies, support was availed in the form of social security grants (on a small scale), spirituality, and social support from family members and friends. Previous researchers found social support to be positively associated with life satisfaction (Chen & Feeley, 2012; Gerard et al., 2006). Social support is a coping mechanism as is confrontational coping, acceptance of responsibility, problem solving, self-control, positive reappraisal, and distancing (Ross & Aday, 2006). The current study, however, did not entirely support previous findings. Overall coping was not associated with well-being, after personal and social assets were entered as blocks into models, even though each of the coping mechanisms was associated with well-being in univariate analysis. The type of family (skipped or multigeneration) could have masked the findings. This question could also have been misinterpreted, however, as coping is a relative term. Some grandmothers stated that they were coping overall because they could get food and were not worried about the other basic needs.

Limitations and Suggestions for Future Research

A limitation of the current study is that it was a cross-sectional survey. A longitudinal study could yield different findings. Another limitation of the current study is that results cannot be generalized to grandfather carers as grandfathers may have different views and perceptions to caregiving. A gendered approach that considers the unique position of older women and not only acknowledges biological differences but also the social, political, and cultural constructs and roles given to women must be adopted (Davidson et al., 2011). Another limitation of the study is that it was carried out in two out of 10 provinces in Zimbabwe, limiting generalizability because of the different ethnic groups in the country.

Future research should explore other potential mediators between enacted support and well-being (Chen & Feeley, 2012). Possible mediators to include are informational support (e.g., advice) and companionship (e.g., sense of belonging) on the health and well-being of carers for orphans using a national sample with diversified ethnicities.

Implications for Health and Well-Being Interventions

Programs need to be designed and implemented to strengthen assets or resources for caregivers of children. Caregivers should be given social security grants so that they can maintain their health and well-being. The monthly grants should be provided from age 50 for unemployed grandparent carers. In addition, free health services should be provided from 50 years for unemployed carers rather than wait until they turn 65 so as to maintain good health. Stakeholders should also empower grandparent carers with coping skills and provide social and environmental assets that enable better health and higher well-being.

In conclusion, grandmothers' personal and social assets are important to their health and well-being. Physical health was significantly associated with personal assets and access to health, suggesting that grandmothers with mobility may have overall better health status. Personal assets and a healthy physical environment were significantly associated with mental health, proving that personal attributes and resources bolster health. Family relationships and spirituality were associated with well-being, suggesting that families should be empowered and encouraged to render support to carers. Grandmothers in carer roles are important community resources for child custody.

Grandmothers in sub-Saharan Africa are increasingly taking up caretaker roles due to high HIV and AIDS prevalence. Grandmother carers' lifestyles are dependent on the opportunities availed to them by their families and local communities. Their health and well-being are affected differently because there are enabling and entrapping social niches in diverse communities. In the absence of adequate social security, the carers in Zimbabwe look to service providers and their families for support. Families cannot render more support because of their own burn out, considering their own needs. More studies that reflect the voices of this elderly generation are required because grandmothers are a diverse group and their experiences vary.

FUNDING

The project was not funded, but we thank International Postgraduate Research Scholarship and Australian Postgraduate Award for paying fees for the student's doctoral studies.

REFERENCES

Bigbee, J. L., Boegh, B. V., Prengaman, M., & Shaklee, H. (2011). Promoting the health of frontier caregiving grandparents: A demonstration project evaluation. *Journal for Specialists in Pediatric Nursing*, *16*(2), 156–161.

Bigbee, J. L., Musil, C., & Kenski, D. (2011). The health of caregiving grandmothers: A rural-urban comparison. *Journal of Rural Health*, *27*(3), 289–296.

Brintnall-Peterson, M., Poehlmann, J., Morgan, K., & Shlafer, R. (2009). A web-based fact sheet series for grandparents raising grandchildren and the professionals who serve them. *Gerontologist*, *49*(2), 276–282.

Chen, Y., & Feeley, T. H. (2012). Enacted support and well-being: A test of the mediating role of perceived control. *Communication Studies*, *63*(5), 608–625.

Craig, A. (2012). Resilience in people with physical disabilities. In P. Kennedy (Ed.), *The Oxford Handbook of Rehabilitation Psychology*. New York, NY: Oxford University Press.

Davidson, P. M., DiGiacomo, M., & McGrath, S. J. (2011). The feminization of aging: How will this impact on health outcomes and services? *Health Care for Women International*, *32*(12), 1031–1045.

Degeneffe, C. E., Chan, F., Dunlap, L., Man, D., & Sung, C. (2011). Development and validation of the caregiver empowerment scale: A resource for working with family caregivers of persons with traumatic brain injury. *Rehabilitation Psychology*, *56*(3), 243–250.

Diener, E., Oishi, S., & Lucas, R. E. (2003). Personality, culture, and subjective well-being: Emotional and cognitive evaluations of life. *Annual Review Psychology*, *54*, 403–425.

Diener, E., & Ryan, K. (2009). Subjective well-being: A general overview. *South African Journal of Psychology*, *39*(4), 391–406.

Fergus, S., & Zimmerman, M. A. (2005). Adolescent resilience: A framework for understanding healthy development in the face of risk. *Annual Reviews of Public Health, 26,* 399–419.

Gaudine, A., Gien, L., Thuan, T. T., & Dung, D. V. (2010). Perspectives of HIV-related stigma in a community in Vietnam: A qualitative study. *International Journal of Nursing Studies, 47*(1), 38–48.

Gerard, J. M., Landry-Meyer, L., & Roe, J. G. (2006). Grandparents raising grandchildren: The role of social support in coping with caregiving challenges. *International Journal of Aging and Human Development, 62*(4), 359–383.

Gupta, N. T., & Simonsen, M. (2007). *Non-cognitive child outcomes and universal high quality child care.* IZA Discussion Papers, No. 3188. Retrieved from http://www.tandfonline.com.

Hayslip (Jr.), B., & Kaminski, P. L. (2005). Grandparents raising their grandchildren: A review of the literature and suggestions for practice. *Gerontologist, 45*(2), 262–269.

Hobfoll, S., Neria, Y., Gross, R., Marshall, R., & Susser, E. (2006). *Guiding community intervention following terrorist attacks: Mental health in the wake of terrorist attacks.* New York, NY: Cambridge Press.

Hodge, D. R., & Horvath, V. E. (2011). Spiritual needs in health care settings: A qualitative meta-synthesis of clients' perspectives. *Social Work, 56*(4), 306–316.

Howard, B. H., Phillips, C. V., Matinhure, N., Goodman, K. J., McCurdy, S. A., & Johnson, C. A. (2006). Barriers and incentives to orphan care in a time of AIDS and economic crisis: A cross-sectional survey of caregivers in rural Zimbabwe. *BioMed Central Public Health, 6,* 11P.

Hughes, M. E., & Waite, L. J. (2002). Health in household context: Living arrangements and health in late middle age. *Journal of Health and Social Behavior, 43*(1), 1–21.

Hughes, M. E., Waite, L. J., LaPierre, T. A., & Luo, Y. (2007). All in the family: The impact of caring for grandchildren on grandparents' health. *Journals of Gerontology—Series B Psychological Sciences and Social Sciences, 62*(2), S108–S119.

Ice, G. H., Heh, V., Yogo, J., & Juma, E. (2011). Caregiving, gender, and nutritional status in Nyanza Province, Kenya: Grandmothers gain, grandfathers lose. *American Journal of Human Biology, 23*(4), 498–508.

Ice, G. H., Sadruddin, A. F. A., Vagedes, A., Yogo, J., & Juma, E. (2012). Stress associated with caregiving: An examination of the stress process model among Kenyan Luo elders. *Social Science and Medicine, 74*(12), 2020–2027.

Kamya, H., & Poindexter, C. C. (2009). Mama Jaja: The stresses and strengths of HIV-affected Ugandan grandmothers. *Social Work in Public Health, 24*(1–2), 4–21.

Killian, B. (2004). *Vulnerable children and security in Southern Africa: A generation at risk of HIV/AIDS.* Pretoria, South Africa: Southern African AIDS Trust (SAFAIDS).

Kipp, W., Tindyebwa, D., Karamagi, E., & Rubaale, T. (2007). How much should we expect? Family caregiving of AIDS patients in rural Uganda. *Journal of Transcultural Nursing, 18*(4), 358–365.

Kuhn, D., Fulton, B., & Edelman, P. (2003). Powerful tools for caregivers: Improving welfare and self-efficacy of family caregivers. *Alzheimer Care Quarterly, 4*(3), 189–200.

Luo, L., LaPierre, T. A., Hughes, M. A., & Waite, L. A. (2012). Grandparents providing care to grandchildren: A population based study of continuity and change. *Journal of family issues, 33*(9), 1143–1167.

Mertler, C., & Vannatta, R. (2005). *Advanced and multivariate statistical methods: Practical application.* Retrieved from www.amazon.com/Advanced-Multi variate-Statistical-Methods-Interpretation/dp/1884585590

Mhaka-Mutepfa, M., Phasha, N., Mpofu, E., Tchombe, T., Mwamwenda, T., Kizito, S., & Jere-Folotiya, J. (2008). Child headed households in sub-Saharan Africa. In T. Maundeni, L. L. Lopez, & G. Jacques (Eds.), *Families in a changing world.* Gaborone, Botswana: Bay Publishing.

Michalos, A. C. (2008). Education, happiness and wellbeing. *Social Indicators Research, 87*(3), 347–366.

Minkler, M., & Fuller-Thomson, E. (2005). African American grandparents raising grandchildren: A national study using the Census 2000 American Community Survey. *The Journals of Gerontology: Series B, Psychological Sciences and Social Sciences, 60*(2), S82–92.

Norris, F. H., Stevens, S. P., Pfefferbaum, B., Wyche, K. F., & Pfefferbaum, R. L. (2008). Community resilience as a metaphor, theory, set of capacities, and strategy for disaster readiness. *American Journal of Community Psychology, 41*(1), 127–150.

Nyambedha, E. O., Wandibba, S., & Aagaard-Hansen, J. (2003a). "Retirement lost"—The new role of the elderly as caretakers for orphans in Western Kenya. *Journal of Cross-Cultural Gerontology, 18*(1), 33–52.

Nyambedha, E. O., Wandibba, S., & Aagaard-Hansen, J. (2003b). Changing patterns of orphan care due to the HIV epidemic in western Kenya. *Social Science and Medicine, 57*(2), 301–311.

Nyasani, E., Sterberg, E., & Smith, H. (2009). Fostering children affected by AIDS in Richards Bay, South Africa: A qualitative study of grandparents' experiences. *African Journal of AIDS Research, 8*(2), 181–192.

Oburu, P. O., & Palmerus, K. (2005). Stress related factors among primary and part-time caregiving grandmothers of Kenyan grandchildren. *International Journal of Aging and Human Development, 60*(4), 273–282.

Ogunmefun, C., Gilbert, L., & Schatz, E. (2011). Older female caregivers and HIV/AIDS-related secondary stigma in rural South Africa. *Journal of Cross-Cultural Gerontology, 26*(1), 85–102.

Poehlmann, J. (2003). An attachment perspective on grandparents raising their very young grandchildren: Implications for intervention and research. *Infant Mental Health Journal, 24*(2), 149–173.

Poehlmann, J., Park, J., Bouffiou, L., Abrahams, J., Shlafer, R., & Hahn, E. (2008). Representations of family relationships in children living with custodial grandparents. *Attachment and Human Development, 10*(2), 165–188.

Ross, M. E. T., & Aday, L. (2006). Stress and coping in African American grandparents who are raising their grandchildren. *Journal of Family Issues, 27*, 912–932.

Rutter, M. (2011). Implications of resilience concepts for scientific understanding and for policy/practice. *European Child and Adolescent Psychiatry, 20*, S114.

Schatz, E., & Ogunmefun, C. (2007). Caring and contributing: The role of older women in rural South African multi-generational households in the HIV era. *World Development, 35*(8), 1390–1403.

Skevington, S. M., & O'Connell, K. A. (2004). Can we identify the poorest quality of life? Assessing the importance of quality of life using the WHOQOL-100. *Quality of Life Research*, *13*(1), 23–34. Retrieved from www.ncbi.nlm.nih.gov/pubmed/15058784

Stockstrom, S. (2008). How pensions reduce poverty: Social pensions. *HelpAge International*, *70*, 4–5.

UNAIDS. (2011). *Global HIV/AIDS response: Epidemic update and health*. Retrieved from http://www.unaids.org/en/media/unaids/contentassets/documents/unaidspublication/2011/20111130_ua_report_en.pdf

U.S. Census Bureau. (2012). *Shades of gray: A cross-country study of health and well-being of the older populations in SAGE countries, 2007–2010*. Washington, DC: Author.

World Health Organization (WHO). (1996). *Introduction, adminstration, scoring and generic version of the assessment*. Retrieved from www.who.int/mental_health/media/68.pdf

World Health Organization (WHO). (2001). *International classification of functioning, disability and health: ICF short version*. Retrieved from http://www.who.int/classifications/icf/en/

Index

Page references in **bold** refer to tables and those in *italics* indicate a figure.

Printed and bound by CPI Group (UK) Ltd, Croydon, CR0 4YY

18/10/2024

01776253-0006